Sex Differences in the Brain

SEX DIFFERENCES IN THE BRAIN
FROM GENES TO BEHAVIOR

Edited by
Jill B. Becker, Karen J. Berkley, Nori Geary,
Elizabeth Hampson, James P. Herman, and Elizabeth A. Young

OXFORD
UNIVERSITY PRESS

2008

OXFORD
UNIVERSITY PRESS

Oxford University Press, Inc., publishes works that further
Oxford University's objective of excellence
in research, scholarship, and education.

Oxford   New York
Auckland   Cape Town   Dar es Salaam   Hong Kong   Karachi
Kuala Lumpur   Madrid   Melbourne   Mexico City   Nairobi
New Delhi   Shanghai   Taipei   Toronto

With offices in
Argentina   Austria   Brazil   Chile   Czech Republic   France   Greece
Guatemala   Hungary   Italy   Japan   Poland   Portugal   Singapore
South Korea   Switzerland   Thailand   Turkey   Ukraine   Vietnam

Published by Oxford University Press, Inc.
198 Madison Avenue, New York, New York 10016
www.oup.com

Oxford is a registered trademark of Oxford University Press

Library of Congress Cataloging-in-Publication Data
Sex differences in the brain : from genes to behavior /
edited by Jill Becker . . . [et al.].
p. cm. Includes bibliographical references.
ISBN 978-0-19-531158-7
1. Sex differences.
2. Sex differences (Psychology)
3. Brain—Sex differences.
4. Human behavior—Physiological aspects.
I. Becker, Jill B.
[DNLM: 1. Brain—physiology.
2. Behavior—physiology.
3. Central Nervous System Diseases—physiopathology.
4. Mental Disorders—physiopathology.
5. Mental Processes—physiology.
6. Sex Factors. WL 300 S5185 2008]
QP81.5.S484 2008   612.8'2—dc22   2007021143

3 5 7 9 8 6 4 2

Printed in the United States of America
on acid-free paper

This book is dedicated to Florence P. Haseltine, Ph.D., M.D., founder of the Society for Women's Health Research. Her unstoppable energy and commitment in support of sex differences research is inspirational to us all.
Florence—thank you for leading the way.

Contents

Foreword

MENTAL DISORDERS ARE BRAIN DISORDERS: WHY SEX MATTERS

There seems to be no end to the debate over sex differences in the brain. When people finally agree that differences exist, there is an even more intense debate over what these differences mean. Do more neurons mean more computing power? Do more connections mean more communication between neurons? Do structural differences correlate with functional differences?

In fact, there are clear, reproducible mean differences in many neuroanatomical variables when groups of male and female brains are compared. But understanding these differences runs directly into a central quandary in neuroscience: How do we link form and function? We are now able to define form at the molecular level by identifying individual cells by their RNA transcripts. In addition, we are able to detect function in individual neurons by measuring physiological signatures of identified cells. Similarly,

we have been able to image physiological changes in brain systems associated with behavior and cognition. However, we have not been able to build the bridge from individual cells to brain systems in a way that allows a seamless understanding that spans from molecules to behavior.

This is one of the ways in which the study of sex differences can make a difference: by understanding how chromosomal sex confers genomic differences, how gonadal hormones and their transcription factor receptors lead to developmental changes in brain systems, and how systems in the brain become associated with differences in cognition and behavior. The study of sex differences is a unique opportunity to elucidate the entire trajectory from genes to behavior, or, as more frequently stated in the clinical realm, from genotype to phenotype.

Why is this important? Aside from answering fundamental questions for neuroscience, the study of sex differences is important for public health. According to the World Health Organization, mental disorders are the leading source of disability in Americans between the ages of 15 and 44. We now understand mental disorders as brain disorders, but we do not understand how brain circuits become abnormal. Part of finding this answer will reside in being able to identify the risk factors for disease and, more importantly, defining the mechanisms by which these factors confer risk.

Among the various risk factors for mental disorders, gender is preeminent. Relative to males, females are at least three times as likely to have anorexia nervosa, twice as likely to have depression, and one fourth as likely to have autism. For schizophrenia and obsessive-compulsive disorder, with roughly equivalent prevalence in males and females, the onset is earlier in males. Moreover, there are gender differences in the clinical features: females with major depressive disorder are more likely to express sadness whereas males present with irritability.

We do not understand the mechanisms for any of these gender differences, but patterns of gonadal hormone action are major candidates. We know that many mental disorders emerge with hormonal transitions at puberty, parturition, and menopause. We also know that the brain is a target organ for gonadal hormones. As we define the mechanisms by which these hormones alter brain function at the molecular, cellular, and systems levels, we should begin to define how gender and hormonal transitions increase risk for mental disorders.

This book results from the visionary leadership of the Society for Women's Health Research and specifically the staff who have sponsored the Isis Fund Network on Sex, Gender, Drugs, and the Brain. By exploring a range of sex differences from genes to behavior, the chapters herein review the latest insights into how sex and gender matter. The findings promise to alter our approach to mental disorders, leading initially to a better understanding of pathophysiology and ultimately to better treatments. Of course sex differences exist, but what really matters for public health is how these differences lead to vulnerability for some individuals and resilience for others.

Thomas R. Insel, MD
Director, National Institute
of Mental Health, NIH

Preface

Differences in the brain between males and females have been observed in behavioral traits, in the anatomy of the brain, and in the physiological responses of the nervous system to outside stimuli and internal perturbation. The brain is sensitive to the effects of gonadal hormones, beginning in fetal development and continuing throughout the lifespan, and there is mounting evidence that some sex differences may result from differences in gene expression that are independent of the effect of gonadal hormones. In humans, these differences are reflected in the differential impact of neurological and mental illness on men and women, including conditions as diverse as multiple sclerosis, major depression, dementia, and chronic pain disorders. This book brings together an international group of experts on sex differences in the brain, writing about critical methodological issues in sex differences research as well as the most recent developments in this rapidly moving field. It is the culmination of the work of many individuals, and has its origins in a meeting at the Cosmos Club in Washington, DC, in 1990.

At that meeting, a group of researchers, clinicians, and activists began work that led to the founding of the Society for Women's Health Research (SWHR) to "advance the health of women through research." This group identified the paucity of women participants in medical research studies as a major barrier to such advancement. By 1993, SWHR had brought about changes in grant guidelines at the US National Institutes of Health, and in guidelines for new drug applications at the US Food and Drug Administration. Researchers are now required to include women in research studies unless there is an adequate scientific reason for doing a study in a single sex. By 1995, scientists on SWHR's Board of Directors had a clear vision of the outcome of the inclusion of women (and female animals) as research subjects: the discovery and elucidation of biological sex differences that have a significant impact on health and disease. The Society turned that vision into a proposal for a study by the Institute of Medicine (IOM) that would address the questions, "Does sex matter?" "When does sex matter?" "How does sex matter?" Once the IOM accepted the report proposal, Society staff raised more than $650,000 in public and private funds to cover the costs of producing a report.

The Institute of Medicine (IOM) published this landmark report in 2001. The book was a product of the IOM Committee on Understanding Sex and Gender Differences, entitled *Exploring the Biological Contributions to Human Health: Does Sex Matter?* (Wizemann & Pardue, 2001) The Committee concluded that sex is a significant and often ignored biological variable, and that understanding sex differences is crucial for improving human health. They found that much of what was known about sex differences came from descriptive findings, and that hypothesis-driven research to study the mechanisms and origins of sex differences is now needed. They identified several barriers to progress in research on sex differences, including the need for more accurate use of the terms "sex" and "gender," and the need for better tools and resources for the study and analysis of sex differences.

Another barrier identified by the IOM committee was the inherently interdisciplinary nature of research on sex differences, the lack of funding for this type of research, and the lack of funding for collaborative opportunities for sex differences research. The report noted that progress in sex-based biology would require "synergy... between and among basic scientists, epidemiologists, social scientists, and clinical researchers." In addition, integration of findings at different levels of biological organization (genes, cells, tissues, organs, whole animals) and better "bench-to-bedside" translational research is needed.

In the six years that it took to raise the funding for and produce the IOM report, SWHR developed and launched a strategic plan for developing interest and capacity in sex differences research among basic and clinical scientists. In addition to the traditional role of SWHR as an advocacy group working with the US Congress and federal agencies, SWHR worked to expand its direct outreach to the scientific community. The Society identified two ways in which it could work to encourage research on sex differences: by providing a venue for researchers to present and discuss their work in this area, and by providing financial support for research.

From 2000–2005 SWHR produced the annual Conference on Sex and Gene Expression (SAGE), a small interdisciplinary meeting that explored all aspects of biological sex differences. The SAGE Conferences brought together researchers working at all levels of biological organization, in animal models from *C. elegans* to primates, and in various physiological systems and clinical disciplines. The SAGE Conferences were designed to allow ample time for informal discussion among the participants, and surveys of attendees found that a significant number of new collaborations and new lines of research were begun at these meetings.

In 1998 SWHR established the Isis Fund for Sex Differences Research, named for the Egyptian Goddess who was the founder of the art of medicine. The Society consulted with staff from the MacArthur Foundation, which had a program of highly successful interdisciplinary research networks to address issues in mental health. Using the MacArthur Networks as a model, funded by unrestricted grant of $1 million over four years from Ortho-McNeil Pharmaceuticals, Society staff assembled a core group of five scientists and posed to them the question "How are sex and gender differences important in the development and testing of neuropharmaceuticals?" At their first meeting in 2002, the network quickly renamed itself the Isis Fund Network on Sex, Gender, Drugs, and the Brain, and established this mission: To develop collaborations for exploratory and hypothesis-driven research on sex differences in nervous system function, and to translate the results of this research into new and/or improved therapies for advancing human health. In addition to the original goal of network members collaborating on pilot projects, the Network established the following goals in support of that mission: to promote research and education in the area of sex/gender differences in brain health and disease, and to educate and advocate among research funders, scientists, reviewers, regulators and the public. They identified three ways to accomplish those goals: through Network publications, by organizing symposia at large scientific meetings, and by seeking funding for new investigator training grants for sex differences research.

By the third meeting of the Network, which had expanded to eight members, a discussion of potential network projects brought out the need for a guideline to "best practices" for research on sex differences. The network members were concerned that the greatest barrier to the study of sex differences (or to simply including females in an experiment) was difficulty of dealing with the ovarian cycle (estrous and menstrual cycles). Many investigators are reluctant to include females in their experiments because they are uncertain how best to account for the female cycle, or how to determine the role of hormones when they observe an effect of the estrous cycle. The Network decided to create a document that described the strategies, methods, and procedures used in sex differences research. The product that resulted was a 24-page review that was published in *Endocrinology* (Becker et al., 2005). Although the review addressed these methodologic issues in the context of central nervous system function, the basic information was widely applicable to research on sex and gender differences in other systems.

Soon after the review appeared in *Endocrinology*, the Network (which by then had 11 members) discovered that the article was only a beginning. Many researchers who read the article appreciated its value, while at the same time mentioning that there was a much wider need for this kind of information. The Network agreed that the next step was to produce an edited volume that would expand on the material presented in the review, and would include chapters on basic and clinical sex differences research in neuroscience. This book is the result of that decision.

The Society for Women's Health Research, and specifically the staff who have had a direct role in the development of the Isis Fund Network on Sex, Gender, Drugs, and the Brain,* are proud of our role in funding and supporting the work of this Network, and of the other Networks supported by the Isis Fund for Sex Differences Research: the Network on Sex Differences in Metabolism, supported by an unrestricted grant from Aventis Pharmaceuticals (now sanofi-aventis); and the Network on Sex Differences in the Musculoskeletal System, supported by an unrestricted donation from Zimmer, Inc.

The Isis Fund Networks have significantly advanced innovative interdisciplinary research on sex differences and, at the same time, have helped launch sex differences as a new field of biomedical research. Network members have organized and participated in symposia on sex differences at meetings of the Society for Neuroscience, the International Society for Psychoneuroendocrinology, and the Congress of the International Union of Physiological Societies. Network members served as guest editors for a special issue of the *American Journal of Physiology* on sex differences in pain and inflammation and a special issue of *Brain Research* featuring papers presented at a joint meeting of the Conference on Sex and Gene Expression and the Workshop on Steroid Hormones and Brain Function held in 2006.

Network members have also been instrumental in founding the Organization for the Study of Sex Differences (OSSD). The OSSD is a new scholarly scientific society for which the Society for Women's Health Research is providing fiscal sponsorship and staff support. The OSSD was founded so that the mission of the Network on Sex, Gender, Drugs, and the Brain, "to promote research and education in the area of sex/gender differences in brain health and disease, and to educate and advocate among research funders, scientists, reviewers, regulators, and the public for the study of sex differences," will continue long after the Network no longer meets.

It is our hope that this volume will prove informative and inspiring, that it will engender curiosity about the role of sex as a factor in the development and function of physiological systems, and that it will fuel the growth of a field of research that is crucial to advancing our knowledge of human biology, and our understanding of human health and disease.

Sherry A. Marts, PhD
Vice President, Scientific Affairs
Society for Women's Health Research
Executive Director
Organization for the Study of Sex Differences

---

* Sherry A. Marts, Ph.D., Vice President for Scientific Affairs; Regina Vidaver, Ph.D., Scientific Programs Manager (now Executive Director, National Lung Cancer Partnership); Viviana Simon, Ph.D., Scientific Programs Director; Eileen Resnick, Ph.D., Scientific Programs Manager.

Introduction

In August 2001, the Institute of Medicine (IOM) published a report called "Exploring the Biological Contributions to Human Health: Does Sex Matter?" The IOM concluded that sex is a variable of significant importance for understanding health and disease, and for understanding human physiology more generally. The IOM report was a wake-up call to basic and clinical researchers in many disciplines. In response, the past few years have witnessed a marked growth in research on the effects of sex, as well as signs of greater awareness among professionals that scientifically and clinically important sex differences can and do exist—in susceptibility, symptom expression, response to drugs, immune responses, and many other domains. Sex-based biology has come into its own!

In this volume, we focus on the neurosciences—a set of disciplines where research on sex differences has a lengthy history. In the 1970s, pioneering studies identified sex differences in brain morphology at both the cellular and macroscopic levels, with some structural differences visible even to the naked eye (Raisman & Field, 1971, 1973; Greenough et al., 1977; Gorski et al., 1978). Outside the laboratory, neuropsychologists studying the effects of brain tumors and strokes in neurological patients noted sex differences in some of the cognitive effects of localized lesions, especially in the language domain (Kimura, 1983; Kimura & Harshman, 1984), an observation that suggested the functional organization of the brain might not be entirely the same in men and women. Now we know that even the basic neurochemistry of the brain can differ according to sex, due to developmental events and the effects of steroid hormones on neuronal and glial activity (e.g., Bazzett & Becker, 1994; Andersen et al., 1997; Auger, 2003; Walker et al., 2006). This book carries on the tradition of highlighting sex differences and illustrates the rich and varied work that is going on in the neuroscience of sex and gender today.

With this volume, we offer food for thought to both novices and experts in the field of sex differences. We open with an overview of the evolution of sex differences (Chapter 1), and the biology of sexual differentiation of the brain (Chapter 2), emphasizing how cutting-edge ideas and discoveries are revolutionizing our concepts of what makes a male or female brain. Some expert readers might be surprised to discover a renewed emphasis on the direct actions of X and Y chromosome genes in bringing about sex differences. The endocrine model, however, is still ascendant, as many of the chapters reflect. Chapters 3 and 4 are both methodological chapters that discuss research methods and strategies for the intelligent study of sex differences. After all, discovering a sex difference is only the first step—identifying the genetic or hormonal pathways by which the sex difference is established, and understanding its significance in the context of an organism's ecology and larger behavioral context are the ultimate goals of the basic neuroscientist. The new science of pharmacogenomics is a promising tool to consider when studying central nervous system disorders, and here, too, sex differences are being discovered as discussed, in Chapter 5.

Several of the chapters in this book were written by basic scientists who study the brain and its outward product behavior, but many of these topics have exciting implications for the clinic. These include chapters on such fundamental topics as a thorough review of steroid hormone receptors and their role in sexual behavior (Chapter 7), sex differences in social bonding and affiliative behavior (Chapter 8), sex differences in the neural organization of movement (Chapter 9), as well as sex differences in motivation (Chapter 10) and sex differences in energy metabolism and eating behavior (Chapter 13). These chapters discuss information important for the understanding of the neural basis of addiction and other disorders related to the function of motivational systems.

In this volume we also discuss topics of importance for understanding the recovery from brain injury, as discussed in sex differences in neuroplasticity (Chapter 11). Three chapters deal with sex differences in cognitive function, either in rodents (Chapter 12) or in humans and other primates (Chapters 15 and 16). This has been an especially active arena for sex differences research over the past 20 years, and these chapters represent timely reviews on the topic. Newer areas of research discussed include sex differences in children's play and affiliation with same-sex and opposite-sex peers (Chapter 14).

Other chapters present sex differences in the neurobiology of disease, and illustrate how the rec-

ognition of sex differences has enlightened our understanding of a wide range of medical conditions. Chapters 17 and 18 offer insights into sex differences in infections and the activity of the immune system. Chapter 19 describes the important area of sex differences in pain, a difference with wide applicability in the medical sciences. Sex differences are a prominent feature of a number of psychiatric disorders, including major depression, and mood and anxiety-related disorders. These differences are described in Chapters 20 and 21, along with Chapter 6, where sex differences in the responsiveness to stress and in the regulation of the hypothalamic-pituitary-adrenal (HPA) axis are discussed. As illustrated in these chapters, dysregulation of the HPA axis is a feature of many psychiatric conditions.

The book concludes with two chapters on aging and degenerative diseases of the nervous system (Chapters 22 and 23), including Alzheimer's (which shows a female predominance) and Parkinson's disease (which shows a male predominance). Understanding sex differences in aging, especially brain aging, will be an important practical issue over the next decades.

Does sex matter? To respond to the question posed by the IOM: of course sex matters! It matters to biology and medicine at every level of organization and function, from gene to behavior. The realization that there are real and identifiable differences between the sexes that can potentially have a major impact in physiology and medicine, and the potential significant applications of sex differences research, are now driving the agenda. We must have a clear understanding of the important role of sex if we are to optimize medical treatments, effectively target rehabilitation methods, and devise the most effective preventative strategies in the two sexes. Yes, sex does matter, and it matters to basic and clinical scientists in ways we can't even foresee—studying how phenomena in the brain might differ according to sex can help to illuminate the basic mechanisms and physiology that are the essential research targets of every neuroscientist.

No introduction is complete without thanking those who helped us. We thank Viviana Simon and her staff at the Society for Women's Health Research for all their assistance and support throughout the project. Without Viviana's valuable time and wonderful positive attitude, we could not have accomplished this in the short time we had. We also thank

Sherry Marts and Phyllis Greenberger, from the Society for Women's Health Research for their inspiration to create the Isis Fund Networks and for their constant efforts on behalf of sex differences research. We would not have come together without them, and we have benefited in many ways, both scientifically and personally, from our association with the Society and from our warm relationships with Sherry and Phyllis. Finally, we dedicate this book to Florence P. Hazeltine, founder of the Society for Women's Health Research, whose unstoppable energy on behalf of sex differences research is an inspiration to us all.

We hope you enjoy the book.

On behalf of the Isis Fund Network on Sex, Gender, Drugs, and the Brain
Jill B. Becker, Karen J. Berkley, Nori Geary, Elizabeth Hampson, James P. Herman, & Elizabeth A. Young
July 2007

References

Andersen SL, Rutstein M, Benzo JM, Hostetter JC, Teicher MH. (1997). Sex differences in dopamine receptor overproduction and elimination. *Neuroreport*, 8:1495–1498.

Auger AP. (2003). Sex differences in the developing brain: crossroads in the phosphorylation of cAMP response element binding protein. *J Neuroendocrinology*, 15:622–627.

Bazzett TJ, Becker JB. (1994). Sex differences in the rapid and acute effects of estrogen on striatal D2 dopamine receptor binding. *Brain Res*, 637:163–172.

Gorski RA, Gordon JH, Shryne JE, Southam AM. (1978). Evidence for a morphological sex difference within the medial preoptic area of the rat brain. *Brain Res*, 148:333–346.

Greenough WT, Carter CS, Steerman C, DeVoogd TJ. (1977). Sex differences in dentritic patterns in hamster preoptic area. *Brain Research*, 126:63–72.

Kimura D. (1983). Sex differences in cerebral organization for speech and praxic functions. *Can J Psychology*, 37:19–35.

Kimura D, Harshman RA. (1984). Sex differences in brain organization for verbal and non-verbal functions. *Prog Brain Research*, 61:423–441.

Raisman G, Field PM. (1971). Sexual dimorphism in the preoptic area of the rat. *Science*, 173:731–733.

Raisman G, Field PM. (1973). Sexual dimorphism in the neuropil of the preoptic area of the rat and its dependence on neonatal androgen. *Brain Research*, 54:1–29.

Walker QD, Ray R, Kuhn CM. (2006). Sex differences in neurochemical effects of dopaminergic drugs in rat striatum. *Neuropsychopharmacology*, 31:1193–1202.

Contributors

Margaret Altemus
Cornell University
Weill Medical College
Department of Psychiatry
USA

Arthur P. Arnold
University of California,
Los Angeles
Department of Physiological Science
Laboratory of Neuroendocrinology
of the Brain Research Institute
USA

Matia Banks-Solomon
University of Cincinnati
Department of Psychiatry
USA

Jill B. Becker
University of Michigan
Molecular and Behavioral
Neuroscience Institute
USA

Sheri A. Berenbaum
The Pennsylvania State University
Department of Psychology
USA

Karen J. Berkley
Florida State University
Program in Neuroscience
USA

Jeffrey D. Blaustein
Center for Neuroendocrine Studies
University of Massachusetts, Amherst
USA

Phillip T. Briggs
Arizona State University
School of Social and Family Dynamics
USA

Ippolita Cantuti-Castelvetri
Harvard Medical School
Massachusetts General Hospital
Institute for Neurodegenerative Disease
USA

C. Sue Carter
University of Illinois at Chicago
Department of Psychiatry
Brain Body Center
USA

David Crews
University of Texas at Austin
School of Biological Sciences
Section of Integrative Biology
USA

Gary Dohanich
Tulane University
Department of Psychology
Program in Neuroscience
USA

Ira Driscoll
National Institute on Aging
Laboratory of Personality and Cognition
USA

Lisa A. Eckel
Florida State University
Department of Psychology
Program in Neuroscience
USA

Laura Epstein
University of California,
San Francisco
School of Medicine
USA

Richard A. Fabes
Arizona State University
School of Social and Family Dynamics
USA

Evelyn F. Field
Department of Physiology and Biophysics
University of Calgary
School of Medicine
Canada

Helmer F. Figueiredo
University of Cincinnati
Department of Psychiatry
USA

Nori Geary
Cornell University
Weill Medical College
Department of Psychiatry
USA

and

ETH Zurich
Institute of Animal Science
Switzerland

Tibor Hajszan
Yale University School of Medicine
Department of Obstetrics, Gynecology,
and Reproductive Sciences
USA

Elizabeth Hampson
University of Western Ontario
Department of Psychology
Program in Neuroscience
Canada

Robert J. Handa
Colorado State University
College of Veterinary Medicine
and Biomedical Sciences
Neurosciences Division
Department of Biomedical Sciences
USA

Laura D. Hanish
Arizona State University
School of Social and Family Dynamics
USA

James P. Herman
University of Cincinnati
Department of Psychiatry
USA

Sabra L. Klein
The Johns Hopkins Bloomberg School of Public Health
The W. Harry Feinstone Department
of Molecular Microbiology and Immunology
USA

Ania Korszun
Centre for Psychiatry
Queen Mary, University of London
United Kingdom

JENNIFER S. LABUS
University of California, Los Angeles
Center for Neurovisceral Sciences & Women's
Health
USA

CSABA LERANTH
Yale University School of Medicine,
Departments of Obstetrics, Gynecology,
and Reproductive Sciences and Neurobiology
USA

JENNIFER LOVEJOY
Bastyr University
School of Nutrition and Exercise Science
USA

VICTORIA LUINE
City University of New York
Hunter College
Department of Psychology
USA

NEIL J. MACLUSKY
University of Guelph
Ontario Veterinary College
Department of Biomedical Sciences
Canada

CAROL LYNN MARTIN
Arizona State University
School of Social and Family Dynamics
USA

EMERAN A. MAYER
University of California, Los Angeles
Center for Neurovisceral Sciences & Women's
Health
USA

MARGARET M. McCARTHY
University of Maryland, Baltimore
Departments of Physiology and Psychiatry
Program in Neuroscience
USA

ROBBIN A. MIRANDA
Georgetown University
Brain and Language Laboratory
Department of Neuroscience
USA

TONI R. PAK
Loyola University
Stritch School of Medicine
Department of Cell Biology,
Neurobiology, and Anatomy
USA

JULIA PINSONNEAULT
The Ohio State University
College of Medicine and Public Health
Department of Pharmacology Program
in Pharmacogenomics
USA

SUSAN RESNICK
National Institute on Aging
Laboratory of Personality and Cognition
USA

TURK RHEN
University of North Dakota
Department of Biology
USA

WOLFGANG SADÉE
The Ohio State University
College of Medicine and Public Health
Department of Pharmacology Program
in Pharmacogenomics
USA

DAVID G. STANDAERT
University of Alabama at Birmingham
Department of Neurology
USA

MEIR STEINER
McMaster University
Psychiatry & Behavioural Neurosciences
and Obstetrics & Gynecology
Canada

JANE R. TAYLOR
Yale University School of Medicine
Associate Professor of Psychiatry
USA

MICHELLE L. TRAVERS
Georgetown University
Brain and Language Laboratory
USA

MICHAEL T. ULLMAN
Georgetown University
Brain and Language Laboratory
Departments of Neuroscience, Linguistics,
Psychology and Neurology
Center for the Study of Sex Differences
USA

IAN Q. WHISHAW
University of Lethbridge
Department of Neuroscience
Canadian Centre for Behavioural Neuroscience
Canada

ELIZABETH A. YOUNG
University of Michigan
Department of Psychiatry
Molecular and Behavioral
Neuroscience Institute
USA

LARRY J. YOUNG
Emory University
Department of Psychiatry and Behavioral Sciences
Center for Behavioral Neuroscience
Yerkes National Primate Research Center
USA

STEVEN S. ZALCMAN
UMDNJ-New Jersey Medical School
Department of Psychiatry
USA

Part I

Strategies, Methods, and Background

Chapter 1

Why Are There Two Sexes?

Turk Rhen and David Crews

One of the most fascinating aspects of life on earth is the myriad of differences between males and females (Judson, 2002). Children and adults alike are captivated when they first learn that males, rather than females, gestate and give birth to offspring in certain species of seahorse. Role reversal is also observed in the red-necked phalarope, a shorebird in which polyandrous females are more brightly colored than their mates and males alone incubate eggs. People are likewise amazed when they hear that ambient temperature determines the sex of many reptiles. While such unusual phenomena capture our curiosity, there are also practical reasons for studying sex differences. For instance, defects in development of the reproductive tract and genitalia are fairly common in humans. Sex differences in physiology and disease affect virtually every organ system in the human body, including the nervous system. Depression, Alzheimer's disease, and schizophrenia are examples of afflictions that differ in incidence, onset, and/or symptoms between males and females. Understanding of the mechanisms underlying sexual differentiation of the body and mind should lead to novel therapies designed to prevent birth defects and cure devastating neurological diseases.

To fully comprehend sex differences in the brain and behavior in humans and to appreciate how animals can be used to model these differences, we need to examine sexual dimorphisms in an evolutionary context. The basic principle that guides biomedical research is that genetic, developmental, physiological, and behavioral mechanisms are conserved in species that have evolved from common ancestors. The unity of life is seen in our hereditary material: the universal genetic code, the enzymes that synthesize DNA, and the proteins that distribute chromosomes to daughter cells during mitosis and meiosis. This principle also permits significant advances in neuroscience. Hodgkin and Huxley, for example, used the giant axon of squid to elucidate action potentials (Clay, 2005). Our knowledge of the mechanisms underlying long-term potentiation and learning has been furthered by studies in sea slugs (Kandel, 2004). Research on guinea pigs has been critical in formation of the concept of organization and activation of sexual behavior by gonadal steroids (Phoenix et al., 1959). Consequently, male seahorses giving birth, polyandrous female phalaropes, and reptiles with temperature-dependent sex determination may not be as esoteric as they seem if conserved genes and biological processes have been co-opted for different uses during evolution. Still, these examples highlight an emerging paradox in studies of sexual differentiation. Reproductive traits in general appear to be evolving more rapidly than other characteristics. Here we provide a three-part introduction to sex differences, stressing both the conserved and the unique as part of Darwin's notion of descent with modification (Darwin, 1859).

In the first section, we step back in time and provide a broad perspective on the evolution of eukaryotes. The evolution of meiosis and syngamy (i.e., the fusion of two cells) was a precondition for the evolution of dimorphic gametes and the subsequent evolution of all other sex differences. We then outline general causes of sex differences in animals by focusing on natural and sexual selection. In particular, we illustrate how sex-specific selection can favor different phenotypes in males and females. This pattern of divergent selection ultimately leads to changes in the neural mechanisms that regulate behavior in the two sexes.

In the second section, we explain the mechanisms that underlie sex differences in gene expression as well as the basic developmental mechanisms that produce sex differences. Despite abundant examples of differential selection on males versus females, there is an inherent constraint to the evolution of sex differences. To be precise, the same genes control homologous traits in both sexes. We describe how several mechanisms relieve this genetic constraint. For instance, genetic differences in the form of sex chromosomes and sex-linked genes have evolved independently in many eukaryotic lineages. Another major mechanism is sex-limited (or differential) expression of autosomal loci, as exemplified by hormonal regulation of gene expression. Environmental factors can also have a large impact on the development of sex differences, a phenomenon commonly referred to as phenotypic plasticity.

Finally, we review some elegant research that links evolutionary causes of and proximate mechanisms for sex differences in the brain and behavior. These examples show how sex-specific selection on behavior

ultimately drives neural evolution. We bring the chapter to a close by briefly outlining what is known about sexual differentiation of neural mechanisms in humans. These mechanisms are undoubtedly related to sex differences in aggressive and sexual behavior and emotional memory, as well as the incidence of affective disorders, anxiety disorders, schizophrenia, and post-traumatic stress disorder (PTSD).

THE EVOLUTION OF EUKARYOTES, MEIOSIS, AND TWO SEXES

Advances in molecular and cellular biology, along with comparative genomics, are allowing reconstruction of the earliest stages in the evolution of life on earth. The first organisms lacked a membrane-bound nucleus, replicated by binary fission, and are survived by today's prokaryotes. Two groups of extant prokaryotes, the eubacteria and the archaebacteria, appear to be as distinct from one another as they are from eukaryotes (Brown & Doolittle, 1997; Bell & Jackson, 2001; Forterre, 2001; Makarova & Koonin, 2003; Robinson & Bell, 2005). This finding makes it difficult to codify the prokaryote-eukaryote transition (Martin, 2005). Yet, research is beginning to elucidate how the first nucleated cells originated and diversified. Some of the most important events in the evolution of eukaryotes involved symbioses (mutually beneficial associations of different species). For instance, the endosymbiotic theory for the origin of mitochondria is well established, even if the timing is in dispute (Embley & Martin, 2006).

One hypothesis has it that the first eukaryotes lacked endosymbionts (currently represented by diplomonads, parabasalids, and microsporidia) and that endosymbionts were acquired in a separate lineage that gave rise to eukaryotes with mitochondria. An alternative hypothesis suggests that endosymbiotic bacteria were acquired concurrent (or nearly so) with the origin of eukaryotes and that these organisms evolved into mitochondria as well as the more derived organelles called hydrogenosomes and mitosomes in eukaryotes that lack prototypical mitochondria (Embley & Martin, 2006). In either case, this ancient event has direct implications for human health because mutations in mitochondrial DNA, which is maternally inherited, cause a number of diseases (Chen & Butow, 2005; Dimauro & Davidzon, 2005). Mitochondria also play a central role in apoptosis, a form of cell death that contributes to normal development and to diverse pathological states (Schafer & Kornbluth, 2006; Garrido et al., 2006). It is especially interesting that vertebrates evolved the capacity for a novel class of molecules (i.e., estrogens and androgens) to influence mitochondia-dependent apoptosis in the nervous system (Nilsen & Brinton, 2004; Forger, 2006; Lin et al., 2006).

There are several hypotheses for the origin of the membrane-bound nucleus (Martin, 2005), but two basic categories can be distinguished. The first group of hypotheses suggests direct evolution of this unique structure in the initial forms of life (Woese, 1998), while the second posits a symbiotic origin for the nucleus (Dolan et al., 2002). Whether the nucleus evolved *de novo* or from an archaebacterial-eubacterial symbiont, it is clear that microtubules played a central role in the evolution of eukaryotes. Microtubules are essential for mitosis and are a key component of the cytoskeleton. Moreover, the first split within the eukaryotic lineage involves a basic difference in the assembly of microtubules (Stechmann & Cavalier-Smith, 2003; Richards & Cavalier-Smith, 2005). While animals, fungi, Choanozoa, and Amoebozoa (unikonts) have a single microtubule-organizing center, plants, chromists, and all other protozoa (bikonts) have two microtubule-organizing centers.

In animals, the microtubule-organizing center or centrosome is composed of two centrioles located near the nucleus. Each centriole replicates during interphase to produce two pair of centrioles. In prophase of mitosis, paired centrioles are pushed apart by microtubule polymerization. Microtubules spanning pole-to-pole (i.e., centriole-to-centriole) form the backbone of the mitotic spindle. Another set of microtubules attaches one pole to one side of the centromere of sister chromatids. An opposing set of microtubules links the other side of the centromere to the other pole. Depolymerization of these microtubules during anaphase pulls the sister chromatids to opposite ends of the cell, which then divides to complete mitosis. In plants, spindle fibers form between two microtubule-organizing centers already located on opposite ends of the cell. Otherwise, mitosis is essentially the same in unikonts and bikonts.

Given the basic role that microtubules play in mitosis, it is amazing that mutations in a few genes that interact with microtubules have a highly specific effect on the size of the mammalian brain (Bond & Woods, 2006). Products of these genes are localized to the centrosome in periventricular cells and are hypothesized to regulate formation and orientation of the mitotic spindle. Proliferation of neural progenitors occurs when spindle fibers run parallel to the ventricular epithelium. In contrast, neurogenesis generally occurs when spindle fibers are perpendicular to the ventricular epithelium. Exactly how orientation of the mitotic spindle relates to commitment to a neuronal fate is unknown, but it is possible that the post-mitotic location of the centrosome (i.e., cell asymmetry and microtubule polarity) is vital, like it is to development of neuronal polarity (de Anda et al., 2005). Again, we see how an ancient event in the evolution of eukaryotes has implications for neural development.

While mitochondria and mitosis are important to human health, the adaptations most salient to our discussion of sex differences are meiosis and syngamy. Three simple molecular changes account for the transition from mitosis to meiosis. The first change was in alignment and crossing over between homologous chromosomes. This process of genetic recombination utilized pre-existing mechanisms for DNA repair found in prokaryotes (Santucci-Darmanin & Paquis-Flucklinger, 2003), further illustrating Darwin's concept of descent with modification. Another change was in attachment of microtubules to sister chromatids. Two kinetochores, which link microtubules to the centromere, are in a bipolar orientation in mitotic cells. The end result of this geometric arrangement is that sister chromatids are attached and pulled to opposite poles. In contrast, kinetochores on sister chromatids are oriented in the same direction during meiosis I (Hauf & Watanabe, 2004). Special proteins also serve to hold sister chromatids together during meiosis I (Kitajima et al., 2004). The natural consequence of unipolar kinetochore geometry, sister chromatid cohesion, and synapsis is that sister chromatids are pulled to the same pole and that homologous chromosomes are pulled to opposite poles. Finally, meiosis II, which is virtually identical to mitosis, completes reduction division. Discussion of the evolution of syngamy is beyond the scope of this chapter (see Cavalier-Smith, 2002), but suffice it to say that alternation between diploid and haploid stages in the life cycle of eukaryotes opened the door for selection to produce sex differences.

The first characteristic that we might broadly consider a sex difference is mating type. Nearly all lower eukaryotes have mating-type loci that prevent syngamy between cells with the same genotype (Charlesworth,

1994; Souza et al., 2003). Yet, most eukaryotic lineages display no other sign of sexual dimorphism (i.e., fungi, Choanozoa, Amoebozoa, chromists and protozoa). The cells that fuse during syngamy in these groups are of the same size, indicating isogamy was the ancestral state in eukaryotes. Because anisogamy (i.e., dimorphic gametes) and more derived sex differences are only found in one lineage on either side of the unikont-bikont split, sexual dimorphism, it is suggested, evolved independently in animals and plants. Until that point, natural selection was the main force driving biological evolution.

Sexual selection only became relevant with the evolution of dimorphic gametes (Levitan, 1996; Levitan & Ferrell, 2006). The key to understanding the evolution of sex differences therefore lies in the fact that each zygote gets half its genome from its father and half from its mother. This means that an individual's reproductive success through male function (i.e., sperm) must be measured relative to the male function of other individuals. The converse applies to fitness through female function (i.e., eggs). Accordingly, traits that benefit one sex can have harmful effects when expressed in the other sex. This pattern of sex-specific selection favors different phenotypes in males and females and the evolution of sexual dimorphism. Elegant experimental work by William Rice (1992) demonstrated that genes with sexually antagonistic effects on male versus female fitness are abundant in fruit flies.

Another important concept is sexual conflict, which occurs when male and female reproductive interests do not coincide. In other words, traits that increase the fitness of the sex expressing the trait can decrease a mate's fitness (Rice, 1996a; Chapman et al., 2003). Male fruit flies, for instance, produce seminal chemicals that induce females to lay more eggs and decrease the likelihood that females will mate again (Wolfner, 1997). These chemicals increase the fitness of polygynous males, but simultaneously decrease the fitness of females by shortening their lifespan (Wigby & Chapman, 2005). Another example of sexual conflict occurs in water striders, a species in which males and females struggle over mating (Rowe et al., 1994; Preziosi & Fairbairn, 2000; Rowe & Arnquist, 2002). Males can prevent their mates from re-mating with other males by clinging to females' backs after copulation. This behavior, while ensuring that a male fertilizes all of his mate's eggs, has a significant energetic cost for females that carry males for a few minutes up to several weeks (Watson et al., 1998). It is not sur-

prising then that males and females physically struggle with each other to control the frequency and duration of mating.

MECHANISMS UNDERLYING SEX DIFFERENCES

Sexual selection occurs in two basic ways: *intrasexual* and *intersexual*. Intrasexual selection results from direct competition for mates or mating opportunities within a sex. For instance, female shore birds, like red-necked phalaropes, spotted sandpipers, and jacanas compete with each other for paternal males (Schamel et al., 2004a,b). Females in these species are physiologically capable of producing two (or more) clutches of eggs in a breeding season, while males can only incubate and care for one clutch. Females able to monopolize two (or more) males therefore have higher fitness than females that are only able to mate with one male or who aren't fortunate enough to mate at all (Andersson, 2005).

Intersexual selection occurs when interactions between the sexes influence reproductive success. A classic example is female mate choice that is based on male characteristics, i.e., the peacock's tail. Conversely, the bright plumage of female phalaropes and the facial ornamentation of female wattled jacanas may be a result of male preferences for these traits (Emlen & Wrege, 2004). Exaggerated traits, be they behavioral or morphological, provide a mating advantage in one sex, but are costly to display for both sexes. Asymmetric benefits and costs once more favor the development of sex differences. Yet, there is an inherent constraint to the evolution of such differences because the same genes control homologous traits in the initially monomorphic sexes. How then do males and females develop different phenotypes?

One way is through the evolution of chromosomes passed exclusively from father to son or from mother to daughter, as in mammals (XY males, XX females) and birds (ZZ males, ZW females). Empirical and theoretical studies support the following model for the evolution of sex chromosomes and sex-linked inheritance. A new sex-determining locus initially evolves on an autosome: i.e., a locus with a dominant allele M for maleness, and a recessive allele m for femaleness. There are two possible genotypes with this sex-determining system: Mm individuals develop as males, while mm individuals develop as females. By chance, genes with antagonistic effects on male versus female fitness may reside on the same chromosome as the novel sex-determining gene. Selection then favors tighter linkage between alleles that benefit males and the male-determining allele M. Selection also favors linkage between alleles that benefit females and the female allele m. Recombination between nascent X and Y chromosomes is suppressed, which in turn leads to progressive deterioration of the Y chromosome (Rice 1996b; Lahn & Page, 1999). An analogous scenario applies to the evolution of W and Z chromosomes.

Sex chromosomes have evolved independently in diverse groups of animals and are even found in some plants (Bull, 1983; Tanurdzic & Banks, 2004). Nevertheless, the importance of sex linkage as a mechanism for phenotypic differentiation between the sexes varies among groups. For example, just 0.15% of all genes (or 45/30,000) are Y-linked in humans. Roughly 4.5% of all genes (or 1,344/30,000) are X-linked in humans. A much higher percentage of genes are found on the X chromosome in fruit flies (~16% or 2,309/14,449), though the Y chromosome carries proportionately fewer genes (0.06% or 9/14,449) (Carvalho et al., 2001). The difference in gene content between the Z and W chromosomes is lower in chickens: 1.4% of all genes are Z-linked (328/23,000), while 0.2% are W-linked (47/23,000). The degree of sex chromosome differentiation even varies within groups: zebrafish have autosomes, platyfish have genotypic sex determination without any distinction between sex chromosomes, and guppies have morphologically distinct X and Y chromosomes (Traut & Winking, 2001). The potential for sex-linked genes to play a direct role in differentiation of the brain has been under appreciated until recently (Arnold, 2004).

The majority of genes, however, do not reside on sex chromosomes. Moreover, many organisms do not have sex chromosomes at all, but still have dimorphic males and females. How do the sexes come to differ in these species? To answer this question, we need to understand what happens when selection favors different autosomal alleles in males versus females (Rhen, 2000). Imagine, for instance, a gene that induces development of a trait that is favored in females, but disfavored in males. A constitutively expressed allele would be advantageous in females while a null allele would benefit males. Neither sex is able to reach its phenotypic optimum with this type of genetic variation. A simple solution to this dilemma is the evolution of a third allele that is only expressed in females.

While sexually antagonistic selection causes the rapid fixation of such sex-limited mutations, other patterns of sex-specific selection can also increase sexual dimorphism (Rhen, 2000).

At least two distinct mechanisms produce differential expression of autosomal loci in males and females. The first involves interactions between sex-linked and autosomal loci (Noonan & Hoffman, 1994; Kreutz et al., 1996; Montagutelli et al., 1996; Paallysaho et al., 2003; Perry et al., 2003; Chase et al., 2005), while the second involves sex steroids (Hughes, 2001; MacLaughlin & Donahoe, 2004, this volume). The first mechanism is not widely recognized, but the latter is well known. In fact, sex steroids, which act independently of sex chromosomes, are the major mechanism regulating the development of sex differences in vertebrates. Despite diversity in the initial trigger for sex determination among amniotic vertebrates, the basic morphogenetic process of gonadal differentiation is conserved. The gonadal anlagen are initially bipotential, consist of a cortical region that gives rise to the ovary, and a medullary region that gives rise to the testis. Moreover, the key somatic cell types in the ovary (granulosa and theca cells) and the testis (sertoli and leydig cells) are conserved, as are the steroids these cells produce: estrogens, progestins, and androgens.

The evolution of this mode of sexual differentiation depended upon the appearance of a receptor that recognized and bound steroidal molecules (Thornton, 2001). Indeed, phylogenetic analyses indicate that the first steroid hormone receptor evolved before the protosome-deuterostome split 600–1000 mya. The ancestral receptor had estrogen receptor-like properties and gave rise to all of the steroid hormone receptors that exist today (Thornton et al., 2003). The putative estrogen receptor co-opted as its ligand the estrogen-like molecules associated with oocyte maturation. This event was significant because estrogen is the terminal hormone in the steroidogenic pathway, thereby making the intermediate hormones, progesterone and androgen, potential ligands. After the first of two genome-wide duplications, one of the duplicated estrogen-receptor genes evolved into a progesterone receptor, which like estrogen, was linked to the ovarian cycle, and in particular ovulation, oviposition, and birth. The second genome-wide duplication occurred after separation of the lamprey lineage from other vertebrates. This event was followed by evolution of the androgen receptor, laying the groundwork for androgen-mediated sex differences. In general, steroids enter cells, bind to cognate receptors, and induce or suppress transcription of target genes (Rhen & Cidlowski, 2004). Research during the last decade has shown that sex steroids also have non-genomic effects that are mediated by second messenger pathways (Rhen & Cidlowski, 2004). Yet, the importance of nongenomic mechanisms of steroid action for sex differences in the brain is currently unclear.

So far we have only discussed the evolution of the intrinsic genetic and hormonal factors responsible for sex differences. The two sexes, however, do not develop in a vacuum. Many environmental factors, including embryonic, ecologic, and social surroundings, are known to influence sexual differentiation. The pivotal role of the environment in development was recognized at the turn of the twentieth century by Hertwig and Woltereck, whose work on *Daphnia*, an organism that reproduces asexually to produce clones of itself, demonstrated that genetically identical individuals would develop very different phenotypes depending upon their environment (Gilbert, 2002); a human counterpart has recently been described in monozygotic twin studies (e.g., Chakravarti & Little, 2003; Fraga et al., 2005). The general phenomenon in which a single genotype (i.e., individual) can produce more than one phenotype in response to specific environmental stimuli is referred to as phenotypic plasticity (Lewontin, 2000). It is also important that individuals with different genotypes often have different responses to the same environmental stimuli. This means that phenotypic plasticity itself has a genetic basis and can evolve adaptively (Pigliucci, 2005; Gluckman et al., 2005; Fordyce, 2006). Genotype-environment interactions of this sort include the processes underlying neural and behavioral development and learning (Duchaine et al., 2001; Dopazo et al., 2003; Egnor & Hauser, 2004).

Phenotypic plasticity has two important implications for our understanding of sex differences. First, males and females may differ in their level of plasticity (Jonasson, 2004; Cahill, 2006; Sherry, 2006). Second, sex differences may be shaped or caused by experiential differences (McCarthy & Konkle, 2005). It is frequently the same genetic and hormonal factors that we have already introduced that mediate environmental effects on phenotype. For instance, exposure to exogenous (i.e., maternally derived) hormones or xenobiotics (i.e., man-made chemicals) early in life can alter responses to hormones later in life (Crews & McLachlan, 2006). Other factors such as stress and

drugs in action during embryogenesis can shape the subsequent behavioral phenotype of the individual, and modify the way the individual responds to adult experiences. The clinical significance of this work resides squarely within the concept identified as the "fetal basis of adult disease." For example, malnutrition in a mother during early pregnancy increases the risk of schizophrenia in the child once the child reaches adulthood (Barker, 2003; Barker et al., 2002; Bateson et al., 2004; Gluckman & Hanson, 2005). These disorders are often precipitated by stress, which alters the endocrine state. Some women who experienced the collapse of the World Trade Center while pregnant developed PTSD. These women and their babies have lower cortisol levels than unaffected mothers and their babies (Yehuda et al., 2005).

Building on a long history of research in developmental psychobiology, Meaney and colleagues (2001; Weaver et al., 2004) have demonstrated that the nature and amount of care a rat pup receives from its mother modulates its reaction to stress later in life through effects on the glucocorticoid receptor (GR) in the hippocampus. This maternal effect can cross generations, but critically depends on the pup's experience in the first week of life. Recently, it was documented by this group that rearing by a high-quality mother results in the expression of the transcription factor NGFI-A, a nerve growth factor-inducible protein, that binds to the first exon of the GR gene, resulting in increased expression of GR. High-quality maternal care during this critical period results in demethylation of the NGFI-A binding site in the GR promoter and increases the acetylation of histones at the promoter. Just as cross fostering pups can reverse these molecular changes, infusion of histone deacetylase inhibitor into the hippocampus can reverse these events. Is there a counterpart in humans? Caspi and colleagues (2002, 2003) have demonstrated how the rearing environment can overcome the influence of genotype in the etiology of violent behavior. It is important to note, however, that this form of epigenetic transmission is not transgenerational, but rather induced in each generation by the parent or the environment.

EXAMPLES OF SEX DIFFERENCES IN THE BRAIN AND BEHAVIOR

Males and females behave differently, and from an evolutionary point of view, this dimorphism results from the influence of behavior on the fitness of the two sexes. From a mechanistic point of view, this leaves us with two questions: What exactly is different about male and female brains? How might sex differences evolve through the mechanisms just outlined?

Enormous progress has been made in answering the first question. We now understand that the same steroid and peptide hormones involved in regulating gamete production, pregnancy (gravidity), birth (oviposition), and parental care, if it occurs, are powerful determinants of brain function. These hormones direct the development of sexually dimorphic brain structures and influence reproductive as well as non-reproductive behaviors (Jonasson, 2004; Cahill, 2006). Although less progress has been made on the second question, two success stories involve closely related sexual and unisexual whiptail lizards and monogamous and polygamous voles.

Whiptail lizards (genus *Cnemidophorus*) exhibit an extremely simple pattern of sexually dimorphic behavior (Crews, 2005). Around the time of ovulation, females allow males to mount them in a fashion characteristic of the genus. Outside of this period, there is essentially no interaction between the sexes; no parental behavior, minimal courtship, no territoriality, and as far as is known, very little social behavior. Perhaps the most significant aspect of whiptail lizards is that a number of species consist only of females that reproduce by obligate parthenogenesis. Further, we know that parthenogenetic species arose through hybrid unions of sexual species. For example, the desert-grasslands whiptail (*C. uniparens*, trans. one parent) arose through an initial hybridization between two sexually reproducing species, the rusty rumped whiptail (*C. burti*) and the little striped whiptail (*C. inornatus*, trans. without ornament, referring to this species' lack of spots), and a subsequent backcross of the hybrid with *C. inornatus*. Hence, the relationship among these species is perhaps best viewed as a snapshot of evolution (representatives of the ancestral and the descendant species).

Equally remarkable is that each parthenogen displays both male-like and female-like copulatory behavior during the reproductive cycle: since these animals are all female and lack intromittent organs, this behavior has been termed *pseudocopulation* (Crews & Fitzgerald, 1980). Thus, unlike the ancestral species in which mating behaviors are sexually dimorphic, with males mounting females who are receptive to this behavior, *C. uniparens* display both male- and female-typical sexual behaviors in alternating fashion, according to ovarian state. The ovarian cycle is characterized by circulating concentrations of estradiol, gradually increasing during follicular development, and then declining sharply following ovulation; whereas, progesterone titer is low during follicular development and increases dramatically around the time of ovulation.

Androgens are undetectable throughout the cycle in female *C. inornatus* and in *C. uniparens*. Female-like receptive behavior is limited to the preovulatory phase of the cycle whereas male-like mounting behavior is displayed most frequently following ovulation. Thus, the behavioral transition occurs at ovulation when there is a parallel transition from estradiol dominance to progesterone dominance, suggesting that changes in hormone levels could underlie changes in behavior.

Clonal reproduction and the retention of sexual behavior allows the investigator to circumvent major confounds in the study of sexual dimorphisms, namely that males and females differ in several ways, and hence sex differences may be due to genotypic differences, hormonal background, or even experiences particular to each sex. In addition to each parthenogen displaying mounting and receptive behaviors, it is possible to create 'males' to compare with the males of the ancestral sexual species. That is, by treating eggs with an aromatase inhibitor one can induce development of *Virago* males (meaning "a man-like woman"). Virago males are genetically identical to parthenogens yet they have fully developed male genitalia, motile sperm, and only display male-like mounting behaviors. Taken together, these whiptail lizards enable study of the neural substrates underlying sex-typical behaviors from an evolutionary standpoint (comparing the ancestral and descendant species).

Species and sex differences are found in hormonal regulation of steroid receptors in the brain. Females, but not males, of the sexual species respond to exogenous estrogen by increasing progesterone receptor (PR) mRNA in the ventromedial hypothalamus (VMH). Males have higher androgenic receptor (AR) mRNA in the medial preoptic area (POA) than do females of the sexual species or the descendant parthenogens. Androgen treatment also increases the expression of PR mRNA in the periventricular preoptic area (PvPOA) in both males and females of the sexual species as well as in the descendant parthenogens. Exogenous estradiol increases PR mRNA expression in the PvPOA of the parthenogen, but not in females of the sexual species. This last finding suggests a possible proximate mechanism underlying species differences in behavior. The POA is a conserved brain area involved in the control of mounting behavior and is normally sensitive to androgen. In the parthenogenetic species, the preovulatory surge in estrogen upregulates PR mRNA in this brain region, enabling the postovulatory progesterone surge to activate pseudocopulatory behavior. In contrast, estradiol does not upregulate PR in the PvPOA during the preovulatory phase in females of the sexual species, and these females do not display male-typical mounting behavior in response to the surge of progesterone following ovulation. Finally, despite their male-like morphology and behavior, Virago C. *uniparens* are female-like in characteristics that are sexually dimorphic in C. *inornatus*. For example, in Virago males the volume of both the POA and VMH is female-typical; they display estrogen-induced upregulation of PR in the POA and testosterone regulation of arginine vasotocin (AVT) expression, which is independent of neuroendocrine history or genetic sex (Hillsman et al., 2007).

Insight into the evolution of more complex social behavior comes from comparative studies of prairie voles, which are monogamous, and in montane voles, which are polygamous (Carter et al., 1995; Young et al., 2005; Nair & Young, 2006; Young & Carter, this volume). In the polygamous species, males and females are solitary, except during mating, and only females care for offspring. In contrast, males and females in the monogamous species display long-term social bonds (regardless of reproductive status), biparental care of offspring, and aggression toward unfamiliar con-specifics. Formation of pair bonds that endure beyond mating in monogamous prairie voles depends on oxytocin signaling in females and arginine vasopressin (AVP) signaling in males (Young & Wang, 2004). In fact, central administration of oxytocin to females and AVP to males enhances formation of a pair bond even if the duo is not allowed to mate. Conversely, antagonists for the oxytocin receptor and the AVP receptor 1a block social attachment in mated female and male prairie voles. A nucleus-specific difference in expression of AVP receptor 1a between prairie and montane voles is responsible for the difference in social behavior in these closely related species (Lim et al., 2004a). In particular, AVP receptor 1a is expressed at a higher level in the ventral pallidum of the prairie vole than in the montane vole.

Transgenic overexpression of the AVP receptor 1a in the ventral pallidum of male montane voles results in attachment of males to their mate. An analogous experiment examining the role of oxytocin in the evolution of social attachment in females has yet to be conducted, but there are differences in oxytocin receptor expression between prairie and montane voles (i.e., higher expression in the nucleus accumbens in the monogamous species). A working model for pair bonding has olfactory cues from a sexual partner activating oxytocin and AVP pathways in females and males, respectively. In turn, these pathways converge on a common dopaminergic reward pathway that is activated during copulation in both sexes, which results in a conditioned preference for the sexual partner (Young & Wang, 2004).

Although there are no sex differences in AVP receptor 1a expression in the prairie vole, males have more AVP positive cells in the bed nucleus of the stria terminalis and the medial amygdala as well as denser AVP projections to nuclei involved in social behavior (Bamshad et al., 1993; Laszlo et al., 1993; Lim et al., 2004b). It is particularly intriguing that male-biased expression of AVP (or its non-mammalian homologue arginine vasotocin AVT) appears to be conserved among vertebrates, even though the mechanism underlying this sex difference varies (De Vries & Panzica, 2006). For example, although testosterone induces AVP/AVT expression in adult male rats and Japanese quail, hormonal organization of this male-typical response is different. Testosterone via aromatization to estrogen during early development masculinizes the AVP system in rats. Conversely, early exposure to estrogen feminizes the AVP system in Japanese quail. There is evidence that sex-linked genes contribute to sex differences in AVP expression in mice (De Vries et al., 2002; Arnold, 2004; Gatewood, et al., 2006), but not in whiptail lizards (see previous).

Humans appear to be different from many other vertebrates in not having a gross sex difference in the AVP system (Fliers et al., 1986). Nevertheless, administration of physiologically relevant levels of AVP has sex-specific effects on social perception of and autonomic responses to other humans (Thompson et al., 2006). Men treated with AVP and allowed to view pictures of men with affiliative facial expressions respond with agonistic facial activity and lower ratings of the friendliness of those faces. Women treated with AVP have just the opposite response to pictures of women with affiliative facial expressions.

The conserved function of AVP/AVT as a modulator of social behavior, in conjunction with changes in the regulation of AVP expression in the brain underscores the notion of descent with modification. This general concept is also evident in the function of certain brain nuclei: the amygdala, for instance, plays a key role in behavioral sex differences in humans and other animals (Hamann, 2005; Cahill, 2006). This particular brain region is involved in regulating social behaviors that have an emotional component, including fear, aggression, and sexual motivation, but the socially relevant input varies (i.e., pheromones in rodents, visual stimuli in humans).

There are many other sex differences in brain structure, gene expression, neurochemistry, reproductive behavior, and nonreproductive behavior in humans (Nopoulos et al., 2000; Hamann, 2005; Rinn & Snyder, 2005; Cahill, 2006; reviewed in this volume). While we are unique in many ways, especially with respect to our brain and behavior, we cannot hope to understand why we have these characteristics without understanding our ecological and evolutionary history (Joseph, 2000; Panter-Brick, 2002; Sherry 2004). Our goal in this chapter was to provide a conceptual overview of the ultimate (natural and sexual selection) and proximate (sex chromosomes, sex steroids, and phenotypic plasticity) causes of sex differences and to illustrate how animals can be used to help us understand these differences in humans.

References

Andersson M. (2005). Evolution of classical polyandry: Three steps to female emancipation. *Ethology*, 111:1–23.

Arnold AP. (2004). Sex chromosomes and brain gender. *Nature Rev Neurosci*, 5:1–8.

Bamshad M, Novak MA, De Vries GJ. (1993). Sex and species differences in the vasopressin innervation of sexually naive and parental prairie voles, Microtus ochrogaster and meadow voles, Microtus pennsylvanicus. *J Neuroendocrinol*, 5:247–255.

Barker DJ, Eriksson JG, Forsen T, Osmond C. (2002). Fetal origins of adult disease: strength of effects and biological basis. *Int J Epidemiol*, 31:1235–1239.

Barker DJ. (2003). The developmental origins of adult disease. *Eur J Epidemiol*, 18:733–736.

Bateson P, Barker D, Clutton-Brock T, Deb D, D'Udine B, Foley RA, et al. (2004). Developmental plasticity and human health. *Nature*, 430:419–421.

Bell SD, Jackson SP. (2001). Mechanism and regulation of transcription in archaea. *Curr Opin Microbiol*, 4:208–213.

Bond J, Woods CG. (2006). Cytoskeletal genes regulating brain size. *Curr Opin Cell Biol*, 18:95–101.

Brown JR, Doolittle WF. (1997). Archaea and the prokaryote-to-eukaryote transition. *Microbiol Mol Biol Rev*, 61:456–502.

Bull JJ. (1983). *Evolution of sex determining mechanisms.* Menlo Park, CA: Benjamin/Cummings.

Cahill L. (2006). Why sex matters for neuroscience. *Nat Rev Neurosci*, 7:477–484.

Carter CS, DeVries AC, Getz LL. (1995). Physiological substrates of mammalian monogamy: the prairie vole model. *Neurosci Biobehav Rev*, 19:303–314.

Carvalho AB, Dobo BA, Vibranovski MD, Clark AG. (2001). Identification of five new genes on the Y chromosome of Drosophila melanogaster. *Proc Natl Acad Sci*, 98:13225–13230.

Caspi A, McClay J, Moffitt TE, Mill J, Martin C, Craig IW, Taylor A, Poulton R. (2002). Role of genotype in the cycle of violence in maltreated children. *Science*, 297:851–854.

Caspi A, Sugden K, Moffitt TE, Taylor A, Craig IW, Harrington H, et al. (2003). Influence of life stress on depression: moderation by a polymorphism in the 5-HTT gene. *Science*, 301:386–389.

Chakravarti A, Little P. (2003). Nature, nurture and human disease. *Nature*, 421:412–414.

Chapman T, Arnqvist G, Bangham J, Rowe L. (2003). Sexual conflict. *Trends in Ecology and Evolution*, 18:41–47.

Cavalier-Smith T. (2002). The phagotrophic origin of eukaryotes and phylogenetic classification of Protozoa. *Int J Syst Evol Microbiol*, 52:297–354.

Charlesworth B. (1994). Evolutionary genetics. The nature and origin of mating types. *Curr Biol*, 4:739–741.

Chase K, Carrier DR, Adler FR, Ostrander EA, Lark KG. (2005). Interaction between the X chromosome and an autosome regulates size sexual dimorphism in Portuguese Water Dogs. *Genome Res*, 15:1820–1824.

Chen XJ, Butow RA. (2005). The organization and inheritance of the mitochondrial genome. *Nat Rev Genet*, 6:815–825.

Clay JR. (2005). Axonal excitability revisited. *Prog Biophys Mol Biol*, 88:59–90.

Crews D. (2005). Evolution of neuroendocrine mechanisms that regulate sexual behavior. *Trends Endocrinol Metab*, 16:354–361.

Crews D, Fitzgerald KT. (1980). "Sexual" behavior in parthenogenetic lizards (Cnemidophorus). *Proc Natl Acad Sci USA*, 77:499–502.

Crews D. McLachlan JA. (2006). Epigenetics, evolution, endocrine disruptors, health and disease. *Endocrinology*, 147(Supplement):S4-S10.

Darwin C. (1859). *On the origin of species.* London: John Murray.

de Anda FC, Pollarolo G, Da Silva JS, Camoletto PG, Feiguin F, Dotti CG. (2005). Centrosome localization determines neuronal polarity. *Nature*, 436:704–708.

De Vries GJ, Panzica GC. (2006). Sexual differentiation of central vasopressin and vasotocin systems in vertebrates: different mechanisms, similar endpoints. *Neuroscience*, 138:947–955.

De Vries GJ, Rissman EF, Simerly RB, Yang LY, Scordalakes EM, Auger CJ, et al. (2002). A model system for study of sex chromosome effects on sexually dimorphic neural and behavioral traits. *J Neurosci*, 22:9005–9014.

Dimauro S, Davidzon G. (2005). Mitochondrial DNA and disease. *Ann Med*, 37:222–232.

Dolan MF, Melnitsky H, Margulis L, Kolnicki R. (2002). Motility proteins and the origin of the nucleus. *Anat Rec*, 268:290–301.

Dopazo H, Gordon MB, Perazzo R, Risau-Gusman S. (2003). A model for the emergence of adaptive subsystems. *Bull Math Biol*, 65:27–56.

Duchaine B, Cosmides L, Tooby J. (2001). Evolutionary psychology and the brain. *Curr Opin Neurobiol*, 11: 225–230.

Egnor SE, Hauser MD. (2004). A paradox in the evolution of primate vocal learning. *Trends Neurosci*, 27:649–654.

Embley TM, Martin W. (2006). Eukaryotic evolution, changes and challenges. *Nature*, 440:623–630.

Emlen ST, Wrege PH. (2004). Size dimorphism, intrasexual competition, and sexual selection in Wattled Jacana (Jacana jacana), a sex-role-reversed shorebird in Panama. *Auk*, 121:391–403.

Fliers E, Guldenaar SE, van de Wal N, Swaab DF. (1986). Extrahypothalamic vasopressin and oxytocin in the human brain; presence of vasopressin cells in the bed nucleus of the stria terminalis. *Brain Res*, 375:363–367.

Fordyce JA. (2006). The evolutionary consequences of ecological interactions mediated through phenotypic plasticity. *J Exp Biol*, 209:2377–2383.

Forger NG. (2006). Cell death and sexual differentiation of the nervous system. *Neuroscience*, 138:929–938.

Forterre P. (2001). Genomics and early cellular evolution. The origin of the DNA world. *C R Acad Sci III*, 324:1067–1076.

Fraga MF, Ballestar E, Paz MF, Ropero S, Setien F, Ballestar ML, et al. (2005). Epigenetic differences arise during the lifetime of monozygotic twins. *Proc Natl Acad Sci USA*, 102:10604–10609.

Garrido C, Galluzzi L, Brunet M, Puig PE, Didelot C, Kroemer G. (2006). Mechanisms of cytochrome c release from mitochondria. Cell Death Differ e-pub ahead of print.

Gatewood JD, Wills A, Shetty S, Xu J, Arnold AP, Burgoyne PS, Rissman EF. (2006). Sex chromosome complement and gonadal sex influence aggressive and parental behaviors in mice. *J Neurosci*, 26:2335–2342.

Gilbert SF. (2002). The genome in its ecological context philosophical perspectives on interspecies epigenesis. *Ann NY Acad Sci*, 981:202–218.

Gluckman PD, Hanson MA. (2005). *The fetal matrix: evolution, development and disease.* Cambridge: Cambridge University Press.

Hamann S. (2005). Sex differences in the responses of the human amygdala. *Neuroscientist*, 11:288–293.

Hauf S, Watanabe Y. (2004). Kinetochore orientation in mitosis and meiosis. *Cell*, 119:317–327.

Hillsman KD, Sanderson NS, Crews D. (2007). Testosterone stimulates mounting behavior and arginine vasotocin expression in the brain of both sexual and unisexual whiptail lizards. *Sexual Development*, 1: 77–84.

Hughes IA. (2001). Minireview: sex differentiation. *Endocrinology*, 142:3281–3287.

Jonasson Z. (2005). Meta-analysis of sex differences in rodent models of learning and memory: a review of behavioral and biological data. *Neurosci Biobehav Rev*, 28:811–825.

Joseph R. (2000). The evolution of sex differences in language, sexuality, and visual-spatial skills. Arch Sex Behav, 29:35–66.

Judson O. (2002). *Dr. Tatiana's sex advice to all creation.* New York: Metropolitan Books.

Kandel ER. (2004). The molecular biology of memory storage: a dialog between genes and synapses. *Biosci Rep*, 24:475–522.

Kitajima TS, Kawashima SA, Watanabe Y. (2004). The conserved kinetochore protein shugoshin protects centromeric cohesion during meiosis. *Nature*, 427:510–517.

Kreutz R, Stock P, Struk B, Lindpaintner K. (1996). The Y chromosome. Epistatic and ecogenetic interactions in genetic hypertension. *Hypertension*, 28: 895–897.

Lahn BT, Page DC. (1999). Four evolutionary strata on the human X chromosome. *Science*, 286:964–967.

Laszlo FA, Varga C, Papp A, Pavo I, Fahrenholz F. (1993). Difference between male and female rats in vasopressor response to arginine vasopressin. *Acta Physiol Hung*, 81:137–145.

Levitan DR. (1996). Effects of gamete traits on fertilization in the sea and the evolution of sexual dimorphism. *Nature*, 382:153–155.

Levitan DR, Ferrell DL. (2006). Selection on gamete recognition proteins depends on sex, density, and genotype frequency. *Science*, 312:267–269.

Lewontin RC. (2000). *The triple helix: gene, organism and environment.* Cambridge, MA: Harvard University Press.

Lim MM, Wang Z, Olazabal DE, Ren X, Terwilliger EF, Young LJ. (2004a). Enhanced partner preference in a promiscuous species by manipulating the expression of a single gene. *Nature*, 429:754–757.

Lim MM, Murphy AZ, Young LJ. (2004b). Ventral striatopallidal oxytocin and vasopressin V1a receptors in the monogamous prairie vole (Microtus ochrogaster). *J Comp Neurol*, 468:555–570.

Lin Y, Kokontis J, Tang F, Godfrey B, Liao S, Lin A, Chen Y, Xiang J. (2006). Androgen and its receptor promote Bax-mediated apoptosis. *Mol Cell Biol*, 26:1908–1916.

MacLaughlin DT, Donahoe PK. (2004). Sex determination and differentiation. *N Engl J Med*, 350:367–378.

Makarova KS, Koonin EV. (2003). Comparative genomics of Archaea: how much have we learned in six years, and what's next? *Genome Biol*, 4:115.

Martin W. (2005). Archaebacteria (Archaea) and the origin of the eukaryotic nucleus. *Curr Opin Microbiol*, 8:630–637.

McCarthy MM, Konkle AT. (2005). When is a sex difference not a sex difference? *Front Neuroendocrinol*, 26:85–102.

Meaney MJ. (2001). Maternal care, gene expression and the transmission of individual differences in stress reactivity across generations. *Ann Rev Neurosci*, 24: 161–192.

Montagutelli X, Turner R, Nadeau JH. (1996). Epistatic control of non-Mendelian inheritance in mouse interspecific crosses. *Genetics*, 143:1739–1752.

Nair HP, Young LJ. (2006). Vasopressin and pair-bond formation: genes to brain to behavior. *Physiology*, 21:146–152.

Nilsen J, Brinton RD. (2004). Mitochondria as therapeutic targets of estrogen action in the central nervous system. *Curr Drug Targets CNS Neurol Disord*, 3:297–313.

Noonan FP, Hoffman HA. (1994). Control of UVB immunosuppression in the mouse by autosomal and sex-linked genes. *Immunogenetics*, 40:247–256.

Nopoulos P, Flaum M, O'Leary D, Andreasen NC. (2000). Sexual dimorphism in the human brain: evaluation of tissue volume, tissue composition and surface anatomy using magnetic resonance imaging. *Psychiatry Res*, 98:1–13.

Paallysaho S, Aspi J, Liimatainen JO, Hoikkala A. (2003). Role of X chromosomal song genes in the evolution of species-specific courtship songs in Drosophila virilis group species. *Behav Genet*, 33: 25–32.

Panter-Brick C. (2002). Sexual division of labor: energetic and evolutionary scenarios. *Am J Hum Biol*, 14:627–640.

Paul, A. (2002). Sexual selection and mate choice. *Int J Primat*, 23:877–904.

Perry GM, Ferguson MM, Danzmann RG. (2003). Effects of genetic sex and genomic background on epistasis in rainbow trout (Oncorhynchus mykiss). *Genetica*, 119:35–50.

Phoenix CH, Goy RW, Gerell AA, Young WC. (1959). Organizing action of prenatally administered testosterone propionate on the tissues mediating behavior in the female guinea pig. *Endocrinology*, 65:369–382.

Pigliucci M. (2005). Evolution of phenotypic plasticity: where are we going now? *Trends Ecol Evol*, 20:481–486.

Preziosi RF, Fairbairn DJ. (2000). Lifetime selection on adult body size and components of body size in a waterstrider: opposing selection and maintenance of sexual size dimorphism. *Evolution*, 54:558–566.

Rhen T. (2000). Sex-limited mutations and the evolution of sexual dimorphism. *Evolution*, 54:37–43.

Rhen T, Cidlowski JA. (2004). *Steroid hormone action.* In Strauss JF, Barbieri R (Eds.), *Yen and Jaffe's reproductive endocrinology*, 5th Edition, (pp. 155–174). Orlando: W.B. Saunders.

Rice WR. (1992). Sexually antagonistic genes: Experimental evidence. *Science*, 256:1436–1439.

Rice WR. (1996a). Sexually antagonistic male adaptation triggered by experimental arrest of female evolution. *Nature*, 381:232–234.

Rice WR. (1996b). Evolution of the Y sex chromosome in animals. *BioScience*, 46:331–343.

Richards TA, Cavalier-Smith T. (2005). Myosin domain evolution and the primary divergence of eukaryotes. *Nature*, 436:1113–1118.

Rinn JL, Snyder M (2005) Sexual dimorphism in mammalian gene expression. *Trends Genet*, 21:298–305.

Robinson NP, Bell SD. (2005). Origins of DNA replication in the three domains of life. *FEBS J* 272:3757–3766.

Rowe L, Arnqvist G, Sih A, Krupa JJ. (1994). Sexual conflict and the evolutionary ecology of mating patterns: water striders as a model system. *Trends Ecol Evol*, 9:289–293.

Rowe L, Arnqvist G. (2002). Sexually antagonistic coevolution in a mating system: combining experimental and comparative approaches to address evolutionary processes. *Evolution*, 56:754–767

Santucci-Darmanin S, Paquis-Flucklinger V. (2003). Les homologues de MutS et de MutL au cours de la méiose chez les mammifères. *Med Sci (Paris)*, 19: 85–91.

Schafer ZT, Kornbluth S. (2006). The apoptosome: physiological, developmental, and regulatory modes of regulation. *Dev Cell*, 10:549–561.

Schamel D, Tracy DM, Lank DB. (2004a). Male mate choice, male availability and egg production as limitations on polyandry in the red-necked phalarope. *Animal Behaviour*, 67:847–853.

Schamel D, Tracy DM, Lank DB, Westneat DF. (2004). Mate guarding, copulation strategies and paternity in the sex-role reversed, socially polyandrous red-necked phalarope Phalaropus lobatus. *Behav Ecol Sociobiol*, 57:110–118.

Sherry DF. (2006). Neuroecology. *Annu Rev Psychol*, 57:167–197.

Souza CA, Silva CC, Ferreira AV. (2003). Sex in fungi: lessons of gene regulation. *Genet Mol Res*, 2:136–147.

Stechmann A, Cavalier-Smith T. (2003). The root of the eukaryote tree pinpointed. *Curr Biol*. 13:R665–R666.

Tanurdzic M, Banks JA. (2004). Sex-determining mechanisms in land plants. *Plant Cell* 16(Supplement): S61–S71.

Thompson RR, George K, Walton JC, Orr SP, Benson J. (2006). Sex-specific influences of vasopressin on human social communication. *Proc Natl Acad Sci USA*, 103:7889–7894.

Thornton JW. (2001). Evolution of vertebrate steroid receptors from an ancestral estrogen receptor by ligand exploitation and serial genome expansions. *Proc Natl Acad Sci USA*, 98:5671–5676.

Thornton JW, Need E, Crews D. (2003). Resurrecting the ancestral steroid receptor: ancient origin of estrogen signaling. *Science*, 301:1714–1717.

Traut W, Winking H. (2001). Meiotic chromosomes and stages of sex chromosome evolution in fish: zebrafish, platyfish and guppy. *Chromosome Res*, 9:659–672.

Watson PJ, Arnqvist G, Stallmann RR. (1998). Sexual conflict and the energetic costs of mating and mate choice in water striders. *Am Nat*, 151:46–58.

Weaver IC, Cervoni N, Champagne FA, D'Allessio AC, Sharma S, Seckl JR, et al. (2004). Epigenetic programming by maternal behavior. *Nature Neurosci*, 7:847–854.

Wigby S, Chapman T. (2005). Sex peptide causes mating costs in female Drosophila melanogaster. *Curr Biol*, 15:316–321.

Woese C. (1998). The universal ancestor. *Proc Natl Acad Sci USA*, 95:6854–6859.

Wolfner MF. (1997). Tokens of love: functions and regulation of Drosophila male accessory gland products. *Insect Biochem Mol Biol*, 27:179–192.

Yehuda R, Engel SM, Brand SR, Seckl J, Marcus SM, Berkowitz GS. (2005). Transgenerational effects of posttraumatic stress disorder in babies of mothers exposed to the World Trade Center attacks during pregnancy. *J Clin Endocrinol Metab*, 90:4115–4118.

Young LJ, Wang. (2004). The neurobiology of pair bonding. *Nat Neurosci*, 7:1048–1054.

Young LJ, Murphy Young AZ, Hammock EA. (2005). Anatomy and neurochemistry of the pair bond. *J Comp Neurol*, 493:51–57.

Chapter 2

Sex Differences in the Brain: What's Old and What's New?

Margaret M. McCarthy
and Arthur P. Arnold

No one will ever win the battle of the sexes;
there is too much fraternizing with the enemy.
—Henry Kissinger

The study of sex differences in the brain has a long, rich history and remains a vibrant and controversial topic that is central to the field of neuroscience both for its obvious relevance and its heuristic value. The goal of this chapter is to provide a brief historical perspective, largely by directing the reader to the many excellent reviews already available, while emphasizing emerging paradigm shifts in our view of the origin and functional significance of brain sex differences. We will highlight two major new initiatives: the direct role of sex chromosome genes in determining brain sex differences, and, the novel theoretical view indicating that sometimes the sexes are striving to be the same.

We will also review 10 recent discoveries that have changed our thinking about sex differences in the brain, but emphasize that the list is not complete nor meant to place relative value on one finding over another. The study of sex differences in the brain is confounded by its biological complexity as well as the social and cultural implications of the findings.

The traditional view of a sex difference is any quantifiable endpoint with a mean value that is significantly different between males and females (Hines, 2004); however, it is becoming increasingly clear that this definition is too restrictive and does not reflect the complex and myriad ways sex differences are manifest. Males and females differ in such traits as their averages, extremes, permanence, temporal qualities, susceptibility to disease, and in their functional impact. Evolutionary processes have created sex differences that are expressed only at one life stage or maybe only at one season. Some sex differences become apparent only under unusual circumstances, such as conditions of extreme stress, or in response to drugs that humans have created but which were not available as animals evolved. Thus, a sex difference in a particular endpoint under one set of circumstances may disappear or even be reversed under a different set of circumstances.

Appreciating this complexity is not only important for a proper approach to the study of sex differences, a topic discussed in detail in Chapter 3 of this volume, but is also important to the interpretation of the relative significance of a sex difference. Understanding the origins of a sex difference also provides insight into the potential cellular and molecular mechanisms determining the phenotype of the trait under study. In the end, all sex differences require an explanation.

It is useful to discriminate between the study of sex differences and the study of sexual differentiation. Sexual differentiation has historically meant the study of permanent, ontogenetic differentiation of tissues in males and females, and the field has focused on adaptive sex differences that produce the normal male and female phenotype required for the two different reproductive roles.

In contrast, the study of sex differences aims to explain *any* sex difference. Many sex differences are assumed to be adaptive, but because of the pleiotropic actions of genes, negative side effects of being male or female, at least in certain contexts, are unavoidable. For example, the greater susceptibility of males to X-linked mental retardation, or of females to autoimmune disease, can hardly be explained as an adaptive difference. Rather, these susceptibilities are each likely disadvantageous side effects of some adaptive sex difference that was selected for its other advantages (i.e., because of other effects on fitness).

All biological sex differences arise from the sex differences carried by the sex chromosomes. In mammals, the male sex chromosomes are XY; and the female, XX. The difference in chromosome complement leads to three genetic sex differences (Arnold & Burgoyne, 2004): male cells have Y genes absent in females (but not many, since the Y chromosome is small and gene-poor), female cells have two genomic doses of X genes (but the difference has relatively little impact at the level of gene expression because each female cell transcriptionally silences, or inactivates, one of the two X chromosomes (Itoh et al., 2006c) and, female cells receive a paternal X chromosome imprint that males lack.

These genetic sex differences cause XX and XY cells to differ. The most important difference occurs in the gonads. The Y-linked gene *Sry* is expressed in the undifferentiated gonad of males causing it to commit irreversibly to a testicular fate. The differentiation of testes in males, and ovaries in females, leads to sex differences in the secretion of gonadal sex steroid hormones. These hormones act on many tissues of the body to cause them to develop differently and function differently in adults. The sex differences caused by gonadal hormones probably represent a continuum in terms of their permanence. At one extreme are the permanent effects of gonadal steroids, the *organizational effects*; at the other extreme are reversible effects, or *activational effects*, which last only as long as the hormone is present (Phoenix et al., 1959; Arnold & Breedlove, 1985). Often activational effects are constrained by previous organizational effects. Both of these types of hormonal effects lead to sex differences in function of tissues.

THE CLASSICAL MODEL OF SEXUAL DIFFERENTIATION

The work of Lillie (1916), Jost (1947), and Phoenix et al. (1959) (Lillie, 1916; Jost, 1947; Phoenix et al., 1959) gave rise to the classic model of brain sexual differentiation, which was elaborated and confirmed by many subsequent works (McEwen, 1980; Arnold & Breedlove, 1985; Breedlove, 1994; McCarthy, 1996; Simerly, 2002; Arnold, 2004). The model states that the sex of the gonads is the primary sex difference caused directly by the presence or absence of the Y chromosome in cells of the male gonad.

The differentiation of the gonads leads to sex differences in the secretion of testosterone perinatally, which induces permanent male-specific patterns of differentiation of the genitalia and brain, and other organs. Other secretions of the testes, especially Müllerian-inhibiting hormone, cause male-specific patterns of differentiation (i.e., involution) of the Müllerian ducts. Testosterone enters the brain of the male mammalian fetus, where it is often converted to estradiol because of the presence of the catalyzing enzyme aromatase. The estradiol acts on estrogen receptors (ERs) to cause masculine differentiation of the hypothalamus and related structures, inducing the formation of circuits that are required for masculine patterns of copulation. It also acts on ERs to suppress the formation of circuits that are required for feminine receptive behaviors such as rodent lordosis and proceptive (solicitous) behaviors. These are actually two separate processes, referred to as *masculinization* and *defeminization*.

In male rodents, estradiol derived from testicular androgens permanently alters the reproductive physiology of the rodent by preventing the capacity for positive feedback effects of estradiol on luteinizing hormone (LH) production and release in adulthood— a necessary prerequisite to ovulation. Female rodents exposed to androgen neonatally lose the capacity to ovulate and are referred to as "androgen sterilized" (Barraclough, 1961). Although the pioneers of this classical model (Lillie, Jost, & the William Young lab) focused originally on tissues and behaviors directly involved in reproduction (external and internal genitalia, copulatory behaviors), where the adaptive differences in males and females are most pronounced, the general model has been repeatedly applied in attempts to explain the many different behavioral systems in which more minor sex differences can be found. These include courtship, cognitive behaviors, the response to stress and pain, etc. A great number of experimental studies support the importance of organizational and activational effects of gonadal steroids in causing sex differences in the brain and behavior; however, in some instances, this framework applies less well, suggesting there are other principles that can guide the development and maintenance of sex differences (discussed further below).

SEX DIFFERENCES IN THE NEW MILLENNIUM: TWO PARADIGM SHIFTS

We live in the age of genetics. Not only does this mean that we have new methods for manipulating and understanding genes that control organizational and activational steroid effects on sex differences, but the exponential increase in information on genomes (including the sex chromosomes and their roles outside of the gonads) has forced us to re-evaluate the apparently complementary or opposing effects of diverse sex-specific factors that sum to produce sex differences or counteract each other to make the sexes more similar. These new ideas have led to two basic paradigm shifts in the field of sex differences.

Sex Chromosome Genes Join Hormonal Effects as Proximal Signals Inducing Sex Differences in Neural Tissues

The sex differences produced in the brain by gonadal steroids are indirect effects of sex chromosome genes—in mammals the Y chromosome gene *Sry* induces sex differences directly in the gonads. This leads to sex-specific secretions that cause sex differences in function of the brain or other tissues. The differences in sex chromosome complement also appear to act directly on the brain and other tissues to cause sex differences directly. In other words, XX and XY cells function differently, before or after they are influenced by gonadal steroids, by virtue of the direct sex-specific effects of X and Y gene expression within the cells themselves (Arnold, 2004). These effects are much less well studied than the effects of sex hormones because of the difficulty of manipulating the sex chromosome complement without also altering the levels of gonadal secretions in experimental animals.

Although the classic model of sexual differentiation has been enormously successful, and withstood many attempts to test it, a few cases do not fit this model. Several of these cases involve sex differences that occur before gonadal differentiation, before the steroid-secreting cells of the gonads have differentiated and begun to express genes leading to steroid synthesis. These include somatic differences (e.g., Renfree & Short, 1988; Burgoyne et al., 1995), but of particular interest are those observed in the nervous system. Shortly after gonadal differentiation, but before testicular secretions have been found to be sexually dimorphic, mesencephalic dopamine neurons exhibit some sexually differentiated characteristics. This appears to be due to the action of sex chromosome genes (Reisert & Pilgrim, 1995; Carruth et al., 2002). Moreover, in mice, sex differences in the expression of genes in the brain are detected prior to the differentiation of the gonads (Dewing et al., 2003), and thus cannot be the result of sex differences in gonadal secretions.

Other sex differences, which occur after the gonads are differentiated, also do not fit the classic model. In the zebra finch (*Taeniopygia guttata*), males sing a courtship song that females do not sing. The brain regions controlling song are much larger in males than females. Although treatment of females with estradiol at hatching causes about half-masculinization of the neural song circuit, the masculinization is never complete, even if different hormonal treatments are used.

The study of intersex individuals suggests a role for direct actions of sex chromosome genes on brain sexual differentiation. For example, genetic zebra finch females induced to grow testes have a feminine neural circuit and do not sing (Wade & Arnold, 1996; Wade et al., 1996; Wade et al., 1999); whereas a genetically male zebra finch with an ovary but lacking testes (presumably a mutation in the gonad-determining pathway), had a male brain and sang. Thus, masculine differentiation of the neural song circuit appears to have occurred in the absence of testes (Itoh et al., 2006b).

Another mutant finch, a spontaneously occurring lateral gynandromorph, was genetically male on the right side of its body (containing a testis), and genetically female on the left side (containing an ovary). Although both sides of the brain would have been exposed to the same levels of gonadal steroids (and hence not differentiated by gonadal steroids), the right side of the brain was more masculine than the left

(Fig. 2.1). It appears that the sex chromosome complement of brain cells contributed to differences in the two sides (Agate et al., 2003). A candidate gene encoded on the sex chromosomes, which might contribute to greater masculinization of the male, is the neurotrophin receptor trkB. The constitutively higher expression of trkB in males could facilitate greater growth of the neural circuit for song if it leads to greater action of neurotrophins (Chen et al., 2005).

Once one adopts the hypothesis that XX and XY cells are different, how does one test for such effects? Since sex chromosome complement normally is confounded by the sex-specific effects of gonadal secretions, how does one untangle the effects of hormones from the effects of sex chromosomes? The first step is

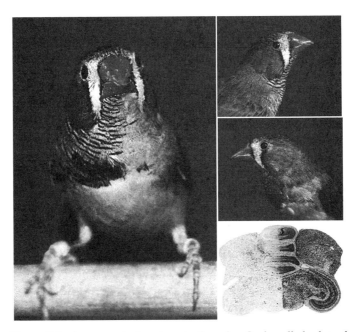

Figure 2.1. An unusual phenotype in the zebra finch, called a lateral gynandromorph, has allowed for a unique comparison of the effects of the gonads versus the genome on brain phenotype. This bird had male plumage (orange cheek patch, chest bar and strips) on one side and female plumage on the other, reflecting a genetic male on one side of the body and a genetic female on the other as demonstrated by expression of the female-specific ASW mRNA on only one side of the brain shown in this autoradiogram (lower right). The presence of testicular tissue would have provided circulating testosterone throughout the body, resulting in equal exposure to both sides of the brain. Quantification of the song nucleus, HVC, found it to be larger on the genetically male side of the brain compared to the female side, consistent with the sex dimorphism observed in the volume of this nucleus in normal males and females (based on data presented in Agate et al., 2003).

to compare animals that differ in the complement or expression of X or Y genes, to determine if this difference has an effect on phenotype. One model is to compare mice that are otherwise genetically the same, but have different strain origins (different alleles) of the Y chromosome. In some cases, for example, mice differing only in Y genes show markedly different levels of aggression (Maxson et al., 1989; Guillot et al., 1995; Monahan & Maxson, 1998), proving that allelic differences on the Y chromosome cause differences in aggression among males.

These differences probably contribute to sex differences in aggression. Is this an example of a direct effect of Y genes on the brain? Such a direct effect is possible, but it is also possible that the allelic differences on the Y chromosome led to differences among males in their levels of testosterone, which then act differently on the brain to modulate aggression. The path to answering the mechanism of Y effects on aggression is to identify the Y gene(s) responsible, and determine the sites and mechanisms of action. Another useful model for investigating sex chromosome effects is the "four core genotypes" model (De Vries et al., 2002). In the mice model, the *Sry* gene is deleted from the Y chromosome, so that the modified Y (called "Y minus," Y^-) does not induce testicular differentiation. Thus, XY^- mice have ovaries and are called females. When a *Sry* transgene is inserted onto an autosome, the mouse develops testes and is called a male (XY^-Sry). Mating XY^-Sry males with XX females produces four genotypes (XX females, XY^- females, XX*Sry* males, XY^-Sry males) in which sex chromosome complement (XX vs. XY) is varied independently of gonadal type (*Sry* present vs. absent; testes vs. ovaries).

This two-by-two comparison allows not only the unusual opportunity to measure separately the effects of testicular versus ovarian secretions on a trait, but also the effect of sex chromosome complement (XX vs. XY). To date, dozens of adult and neonatal phenotypes have been measured in these mice. Some of the classic morphological sex differences in the central nervous system (CNS) show no sex chromosome effect because gonadal males are masculine and gonadal females are feminine in these traits, regardless of chromosomal complement. That result confirms the classic model for those specific traits.

In other cases, however, sex chromosome complement has an effect. For example, XX and XY mice differ in aggression, parental behavior, and density of arginine vasopressin in the lateral septum (De Vries et al., 2002; Gatewood et al., 2006). Because the sex chromosome effects were measured in mice that had the same level of gonadal hormones in adulthood, the sex chromosome effects cannot be attributed to an indirect effect of sex chromosome complement on levels of circulating sex hormones at the time of testing (i.e., differences in activational effects of hormones). It is possible, however, that XX and XY mice of the same gonadal type experienced differences in gonadal hormone levels at earlier times of life, so an indirect organizational effect is not excluded. However, such effects seem unlikely based on the pattern of the results. For example, sometimes an XY mouse is more masculine, sometimes less masculine than an XX mouse of the same gonadal type (e.g., Carruth et al., 2002; Gatewood et al., 2006; Palaszynski et al., 2005).

Other models compare mice with different genomic imprints on the X chromosome. For example, XmO versus XpO female mice (i.e., those with a maternal vs. paternal X chromosome imprint on the single X chromosome) show differences in tests of reversal learning, suggesting that one or more X genes show different expression if the genes are inherited from the farther versus the mother. A candidate X gene has been identified which shows imprinting that causes differences in expression in the brain. Because only females receive an X chromosome with a paternal imprint, imprinting effects could contribute to sex differences in brain and behavioral traits (Davies et al., 2006).

A fourth method for studying sex chromosome effects is by observing the effects of X or Y gene-specific manipulations on traits. For example, the Y gene *Sry* is expressed in the substantia nigra of the midbrain (Dewing et al., 2006), the origin of dopamine neurons that innervate the striatum. Mice receiving unilateral injections of antisense oligonucleotides that reduce expression of *Sry* show a loss of tyrosine hydroxylase expression on the antisense side. Asymmetries in motor behavior indicate that *Sry* expression influences those behaviors. Rodents show sex differences in expression of midbrain TH. The results indicate that *Sry* has male-specific effects in the midbrain. Indeed, this is the first demonstration of a direct male-specific effect of a specific Y gene in the brain. It is not yet clear if the *Sry* effect produces sex differences in phenotypes, because its effects may be compensated by the female-specific effect of a factor operating only in females (see next section).

Sometimes the Sexes Strive
to be the Same

Although it seems like almost any trait is in some way impacted by sex, in reality, there just isn't a difference in traits, in some instances, between males and females. A specific cellular or physiological process may simply be outside the sphere of influence of hormones and/or sex-specific genes. In other cases, the two sexes are similar because one sex difference is canceled by another, or because males and females reach the same end result by two different paths. Because several different factors (different hormones, different times of action, different X or Y genes) contribute to sex differences in the function of the brain and other non-gonadal tissues, they can interact to modulate, enhance, or block each other. For example, testosterone has organizational and activational effects that both contribute to making the male more likely to show masculine copulatory behaviors. In other cases, however, two male-specific factors might counteract and cancel each other, reducing rather than producing sex differences (De Vries & Boyle, 1998; Voskuhl & Palaszynski, 2001; De Vries, 2004; Palaszynski et al., 2005). For example, Y genes and testosterone may work in opposition.

The compensatory effects of two sex-specific factors can be seen as adaptive if some sex-specific factor has disadvantageous side effects which are then reduced by the evolution of a compensatory process. One of the best examples of this is that the sex difference in genomic dose of X-chromosome genes (double dose in XX females, single dose in XY males) has evolved because of inevitable forces that make the X and Y chromosomes different (Charlesworth, 1991; Graves, 2006).

However, the different dose of X genes is thought to be highly maladaptive for one or both sexes, because gene dose can have a critical effect on cell function and cannot be optimal in both sexes if they have a permanent twofold difference in expression. The evolution of a female-specific mechanism of X inactivation effectively reduces the sexual disparity in X gene expression (Itoh et al., 2006a) and avoids a host of problematic sex differences in gene expression in metabolic pathways that must function equivalently in the two sexes. X inactivation is one of the best studied sex-specific mechanisms that allows the sexes to be more equal, not less.

Alternatively, the sexes may converge on the same behavioral endpoint from different origins. In mammals, the female's large investment in individual gametes, including a long gestation and period of lactation, leads to a strong maternal involvement in parental care. Maternal behavior by females is a tightly controlled hormonally-regulated process that probably evolved in the context of hormonal changes at the end of pregnancy, causing the female to become influenced by those changes. Males are less constrained in their choices regarding parenting and when the choice for parenting does appear, it must have evolved outside of the hormonal parameters that likely influenced females. Thus, parental behavior in males represents a convergence in behavior with females using divergent physiological mechanisms (De Vries, 2004) (Fig.2.2).

One system that appears to have been exploited to that end is the neurohormone, vasopressin, which is important for parental behavior and for related affiliative behaviors across a wide range of species including birds, rodents, and primates (Wang & De Vries, 1995; Lim & Young, 2006; Nair & Young, 2006). Vasopressin innervation is among the most sexually dimorphic in the brain (De Vries et al., 1994; De Vries & Panzica, 2006) and appears to have been co-opted to regulate parental behavior in males. The cellular and molecular mechanisms by which the vasopressin system is modulated developmentally to direct appropriate adult behavior in response to specific stimuli, such as neonates, is not well established.

Sometimes the sexes try to be the same, literally by using different strategies to solve the same problem. Studies of sex differences in cognition in animal models focus almost exclusively on spatial learning ability. There are a variety of experimental paradigms for assessing learning in rats, but the only model routinely employed for sex differences is the Morris Water Maze. This not because it is the best test for learning, but because it is the only test that reliably shows any sex differences in performance (Jonasson, 2005).

Performance in this instance is the amount of time in seconds (i.e. latency) for a subject animal to find a hidden platform from which to escape the aversive water. Males routinely find the platform faster than females and are thereby considered to have superior spatial learning (Jonasson, 2005). This may very well be true. Human males are also consistently better than females in some spatial tasks (Hamilton et al., 2002;

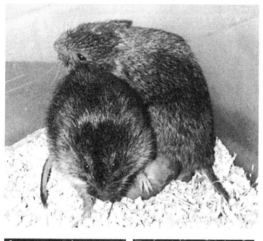

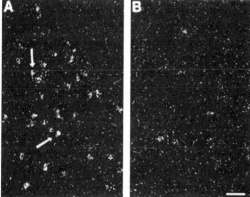

Hines, 2004; Driscoll et al., 2005). However, recent studies in rodents have re-examined the Morris Water Maze and the conditions associated with the test.

Two important and related principles emerged. One is that females use a different strategy than males to solve the problem (Perrot-Sinal, 1996; Beiko et al., 2004). When the platform is raised above the water so that the animals can readily see it, males will swim the most direct path; whereas females exhibit a strong thigmotaxis, swimming close to the walls of the tank before darting out into the open water to reach the platform (Fig. 2.3). Importantly, both males and females learn the task, but the rate at which it is learned differs. Moreover, males and females differ in their

Figure 2.2. An emerging principle in sex differences research is that sometimes males and females strive to be the same. This can occur at the neuronal level in order to converge on the same behavior and is best exemplified in the parental behavior of the prairie vole. In most rodent species, including most voles, the male provides little to no parental care of his own offspring. In the prairie vole, however, the male actively takes care of and protects his young. This is correlated with an increased expression of vasopressin, a neuropetide that fosters affiliative behavior. The top panel shows a male and female prairie vole taking care of their young, and the bottom panel is a dark field image of in situ hybridization detection of mRNA for vasopressin in the bed nucleus of the stria terminalis of a male (A) and female (B). Note the much higher level of expression in males. Reprinted with permission from De Vries GJ (2004). Minireview: Sex differences in adult and developing brains: compensation, compensation, compensation. *Endocrinology*, 145:1063–1068.

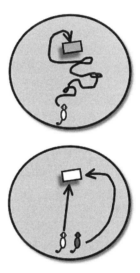

Figure 2.3. Males and females may also strive to reach the same endpoint by using different behavioral strategies. The Morris Water Maze is a well known test for spatial learning and males are consistently reported to outperform females. Performance on the task is a function of the latency to find a platform hidden beneath the surface of the water. Animals often spend considerable time searching for the platform as illustrated in the top panel. However, when the platform is raised above the surface of the water, male and female rats adopt different strategies for approaching it. Males swim directly, while females take a more circuitous, and presumably less anxiety-provoking, route that takes longer. When the stress of the task is reduced, male and female rats both swim directly to the platform. Based on studies by Beiko et al., 2004.

sensitivity to variables that impact on learning, such as stress. In general, females seem to suffer from greater "test anxiety," and are more severely impaired in their ability to learn if there is stress associated with the task (Shors et al., 2001).

Thus, with this one cognitive task we have an example of the sexes using different strategies to solve the same problem; and a situation in which the sexes perform the same unless there is an extrinsic variable, such as stress, introduced into the situation. An important point is that neither of these necessarily represents a sex difference in learning *per se*. Similar arguments have been made regarding evidence for sex differences in human cognitive ability (Spelke, 2005) and highlight the continuing gaps in our understanding of what is or is not different between males and females.

SEX DIFFERENCES IN THE NEW MILLENIUM: 10 FINDINGS THAT ARE CHANGING OUR THINKING

Despite the risks inherent in making any list, we present one here in an attempt to emphasize both major recent advances and the reemergence of decades-old problems that still lack clarification. Our goal is not to applaud some of these advances while ignoring others, but hopefully to provide a framework for determining the best avenues for future work. The topics are loosely organized along conceptual themes to highlight how they might support or contradict each other, with no intention of suggesting relative importance.

Growth Factors Mediate Effects of Gonadal Hormones

Hormonal induction of neurotrophic factors seems a fairly obvious mechanism that nature might have utilized to differentiate particular brain structures, but evidence for this mechanism is not abundant. Estradiol increases the amount of brain derived nerve growth factor (BDNF) in the developing hippocampus (Solum & Handa, 2002), midbrain (Ivanova et al., 2001), and vocal nuclei of songbirds (Dittrich et al., 1999; Fusani et al., 2003), but seems to have little effect on the primary receptor, trkB. Conversely, estradiol increases binding of nerve growth factor (NGF), and thereby, presumably, the amount of receptor in

the developing telencephalon of the zebra finch (Contreras & Wade, 1999).

Estradiol and insulin have long been known to have a synergistic effect on neurite growth in fetal hippocampal explants (Toran-Allerand et al., 1991; Toran-Allerand, 1996), an effect now known to be the result of an interaction between insulin-like growth factor (IGF-1) receptors and estrogen receptors, presumably at the membrane (Toran-Allerand et al., 1999). These two receptors appear to act in tandem to promote cell survival and neurite outgrowth in a variety of brain regions, with considerable emphasis placed on a potential neuroprotective effect in the adult (Cardona-Gomez et al., 2002).

In only one sexually dimorphic system, the spinal nucleus of the bulbocavernosus (SNB), has a clear functional impact of elevated growth factor been found. In this system, ciliary neurotropic factor (CNTF) is upregulated in the bulbocavernosus muscle by androgens, and then retrogradely acts on the CNTF receptors on the motoneurons of the SNB, promoting their survival (Forger, 2006). Mutant mice lacking receptors for CNTF have no sex difference in the size of the SNB. Because the SNB motoneurons innervate muscles that attach to the penis, the functional significance of the male's greater number of neurons is evident.

When CNTF is administered to females, it rescues the motoneurons in females; and treating males with antagonists to CNTF receptor, reduces the number of motoneurons in males. Why then has it been difficult to find similar functional significance for growth factor signaling in sexual differentiation of diencephalic or telencephalic brain structures? One reason is technical. There are no receptor antagonists for BDNF, and trkB knock-out mice have only recently been developed. Moreover, BDNF signaling is so pervasively important to normal brain development, that it is difficult to interfere selectively with its putative role in hormonally induced sexual differentiation.

For instance, estradiol is a potent inducer of BDNF in the developing hippocampus (Solum & Handa, 2002), yet BDNF is fundamental to the balance of glutamatergic versus GABAergic synapses in this region (Singh et al., 2006), making it difficult to dissect out the role of estradiol-induced BDNF from BDNF in general. Nonetheless, there is good reason to suspect that growth factors are critical players in the sex differentiation process, and that this role extends beyond the spinal cord.

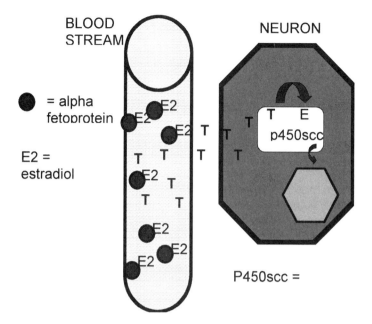

BLOOD STREAM

● = alpha fetoprotein

E2 = estradiol

NEURON

T   E
p450scc

P450scc =

Figure 2.4. Estradiol is a major regulator of brain masculinization and defeminization. This is achieved by testicularly-derived androgen gaining access to neurons where it is locally converted to estradiol by the P450scc enzyme, aromatase. High levels of estradiol in maternal circulation also gain access to the fetal circulation, but are sequestered there by the steroid binding globulin, alpha-fetoprotein, preventing masculinization and defeminization from occurring in developing females. Testosterone is not bound to alpha-fetoprotein and so selectively gains access to the neurons, where it is aromatized to estradiol. Together, these observations form the basis of the Aromatization Hypothesis of sex differentiation of the brain.

Estradiol Induces a Target-Derived Diffusible Axonal Growth Factor

In addition to steroid-induced regulation of neurotrophins that regulate cell survival, steroids appear to alter trophic factors that control axonal outgrowth. The principle nucleus of the bed nucleus of the stria terminalis (pBNST) projects to the anteroventral periventricular (AVPV) nucleus as part of a neural circuit controlling gonadotropin secretion from the anterior pituitary.

One of the most robust morphological and functionally significant sex differences in the brain is the 10-fold larger pBNST to AVPV projection in the male. Clever use of explant cultures, in which male and female pBNST and AVPV could be mixed and matched, definitively revealed that estradiol was acting in the AVPV to produce a signal to attract the growing axons of the pBNST neurons (Ibanez et al., 2001) (Fig. 2.4).

The identity of the diffusible factor remains to be determined. The AVPV appears to be a critical node for the induction of the surge in LH release that is required for ovulation. AVPV neurons are largely glutamatergic and project to the vicinity of the LHRH neurons, which in turn project to the anterior pituitary and regulate LH release. No compelling evidence exists for sex differences in the LHRH neurons themselves. When placed in a circuit context, one can envision the inhibitory pBNST projecting to and clamping the excitatory AVPV in males, preventing the induction of an LH surge in response to elevated estradiol, one of the hallmarks of the masculinized brain.

Steroid-Mediated Sex Differences in Cell Death are Independent of Steroid-Mediated Neurochemical Phenotype

Up to this point, we have not discussed the most well-established and intensely studied sex difference in the brain, the overall size of specific brain regions. In rats, the sexually dimorphic nucleus of the POA (SDN-POA) is 5 to 7 times larger in males and the AVPV of the POA is 3 to 5 times larger in females (Simerly, 2000, 2002; Morris et al., 2004). The SNB of females has one third the number of neurons as in males (Forger, 2006) and several of the song control nuclei in birds are 5 to 6 times larger in males than females (Ball & MacDougall-Shackleton, 2001).

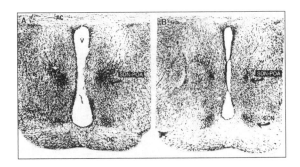

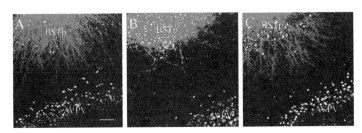

Figure 2.5. Many sex differences in the brain are characterized as the size of a structure being larger in one sex versus another. These structures include entire brain regions, major projections, and subnuclei. Work in bird brains demonstrated that differential cell death in one sex versus the other can contribute to volumetric sex differences, and this was subsequently confirmed in the mammalian brain for the sexually dimorphic nucleus (SDN) of the preoptic area, shown here in the upper panel and visualized by cresyl violet. More cells die in females than males during the perinatal sensitive period, resulting in a smaller SDN volume in females (right) compared to males (left). Alternatively, in the AVPV, more cells die in the male than in the female, resulting in the opposite volumetric difference. However, a target-derived factor from the male AVPV encourages a much larger innervation by BNST neuronal axons, resulting in a larger male projection than in females. This is illustrated in the lower panel illustrating explant cultures of the BNST (red) and the AVPV (green). More fibers grow toward the AVPV from a male BNST (left) and a female BNST treated with testosterone (right) than in an untreated female (middle). Reprinted with permission from Ibanez MA, Gu G, Simerly RB. (2001) Target-dependent sexual differentiation of a limbic-hypothalamic neural pathway. *J Neurosci*, 21:5652–5659.

The SDN-POA is arguably the most intensively studied of these, with literally hundreds of published studies since its discovery in the 1970s (Gorski et al., 1978) (Fig. 2.5). Study of various systems, including birds and mammals, demonstrate that volumetric sex differences can be established when males and females begin with the same number of neurons, but that differential hormonal exposure results in sex differences in cell death (e.g., Konishi & Akutagawa, 1985; Nordeen et al., 1985). We know very little about

how steroids regulate which cells live and which cells die, however, this does not exclude other contributing variables such as differential migration or neurogenesis, in the establishment of volumetric sex differences.

Recent studies of knock-out mice provide important new information on sex differences in cell death. Studies of neuronal death during a developmental window are inherently limited by the difficulty in detecting the cell while it is dying. Dying itself occurs quickly, in the course of a few hours (see Forger, 2006, for review). Markers for dying cells disappear with the cell and do not predict which cells might die in the future. Recognizing this limitation, Nancy Forger has exploited the benefits offered by mice that have a null mutation in the Bcl-2 gene, a potent inhibitor of cell death, or in Bax, a promoter of cell death. In the case of the latter, Forger and colleagues found that sex differences in the SNB, AVPV, and pBNST were all eliminated in Bax−/−mice (Forger et al., 2004), indicating Bax is required for sexually dimorphic cell death in the mouse forebrain and spinal cord.

Interestingly, Bax is involved in cell death that is increased by estradiol (AVPV) as well as that decreased by testosterone (SNB). One advantage of this approach is that the number of neurons observed in Bax−/−adults represents the original number generated in each sex, whereas the difference in cell number between Bax−/−and Bax +/+ adults reveals the total number of neurons lost or "integrated over the entire developmental cell death period" (Forger, 2006), further supporting the notion that sex differences in cell death contribute to volume differences in multiple brain regions.

However, there is more to the story. Within the AVPV, a heterogeneity of cell type exists, and females have 3 to 4 times more dopaminergic neurons than males (Simerly et al., 1997). In Bax−/−mice, there is no sex difference in the size of the AVPV, and AVPV is markedly larger in both sexes than in Bax +/+ mice. When one examines only the dopaminergic neurons, there is a robust sex difference and no effect of the Bax mutation (Forger et al., 2004), suggesting that estradiol directs the phenotype of a subset of neurons in the AVPV. A similar phenomenon may be occurring in regards to the vasopressin phenotype in the pBNST (Han & De Vries, 2003). Integrating these findings with the apparent role of Sry in differentiating midbrain dopaminergic neurons (Dewing et al., 2003; Dewing et al., 2006) will also be a fruitful area for future investigation.

A Prostaglandin Mediates Masculinization of Sex Behavior in Rats

The ability of gonadal steroids to sexually differentiate the brain during a defined sensitive period of development has been established for almost 50 years. During that time, there has been considerable effort to find the cellular mechanisms of hormone action. Early studies focused on neurotransmitters such as noradrenaline, dopamine and serotonin. These have all been proposed by various groups as important mediators of steroid-induced masculinization of the brain and important sex differences in these systems have been reported (Ani, 1978; Simerly et al., 1985; Simerly, 1998). Some differences occur very early in development and perhaps prior to the influence of gonadal steroids (Reisert & Pilgrim, 1995). Manipulation of these transmitter systems during the critical period for masculinization has deleterious effects on adult behavior. However, the converse is not true; administering serotonin, dopamine or noradrenalin analogs or antagonists to newborn females does not initiate masculinization, suggesting some important element of the story was missing.

A recent and surprising finding reveals that the missing element appears to be the prostaglandin, PGE$_2$. The synthesis of all the prostanoids begins with the oxygenative cyclization of arachidonic acid by cyclooxygenase. The inducible isoform of cyclooxygenase, COX-2, is an immediate early gene responsive to a variety of stimuli including fever, injury, and stimuli associated with neuronal plasticity (Hoffmann, 2000; Camu et al., 2003; Giovannini et al., 2003). COX-2 mRNA and protein are higher in the POA of newborn males than females and treating females with estradiol increases COX levels to that of males. Increased COX-2 is directly correlated with increased PGE$_2$ production. Treating newborn females with estradiol increases PGE$_2$ levels in the POA almost sevenfold.

Moreover, administration of PGE$_2$ to newborn females has two striking and presumably associated effects: a two- to threefold increase in dendritic spines (the primary site of excitatory glutamatergic synapses) in the POA, and a dramatic induction of masculine sexual behavior in adulthood. Conversely, blocking PGE$_2$ synthesis temporarily in newborn males significantly reduces POA dendritic spines, to the level seen in normal females, and severely impairs the expression of male sexual behavior in adulthood (Amateau & McCarthy, 2002b; Amateau & McCarthy, 2004). Thus, PGE$_2$ satisfies the criteria of being an essential mediator of steroid hormone-induced masculinization of sexual behavior in the rat in that it can both induce the masculinization process, and when blocked, disrupt the same process.

Masculinization and Defeminization are Determined by Different Cellular Mechanisms

If one takes a rodent-centric, steroid-mediated, sex-behavior-focused view of sexual differentiation of the brain (which many do, including one of the authors), sexual differentiation of sex behavior involves three independent processes: feminization, masculinization, and defeminization, but no naturally occurring demasculinization. *Feminization* is the default (yet active) pathway leading to expression of lordosis under the proper hormonal conditions in adulthood. *Masculinization* is the active developmental process initiated by testosterone during the perinatal sensitive period resulting in normal male copulatory behavior in adulthood. *Defeminization* is also an active and natural process whereby the ability to express female sexual behavior or reproductive function is lost in males. Defeminization normally occurs in tandem with masculinization in males. Thus, both masculinization and defeminization are active steroid-driven processes that can be initiated in females by exogenous treatment with steroids.

Early studies established that the two processes can be manipulated independently. There is a differential sensitivity to androgen, with masculinization being more potently induced than defeminization in females administered weak androgens. There is also a difference in the duration of the precise parameters of the critical period for each process (Whalen & Edwards, 1967) and reducing the steroid receptor co-activator, CBP, with antisense oligonucleotides, selectively impairs defeminization, however, does not effect masculinization (Auger et al., 2002). Yet all of these studies involve some sort of manipulation involving steroids. As a result, it has been difficult to clearly delineate both the anatomical region critical to defeminization of behavior (the POA is central to masculinization), and the cellular processes being regulated by estradiol or androgens that mediate each process independently of the other.

Two recent findings provide potential insight for solving this problem. The first is based on the estrogen receptors ERalpha and ERbeta. Male mice bearing a null mutation for ERbeta exhibit essentially normal male sexual behavior, but also exhibit robust female sexual behavior, suggesting normal masculinization, but impaired defeminization (Kudwa et al., 2005). Thus, the divergence in mechanisms of estradiol's

effects may begin at its receptors. Still, it begs the question: What is the cellular pathway initiated to defeminize the brain?

The cellular mediator of masculinization is PGE_2, which may provide the needed tool to begin to identify the mediator of defeminization. As they exhibit normal female sex behavior as adults, females masculinized with neonatal PGE_2 are not defeminized. Likewise, males in which masculinization has been blocked by preventing PGE_2 synthesis, are still defeminized by their own gonadal steroids, reaffirming the maxim that defeminization is a hormonally driven process independent of masculinization (Todd et al., 2005). Thus, PGE_2 is both necessary and sufficient for behavioral masculinization, but plays no role in defeminization.

Any cellular process induced by estradiol (or androgen) during the sensitive period would be a logical candidate for mediating defeminization. For instance, there is a sex difference in the number of dendritic spines and the length of dendrites on neurons in the mediobasal hypothalamus, a critical brain region controlling lordosis, and therefore a logical candidate for the anatomical site of defeminization. Neonatal testosterone or estradiol treatment increases dendritic spine levels in females to that of males (Mong et al., 1999; Todd et al., 2006), but PGE_2 has no effect in this brain region. However, the actions of estradiol can be either blocked or mimicked by antagonizing or activating the NMDA glutamate receptor.

In fact, estradiol promotes the synaptic release of glutamate from immature hypothalamic neurons, leading to activation of mitogen-activated protein (MAP) kinase and the induction of dendritic spine formation (Schwarz et al., 2006). This series of cellular events has not yet been directly linked to behavioral defeminization, but highlights the utility of this approach by illustrating the general principle that the same hormone can simultaneously activate multiple cellular mechanisms to induce masculinization and defeminization to achieve a coordinated whole male brain.

Glial–Neuronal Crosstalk Is Involved in Establishment of Sex Differences

Although much attention has focused on sex differences in the shape, size, and number of neurons, there are equally robust morphological differences in the astrocytes of males versus females in several brain regions, including the preoptic area (Amateau & McCarthy, 2002a), arcuate nucleus (Mong et al., 1999), and hippocampus (Day et al., 1993). It is not clear whether the changing shape of astrocytes causes or is caused by changes in neurons.

The communication between neurons and glia must, however, be important during the process of sexual differentiation in some brain regions. This is perhaps most clearly established in the arcuate nucleus, where a neuronal factor, GABA, is upregulated in response to estradiol released from neurons and then acts on astrocytes to increase the number of processes and frequency of branching (Mong et al., 2002). These early effects on astrocytes in the arcuate nucleus follow the organizational principle of sexual differentiation in that the effects are permanent and occur in response to active hormonal induction in males.

A similar process, but mediated by a different messenger, occurs in the preoptic area where PGE_2 increases both the number and branching frequency of astrocyte processes (Amateau & McCarthy, 2002a). Sex differences in glia appear to precede sex differences in neurons in the songbird system (Nordeen & Nordeen, 1996; Nordeen et al., 1998). The detection of estrogen receptors and the appearance of aromatase enzyme in astrocytes following traumatic injury (Garcia-Segura et al., 1996; Garcia-Segura et al., 1999; Jordan, 1999; Peterson et al., 2004), has further increased attention on this previously neglected cell type.

The Brain Is its Own Gonad—*de novo* Estradiol Synthesis

In zebra finches, sex steroid hormones seem to be important for developing a masculine neural circuit for song. For example, females treated at hatch with estradiol are more masculine in the song circuit than a normal female, but about half as masculine as a normal male; and they also sing (Wade & Arnold, 2004). Thus, although sex chromosome genes may control the sexual differentiation process, estradiol seems to play an important role. Androgens may also be necessary for fully masculine development (Bottjer & Hewer, 1992; Grisham et al., 2002; Kim et al., 2004).

However, several findings suggest that the steroids come from the brain itself, not from the gonads. In zebra finches, the brain has exceptionally high expression of aromatase, and it converts androgens from the systemic blood into estrogens and releases the estrogens into general circulation (Schlinger & Arnold, 1992). Moreover, slice cultures of juvenile zebra finch forebrain synthesize estradiol *de novo*, and male slices release more estradiol than female slices. The estradiol directly masculinzes the slices *in vitro* (Holloway & Clayton, 2001). These results suggest that all of the synthetic enzymes required to produce estrogens are present in the forebrain, and that they contribute to brain sexual differentiation. The enzymes have been cloned and their expression studied (London et al., 2006). Interestingly, several of the enzymes are expressed along the germinal zone near the ventricle, where androgen receptors are also expressed in the embryo (Perlman & Arnold, 2003; Perlman et al., 2003), so a role for androgens or estrogens in cell proliferation or differentiation is possible.

Sex chromosome genes might cause sex differences in steroid synthesis leading to morphological and functional sex differences in the circuit. Evidence for *de novo* sex steroidogenesis by avian brains suggested that the same might occur in mammals. The evidence in mammals is scant partly because of the small number of studies, and partly because of the difficulty of definitively identifying the relevant steroidogenic enzymes in the mammalian brain. There is considerable evidence for *de novo* synthesis of progesterone and its metabolites (Schumacher et al., 2003). Independent observation by several laboratories (Prange-Kiel et al., 2003; Amateau et al., 2004; Hojo et al., 2004) provides reasonable confidence that there is some capacity for *de novo* estradiol synthesis by the rat brain. Unlike the situation for songbirds, however, for mammals there is little confidence that *de novo* estradiol synthesis in the brain plays a role in sexual differentiation. Indeed, the opposite may be true.

High levels of estradiol were detected in the hippocampus and cortex of newborn females rats and were on par with those found in males. *De novo* synthesis by telencephalic neurons or glia remains the most plausible explanation (Amateau et al., 2004). An underlying assumption of any studies of gonadal steroids in the developing brain is the establishment of sex differences, but if endogenous levels of estradiol do not differ in developing males and females, it is difficult to envision this as the basis for a sex difference. That estradiol is a general trophic factor needed by both male and female brains, or that is made selectively in specific brain regions in one or both sexes in order to reduce, not produce, sex differences are all possibilities that need to be considered (McCarthy & Konkle, 2005).

Receptor ER-X and the Ligand 17-alpha-estradiol

An interesting potential novel membrane estrogen receptor, called ER-X, is distinguished from other ERs by its distinct molecular weight and high affinity for 17-alpha-estradiol. ER-X is associated with caveolar-like microdomains, increasing its proximity to membrane anchored kinases. Peak levels are found in the neocortex beginning about one week after birth (Toran-Allerand et al., 2002; Toran-Allerand et al., 2005). Whether ER-X is present in highly sexually differentiated regions of the rodent brain, such as the diencephalon, remains unknown, as does the functional significance to cortical development. Studies of ER-X have not addressed whether there is a sex difference in its expression.

One of the more interesting and usual aspects of ER-X is the preferred ligand of 17-alpha-estradiol, the naturally occurring stereoisomer of 17-beta-estradiol. Traditionally, 17-alpha has been considered an inactive form of the steroid, but this is being re-evaluated in light of evidence that it provides neuroprotection, possibly via rapid activation of MAP kinase and the PI3-Akt signaling pathway. From a developmental standpoint, 17-alpha-estradiol is of particular interest: it does not bind to alpha-fetoprotein, it's found at very high levels early in development, and it appears to be made *de novo* by the brain (Toran-Allerand et al., 2005).

To detect 17-alpha estradiol in the brain, and distinguish it from 17-beta-estradiol, requires mass spectrometry of samples after either liquid or gas chromatography, a difficult technique. The findings of Toran-Allerand and colleagues highlight the need for more quantitative techniques to measure brain steroids. These techniques need to be applied to a large number of brain regions across a wide range of development. Moreover, recent developments in rapid synthesis of estradiol via aromatization raise the specter of highly local neurotransmitter-like actions of this steroid, further highlighting the importance of knowing the actual steroid concentrations in a given time and place (Balthazart & Ball, 2006).

Alpha-fetoprotein Really *Is* a Critical Barrier to Maternal Estrogens

A developing mammalian fetus is in a soup of maternal steroids, most prevalent being estradiol. Why is the female rodent fetus not masculinized by this estradiol? A long-standing explanation was that the liver protein, alpha-fetoprotein (AFP), prevents maternal estradiol entry into the brain because it binds estradiol (but not testosterone). In rats and mice AFP is found at very high levels in the circulation prior to and shortly after birth (Fig. 2.4). The end result is that maternal estradiol is sequestered in the circulation (of both sexes) while testosterone (in the male) gains access to the brain where it is locally converted to estradiol in neurons during the critical period for sexual differentiation.

A corollary of this scenario is that the female brain develops as a result of the absence of testosterone and estradiol. Although this scenario made good sense, it had not been actually tested critically until mice were developed bearing a null mutation for AFP. Female offspring of AFP knock-out dams are behaviorally and morphologically masculinized in regard to sex behavior because of the loss of protection against maternal estrogens (Bakker et al., 2006). This finding shows that sufficient estradiol is present in the womb to masculinize the fetus, and it draws attention to the question of the role of estradiol in feminization. There has long been lingering evidence that estradiol might play a role in active feminization and it has been proposed that AFP is a selective carrier that delivers estradiol to specific cells (Toran-Allerand, 1980, 1987). This still might be true but requires further examination.

Estradiol Is Required for Female Brain Development

Recently, mice were produced that lack the aromatase (estrogen synthase) gene, which is responsible for all estrogen synthesis from androgenic precursors. Female ArKO mice show less female sexual receptivity, and less sensitivity to olfactory stimuli (Bakker et al., 2002). Estradiol treatment of adult ArKOs restores much of the olfactory impairment, but not sexual behavior. These results suggest that normal development of the female neural and behavioral phenotype requires some estradiol. That result conflicts with the classic view of the female as the "default condition," the state that occurs in the complete absence of gonadal secretions.

The classical view of the female as the default has been met with skepticism over the years, based on a variety of evidence that estradiol or other ovarian secretions contribute to the differentiation of females (e.g., Fitch & Denenberg, 1995). However, the study by Bakker et al. (2002) provides strong new support for the importance of estradiol for feminization because the null mutation of the aromatase gene is thought to eliminate the synthesis of estrogens completely. A particular advantage of this mouse model is that exogenous estradiol can be re-introduced into the mouse at any stage of development, allowing for dissection of estradiol effects during specific life stages. The disadvantage of the model, as usual for transgenic mice, is that findings are limited to mice.

THE CHALLENGES AHEAD: WHAT REMAINS TO BE LEARNED

The challenge in discussing this topic is trying to limit the list. There are several major questions: How does brain feminization occur? How do gonadal steroid and chromosomal sex differences interact? What gene(s) are activated by steroids during brain development?

Each of these presents unique theoretical and technical challenges. Finding a tractable experimental approach to female brain development is difficult in the absence of the clear hormonal trigger that occurs in males. Separating steroidal from chromosomal effects, and understanding their interactions, is made difficult because of the profound effects of chromosomal sex on gonadal sex. And lastly, expression microarrays have been employed to search for and identify genes that are expressed during the critical period for sexual differentiation (Wade et al., 2004; Yang et al., 2006), and to identify sex-specific genes NOT induced by steroids (Dewing et al., 2003). However, in the most commonly studied model system, the laboratory rat, this approach has been largely disappointing, with the exception of the discovery of hormonal induction of granulin (Suzuki & Nishiahara, 2002). This may be in part due to nontranscription factor-related effects of steroids, such as by ER-X, or may be confounded by the multiplicative cascading effect of initiating low-level transcription of a large number of genes. At this point, we simply don't know.

There are also any number of more detailed questions to ask, most important being how specific cellular processes are determined by species, brain region, developmental time point and genetic sex. Finding the commonalities and the unique situations will require meticulous and expansive study of the developing brain with direct comparison between males and females. This goal will only be achieved if the best and brightest young scientists continue to turn their attention to this fascinating and pervasively important topic.

References

Agate RJ, Grisham W, Wade J, Mann S, Wingfield J, Schanen C, et al. (2003). Neural, not gonadal, origin of brain sex differences in a gynandromorphic finch. *Proc Natl Acad Sci U S A*, 100:4873–4878.

Amateau SK, McCarthy MM. (2002a). Sexual differentiation of astrocyte morphology in the developing rat preoptic area. *J Neuroendo*, 14:904–910.

Amateau SK, McCarthy MM. (2002b). A novel mechanism of dendritic spine plasticity involving estradiol induction of prostglandin-E2. *J Neurosci*, 22: 8586–8596.

Amateau SK, McCarthy MM. (2004). Induction of PGE(2) by estradiol mediates developmental masculinization of sex behavior. *Nat Neurosci*, 7:643–650.

Amateau SK, Alt JJ, Stamps CL, McCarthy MM. (2004). Brain estradiol content in newborn rats: sex differences, regional heterogeneity, and possible de novo synthesis by the female telencephalon. *Endocrinology*, 145:2906–2917.

Ani M, Butterworth, PJ, Thomas, PJ. (1978). Sexual dimorphism in the adenylate cyclase activity in the hypothalamus of newborn rats. *Brain Res*, 151:615–618.

Arnold AP. (2004). Sex chromosomes and brain gender. *Nat Rev Neurosci*, 5:701–708.

Arnold AP, Breedlove SM. (1985). Organizational and activational effects of sex steroids on brain and behavior: a reanalysis. *Horm Behav*, 19:469–498.

Arnold AP, Burgoyne PS. (2004). Are XX and XY brain cells intrinsically different? *Trends Endocrinol Metab*, 15:6–11.

Auger AP, Perrot-Sinal TS, Auger CJ, A. EL, Tetel MJ, McCarthy MM. (2002). Expression of the nuclear receptor coactivator, cAMP response element-binding proteins, is sexually dimorphic and modulates sexual differentiation of neonatal rat brain. *Endocrinology*, 143:3009–3016.

Bakker J, De Mees C, Douhard Q, Balthazart J, Gabant P, Szpirer J, Szpirer C. (2006). Alpha-fetoprotein protects the developing female mouse brain from masculinization and defeminization by estrogens. *Nat Neurosci*, 9:220–226.

Ball GF, MacDougall-Shackleton SA. (2001). Sex differences in songbirds 25 years later: what have we learned and where do we go? *Microsc Res Tech*, 54: 327–334.

Balthazart J, Ball GF. (2006). Is brain estradiol a hormone or a neurotransmitter? Trends *Neurosci*, 29:241–249.

Barraclough CA. (1961). Production of anovulatory, sterile rats by single injections of testosterone propionate. *Endocrinology*, 68:62–67.

Beiko J, Lander R, Hampson E, Boon F, Cain DP. (2004). Contribution of sex differences in the acute stress response to sex differrnces in water maze performance. *Behav Brain Res*, 151:239–253.

Bottjer SW, Hewer SJ. (1992). Castration and antisteroid treatment impair vocal learning in male zebra finches. *J Neurobiol*, 23:337–353.

Breedlove SM. (1994). Sexual differentiation of the human nervous system. *Annu Rev Psychol*, 45:389–418.

Burgoyne PS, Thornhill AR, Boudrean SK, Darling SM, Bishop CE, Evans EP. (1995). The genetic basis of XX-XY differences present before gonadal sex differentiation in the mouse. *Philos Trans R Soc Lond B Biol Sci*, 350:253–260.

Camu F, Shi L, Vanlersberghe C. (2003). The role of COX-2 inhibitors in pain modulation. *Drugs*, 63(Suppl 1):1–7.

Cardona-Gomez GP, Mendez P, DonCarlos LL, Azcoitia I, Garcia-Segura LM. (2002). Interactions of estrogen and insulin-like growth factor-I in the brain: molecular mechanisms and functional implications. *J Steroid Biochem Mol Biol*, 83:211–217.

Carruth LL, Reisert I, Arnold AP. (2002). Sex chromosome genes directly affect brain sexual differentiation. *Nat Neurosci*, 5:933–934.

Charlesworth B. (1991). The evolution of sex chromosomes. *Science*, 251:1030–1033.

Chen X, Agate RJ, Itoh Y, Arnold AP. (2005). Sexually dimorphic expression of trkB, a Z-linked gene, in early posthatch zebra finch brain. *Proc Natl Acad Sci U S A*, 102:7730–7735.

Contreras ML, Wade J. (1999). Interactions between nerve growth factor binding and estradiol in early development of the zebra finch telencephalon. *J Neurobiol*, 40:149–157.

Davies W, Isles AR, Burgoyne PS, Wilkinson LS. (2006). X-linked imprinting: effects on brain and behaviour. *Bioessays*, 28:35.

Day JR, Laping NJ, Lampert-Etchells M, Brown SA, O'Callaghan JP, McNeill TH, et al. (1993). Gonadal steroids regulate the expression of glial fibrillary acidic protein in the adult male rat hippocampus. *Neuroscience*, 55:435–443.

De Vries GJ. (2004). Minireview: Sex differences in adult and developing brains: compensation, compensation, compensation. *Endocrinology*, 145: 1063–1068.

De Vries GJ, Boyle PA. (1998). Double duty for sex differences in the brain. *Behav Brain Res*, 92: 205–213.

De Vries GJ, Panzica GC. (2006). Sexual differentiation of central vasopressin and vasotocin systems in vertebrates: different mechanisms, similar endpoints. *Neuroscience*, 138:947–955.

De Vries GJ, al-Shamma HA, Zhou L. (1994). The sexually dimorphic vasopressin innervation of the brain as a model for steroid modulation of neuropeptide transmission. *Ann N Y Acad Sci*, 743:95–120.

De Vries GJ, Rissman EF, Simerly RB, Yang LY, Scordalakes EM, Auger CJ, et al. (2002). A model system for study of sex chromosome effects on sexually dimorphic neural and behavioral traits. *J Neurosci*, 22:9005–9014.

Dewing P, Shi T, Horvath S, Vilain E. (2003). Sexually dimorphic gene expression in mouse brain precedes gonadal differentiation. *Brain Res Mol Brain Res*, 118:82–90.

Dewing P, Chiang CW, Sinchak K, Sim H, Fernagut PO, Kelly S, et al. (2006). Direct regulation of adult brain function by the male-specific factor SRY. *Curr Biol*, 16:415–420.

Dittrich F, Feng Y, Metzdorf R, Gahr M. (1999). Estrogen-inducible, sex-specific expression of brain-derived neurotrophic factor mRNA in a forebrain song control nucleus of the juvenile zebra finch. *Proc Natl Acad Sci U S A*, 96:8241–8246.

Driscoll I, Hamilton DA, Yeo RA, Brooks WM, Sutherland RJ. (2005). Virtual navigation in humans: the impact of age, sex, and hormones on place learning. *Horm Behav*, 47:326–335.

Fitch RH, Denenberg VH. (1995). A role for ovarian hormones in sexual differentiation of the brain. psycloquy 95.6.05.sex-brain.1.fitch.

Forger NG. (2006). Cell death and sexual differentiation of the nervous system. *Neuroscience*, 138:929–938.

Forger NG, Rosen GJ, Waters EM, Jacob D, Simerly RB, De Vries GJ. (2004). Deletion of Bax eliminates sex differences in the mouse forebrain. *PNAS*, 101: 13666–13671.

Fusani L, Metzdorf R, Hutchison JB, Gahr M. (2003). Aromatase inhibition affects testosterone-induced masculinization of song and the neural song system in female canaries. *J Neurobiol*, 54:370–379.

Garcia-Segura LM, Chowen JA, Naftolin F. (1996). Endocrine glia: roles of glial cells in the brain actions of steroid and thyroid hormones and in the regulation of hormone secretion. *Front Neuroendocrinol*, 17:180–211.

Garcia-Segura LM, Wozniak A, Azcoitia I, Rodriguez JR, Hutchison RE, Hutchison JB. (1999). Aromatase expression by astrocytes after brain injury: implications for local estrogen formation in brain repair. *Neuroscience*, 89:567–578.

Gatewood JD, Wills A, Shetty S, Xu J, Arnold AP, Burgoyne PS, Rissman EF. (2006). Sex chromosome complement and gonadal sex influence aggressive and parental behaviors in mice. *J Neurosci*, 26:2335–2342.

Giovannini MG, Scali C, Prosperi C, Bellucci A, Pepeu G, Casamenti F. (2003). Experimental brain inflammation and neurodegeneration as model of Alzheimer's disease: protective effects of selective COX-2 inhibitors. *Int J Immunopathol Pharmacol*, 16:31–40.

Gorski RA, Gordon JH, Shryne JE, Southam AM. (1978). Evidence for a morphological sex difference within the medial preoptic area of the rat brain. *Brain Res*, 148:333–346.

Graves JA. (2006). Sex chromosome specialization and degeneration in mammals. *Cell*, 124:901–914.

Grisham W, Lee J, McCormick ME, Yang-Stayner K, Arnold AP. (2002). Related antiandrogen blocks estrogen-induced masculinization of the song system in female zebra finches. *J Neurobiol*, 5:1–8.

Guillot PV, Carlier M, Maxson SC, Roubertoux PL. (1995). Intermale aggression tested in two procedures, using four inbred strains of mice and their reciprocal congenics: Y chromosomal implications. *Behav Genet*, 25:357–360.

Hamilton DA, Driscoll I, Sutherland RJ. (2002). Human place learning in a virtual Morris water task: some important constraints on the flexibility of place navigation. *Behav Brain Res*, 129:159–170.

Han TM, De Vries GJ. (2003). Organizational effects of testosterone, estradiol, and dihydrotestosterone on vasopressin mRNA expression in the bed nucleus of the stria terminalis. *J Neurobiol*, 54:502–510.

Hines M. (2004). *Brain Gender*. New York: Oxford University Press.

Hoffmann C. (2000). COX-2 in brain and spinal cord implications for therapeutic use. *Curr Med Chem*, 7:1113–1120.

Hojo Y, Hattori TA, Enami T, Furukawa A, Suzuki K, Ishii HT, et al. (2004). Adult male rat hippocampus synthesizes estradiol from pregnenolone by cytochromes P45017alpha and P450 aromatase localized in neurons. *Proc Natl Acad Sci U S A*, 101:865–870.

Holloway CC, Clayton DF. (2001). Estrogen synthesis in the male brain triggers development of the avian song control pathway in vitro. *Nat Neurosci*, 4:170–175.

Ibanez MA, Gu G, Simerly RB. (2001). Target-dependent sexual differentiation of a limbic-hypothalamic neural pathway. *J Neurosci*, 21:5652–5659.

Itoh Y, Kampf K, Arnold AP. (2006a). Assignment of human X-linked genes to a zebra finch microchromosome by in situ hybridization of BAC clones. *Cytogenet Genome Res*, 112:342M.

Itoh Y, Chen X, Kim Y-H, Grisham W, Agate R, Wingfield J, Wade J, Arnold AP. (2006b). Brain masculinization in the absence of testes in a mutant zebra finch. In: Society for Behavioral Endocrinology Meeting, Pittsburgh PA, June 2006.

Itoh Y, Melamed E, Yang X, Kampf K, Wang S, Yehya N, et al. (2006c). Dosage compensation in birds versus mammals. *Journal of Biology*, submitted.

Ivanova T, Kuppers E, Engele J, Beyer C. (2001). Estrogen stimulates brain-derived neurotrophic factor expression in embryonic mouse midbrain neurons through a membrane-mediated and calcium-dependent mechanism. *J Neurosci Res*, 66:221–230.

Jonasson Z. (2005). Meta-analysis of sex differences in rodent models of learning and memory: a review of behavioral and biological data. *Neurosci Biobehav Rev*, 28:811–825.

Jordan CL. (1999). Glia as mediators of steroid hormone action on the nervous system: An overview. *J Neurobiol*, 40:434–445.

Jost A. (1947). Reserches sur la différenciation sexuelle de l'embryon de lapin. *Arch Anat Microsc Morphol Exp*, 36:271–315.

Kim YH, Perlman WR, Arnold AP. (2004). Expression of androgen receptor mRNA in zebra finch song system: developmental regulation by estrogen. *J Comp Neurol*, 469(4):535–547.

Konishi M, Akutagawa E. (1985). Neuronal growth, atrophy and death in a sexually dimorphic song nucleus in the zebra finch brain. *Nature*, 315:145–147.

Kudwa AE, Bodo C, Gustafsson JA, Rissman EF. (2005). A previously uncharacterized role for estrogen receptor beta: defeminization of male brain and behavior. *Proc Natl Acad Sci U S A*, 102:4608–4612.

Lillie FR. (1916). The theory of the freemartin. *Science*, 43:611–613.

Lim MM, Young LJ. (2006). Neuropeptidergic regulation of affiliative behavior and social bonding in animals. *Horm Behav*, 50:506–517.

London SE, Monks DA, Wade J, Schlinger BA. (2006). Widespread capacity for steroid synthesis in the avian brain and song system. *Endocrinology*, 147(12):5975–5987.

Maxson SC, Didier-Erickson A, Ogawa S. (1989). The Y chromosome, social signals, and offense in mice. *Behav Neural Biol*, 52:251–259.

McCarthy MM. (1996). Molecular approaches to control of reproductive behavior and sexual differentiation of brain in rodents. In Palumbi JDFaSR, (Ed), *Molecular Zoology* (Chapter 21; pp. 387–400). New York: Wiley Press.

McCarthy MM, Konkle AT. (2005). When is a sex difference not a sex difference? *Front Neuroendocrinol*, 26:85–102.

McEwen BS. (1980). Gonadal steroids and brain development. *Biol Reprod*, 22:43–48.

Monahan EJ, Maxson SC. (1998). Y chromosome, urinary chemosignals, and an agonistic behavior (offense) of mice. *Physiol Behav*, 64:123–132.

Mong JA, Glaser E, McCarthy MM. (1999). Gonadal steroids promote glial differentiation and alter neuronal morphology in the developing hypothalamus in a regionally specific manner. *J Neurosci*, 19:1464–1472.

Mong JA, Nunez JL, McCarthy MM. (2002). GABA mediates steroid-induced astrocyte differentiation in the neonatal rat hypothalamus. *J Neuroend*, 14:1–16.

Morris JA, Jordan CL, Breedlove SM. (2004). Sexual differentiation of the vertebrate nervous system. *Nat Neurosci*, 7:1034–1039.

Nair HP, Young LJ. (2006). Vasopressin and pair-bond formation: genes to brain to behavior. *Physiology*, (Bethesda) 21:146–152.

Nordeen EJ, Nordeen KW. (1996). Sex difference among nonneuronal cells precedes sexually dimorphic neuron growth and survival in an avian song control nucleus. *J Neurobiol*, 30:531–542.

Nordeen EJ, Voelkel L, Nordeen KW. (1998). Fibroblast growth factor-2 stimulates cell proliferation and decreases sexually dimorphic cell death in an avian song control nucleus. *J Neurobiol*, 37:573–581.

Nordeen EJ, Nordeen KW, Sengelaub DR, Arnold AP. (1985). Androgens prevent normally occurring cell death in a sexually dimorphic spinal nucleus. *Science*, 229:671–673.

Palaszynski KM, Smith DL, Kamrava S, Burgoyne PS, Arnold AP, Voskuhl RR. (2005). A yin-yang effect between sex chromosome complement and sex hormones on the immune response. *Endocrinology*, 146:3280–3285.

Perlman WR, Arnold AP. (2003). Expression of estrogen receptor and aromatase mRNAs in embryonic and posthatch zebra finch brain. *J Neurobiol*, 55:204–219.

Perlman WR, Ramachandran B, Arnold AP. (2003). Expression of androgen receptor mRNA in the late embryonic and early posthatch zebra finch brain. *J Comp Neurol*, 455:513–530.

Perrot-Sinal TS. (1996). Sex differences in performance in the Morris water maze and the effects of initial nonstationary hidden platform training. *Behav Neurosci*, 110:1309–1320.

Peterson RS, Lee DW, Fernando G, Schlinger BA. (2004). Radial glia express aromatase in the injured zebra finch brain. *J Comp Neurol*, 475:261–269.

Phoenix CH, Goy RW, Gerall AA, Young WC. (1959). Organizing action of prenatally administered testosterone proprionate on the tissues mediating mating behavior in the female guinea pig. *Endocrinology*, 65:369–382.

Prange-Kiel J, Wehrenberg U, Jarry H, Rune GM. (2003). Para/autocrine regulation of estrogen receptors in hippocampal neurons. *Hippocampus*, 13:226–234.

Reisert I, Pilgrim C. (1995). Catecholaminergic systems and the sexual differentiation of the brain. Cellular mechanisms and clinical implications. In Segawa M, Nomura, Y. (Ed.), *Age-Related Dopamine-Dependent Disorders.*(pp 216–224). Basel, Switzerland: Karger.

Renfree MB, Short RV. (1988). Sex determination in marsupials: evidence for a marsupial-eutherian dichotomy. *Philosophical Transactions of the Royal Society of London B: Biological Sciences*, 322:41–53.

Schlinger BA, Arnold AP. (1992). Circulating estrogens in a male songbird originate in the brain. *Proc Natl Acad Sci*, 89:7650–7653.

Schumacher M, Weill-Engerer S, Liere P, Robert F, Franklin RJ, Garcia-Segura LM, et al. (2003). Steroid hormones and neurosteroids in normal and pathological aging of the nervous system. *Prog Neurobiol*, 71:3–29.

Schwarz JM, Thompson S, McCarthy MM. (2006). Estradiol promotes glutamate release from immature hypothalamic neurons. In: *Society for Behavioral Neuroendocrinology*. Pittsburgh PA.

Shors TJ, Chua C, Falduto J. (2001). Sex differences and opposite effects of stress on dendritic spine density in the male versus female hippocampus. *J Neurosci*, 21:6292–6297.

Simerly RB. (1998). Organization and regulation of sexually dimorphic neuroendocrine pathways. *Behav Brain Res*, 92:195–203.

Simerly RB. (2000). Development of sexually dimorphic forebrain pathways. In Matsumoto A, (Ed.), *Sexual Differentiation of the Brain* (pp. 175–202). Boca Ratan, FL: CRC Press.

Simerly RB. (2002). Wired for reproduction: organization and development of sexually dimorphic circuits in the mammalian forebrain. *Annu Rev Neurosci*, 25:507–536.

Simerly RB, Swanson LW, Gorski RA. (1985). The distribution of monoaminergic cells and fibers in a periventricular preoptic nucleus involved in the control of gonadotropin release: immunohistochemical evidence for a dopaminergic sexual dimorphism. *Brain Res*, 330:55–62.

Simerly RB, Zee MC, Pendleton JW, Lubahn DB, Korach KS. (1997). Estrogen receptor-dependent sexual differentiation of dopaminergic neurons in the preoptic region of the mouse. *Proc Natl Acad Sci U S A*, 94:14077–14082.

Singh B, Henneberger C, Betances D, Arevalo MA, Rodriguez-Tebar A, et al. (2006). Altered balance of glutamatergic/GABAergic synaptic input and associated changes in dendrite morphology after BDNF expression in BDNF-deficient hippocampal neurons. *J Neurosci*, 26:7189–7200.

Solum DT, Handa RJ. (2002). Estrogen regulates the development of brain-derived neurtrophic factor protein in the rat hippocampus. *J Neuroscience*, 22:2650–2659.

Spelke ES. (2005). Sex differences in intrinsic aptitude for mathematics and science: a critical review. *Am Psychol*, 60:950–958.

Suzuki M, Nishiahara M. (2002). Granulin precursor gene: a sex steroid-inducible gene involved in sexual differentiation of the rat brain. *Mol Genet Metab*, 75:31–37.

Todd BJ, Schwarz JM, McCarthy MM. (2005). Prostaglandin-E2: a point of divergence in estradiol-mediated sexual differentiation. *Horm Behav*, 48: 512–521.

Todd BJ, Schwarz JM, Mong JA, McCarthy MM. (2006). Glutamate AMPA/kainate receptors, not GABAA receptors, mediate estradiol-induced sex differences in the hypothalamus. *J Neurobio*, in press.

Toran-Allerand CD. (1980). Coexistence of alpha-fetoprotein, albumin and transferrin immunoreactivity in neurones of the developing mouse brain. *Nature*, 286:733–735.

Toran-Allerand CD. (1987). Neuronal uptake of alpha-fetoprotein (AFP) synthesized and secreted by hepatocytes in liver/brain co-cultures. *Neurosci Lett*, 83: 35–40.

Toran-Allerand CD. (1996). The estrogen/neurotrophin connection during neural development: is co-localization of estrogen receptors with the neurotrophins and their receptors biologically relevant? *Dev Neurosci*, 18:36–48.

Toran-Allerand CD, M. S, Jr. SG. (1999). Novel mechanisms of estrogen action in the brain: new players in an old story. *Frontiers in Neuroendocrinology*, 20:97–121.

Toran-Allerand CD, Bentham W, Miranda RC, Anderson JP. (1991). Insulin influences astroglial morphology and glial fibrillary acidic protein (GFAP) expression in organotypic cultures. *Brain Res*, 558: 296–304.

Toran-Allerand CD, Tinnikov AA, Singh RJ, Nethrapalli IS. (2005). 17alpha-estradiol: a brain-active estrogen? *Endocrinology*, 146:3843–3850.

Toran-Allerand CD, Guan X, MacLusky NJ, Horvath TL, Diano S, Singh M, et al. (2002). ER-X: a novel, plasma membrane-associated, putative estrogen receptor that is regulated during development and after ischemic brain injury. *J Neurosci*, 22:8391–8401.

Voskuhl RR, Palaszynski K. (2001). Sex hormones in experimental autoimmune encephalomyelitis: implications for multiple sclerosis. *Neuroscientist*,7: 258–270.

Wade J, Arnold AP. (1996). Functional testicular tissue does not masculinize development of the zebra finch song system. *Proc Natl Acad Sci U S A*, 93: 5264–5268.

Wade J, Arnold AP. (2004). Sexual differentiation of the zebra finch song system. *Ann N Y Acad Sci*, 1016: 540–559.

Wade J, Swender DA, McElhinny TL. (1999). Sexual differentiation of the zebra finch song system parallels genetic, not gonadal, sex. *Horm Behav*, 36:141–152.

Wade J, Springer ML, Wingfield JC, Arnold AP. (1996). Neither testicular androgens nor embryonic aromatase activity alters morphology of the neural song system in zebra finches. *Biol Reprod*, 55:1126–1132.

Wade J, Peabody C, Coussens P, Tempelman RJ, Clayton DF, Liu L, et al. (2004). A cDNA microarray from the telencephalon of juvenile male and female zebra finches. *J Neurosci Methods*, 138:199–206.

Wang Z, De Vries GJ. (1995). Androgen and estrogen effects on vasopressin messenger RNA expression in the medial amygdaloid nucleus in male and female rats. *J Neuroendocrinol*, 7:827–831.

Whalen R, Edwards D. (1967). Hormonal determinants of the development of masculine and feminine behavior in male and female rats. *Anat Rec*, 157: 173–180.

Yang X, Schadt EE, Wang S, Wang H, Arnold AP, Ingram-Drake L, et al. (2006). Tissue-specific expression and regulation of sexually dimorphic genes in mice. *Genome Res*, 16:995–1004.

Chapter 3

Research and Methodological Issues in the Study of Sex Differences and Hormone-Behavior Relations

Lisa A. Eckel, Arthur P. Arnold, Elizabeth Hampson, Jill B. Becker, Jeffrey D. Blaustein, and James P. Herman

The study of sex differences requires the investigator to consider a number of factors before beginning. Here we discuss what is meant by the term *sex differences* as well as approaches that can be used. First, some definitions may need to be explained. Most vertebrate species have two sexes: males and females which are defined by their ability to produce sperm or eggs. Males and females have evolved different phenotypes. Usually, "typical" or modal male and female traits are discernible, but each form is variable, and there are intermediates. For example, in humans the breast of women has a different form and size than the breast of men. Within a population, there are people with larger or smaller breasts that are intermediate between the two modal forms. The number of intermediate individuals is much smaller than the number of modal cases, so most people are comfortable defining typical male or female forms as a true dichotomy as opposed to two extremes along a continuum.

Once individuals are dichotomized by their sex, however, one finds that males and females differ rather continuously in numerous other traits. The term *sexually dimorphic* was originally coined to refer to traits in which modal males and modal females express in two distinctly different forms. The use of this term has been expanded to include any sex difference, even if the difference is not a modal male and female form. For example, some might say that verbal fluency scores are sexually dimorphic if the mean score differs in the two sexes despite the fact that the male and female distributions overlap extensively.

THE DIFFERENCE BETWEEN SEX AND GENDER

In humans, the existence of two sexes leads to the recognition of two genders. Sex is determined by whether the person is biologically male or female.

The gender of the person is a social or cognitive construct, i.e., what the person or the person's social community considers is his/her gender. Even these simple definitions of sex and gender are not without ambiguities. For example, because numerous body tissues differ in males and females, an individual may be a mixture of masculine and feminine traits. A person with a Y chromosome can have a vagina as in androgen insensitivity syndrome (AIS), where the androgen receptor is not functional. Thus, the biological sex of an individual may be measured in many ways. The gender of a person is generally what that person reports as his/her sex/gender.

In some circles, the terms *sex* and *gender* are used interchangeably. A physician discussing sex/gender issues with a patient may wish to avoid the undesirable connotations of the word sex (i.e., copulation) and therefore use gender when discussing sex differences or the implications of being biologically male or female. For example, "Your gender influences your susceptibility to disease" usually is meant such that gender refers to biological sex.

A person discussing sex differences in animals may use the two terms interchangeably because separate meanings do not normally apply to non-human animals. On the other hand, many scientists working with non-human animals argue that gender is a social or cognitive construct that is uniquely human and that sex is the appropriate term to be used when referring to male-female differences in non-humans.

What Is a Sex Difference?

We define a sex difference as *anything* that is found to be reliably different in males and females. The two sexes may differ in the mean of a trait, its variance, range, 10th percentile value, ratio, etc. Males and females may differ in the incidence of a trait, in the number of population outliers for a trait, in the correlation of two or more traits, in the timing of the trait, etc., even when there is no sex difference in the mean of the trait. For example, males and females may exhibit some traits at the same mean level, but in one sex the trait is more variable than the other, or the trait varies with reproductive cycle. Alternatively, both sexes may show the trait, but at different stages of development. These sex differences all require an explanation.

Origins of Sex Differences

All sex differences originate because of factor(s) that act in a sex-specific fashion. The factors can be biological or social. Factors may act exclusively in one sex, or be more prevalent in one sex, or in more individuals of one sex than the other.

The sex chromosomes are the origin of all sex differences (at least in species, such as mammals and birds, with heteromorphic sex chromosomes and genetic sex determination). To our knowledge, in mammals and birds, the only factors that discriminate a male and female zygote are those that are encoded on the sex chromosomes. In mammals, for example, XY males have Y-encoded genes that females do not. Moreover, females have a double genomic dose of X genes in contrast to the single genomic dose in males. Females also possess a paternal genomic imprint on one of their X chromosomes, and this imprint is absent in males who receive their X chromosome exclusively from the mother (Arnold & Burgoyne, 2004). All other factors (e.g., cytoplasmic factors inherited from the mother) are currently not thought to carry any sex-specific information (Arnold, 2002). These genetic sex differences lead to several classes of factors that induce sex differences in traits:

1. **Direct genetic effects of sex chromosome genes on the gonads**. The Y-linked gene *Sry* is expressed in the undifferentiated gonadal ridge, where it induces the formation of testes in males (Tilmann & Capel, 2002). In the absence of *Sry* in females, ovaries differentiate. The action of *Sry* in the gonadal ridge is the primary example of what is sometimes called *direct genetic* control of sexual differentiation of a tissue: the tissue develops differently in males and females because of the sex-specific expression within the tissue of a gene that is differentially represented in the male and female genome.

2. **Organizational actions of gonadal hormones**. The newly differentiated testes soon begin to secrete hormones that act directly on other tissues to cause them to develop differently than those in females. For example, testosterone from the testes acts on the genitalia to induce differentiation of the penis and scrotum, on the Wolffian duct structures to induce formation of the sperm ducts and associated glands, and on the brain to induce the formation of male structures and functions. In some cases, testosterone

is metabolized in target tissues to other hormones, such as dihydrotestosterone and estradiol, which then act to carry out masculinization in those tissues. The actions of testosterone and its metabolites early in development are often permanent because they involve irreversible commitment of a tissue to a masculine fate. For example, once the penis forms in response to testosterone, the removal of testosterone does not reverse its effect: the penis remains differentiated. The same process occurs in the brain. For example, testosterone causes the commitment of hypothalamic or spinal circuits to a masculine fate, a masculine pattern of organization. These permanent actions of testosterone are called *organizational* actions (Phoenix et al., 1959; Arnold & Breedlove, 1985). Organizational actions typically occur during the initial differentiation of tissues, often during critical periods of fetal and neonatal life in mammals.

3. **Activational actions of gonadal hormones.** The sex-specific differentiation of the gonads also sets up a life-long sex difference in the pattern of secretion of gonadal hormones. The testes and ovaries differ in the types of hormones secreted, and in their temporal pattern. These sex differences in the levels of hormones cause sex differences in a variety of tissues throughout life. For example, male quail have a larger nucleus in the preoptic area of the hypothalamus than female quail. This sex difference is abolished by adult gonadectomy, indicating that it is caused by sex differences in the adult levels of gonadal hormones (Panzica et al., 2001). Sex differences caused by differences in the levels or types of gonadal secretions in this manner are known as *activational* effects of hormones because the hormones act on fully differentiated tissues. In contrast to organizational effects, activational effects are reversible. Any reversible change in the female caused by cyclic secretion of estradiol during the estrous cycle creates a sex difference, because males do not experience the cyclic secretion of estradiol.

4. **Sex-specific actions of non-gonadal hormones.** Gonadal hormones are not the only hormones that cause sex differences in fully differentiated tissues. For example, the fetal or neonatal surge of testosterone from the testes masculinizes the hypothalamic circuits that control growth hormone (GH) secretion from the

pituitary. This establishes a life-long sex difference in the pattern of GH secretion in rodents. Males have larger daily swings in the level of GH, whereas females have lower GH levels that vary less. The sex differences in the pattern of GH secretion induce sex differences in gene expression in the liver (e.g., Furukawa et al., 1999). Other non-gonadal hormones that are secreted in a sexually dimorphic pattern or which produce a sexually dimorphic response in target tissues include: the adrenal hormones, thyroid hormones, and pancreatic hormones.

5. **Sex-specific effects of the environment.** The formation of the penis and other external genital tissues induced by testosterone leads to major sex differences in the social environment of animals and humans. Human babies are immediately sex-typed at birth (or earlier) based on their genitals, and the parents and others treat a baby differently depending on the apparent sex of the child. Different behaviors are encouraged or tolerated in boys than in girls. These social influences are powerful determinants of the individual's behavior and biology.

6. **Direct sex chromosome effects on brain and somatic tissues.** Although many differences in the brain and rest of the body are caused by organizational and activational effects of gonadal hormones, some sex differences stem from the differences in expression of sex chromosome genes within cells themselves. The primary example was already mentioned above: *Sry* induces formation of the testes. *Sry* is also expressed in the brain where it has male-specific effects (Dewing et al, 2006). Other sex differences also appear to be caused by non-*Sry* sex chromosome effects (De Vries et al., 2002; Carruth et al., 2002; Palaszynski et al., 2005; Gatewood et al., 2006; Arnold & Burgoyne, 2004). Sex chromosome complement and gonadal sex influence aggressive and parental behaviors in mice (Gatewood et al., 2006).

Sex Differences versus Sexual Differentiation

The term *sexual differentiation*—the process of becoming sexually different—has developmental overtones and is generally used to refer to permanent sex differences. This use of the term involves the concepts from developmental biology of irreversible commitment to a fate, and progressive loss of developmental potential. Sexual differentiation implies the developmental divergence of all individuals of one sex from all individuals of the other sex.

However, if a sex difference in expression of a gene in the brain is abolished by gonadectomy in adulthood, we say that the sex difference is caused by activational hormonal effects. One would typically not say that the gonadal hormones caused sexual differentiation of this trait, since the hormone action is impermanent. Viewed from a different perspective, however, the trait, by virtue of its dependence on gonadal steroid levels, is still sexually differentiated because of the permanent differentiation of the gonads.

Some sex differences represent population-level differences in the incidence of a trait. Consider color blindness and color perception. More males have red-green color blindness than females. This is an example of a sex difference at the population level. The color blindness is caused by mutations of opsin genes encoded on the X chromosome. The mutation is less apparent in females, because a mutation on one X chromosome is often mitigated by the effects of a non-mutant allele on the other X chromosome. Males are not protected because they lack a second X chromosome. Therefore, sex differences in colorblindness are due to differences in the number of X chromosomes in males and females.

On the other hand, females can have more types of opsin alleles than males, and this may lead to sex differences in color perception (Jameson et al., 2001). Normally we would not say sexual differentiation has occurred in this case, because there is no sex-typical irreversible commitment to a masculine or feminine fate. Rather, the population of males (or females) includes more individuals of a specific type, compared to the population of females.

Although the sex difference is a response to the action of sex-specific factors (here, encoded on the X chromosome), we do not put this type of process in the same category as sexual differentiation of the penis or clitoris. A *priori* it is not always easy to discriminate this sort of population sex difference in frequencies of specific traits from sexual differentiation in the traditional sense. For example, women may be more susceptible to a disease either because all women are differentiated from all men, or because a particular trait is more prevalent among women than men. An example is Rett's Syndrome, a disease that predominates in females and is caused by a mutation on the X chromosome. It is usually lethal in males, so that many more females are found to be affected (Dragich et al., 2000). In contrast, multiple sclerosis is more prevalent in females, probably because of the acute and differentiating (both organizational and activational) effects of testosterone (Voskuhl, 2002; see also Palaszynski et al., 2005). In all cases of sex differences, some sex-specific factor initiates the sex difference.

Sex-Specific Forces that Reduce Rather than Induce Sex Differences

Because some sex-specific factors may not be adaptive, evolution has provided sex-specific corrections that reduce the problem. For example, the evolution of heteromorphic sex chromosomes has led inexorably to a maladaptive imbalance in the dose of sex chromosome genes. In mammals, females have two X chromosomes, and males have one. This sex difference causes a problem in that females are at risk for having too high a dose of X genes relative to autosomal genes with which they interact, or that males lack sufficient X gene dosage, or both.

Mammals have evolved X *inactivation*—a female-specific process that transcriptionally silences one of the two X chromosomes in each non-germline cell. This process makes males and females more equivalent, each with one active X chromosome. The dose of genes on the single active X chromosome in each sex is also increased to be on a par with the dose of genes encoded on the other chromosomes, with which they interact (Nguyen & Disteche, 2004). In other systems, sex-specific factors also offset each other. For example, the male complement of sex chromosomes causes effects on the immune system that are reduced in males by the action of testosterone (Palaszynski et al., 2005; De Vries et al., 2005).

TESTING ORGANIZATIONAL EFFECTS OF GONADAL STEROIDS

Organizational effects of gonadal hormones are those that are permanent, or at least long-acting. For example, the fetal and neonatal testes in rodents are known to secrete testosterone, which acts during critical periods of development to influence permanently the development of specific tissues including the brain. To test whether a sex difference is caused by an organizational effect, the general approach is to manipulate the level of a hormone (increase it in individuals that have low levels, decrease it in individuals that have high levels) and then measure the effects of the manipulation on the sexually dimorphic trait later in life.

Research Strategies Used in Rodent Studies

The classic approach is to remove gonadal secretions of male rats pre- or postnatally (controls have sham treatments that do not remove gonadal secretions). The rats are then allowed to mature. As adults, animals are tested for the occurrence of a sexually dimorphic trait long after the endocrine manipulation. The actions of neonatal gonadal secretions can be disrupted by treatment with drugs that block androgen or estrogen receptors, or block the synthesis of estrogens from androgens. Postnatally in rodents, gonadal secretions can be removed by gonadectomy. When measuring a sexually dimorphic trait in adulthood, it is important to test the animals under identical conditions (identical levels of hormones, etc.), so that conditions at testing do not produce sex differences themselves (e.g., Breedlove & Arnold, 1983a).

Alternatively, one can administer androgens or estrogens to prenatal or neonatal rats (controls receive placebo treatments), let them mature, then measure the trait of interest in adulthood. Again, the measurement of the adults must be done under identical conditions. Female rats treated with testosterone after birth have more perineal motoneurons (are more masculine in this trait) than females receiving placebo treatments (Breedlove & Arnold, 1983b). Organizational effects of gonadal hormones are often detected only under specific conditions of testing. For example, testosterone acts early in development to masculinize the circuits controlling male rat copulatory behavior, but the neonatal effect can be seen only if the adult animals have sufficient levels of testosterone (Whalen, 1968). If one were to manipulate the level of testosterone in neonatal male rats and test them in the absence of testosterone in adulthood, one would detect no effect of the neonatal testosterone.

Mice with knock-outs of specific genes also reveal information concerning organizational effects of gonadal hormones. For example, male mice with a knock-out of the estrogen receptor alpha (ERα) show less masculine copulatory behavior as adults, indicating that ligands of this receptor (i.e., estrogens) are required for full masculine expression of this behavior (Ogawa et al., 2000). In this case, however, it is not clear whether the effects of estrogens are organizational, acting early in development, or activational, acting in adulthood, or both, since the gene is absent throughout life. In other cases, an organizational effect can be discerned. When the estrogen synthase (aromatase) gene is knocked-out, it prevents normal development of female traits, even when an estrogen is replaced in adulthood (Bakker et al., 2002). In this case, the effects of the knock-out persist when an estrogen is provided to adult females, indicating that aromatase (and therefore an estrogen) is required at times before adulthood for the emergence of a full feminine phenotype.

Research Strategies Used in Human Studies

Designing studies to explore the origins of sex differences in humans poses a challenge. Manipulating hormones exclusively for research purposes is prohibited, for ethical reasons. This means the tools and designs discussed elsewhere in this chapter cannot be applied in human investigations, even when an endocrine basis for a sex difference is suspected. In addition, in human studies, the environment cannot be controlled leaving the possibility open that sex differences might arise from differential exposure to influential environmental variables. This is of particular concern in developmental studies: by changing the sexual phenotype of the brain, organizational effects have the potential to interact with environmental factors, perhaps changing the probability that a person will seek out or encounter particular types of learning experiences.

Using Naturally Occurring Syndromes to Study Organizational Effects

One method used to investigate organizational effects is to study people who have had atypical exposure to specific hormones before birth or during the early postnatal period. The usual cause is genetic errors that lead to anomalies in the synthesis, metabolism, or sensitivity to particular hormones. Another cause of atypical exposure is maternal ingestion of hormones during pregnancy. Until the mid-1970s, synthetic estrogens and progestins were widely prescribed to prevent miscarriage in at-risk pregnancies (e.g., diethylstil-bestrol [DES]). This practice was discontinued once it was discovered that the medications had undesir-able side-effects (in the case of DES, an increased risk of cervical and/or vaginal cancer was identified among female offspring of DES-treated pregnancies [Herbst et al, 1971]).

An advantage of studying naturally occurring syn-dromes is that the hormonal anomalies are usually quite marked, and so constitute a good *natural* ma-nipulation of the hormones. But, there are pitfalls, starting with the rarity of the syndromes which can make it difficult to acquire adequate sample sizes. Because of the sensitive nature of sexual anomalies, recruitment is a delicate issue: patients are often not willing to participate in research that emphasizes the non-normative nature of their condition, or some patients may not be aware of their own condition in which case making contact can be an ethical di-lemma. Scientific and practical issues also limit the conclusions that can be drawn. A single hormone is seldom changed in isolation; multiple parallel chan-ges in other hormones are involved in many clinical conditions. Next, we describe a few of the disorders of sexual differentiation that have been used successfully to study organizational effects in humans. For an ex-ample of the use of DES-exposed subjects to test for organizational effects, and a discussion of some rele-vant issues, see Hines and Sandberg (1996).

1. **Congenital adrenal hyperplasia (CAH).** The classical form of CAH due to 21-hydroxylase deficiency is characterized by overproduction of androgens by the adrenal cortex. It is the syndrome studied most among researchers in-vestigating organizational effects. The androgen excess begins in the third month of gestation and continues until a diagnosis is made, usually at birth or shortly afterward. Because the defec-tive allele is carried on an autosome, CAH can occur in individuals of either sex. Once it is identified, androgen production can be nor-malized with medication taken on a daily basis. The androgen excess that occurs prenatally in CAH overlaps with the period of genital differ-entiation, and thus produces genital malforma-tions in females. Typically, genetic females with CAH are raised as females despite their atypical hormone exposure, and therefore psy-chosocial and hormonal influences on devel-opment are dissociated in girls with CAH.

If the organizational effects of androgens are important in generating a sex difference, a more male-typical pattern would be expected in girls with CAH. An important proviso is that this expectation only holds if the critical period for the initiation of the sex difference falls during the period when androgen is produced in excess. Therefore, studies of females with CAH can be instructive, not only for iden-tifying an organizational effect, but for trac-ing the timing of the effect to the prenatal period (or newborn period before treatment begins).

Though a useful technique, the study of CAH is complicated. The incidence in most of North America is about 1:15,000 live births, of which only half are females, and the preva-lence is further reduced by loss of life in the newborn period. Though often described as a syndrome of androgen excess, this is not the only hormone anomaly; a constellation of hor-monal changes occurs in CAH. Patients are invariably deficient in cortisol and in the ~75% who have the *salt-wasting* variant of CAH, aldosterone is seriously deficient as well. Pro-gesterone and 17-hydroxyprogesterone, plus sev-eral other hormones, are produced in excess. Among infants who survive, there may be neuro-logical sequelae attributable to early salt-wast-ing episodes. Finally, because of the lack of coherent hypotheses for what might be expected in males with CAH and ambiguities about the extent of the androgen anomaly in affected males, most studies of organizational effects are restric-ted to females only, where a clearer hypothesis can be derived.

Advances in treatment have reduced the phe-notypic consequences of CAH since prenatal diagnosis and treatment is now possible. This involves administering dexamethasone during pregnancy to the mother carrying a fetus with CAH to normalize fetal androgen levels. While it is a significant advance in medical manage-ment, the advent of prenatal interventions has reduced the availability of patients with CAH for studies of organizational effects.

2. **Androgen insensitivity syndrome (AIS).** An-other option for studying organizational effects in humans is to study individuals who were deprived of the effects of androgens during de-velopment. This situation occurs in patients with complete androgen insensitivity. AIS is an X-linked disorder in which affected males have a 46,XY karyotype and produce testosterone in

normal or even elevated quantities, but have feminine external genitalia due to the inability of the androgen receptor to properly bind its normal ligands, testosterone and dihydrotestosterone. Patients with complete AIS are reared as females and usually do not come to medical attention until adolescence, when they are detected by a failure to menstruate. The prevalence of AIS is about 1:50,000 live male births. Some patients have incomplete androgen insensitivity (if the mutation in the androgen receptor reduces rather than eliminates the effect of androgens), in which case the external genitalia may not be fully feminine.

Though impaired in the ability of their tissues to respond to androgens, patients with AIS show normal responsiveness to estrogens (i.e., estrogen receptors are intact). Of relevance to some types of research studies, the gonads need to be removed owing to an increased malignancy rate; thereafter, patients are maintained on exogenous estrogen. Since both female sex of rearing and failure to respond to androgens would predict feminization in a range of sex-typed variables, any evidence of masculinization in patients with complete AIS suggests (a) cell-autonomous effects of sex chromosome complement (see discussion of direct sex chromosome effects above), (b) masculinization by the estrogenic metabolites of androgens, acting on estrogen receptors, or (c) a subtle effect of the social environment of the person (parents, self-image, etc.) if the individual's intersex condition is known or suspected, for example if the external genitalia are perceptibly different from that of a normal male.

3. **Gonadal dysgenesis: Turner's syndrome and its variants.** Turner's syndrome is one of the most common disorders of sexual differentiation. Because it involves partial or complete absence of a sex chromosome, it is of interest to researchers studying haploinsufficiency, genetic imprinting, or the contributions of the X chromosome to sexual differentiation. The phenotype is female. Turner's syndrome is associated with a wide variety of somatic anomalies, including bilateral "streak" gonads that are devoid of germ cells. Germ cells are present in the ovaries *in utero,* but undergo an accelerated rate of atresia showing clear differences from controls as early as the fourth month of gestation (Singh & Carr, 1966). It is not known whether the Turner's fetus is steroid-deficient *in utero,* but there is evidence of elevated fol-

licle stimulating hormone (FSH) and decreased estradiol in patients as young as 5 days of age (Conte et al., 1975), implying a lack of feedback inhibition by the gonads.

Turner's syndrome is relevant to studies of organizational effects by virtue of the deficiency in ovarian steroid production. The postnatal rise in estradiol that occurs in the first year of life in control females (Forest et al., 1976) is likely to be absent or attenuated in most females with Turner's syndrome. This is potentially significant from an organizational point of view.

Turner's syndrome occurs in about 1:2000 live female births, of which ~50% have the classic 45,X karyotype. The condition is usually lethal in embryos (greater than 99% of 45,X conceptions are eliminated before birth [Robinson, 1990]), so the few surviving XO individuals probably represent a highly selected group that may differ from normal females not only in the number of sex chromosomes, but also in the complement of autosomal alleles. About 25% of Turner's females are mosaic (mixture of XX and XO cells), but with no structural abnormality of the X chromosome (i.e., 46,XX/45X); and 25% have an X chromosome that is only partially deleted or malformed, with or without mosaicism. Turner's patients typically begin replacement therapy with estrogen at about 13–14 years of age to stimulate the development of female secondary sex characteristics.

Other Methods for Studying Organizational Effects in Humans

1. **Studies of dizygotic twins.** In other species, behavior and physiology can be influenced by natural variations in hormone exposure that result from an animal's position in the uterus, i.e., its placement with respect to adjacent male fetuses (intrauterine position). Female rodents that developed between two male fetuses *in utero* are less female-typical in their postnatal behavior, genital anatomy, and reproductive characteristics than females that develop between two female fetuses. These effects are believed to be due to the transfer of testosterone, in minute amounts, by diffusion from the male to the female fetus.

On the assumption that human twins, also, might be affected by the sex of a co-twin, organizational effects are beginning to be explored in female members of opposite-sex (OS) twin pairs (i.e., females who developed with a male co-twin). If they received small amounts of androgens by diffusion, OS females should be more male-typical and less female-typical than female members of same-sex dizygotic pairs on some traits.

Masculinization of the auditory system has been reported in human females having male co-twins (McFadden, 1993); however, behavioral studies have been equivocal (Cohen-Bendahan et al., 2005). It needs to be stressed that co-twin effects are not well-validated in humans because of technical difficulties inherent in trying to demonstrate fetal transfer of hormones. Genital masculinization is not evident in OS females and the level of androgen diffusion is presumably small. If this method is validated, it will greatly facilitate studies of organizational effects, because the frequency of fraternal twinning is about 1 in 150 births worldwide (Cohen-Bendahan et al., 2005).

2. **Retrospective measurement of hormones in amniotic fluid.** Organizational effects can also be studied by the direct measurement of androgens (or other hormones) in amniotic fluid collected during routine amniocentesis. Although the fluid can be sampled only at highly specific time points, those times coincide with a hypothetical critical period (weeks 8–24) when there is normally a rise in testosterone in the male fetus and when many testosterone-dependent traits are hypothesized to be organized. The origin of estradiol and progesterone in amniotic fluid is debated, but the placenta, not the fetus, is probably the principal source of these hormones. In theory, the amniotic method could be used prospectively, but few investigators can afford to wait many years until the child or adult is old enough for sex differences to be evaluated. Therefore, those studies that have employed this method have retrospectively analyzed archival specimens of amniotic fluid (e.g., Finegan et al., 1989).

A great advantage of the technique is that it allows normal healthy individuals to be assessed, increasing the validity of any relationships found. It also circumvents the problem of small sample sizes endemic to clinical studies. Of course, any associations discovered between brain or behavioral variables and amniotic hormones constitute correlational evidence only for an organizational effect.

TESTING ACTIVATIONAL EFFECTS OF GONADAL HORMONES

Activational effects of gonadal hormones can be studied in two different ways. One can measure the natural variation in hormones across the estrous/menstrual cycle of females or the circannual cycle of hormones in males and females that are seasonal breeders. Alternatively, in non-human animals one can remove the source of gonadal hormones by gonadectomy and then selectively replace hormones of interest to determine causal relations between the hormone's action and various dependent measures.

Using Naturally Occurring Endocrine Changes to Test Activational Effects in Humans

Activational effects are easier to study in humans than organizational effects, and avoid many of the pitfalls associated with organizational studies. However, researchers must contend with the fact that manipulating reproductive hormones purely for research, even on a temporary basis, is disallowed. For this reason, most studies of activational effects use quasi-experimental designs. True experiments are possible if treatments can be justified as part of a randomized trial targeted at improving health care or alleviating a health problem.

One commonly used method is the *naturalistic* one, which involves measuring outcomes under high and low hormone conditions brought about by naturally occurring biological rhythms in hormone production. If one suspects that estradiol exerts an activational effect, for example, it is possible to use the menstrual cycle to evaluate women during carefully timed periods of lowest estradiol production (e.g., at menses) and at highest estradiol production (e.g., during the peak in estradiol that precedes ovulation). In many situations, the optimal hormone conditions will be fairly brief (only hours or days), therefore, careful control of timing is important. In some situations, it is also possible to control the *dose* of the hormone by accurate timing of the assessments. Examples of biological rhythms that have been used to *manipulate* hormones are the diurnal and seasonal changes in testosterone in men, diurnal changes in cortisol secretion, or the menstrual cycle in women.

The naturalistic method requires a thorough knowledge of the hormone systems being studied and external verification of the actual levels of hormones present at time of testing (e.g., immunoassays to quantify levels of circulating hormone). A major advantage of the method is its naturalism—naturally occurring hormones are studied under natural conditions and exhibit true physiological variations (in dose, timing), so that insights can be generated into activational effects in the state under which nature devised them to occur. Major disadvantages are the correlational nature of the data obtained (a common problem in nearly all human studies), and the possibility of co-variation in other variables that might influence outcomes, which requires imaginative and thorough controls to be employed. See Chapter 4 for a more detailed discussion of research methods in menstrual cycle research.

Testing Activational Effects Through Hormone Replacement/Deprivation Methods in Humans

Another quasi-experimental method is to study activational effects by capitalizing upon variations in hormones that result from treatments administered as part of a patient's health care. Examples include postmenopausal women being treated with hormone replacement therapy or men with prostate cancer who are undergoing anti-androgen therapy. Patients can be evaluated pre- and post-treatment or at different time points during the treatment at which hormone concentrations are known to differ. This approach can help to solidify findings obtained using naturalistic methods.

In ideal conditions, studies of activational effects can occur in the context of clinical trials where different treatment options are being tested and subjects are randomly assigned to groups. Otherwise, if researchers merely observe patients receiving routine health care, studies involving hormone replacement/deprivation involve the same logic as strictly naturalistic designs: both are observational designs, but differ in whether variations in hormones are endogenously or exogenously induced. Disadvantages of the latter approach are: subjects are not randomly selected nor randomly assigned to the treatments (if these are prescribed by physicians based on symptoms and patient preferences); the medical conditions being treated may themselves have effects on outcomes; the synthetic hormones that are customarily used in hormone replacement or deprivation studies are different

in chemical structure from the naturally occurring forms of the hormones and have different (though overlapping) biological effects; hormones are typically administered on a non-physiological schedule and in pharmacological doses; even though, in theory, only a single hormone is directly affected by the treatment, there may be secondary changes induced in other hormones.

Despite the disadvantages, medical treatments can provide opportunities for insights into activational effects that would not be possible under normal conditions. As one example, there are several different methods for suppressing androgen activity in men with prostate cancer. If there is a different effect associated with estrogen treatment versus androgen deprivation therapy, it speaks to the mechanisms by which activational effects may be generated.

Using Naturally Occurring Endocrine Changes to Test Activational Effects in Rodents: The Estrous Cycle

1. **Changes in vaginal cytology during the estrous cycle.** In female rodents, ovulation generally occurs at either 4- or 5-day intervals, except when disrupted by pregnancy, pseudopregnancy, or lactation. This produces either a 4-day (more common) or 5-day (less common) estrous cycle. Stages of the estrous cycle are often determined by the appearance of vaginal cytology samples, viewed under low magnification with a light microscope. The types of cells observed during each stage of a typical 4-day estrous cycle are shown in Figure 3.1. Although examination of vaginal cytology samples reveals that the length of individual stages of the estrous cycle ranges from 8–54 h (Freeman, 2006; Long & Evans, 1922), it is conventional to report cycle stage in relation to our circadian day. For example, when rats are housed on a 12–12 h light-dark cycle, each successive 24-h, mid-dark interval is named for 1 stage (Fig. 3.1A).

Using this traditional strategy, ovulation occurs around the transition from proestrus to estrus. During this periovulatory period, rodents display striking changes in many behavioral traits, including increased sexual receptivity, decreased food intake, and increased locomotor activity (Anantharaman-Barr & Decombaz, 1989; Finger, 1969; Eckel et al., 2000; Tarttelin & Gorski, 1971; Long & Evans, 1922;

Richter, 1922). Unfortunately, when using traditional stage assignment, these behavioral changes span two estrous cycle stages (i.e., proestrus and estrus).

To minimize confusion in the literature, those scientists with a primary interest in studying behavioral changes during the periovulatory period have adopted an alternative strategy for assigning estrous cycle stage in which each successive 24-h interval, beginning at the start of each dark period, is named for 1 stage (Fig. 3.1B). With this behavioral strategy, the 12-h dark period, coincident with ovulation, is referred to as *behavioral estrus* (Becker et al., 2005). While the research question dictates which of these strategies should be used in

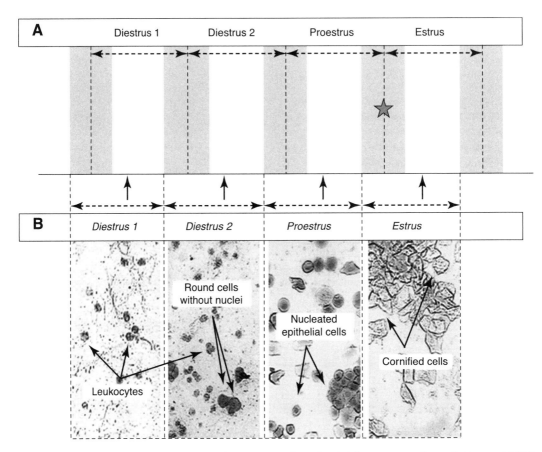

Figure 3.1. Two strategies for assigning cycle stage across the rodent's 4-day estrous cycle in relation to a 12-12 h light-dark cycle and daily samples of vaginal cytology. Successive 12-h dark periods are depicted by the shaded bars in the upper portion of the figure. Short, vertical arrows depict the time in which vaginal cytology is sampled. The gray star denotes the time in which ovulation commences (i.e., 4–6 h into the dark phase). (A). Traditional stage assignment: each successive 24-h interval from mid-dark phase to mid-dark phase is named for 1 cycle stage. (B). Behavioral stage assignment: each successive 24-h interval from dark onset to dark onset is named for 1 cycle stage. The lower potion of the figure contains representative photomicrographs depicting the type(s) of cells that predominate during each cycle stage. Day 1 of the cycle (diestrus 1), is characterized by a progression from leukocytes interspersed with small clusters of cornified cells (sometimes referred to as metesrus, lasting ~10 h) to leukocytes interspersed with larger round cells without nuclei. Day 2 (diestrus 2) is characterized by leukocytes interspersed with larger round cells without nuclei. Day 3 (proestrus) is characterized by large clumps of round, nucleated epithelial cells. Day 4 (estrus) is characterized by large clumps of cornified cells. Adapted with permission from Becker et al. (2005). Strategies and methods for research on sex differences in brain and behavior. *Endocrinology*, 146(4):1650–1673.

assessing estrous cycle stage, comparison across studies relies upon accurate reporting of estrous stage assignment in relation to the light-dark cycle as well as the endocrine events occurring during the time of experimental investigation.

2. **Changes in the ovary.** Each day of the estrous cycle, a number of oocytes (immature ova) are selected for maturation within individual ovarian follicles. This process, known as *folliculogenesis*, is well characterized in the rat. Here, we provide a brief overview of the structural changes in the ovary that occur during this process (for a detailed review, see Freeman, 2006).

Initially, epithelial cells within a primary follicle divide to form a stratified cuboidal epithelium comprised of granulosa cells. The granulosa cells of this secondary follicle induce the surrounding connective tissue of the ovary to differentiate into the theca interna, which becomes a major source of ovarian hormone production and release during the estrous cycle. The connective tissue surrounding the theca interna forms a thin layer of cells, the theca externa, which is thought to play a role in ovulation. As the secondary follicle matures, a clear liquid fills the spaces between cumulus granulosa cells surrounding the oocyte and mural granulosa cells on the follicular wall. Coalescence of the fluid-filled spaces produces a single fluid-filled antrum, resulting in the formation of a tertiary follicle. Follicular cumulus granulosa cells then form a hillock, called the cumulus oophorus, which is attached to one side of the follicular wall. As proestrus approaches, developing follicles are selected to either ovulate or become atretic. Follicles that mature in synchrony with the preovulatory surge in gonadotropin secretion will become committed to the preovulatory pool of maturing follicles. However, a larger number of asynchronous follicles will become atretic.

Secondary and tertiary follicles not committed to the ovulatory pool undergo a shrinking of the nucleus, followed by degeneration of the zona pellucida (outer wall of the ovum) and granulosa cells. Ovulatory follicles undergo additional growth, developing into a Graafian follicle containing a mature ovum consisting of a haploid number of chromosomes. The cumulus granulosa cells then form a ring (the corona radiata) and the volume of antral fluid increases as ovulation approaches. The mature, vascularized Graafian follicle protrudes from the surface of the ovary. Cumulus granulosa cells, the ovum, and follicular fluid are then extruded from the ruptured follicle. Within 1 h following follicular rupture, ova can be found within the rat's oviduct.

The site of the ruptured follicle is occupied by the corpus luteum, a glandular structure arising from growth of the granulosa and thecal cells of preovulatory follicular epithelium. The corpus luteum secretes progesterone. By 12 h following ovulation, the ruptured follicle consists of a wall of glandular luteal cells surrounding a fluid-filled cavity. By 36 h following ovulation, coincident with diestrus, the glandular luteal cells have grown to occupy most of the follicular cavity.

The corpus luteum is maintained at this stage of development through early diestrus of the following cycle. The glandular cells of the corpus luteum then begin to regress during the subsequent 12 h. At this time, another group of preovulatory follicles ruptures, forming a new set of corpora lutea. The regressing corpora lutea continue to decline over the next two estrous cycles until they are reduced to small masses of connective tissue called corpora albicantia.

If mating does not occur, the corpora lutea are considered non-functional as they fail to secrete sufficient progesterone to support a decidual reaction (thickening) of the uterine endometrium. The low secretion of progesterone over 1–2 days results in a *luteal* phase that is considerably abbreviated relative to the 11–14 day luteal phase of other mammals. However, in response to either mating or artificial stimulation of the uterine cervix, the pituitary gland secretes a sufficient quantity of a luteotrophic hormone (prolactin) to allow the corpus luteum to persist for a period of time that more closely resembles a typical mammalian luteal phase.

If mating results in fertilization, the corpus luteum will be rescued for the duration of the 20–22 day pregnancy. In the case of either an infertile mating stimulus or artificial stimulation of the cervix, the latter of which could arise if care is not taken while obtaining a sample of vaginal cytology for characterization of cycle stage as described above, the corpus luteum will persist for 12–14 days, a period of time referred to as pseudopregnancy.

3. **Pattern of endocrine changes.** Radioimmunoassays provide a sensitive technique for measuring the release of ovarian hormones in the

peripheral circulation of cycling rodents (see Freeman, 2006; Butcher et al., 1974). Studies in rats, using traditional nomenclature for assigning estrous cycle stage, reveal that plasma levels of estradiol, the major source of estrogen in the circulation, begin to rise from baseline concentrations of about 3–10 pg/ml during late diestrus 1, continue to rise during diestrus 2, and reach maximum concentration (~40–80 pg/ml) by the afternoon of proestrus, approximately 18 h prior to ovulation. Plasma estradiol then drops precipitously, resulting in very low levels (<5 pg/ml during estrus [Fig. 3.2].

A study examining changes in peripheral plasma estradiol concentration across the estrous cycle revealed that plasma estradiol levels on the first three days following ovulation were similar between groups of 4- and 5-day cycling rats (Nequin et al., 1979). This suggests that differences in cycle length are not attributed to differences in estradiol secretion.

In cycling rats, the pattern of progesterone secretion is characterized by two peaks above the basal concentration of 3–10 ng/ml (Fig. 3.2). The first, smaller peak occurs during the transition between diestrus 1 and diestrus 2,

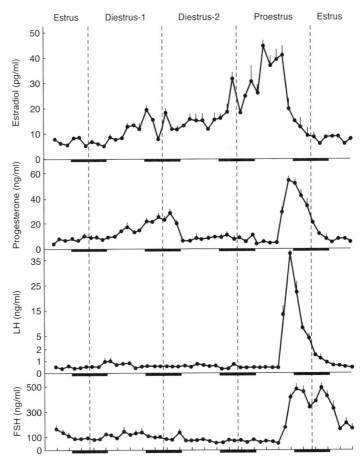

Figure 3.2. Patterns of estradiol, progesterone, LH, and FSH secretion across the rat's 4-day estrous cycle. Successive 12-h dark periods are depicted by the black bars. Cycle stage labels are assigned using traditional stage assignment. Note that peak concentrations of each of these hormones occur during proestrus. Adapted with permission from Smith MS, Freeman ME, Neill JD (1975). The control of progesterone secretion during the estrous cycle and early pseudopregnancy in the rat: prolactin, gonadotropin and steroid levels associated with rescue of the corpus luteum of pseudopregnancy. *Endocrinology*, 96:219–226.

when plasma progesterone concentration reaches 12–22 ng/ml. A second, larger peak occurs near the end of proestrus, when plasma progesterone concentration reaches 40–60 ng/ml, approximately twice the level observed during the first peak. It is believed that the fall in plasma progesterone concentration following the first peak signals regression of the corpus luteum in the non-pregnant rat.

Differences in plasma progesterone concentration during diestrus 2 have been reported in 4- versus 5-day cyclic rats, with greater concentrations reported in the latter condition (Nequin et al., 1979). Thus, differences in plasma progesterone concentration may account for differences in estrous cycle length.

In addition to the ovary, the anterior pituitary gland plays an important role in the control of reproductive function in rodents. For example, hypophysectomy promotes ovarian atrophy and disruption of estrous cyclicity, and small implants of anterior pituitary tissue can reverse these effects in hypophysectomized rats (Smith, 1926). This classic study provided the first evidence that hormones secreted from the anterior pituitary gland, later identified as luteinizing hormone (LH) and follicle stimulating hormone (FSH), stimulate the ovaries and, thereby, regulate reproductive function and estrous cyclicity.

The patterns of LH and FSH secretion from the anterior pituitary gland are well established (Figure 3.2). Serum concentration of LH is low throughout most of the 4-day estrous cycle (<1 ng/ml). However, on the afternoon of proestrus, serum concentration of LH rapidly begins to rise, reaching peak concentration (35–40 ng/ml) near the end of proestrus. Serum LH then falls to basal levels by the morning of estrus. The pattern of FSH secretion is quite similar to that of LH secretion. Basal levels of FSH (80–120 ng/ml) are secreted during diestrus 1 and diestrus 2. On the afternoon of proestrus, FSH concentration rises rapidly in a manner that parallels LH secretion. Peak FSH concentration (440–480 ng/ml) is sustained throughout the transition from proestrus to estrus and then declines to basal levels by the end of estrus. There appears to be little difference in either LH or FSH secretion patterns between 4-day and 5-day cycling rats.

4. **Vaginal cytology: to lavage or not.** If one wants to determine hormone-behavior relations in a rodent, there is no substitute for examination of the vaginal cytology on a daily basis.

Measuring vaginal impedance has gained in popularity recently, but the reliability of this method is still in question (Singletary et al., 2005). The primary problems with this method are that it does not differentiate between all days of the cycle and the data from impedance measures do not correlate with the results of vaginal cytology or hormone measurements (Singletary et al., 2005).

In one study, repeated vaginal lavage was reported to induce conditioned place preference and attenuate the effect of estrous cycle on the behavioral response to cocaine relative to non–lavage-treated rats (Walker et al., 2002). Given the effect on conditioned place preference, it is possible that the lavage technique used in this study produced more stimulation than is necessary in order to obtain a sample sufficient to determine estrous cycle stage. Another possible side effect of daily vaginal lavage in intact female rats is pseudopregnancy which occurs when vaginocervical stimulation reaches a threshold level (Lehmann & Erskine, 2004).

In many systems, the effect of estrous cycle on the dependent measure is small compared to the effect of the independent measure. It is probably not necessary to take vaginal cytology samples under such conditions, but we recommend that the results first be published with the stage of estrous cycle determined, before eliminating this important piece of data from the protocol.

CONDITIONS THAT CAN AFFECT THE ENDOCRINOLOGY OF THE ESTROUS CYCLE

1. **Age.** Unlike humans, rodents experience reproductive failure at an age when there are few, if any, primary changes in the ovary or decreases in ovarian follicular stores. For example, transplantation of the ovaries from aged rats to younger OVX rats frequently results in the resumption of regular estrous cycles (Huang et al., 1976). Despite considerable evidence that the ovaries of aged rats remain capable of normal function throughout their lifespan, it is widely recognized that rats undergo a midlife transition in reproductive function that has been called *estropause* (Chakraborty & Gore, 2004).

In rats, the beginning of this transition is characterized by irregular, typically prolonged rather than shortened, estrous cycles. This is followed by constant estrus, which is characterized by continual cornified vaginal cytology, chronically high estradiol levels, well-developed follicles, an absence of corpora lutea, and uterine proliferation (Chakraborty & Gore, 2004; LeFevre & McClintock, 1988; Huang & Meites, 1975).

A period of irregular cycles then gives way to persistent diestrus, which is characterized by continual leukocytic vaginal cytology, chronically low estradiol levels, and anterior pituitaries with some hemorrhagic or tumorous areas (LeFevre & McClintock, 1988; Huang & Meites, 1975). During this transition rats display decreased fertility, smaller litter sizes, and increased fetal resorptions during pregnancy (Chakraborty & Gore, 2004). Eventually, rats enter an anestrous state, which is characterized by atrophic ovaries and uteri, little follicular development, and large pituitary tumors (Huang & Meites, 1975). Although less well-characterized, female mice undergo a similar transition in which estrous cycles become more prolonged and eventually cease.

In rodents, the cessation of estrous cycling appears to be mediated by age-related alterations in the capacity of the hypothalamic-pituitary system to secrete gonadotropins in response to physiological stimuli. For example, Meites and colleagues (Huang et al., 1976) demonstrated that serum LH in old, constant estrous rats was significantly elevated compared to young, cycling rats on the day of estrus. In contrast, serum LH in old, persistent diestrous rats was similar to that observed in younger, cycling rats on the day of diestrus. In very old, anestrous rats, serum LH levels were undetectable. Moreover, the large increase in serum LH following ovariectomy in young rats was severely blunted in constant estrous and, to a lesser extent, in persistent diestrous rats. When estradiol was administered following ovariectomy, the subsequent fall in LH was much more pronounced in the younger rats, compared to both constant estrous and persistent diestrous rats. A similar pattern of basal and OVX-induced changes in serum FSH were observed in constant estrous and persistent diestrous rats.

2. **Exercise.** Laboratory rodents readily engage in voluntary exercise when given access to running wheels. Like many other behaviors, exercise is influenced by stage of the estrous cycle (e.g., Anantharaman-Barr & Decombaz, 1989; Fin-ger, 1969; Eckel et al., 2000; Richter, 1922). Specifically, female rats display reliable increases in running wheel activity during behavioral estrus, relative to other cycle stages (Fig. 3.3).

This increase in wheel running during behavioral estrus appears to be mediated by estradiol, since cyclic estradiol replacement alone following ovariectomy is sufficient to restore the estrous increase in wheel running observed in ovarian-intact cycling rats (Fig. 3.4).

At present, there is no evidence that voluntary exercise exerts a negative impact on either follicular growth or ovulation in female rats. In one study, four weeks of voluntary exercise in running wheels failed to alter either the number of non-atretic follicles or the number of ova in the oviducts of either superovulated or estrous rats, relative to sedentary control rats (Kagabu et al., 1997). In other studies involving female rats, wheel running did not disrupt estrous cyclicity, provided that access to food was not restricted (Eckel et al., 2000; Dixon et al., 2003). There is also some evidence that voluntary exercise can have a beneficial effect on the reproductive axis. For example, voluntary wheel running restores estrous cyclicity in anestrous golden hamsters maintained

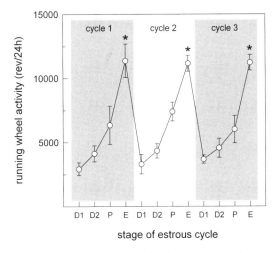

Figure 3.3. Daily running wheel activity across 3 consecutive estrous cycles in the rat. Female rats display a reliable increase in wheel running during behavioral estrus, relative to other cycle stages. *Abbreviations:* D1 = diestrus 1, D2 = diestrus 2, P = proestrus, E = estrus, rev = revolutions. *Greater than D1, D2, and P ($P < .01$).

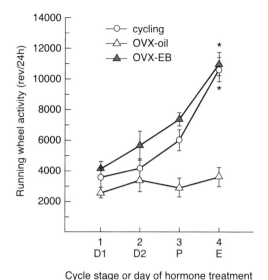

Figure 3.4. Daily running wheel activity in cycling and ovariectomized rats treated with either estradiol benzoate (EB) or sesame oil vehicle. Cycling rats display a prominent increase in wheel running during behavioral estrus. This effect is abolished in ovariectomized rats treated with vehicle. A cyclic regimen of estradiol treatment (daily injection of 4 μg EB on days 1 and 2) restores the estrous-related increase in wheel running observed in cycling rats. *Abbreviations:* D1 = diestrus 1, D2 = diestrus 2, P = proestrus, E = estrus, rev = revolutions, OVX = ovariectomized *Greater than D1, D2, and P ($P<.01$).

on a short-day, non-breeding photoperiod (Nequin et al., 1979).

Unlike voluntary exercise, intensive exercise training programs can disrupt reproductive function in laboratory rodents. In studies involving extended periods of either forced treadmill running or swimming, female rats displayed prolonged, continual diestrous vaginal cytology and delayed ovulation (Chatterton et al., 1990), fewer days of vaginal cornification consistent with an anestrous state (Carlberg & Fregly, 1985), fewer corpora lutea in their ovaries (Chatterton et al., 1995), and decreased circulating levels of estradiol and progesterone accompanied by irregular vaginal cytology (Axelson, 1987). In addition, disruptions in LH secretion and, therefore, ovulation, were observed in female rats exposed to 12 weeks of intensive treadmill running (Caston et al., 1995). Thus, forced exercise can induce changes in anterior pituitary gonadotropin secretion that could

account for the complete cessation of estrous cyclicity observed in many studies of forced exercise training.

3. **Lighting conditions.** It has long been known that the events of the estrous cycle are temporally related to the 24-h light-dark cycle. That is, ovulation generally occurs once every 4 or 5 days in rodents exposed to either a 14:10 or 12:12 alternating light-dark cycle (see Figure 3.1). The pioneering work of Everett and Sawyer (1950) revealed that the LH release mechanism, which is ultimately responsible for this cyclic pattern of ovulation in the rodent, is governed by a circadian rhythm under 24-h photoperiodic control. In their classic experiment involving traditional cycle stage assignment, administration of a centrally acting anesthetic, 5 h prior to dark onset on the afternoon of proestrus, delayed ovulation by 24 h in normally cycling rats exposed to a 14:10 alternating light-dark cycle. Injections of the anesthetic either at this same time during diestrus or estrus or at different times during proestrus failed to delay ovulation. This led to the concept of a critical period during which time a neural event stimulates increased LH release and subsequent ovulation. It was later shown that this critical period can be shifted in the phase, but not in the duration of lighting (Hoffman, 1969). Thus, light-dark cycles appear to regulate the rodent's estrous cycle via entrainment of their circadian system. This concept is further reinforced by the observation that prolonged exposure to constant bright light induces an anestrous state characterized by vaginal cornification (i.e., a constant estrous state), and a disruption in ovulation as well as the behavioral traits associated with estrus (Schwartz & McCormack, 1972; Weber & Adler, 1979; Takeo, 1984; Campbell & Schwartz, 1980). Finally, it should also be noted that brief exposures to light during the dark phase, or brief exposures to dark during the light phase can have a disruptive effect on the rat's estrous cycle.

Changes in levels of gonadotropins and ovarian steroids have also been documented in rodents exposed to constant illumination. In one study (Takeo, 1984), the mean concentration of FSH rats in constant estrous exposed to constant bright light was lower than that observed in control rats (exposed to an alternating light-dark cycle) on the morning of proestrus. In addition, the concentrations of estradiol and estrone in constant estrous rats were elevated, whereas progesterone levels were reduced compared to control rats.

While considerable evidence suggests that the neural mechanism controlling cyclic LH release and subsequent ovulation is photoperiodic, there is some evidence that LH release may also be regulated by non-photoperiodic cues. In an interesting study, constant illumination beginning at 22 days of age shortened the time-to-vaginal opening and the first day of estrus, compared to similarly aged control rats exposed to an alternating light-dark cycle (Hagino et al., 1983). Upon continued exposure to constant light, this precocious puberty was followed by constant estrus and anovulation, but only in those female offspring originating from mothers exposed to a 14:10 alternating light-dark cycle. Other female offspring, reared under constant light but originating from mothers exposed to constant light prior to and during pregnancy, displayed normal onset of puberty, regular 4-day estrous cycles, and cyclic ovulation while continuously exposed to constant light (Hagino et al., 1983). These findings suggest that mothers exposed to constant light produce offspring that are insensitive to the deleterious effects of constant light on estrous cyclicity. The authors concluded that in the absence of alternating light-dark cues, an endogenous clock, perhaps sensitive to daily laboratory cues including temperature, noise, or the sampling of vaginal cytology, may provide important time cues for cyclic release of LH.

4. **Stress.** In rodents, chronic exposure to physical stressors, including tail pinch, electrical foot shock, forced exercise, and cold temperatures, produce reliable disruptions in estrous cyclicity that are usually characterized by a persistent diestrous state (Gonzalez et al., 1994). Rats exposed to milder forms of daily stress, including brief periods of restraint or exposure to wet bedding, often become stalled in a particular estrous stage. However, normal cycles resume once the stressor is removed (Konkle et al., 2003). Interestingly, the response to mild stress is influenced by stage of the estrous cycle. While diestrous rats are typically quite resistant to the effects of brief restraint stress, the same stressor administered to proestrous rats typically prolongs the estrous cycle and delays ovulation (Matysek, 1989). Such mild stress-induced delays in ovulation appear to be mediated by suppressed, preovulatory release of LH and FSH (Roozendaal et al., 1995).

Severe food restriction is another stressor that can have adverse effects on reproduction. In the rat, estrous cycles are reliably disrupted when food is restricted to 50% of normal daily consumption (Cooper et al., 1970). Such disruptions in estrous cyclicity are accompanied by decreased pituitary, ovarian, and uterine weights, as well as increased FSH secretion (Nakanishi et al., 1976). Upon cessation of the severely restricted feeding schedule, rats display regular estrous cycles within 3–5 days of *ad libitum* feeding, regardless of the total amount of weight lost while food restricted. Within a few days of the resumption of normal estrous cycles, pituitary, ovarian and uterine weights are restored and FSH levels are lowered to that observed in control rats during diestrus (Nakanishi et al., 1976).

It is important to note that milder forms of food restriction, like those commonly used in studies of motivated behavior, do not appear to disrupt the estrous cycle of many rat strains. For example, when food is restricted to 85% of normal daily consumption, both Long-Evans and Sprague-Dawley rats continue to display regular estrous cycles, whereas Fischer 344 rats stop cycling by the fifth day of food restriction (Tropp & Markus, 2001). Interestingly, enriching the restricted diet with either sugar or fat delays disruption of the estrous cycle, but does not prevent anestrus, in Fischer rats (Tropp & Markus, 2001).

HORMONE REPLACEMENT OR TREATMENTS: FEMALE RATS

1. **Dose of estradiol.** In rodents and other vertebrates, 17ß-estradiol (often simply referred to as estradiol) is the most prevalent form of estrogen within the circulation. For this reason, it is commonly used in endocrine and neuroendocrine research involving estrogen replacement paradigms. For studies in which short-term treatment is desired, 17ß-estradiol can be administered as an acute injection via the subcutaneous, intravenous, intramuscular, intraperitoneal, or intracranial route (Asarian & Geary, 2002; Rivera & Eckel, 2005). For long-term treatment, either crystalline 17ß-estradiol or 17ß-estradiol dissolved in sesame or peanut

oil vehicle can be enclosed in a length of silas-tic™ tubing that is implanted subcutaneously for as long as estradiol treatment is desired (Wade & Zucker, 1970). For prolonged central administration, crystalline estradiol can also be packed in a cannula that is then implanted into a particular brain region (Butera & Beikirch, 1989). Specific concentrations of 17ß-estradiol can also be delivered, both peripherally and centrally, over a pre-determined period of days to weeks via Alzet minipumps (Martucci & Fishman, 1979).

Because systemic injection of 17ß-estradiol produces only a transient increase in circulat-ing estradiol, it is common practice to use slower-release, esterified forms of 17ß-estradiol. While several modified forms of 17ß-estradiol are available, the most commonly used form is estradiol-3-benzoate (EB), a hormone that is rapidly hydrolyzed in vivo to the physiologi-cally active 17ß-estradiol following its sys-temic administration in oil. Because EB was used in many of the pioneering studies of the role of estrogens in the control of female sexual behavior, its use is now widespread in the field of behavioral endocrinology. For example, it is well established that one or two daily injections of EB (typical dose range = 1–10 µg, s.c.) followed by progesterone in-jection in ovariectomized rats is sufficient to reinstate many of the behavioral changes seen during estrus in cycling rats (e.g., in-creased proceptive behaviors, increased loco-motor activity, decreased food intake) (Powers, 1970).

Although one or two daily injections of EB can reinstate many of the behavioral changes seen during estrus in cycling rats, it fails to model the changes in estradiol secretion across the estrous cycle. As depicted in Figure 3.1, the preovulatory surge in 17ß-estradiol secretion, which peaks on the afternoon of proestrus, is followed by a rapid drop in 17ß-estradiol secre-tion to basal levels by the morning of estrus. In contrast, traditional EB replacement para-digms, like those described above, produce a slower rise in plasma 17ß-estradiol concentra-tion that is sustained for at least 24–48 h following treatment (Tapper et al., 1974). How-ever, Asarian and Geary (2002) have devised an alternate EB replacement protocol, which in-volves injecting rats with 2 µg EB once every four days. This pattern of EB treatment closely mimics the changes in 17ß-estradiol secretion

across the estrous cycle, and reinstates several estrous-related changes in behavior including increased proceptive behavior and decreased food intake.

2. **Dose of progesterone.** Progesterone is the prin-cipal circulating form of the class of hormones known as progestins. In rodents, progesterone, like 17ß-estradiol, can be administered via mul-tiple routes, as described. Unlike 17ß-estradiol, progesterone is only injected in an unmodified form. In order to reinstate the full complement of female reproductive behaviors in ovariecto-mized rats, one must combine injections of both 17ß-estradiol and progesterone. Common pro-tocols involve administering two daily injec-tions of 10 µg 17ß-estradiol (s.c. in oil), or a single injection of 2 µg estradiol benzoate, followed by a single injection of 500 µg pro-gesterone (Xiao & Becker, 1997; Blaustein & Wade, 1977). In the ovariectomized rat, this regimen of ovarian hormone replacement is essential for the full facilitation of sexual recep-tivity, similar to that observed during estrus in cycling rats (Powers, 1970).

3. **Caveats of ovarian hormone replacement.** There are multiple caveats associated with ovar-ian hormone replacement. First, it should be noted that the decrease in blood concentration of 17ß-estradiol following ovariectomy does not necessarily indicate the cessation of 17ß-estradiol activity. This is because cell nuclear ERs, functioning as transcription factors, can retain 17ß-estradiol for a considerable time following the decline in blood concentration. In rats, this interval can range from 18–24 h following intravenous administration of 17ß-estradiol (Blaustein et al., 1979), and for 24–48 h following subcutaneous injection of EB (Schwartz et al., 1979). Thus, the cellular and behavioral consequences of acute estradiol treat-ment may persist for several days, despite an inability to detect the hormone in peripheral circulation.

Second, the neuroendocrine response to ovariectomy and subsequent ovarian hormone replacement is influenced by age. For exam-ple, middle-aged and old rats (9–14 months and 18–30 months, respectively) show a slower decline in ovarian hormone concentrations following ovariectomy, compared to younger rats. In addition, the negative feedback re-sponse to ovarian hormone replacement fol-lowing ovariectomy is greater and occurs more rapidly in young rats (2–6 months) compared to older rats. Finally, fewer days of ovarian hormone replacement are required to induce a surge in LH secretion in young OVX rats compared to middle-aged OVX rats. Thus, the slower neuroendocrine response of older rats should be considered in studies involving OVX and hormone replacement.

Finally, it should be noted that most plant-based oils that are used as the vehicle for injection of most steroid hormone have some estrogenic activity (i.e., phytoestrogens). This means it is important to include injections of the same oil as a control, and if following a protocol from another laboratory make sure the same oil is used for replication.

4. **Estrogen agonists and antagonists (ERα and ERß selective drugs).** Estrogens exert many of their physiological and behavioral effects through two nuclear protein receptors, ERα and ERß. That estrogens exert diverse actions is not surprising, given that ERs are transcription factors that are activated by binding of ligand and modulate target gene expression. This occurs when the receptor-ligand complex dimerizes and binds to estrogen-responsive elements upstream of estrogen-regulated genes. The induction of gene transcription can then influence specific responses within target cells (reviewed in Korach, 1994). In contrast to this well-characterized genomic effect of estrogens, a more rapid, non-genomic mechanism of estrogen action, which likely involves a membrane ER that is not a transcription factor, has also been described (Moriarty et al., 2006). Currently, only the genomic ER has been well studied in the context of the hypothalamic-pituitary-ovarian axis. Thus, our discussion of estrogen agonists is limited to ERα and ERß selective drugs.

In recent years, selective ERα and ERß receptor agonists have been developed to study the relative contribution of each ER subtype to estrogen's diverse actions. Propylpryazole-triol (PPT) is a synthetic, non-steroidal ERα receptor agonist that displays ~1000-fold selectivity for ERα over ERß (Kraichely et al., 2000), and diarylpropionitrile (DPN) is a synthetic, non-steroidal ERß receptor agonist that displays ~200-fold selectivity for ERß over ERα (Sun et al., 1999).

There is some evidence that both of these receptor agonists cross the blood-brain barrier. For example, peripheral administration of PPT increases mRNA expression of the progestin receptor within the hypothalamus of ovariectomized rats (Harris et al., 2002), and peripheral administration of DPN influences anxiety-like behaviors in ovariectomized rats (Walf & Frye, 2005). These receptor agonists have been used to differentiate the roles of ERα and ERß in mediating 17ß-estradiol-induced uterine growth (Harris et al., 2002; Frasor et al., 2003). More recently, each of these receptor agonists has been used to assess the relative contribution of ERα and ERß in mediating 17ß-estradiol's inhibitory effect on food intake.

HORMONE REPLACEMENT OR TREATMENTS: MALE RATS

1. **Dose of testosterone.** As was the case for estrogen treatments, there are acute and chronic dosing strategies for testosterone replacement. Since levels of testosterone do not show large cyclical variations typical of the estrous cycle in females (however, see Caveats, below), constant replacement strategies are used extensively to achieve physiological replacement. Physiological replacement is accomplished using Silastic© capsules containing crystalline testosterone, with internal diameter and length appropriate for long-term maintenance of plasma testosterone in the 1–7 ng/ml range (e.g., see Chen & Zirkin, 1999; Chen et al., 2002; Shetty et al., 2002). Long-term replacement can also be achieved by miniosmotic pump. As was the case for replacement with estrogens, repeated injections can also be used, generally requiring 100–500 µg/day (van Roijen et al., 1997). Doses used for acute physiological replacement vary widely between studies (200–1000 µg/kg).

2. **Doses of dihydrotestosterone.** It is well established that testosterone can be converted to estradiol in tissues that express the aromatase enzyme. In such tissues, the actions of testosterone can be partially or wholly attributed to estrogenic activity. If the presence of aromatase is expected, it is advisable to use the non-aromatizable androgen 5-alpha-dihydrotestosterone (DHT) to distinguish among androgenic and estrogenic actions. Replacement procedures using DHT parallel those of testosterone, e.g., implantation of crystalline DHT in Silastic™ tubing, with appropriate adjustment of dosing (DHT is a more

potent androgen than testosterone) (Shetty et al., 2002).

3. **Androgen receptor antagonists.** Androgen receptor antagonists can be used to directly assess possible effect of testosterone at the androgen receptor. Flutamide is an effective and commonly used androgen receptor antagonist, capable of blocking the actions of testosterone on a variety of endpoints (Labrie, 1993) in many species.

4. **Aromatase inhibitors.** Aromatase inhibitors are commonly used as an anti-cancer treatment, as blocking conversion of endogenous testosterone to estradiol is thought to be beneficial in the treatment of estrogen-sensitive tumors (Brodie & Long, 2001). Compounds such as fadrazole and anastrozole have been used to test the role of the estrogenic metabolites of testosterone in males (Roselli et al., 2003; Moradpour et al., 2006) as well as female rats (Roselli & Resko, 1993).

5. **Caveats.** The above regimens replace steroids at physiological levels, but do not account for the pulsatile and variable nature of endogenous testosterone release. For example, there is evidence for marked circadian variation in testosterone in rats as well as mice (Bartke et al., 1973). Thus, it should be acknowledged that simple replacement does not mimic the normal daily pattern of testosterone exposure in males.

As was the case for estradiol, testosterone levels also decline with age in male rats, as they do in humans. Reduced testosterone secretion and blunting of the circadian testosterone rhythm are evident in middle-aged as well as aged rats (Bonavera et al., 1997). This necessitates that age be considered in designs investigating the effects of testosterone on given endpoints.

HORMONE REPLACEMENT OR TREATMENTS: MICE

Although they have not been studied as extensively as rats, hormone replacement procedures used in the testing of feminine sexual behavior in mice are generally similar to those used in rats (Ring, 1944; Edwards, 1970). There are however, some important differences. First, rats, like other typical laboratory rodent species typically respond readily to injections of estradiol and progesterone after ovariectomy with the expression of feminine sexual behavior. Although there are quite dramatic strain differences that must

be considered, mice tend to require multiple tests (often four to six), before they are fully responsive (e.g., Thompson & Edwards, 1971; Mani et al., 1997; Kudwa & Rissman, 2003). Second, rats have an obvious lordosis response, which can be quantified in terms of the degree of spinal dorsiflexion (Pfaff & Lewis, 1974). In contrast, sexually receptive mice will adopt an immobile posture (McGill, 1961) which allows intromission and ejaculation by the male, but they do not display this characteristic dorsiflexion.

Thompson and Edwards (Thompson & Edwards, 1971) asked the question of whether the repeated hormone injections or the repeated experience of testing were essential. Mice that were only injected with hormones for four weeks without testing showed markedly lower levels of sexual receptivity when tested at five weeks when compared with mice that were injected and tested weekly, suggesting that previous mating experience has a facilitating effect on sexual response to hormone treatments.

The differences in response of females among different strains of mice can be quite dramatic (Thompson & Edwards, 1971; Gorzalka & Whalen, 1974). In a comparison between two strains of mice, Thompson and Edwards (1971) found that females of the C57BL/6J strain showed high levels of response after considerably fewer trials than the Swiss Webster strain. In this experiment, the investigators observed quite high levels of sexual receptivity in C57BL/6J mice after only two weeks. In contrast, in more recent experiments, others typically do not find high levels of receptivity until four to six weeks (e.g., Mani et al., 1997; Kudwa & Rissman, 2003, Laroche & Blaustein, unpublished obs.). The reason for this discrepancy with the earlier work in this strain is not understood, although possible genetic differences even among mice of the same strain cannot be discounted.

Oddly, doses typically required for the induction of feminine sexual behavior in ovariectomized mice are not dramatically different from those used in ovariectomized rats (e.g., Edwards, 1970). Although we are not aware of an extensive dose response study in the commonly used C57BL/6J strain of mice, typical doses of subcutaneously injected hormones are 0.5–2 μg estradiol benzoate followed by 100 μg progesterone two days later. An alternative means of administering estradiol that has been used in mice is the chronic implantation of Silastic© capsules containing estradiol (e.g., Kudwa and Rissman, 2003); in this case, progesterone is injected and subsequent testing is conducted at various intervals, such as weekly. In all cases, because mice are typically tested repeatedly, choice of progesterone dose must be carefully considered, since doses of progesterone that are too high can decrease response to the hormone treatments on successive tests (Laroche & Blaustein, unpublished observations).

TESTING SEX-SPECIFIC EFFECTS OF SEX CHROMOSOME GENES

There is now evidence that not all sex differences are due to hormone-driven events. The hypothesis is that the genetic sex of cells directly determines the sexual phenotype of those cells, or of emergent phenotypes (e.g., behavior) influenced by those cells. In other words, genes encoded on the sex chromosomes are expressed differentially in XX and XY cells because of their different genomic dose (or differences in genomic imprinting), and they cause XX and XY cells to be intrinsically different (Arnold & Burgoyne, 2004). For example, X genes may be expressed more highly in females (XX) than males (XY), or be imprinted differently in males and females, resulting in sex differences in the expression of X genes. Y genes, present only in males, may have a male-specific effect. To test this hypothesis, the approach is fundamentally the same as for testing hormone effects: one manipulates the independent variable (in this case expression of X or Y genes) and measures the effects on the sexually dimorphic traits. Several methods have been used.

Mice with Allelic Differences in the Y Chromosome

Maxson et al. (1989) found that DBA/1 male mice that differed only in the strain origin of the Y chromosome showed group differences in aggression. The conclusion is that differences in Y chromosomes lead to strain differences in male aggression, and that some Y genes influence aggression. The corollary is that allelic differences in the Y genes could, therefore, contribute to sex differences in aggression. Without further work this conclusion leaves open the site of action of the Y genes. For example, it is possible that different Y alleles act on the testes to influence the level of testosterone at some time in life, leading to differences in aggression via organizational or activational effects.

Mice with Different Complements of X and Y Genes

The Four Core Genotypes mouse model (De Vries et al., 2002; Arnold & Burgoyne, 2004) utilizes mice that have a Y *minus* (Y$^-$) chromosome, which is deleted for *Sry*, the testis-determining gene. XY$^-$ mice therefore have ovaries. Some mice receive an autosomal *Sry* transgene, which makes that autosome testis-determining. In this manner testis determination is moved from the Y chromosome to an autosome, so that the complement of sex chromosomes is no longer related to the gonadal sex of the animal. When XY$^-$*Sry* males (possessing the *Sry* transgene) are mated to XX females, four genotypes are produced: XY$^-$*Sry* males, XX*Sry* males, XY$^-$ females, and XX females (where 'male' and 'female' are defined by gonadal type).

This model allows one to compare mice that differ in gonadal type but have the same complement of sex chromosomes (XX*Sry* males vs. XX females; XY$^-$*Sry* males vs. XY$^-$ females) or to compare mice with the same gonadal type, but with a different complement of sex chromosomes (XY$^-$*Sry* males vs. XX*Sry* males; XY$^-$ females vs. XX females). If mice differing in the complement of sex chromosomes differ in a trait, the difference can be attributed to the differences in the sex chromosomes. Differences between XX and XY$^-$ females, for example, can be attributed to differences in the presence of Y genes, differences in the dose of X genes, or differences in genomic imprinting (only XX animals receive a paternal X imprint).

Numerous sex chromosome effects have been reported from this model (De Vries et al., 2002; Carruth et al., 2002; Xu et al., 2002, 2005; Gatewood et al., 2006). For example, XY mice are more immunoreactive than XX mice (Palaszynski et al., 2005). The genes accounting for the sex chromosome effects have so far not been identified. Until the genes are identified, the mechanisms of action of the genes will be undecided. One hypothesis is that the sex chromosome genes cause group differences in the levels of gonadal steroids, which then induce the differences observed. This hypothesis has not been ruled out, but in some cases is not likely, because the differences between XX and XY mice are in both directions (sometimes making XY mice more masculine than XX, sometimes less masculine), and because the XX-XY differences are observed in both gonadal males and females. In most of the studies, the sex chromosome effects are observed in gonadectomized adult mice, so that the XX-XY difference cannot be attributed to group differences in gonadal hormones at the time of testing.

Sex Chromosome Aneuploid Mice (XO, XXY, XYY, etc.)

These mice also differ in the complement of sex chromosomes. Comparison of XO with XX tests for the effect of X gene dosage. XO mice are more fearful than XX mice because of haploinsufficiency of an X-linked gene in XO mice (Isles et al., 2004). Other aneuploid comparisons have been useful in studies of sex differences in non-gonadal phenotypes, but have not yet been applied to studies of brain and behavior. For example, comparing XO females with XY females (or XXY⁻ females with XX females) tests for Y chromosome effects not confounded by the differences in X gene dosage; comparing XXY males with XY males tests for X gene dosage while keeping the number of Y chromosomes constant; comparing XYY with XY tests for the effect of an overdose of Y genes.

Sex chromosome aneuploid mice have been used successfully by Burgoyne and others to show sex chromosome effects on non-brain phenotypes (e.g., Burgoyne et al., 1995; Thornhill & Burgoyne, 1993).

Mice with Altered Sex Chromosomes

Various spontaneous mouse mutants are available with disruptions, fusions, or translocations of the X or Y chromosome. Most of these mouse strains have not yet been used for studies of the brain, however, because the mutations involve the duplication or deletion of numerous X or Y genes. The behavior or *Sxr* mice, with a translocation of numerous Y genes including *Sry* to the X chromosome, has been investigated (Reisert et al., 2002), although that study used gonadally intact mice in which the chromosomal differences were potentially confounded with group differences in circulating gonadal hormones.

Mice Differing in Imprint of the X Chromosome

Recently mice with a paternal versus maternal genomic imprint on the X chromosome have been found to differ in reversal learning (Davies et al., 2005). The X-linked gene Xlr3 is the candidate imprinted gene for this effect (Davies et al., 2006).

Mice Transgenic for X or Y Genes

Mice with deletions of X and Y genes, or with transgenic insertion of X or Y genes, also allow one to construct groups that differ in the expression of Y genes. The Four Core Genotypes model is one example of this approach. Other knock-outs or transgenic mice have so far not been used to evaluate the role of specific X and Y genes in causing sex differences in the brain, although they have been used for studies in other systems (e.g., Mazeyrat et al., 2001).

Gonadless Mice

Gonadless mice have been created by deletion of genes required for gonadal development (Parker et al., 1999; Birk et al., 2000). These mice are potentially useful for comparing XX and XY mice that have never been exposed to gonadal secretions. So far there are no published reports using these models to assess sex differences in the brain.

COMPLICATING FACTORS IN SEX DIFFERENCES RESEARCH

When planning studies of sex differences, it is important to consider the potential impact of intervening factors that themselves differ between the sexes. Male-female differences in responses to extraneous factors have the potential to produce effects that may obscure true actions of chromosomes or steroids, or in fact produce effects that are independent of them. It is important to consider such intervening factors in the design of sex differences studies, and take efforts to minimize their impact. Some relevant factors that may influence sex differences include:

1. **Stress.** Stress can be a major complicating factor in sex differences studies, playing a role above and beyond effects on cyclity, mentioned previously. Stress responses are quite different in males and females. Glucocorticoid secretion is exquisitely yet differentially sensitive to both androgens and estrogens. For example, in rats, stress-induced corticosterone secretion is more pronounced in females than in males (Viau &

Meaney, 1991; Carey et al., 1995). In addition, HPA (hypothalamo-pituitary adrenocortical axis) stress responsivity varies across the estrous cycle in the rat (Viau & Meaney, 1991; Carey et al., 1995) raising the possibility that unintended stress exposure will have different consequences at different points in the cycle. Glucocorticoids modulate multiple processes in the body and brain (Munck et al., 1984), and accordingly differential glucocorticoid levels induced by extraneous stress can confound studies of sex differences.

2. **Pharmacokinetics.** There is some evidence to suggest that sex differences in pharmacokinetics can contribute to sex differences in drug responses in humans. Drug clearance can cause higher plasma concentrations and longer half-lives of certain medications in women than men, which can perhaps be related to increased incidence of side effects (Kornstein & Kirkwood, 2003). Differences in drug metabolism are often encountered in animal models (Czerniak, 2001), and in many cases can account for sex differences in drug responses (c.f., Tseng et al., 2004). Thus, it is critical to consider drug metabolism as a possible factor in studying sex differences in pharmacological responses.

3. **Metabolism.** Males and females differ widely in metabolism and body composition. These differences are addressed in detail elsewhere in this volume (Chapter 13). Body composition can contribute to differential drug response, as noted previously. In addition, sex differences in adiposity can alter circulating factors (e.g., leptin, insulin) that control a variety of metabolic signaling pathways in the body and brain.

4. **Immunity.** There are numerous sex differences in susceptibility to immunological challenge. Infectious diseases tend to preferentially affect males, which may impact sex differences studies under some circumstances (e.g., parasitic or viral infections; see Chapter 17). Thus, opportunistic exposure to environmental antigens may differentially affect males versus females, dependent on pathogen, and should thus be controlled as tightly as possible when studying sex differences.

Many of these factors cannot be completely avoided. However, careful control of housing conditions and environment can obviate the influence of intervening stressors or pathogen exposure on sex differences experiments. In addition, careful consideration of route of administration (e.g., ICV vs. IV vs. IP) can minimize the influence of drug metabolism in pharmacological analyses. Overall, an understanding of how sex differences in extraneous factors can influence dependent variables under study is key to the design of experiments exploring organizational or activational effects of gonadal hormones within or between sexes.

SUMMARY AND CONCLUSIONS

As attested to by this volume, sex differences occur in a variety of physiological and behavioral functions, as well as a number of important clinical disorders. Thus, it is critical to develop an understanding of the biological mechanisms underlying sex differences that are relevant to treatment and prevention. While the designs used to assess sex differences can be relatively simple, there are numerous traps and pitfalls that can cloud interpretation of such studies. Several key factors emerge when assessing sex differences in physiology and behavior. Among the most important considerations are the following, which are relevant to the accurate design and interpretation of sex difference studies:

First, it is important to distinguish 'sex differences' from 'sexual differentiation.' The former implies a difference related to sex that may or may not be reversible by modulation of gonadal hormones or gonadal status. Sexual differentiation implies 'permanent,' developmental changes that cannot be easily altered later in life.

Second, activational versus organizational effects of sex hormones need to be clearly distinguished. Activational effects of gonadal steroids can be observed upon manipulation of hormone levels after the period of sexual differentiation. In contrast, organizational effects result from permanent actions of steroids on given bodily systems that cannot be readily reversed by hormonal interventions, except those that occur during the sex steroid-sensitive critical period in development. There may also be organizational effects of the sex chromosomes that result in sex differences in the brain and body.

Third, when testing sex differences or gonadal steroid action in females, it is important to consider strategies for establishing the stage of estrus, as the hormonal milieu present across the cycle varies widely with obvious implications for experimental endpoints under study.

Finally, the design of replacement regimens should be considered carefully. Replacement with estradiol only may be sufficient to assay the influence of estrogens on a given function, but additional replacement with progesterone may be required for restoration of some sex-related functions, especially those pertaining to sexual behavior.

Overall, this chapter is designed to provide a conceptual and methodological overview of relevant issues in sex differences/sexual differentiation research, and provide guidance to investigators studying the role of sex and/or gonadal steroids in a variety of physiological or behavioral functions in experimental animals and man. It is hoped that the information provided will be of assistance in furthering and facilitating research in this very important and oft-neglected realm of biological research.

References

Anantharaman-Barr HG, Decombaz J. (1989). The effect of wheel running and the estrous cycle on energy expenditure in female rats. *Physiol Behav*, 46:259–263.

Arnold AP. (2002). Concepts of genetic and hormonal induction of vertebrate sexual differentiation in the twentieth century, with special reference to the brain. In Pfaff DW, Arnold AP, Etgen A, Fahrbach S, Rubin R (Eds), *Hormones, brain, and behavior*, (pp. 105–135). San Diego: Academic Press.

Arnold AP, Breedlove SM. (1985). Organizational and activational effects of sex steroid hormones on vertebrate brain and behavior: a re-analysis. *Horm Behav*, 19:469–498.

Arnold AP, Burgoyne PS. (2004). Are XX and XY brain cells intrinsically different? *Trends in Endocrinol Metab*, 15:6–11.

Asarian L, Geary N. (2002). Cyclic estradiol treatment normalizes body weight and restores physiological patterns of spontaneous feeding and sexual receptivity in ovariectomized rats. *Horm Behav*, 42:461–471.

Axelson JF. (1987). Forced swimming alters vaginal estrous cycles, body composition, and steroid levels without disrupting lordosis behavior or fertility in rats. *Physiol Behav*, 41:471–479.

Bakker J, Honda S, Harada N, Balthazart J. (2002). The aromatase knock-out mouse provides new evidence that estradiol is required during development in the female for the expression of sociosexual behaviors in adulthood. *J Neurosci*, 22:9104–9112.

Bartke A, Steele RE, Musto N, Caldwell BV. (1973). Fluctuations in plasma testosterone levels in adult male rats and mice. *Endocrinology*, 92:1223–1228.

Becker JB, Arnold AP, Berkley KB, Blaustein JD, Eckel LA, Hampson E, et al. (2005). Strategies and methods for research on sex differences in brain and behavior. *Endocrinology*, 146:1650–1673.

Birk OS, Casiano DE, Wassif CA, Cogliati T, Zhao L, Zhao Y, et al. (2000). The LIM homeobox gene Lhx9 is essential for mouse gonad formation. *Nature*, 403:909–913.

Blaustein, JD, Wade, GN. (1977). Sequential inhibition of sexual behaviour by progesterone in female rats: comparison with synthetic antiestrogen. *J Comp Physiol Psych*, 91:752–760.

Blaustein JD, Dudley SD, Gray JM, Roy EJ, Wade GN. (1979). Long-term retention of estradiol by brain cell nuclei and female rat sexual behavior. *Brain Res*, 173:355–359.

Bonavera JJ, Swerdloff RS, Leung A, Lue YH, Baravarian S, Superlano L, et al. (1997). In the male brown-Norway (BN) male rat, reproductive aging is associated with decreased LH-pulse amplitude and area. *J Androl*, 18:359–365.

Breedlove SM, Arnold AP. (1983a). Hormonal control of a developing neuromuscular system: I. Complete demasculinization of the male rat spinal nucleus of the bulbocavernosus using the antiandrogen flutamide. *J Neurosci*, 3:417–423.

Breedlove SM, Arnold AP. (1983b). Hormonal control of a developing neuromuscular system: II. Sensitive periods for the androgen induced masculinization of the rat spinal nucleus of the bulbocavernosus. *J Neurosci*, 3:424–432.

Brodie A, Long B. (2001). Aromatase inhibition and inactivation. *Clin Cancer Res*, 7:4343s-4349s; discussion 4411s-4412s.

Burgoyne PS, Thornhill AR, Boudrean SK, Darling SM, Bishop CE, Evans EP. (1995). The genetic basis of XX-XY differences present before gonadal sex differentiation in the mouse. *Philos Trans R Soc Lond B Biol Sci*, 350:253–260.

Butcher RL, Collins WE, Fugo NW. (1974). Plasma concentrations of LH, FSH, prolactin, progesterone, and estradiol-17b throughout the 4-day estrous cycle of the rat. *Endocrinology*, 94:1704–1708.

Butera PC, Beikirch RJ. (1989). Central implants of diluted estradiol: independent effects on ingestive and reproductive behaviors of ovariectomized rats. *Brain Res*, 491:266–273.

Campbell CS, Schwartz NB. (1980). The impact of constant light on the estrous cycle of the rat. *Endocrinology*, 106:1230–1238.

Carey MP, Deterd CH, de Koning J, Helmerhorst F, de Kloet ER. (1995). The influence of ovarian steroids on hypothalamic-pituitary-adrenal regulation in the female rat. *J Endocrinol*, 144:311–321.

Carlberg KA, Fregly MJ. (1985). Disruptions of estrous cycles in exercise-trained rats. *Proc Soc Exp Biol Med*, 179:21–24.

Carruth LL, Reisert I, Arnold AP. (2002). Sex chromosome genes directly affect brain sexual differentiation. *Nat Neurosci*, 5:933–934.

Caston AL, Farrell PA, Deaver DR. (1995). Exercise training-induced changes in anterior pituitary gonadotrope of the female rat. *J Appl Physiol*, 79:194–201.

Chakraborty TR, Gore AC. (2004). Aging-related changes in ovarian hormones, their receptors, and neuroendocrine function. *Exp Biol Med*, 230:49–56.

Chatterton RT, Hartman AL, Lynn DE, Hickson RC. (1990). Exercise-induced ovarian dysfunction in the rat. *Proc Soc Exp Biol Med*,193:220–224.

Chatterton RT, Hrycyk L, Hickson RC. (1995). Effect of endurance exercise on ovulation in the rat. *Med Sci Sports Exerc*, 27:1509–1515.

Chen H, Zirkin BR. (1999). Long-term suppression of Leydig cell steroidogenesis prevents Leydig cell aging. *Proc Natl Acad Sci USA*, 96:14877–14881.

Chen H, Hardy MP, Zirkin BR. (2002). Age-related decreases in Leydig cell testosterone production are not restored by exposure to LH in vitro. *Endocrinology*, 143:1637–1642.

Cohen-Bendahan CC, van de Beek C, Berenbaum SA. (2005). Prenatal sex hormone effects on child and adult sex-typed behavior: Methods and findings. *Neurosci Biobehav Rev*, 29:353–384.

Conte FA, Grumbach MM, Kaplan SL. (1975). A diphasic pattern of gonadotropin secretion in patients with the syndrome of gonadal dysgenesis. *J Clin Endocrinol Metab*, 40:670–674.

Cooper KJ, Haynes NB, Lamming GE. (1970). Effects of unrestricted feeding during oestrus on reproduction in the underfed rat. *J Reprod Fertil*, 22:293–301.

Czerniak R. (2001). Gender-based differences in pharmacokinetics in laboratory animal models. *Int J Toxicol*, 20: 161–163.

Davies W, Isles AR, Burgoyne PS, Wilkinson LS. (2006). X-linked imprinting: effects on brain and behaviour. *Bioessays*, 28:35–44.

Davies W, Isles A, Smith R, Karunadasa D, Burrmann D, Humby T, et al. (2005). Xlr3b is a new imprinted candidate for X-linked parent-of-origin effects on cognitive function in mice. *Nat Genet*, 37:625–629.

De Vries GJ, Rissman EF, Simerly RB, Yang LY, Scordalakes EM, Auger CJ, et al. (2002). A model system for study of sex chromosome effects on sexually dimorphic neural and behavioral traits. *J Neurosci*, 22:9005–9014.

De Vries GJ. (2005). Minireview: Sex differences in adult and developing brains: compensation, compensation, compensation. *Endocrinology*, 145:1063–1068.

Dewing P, Chiang CW, Sinchak K, Sim H, Fernagut PO, Kelly S, et al. (2006). Direct regulation of adult brain function by the male-specific factor SRY. *Curr Biol*, 16:415–420.

Dixon DP, Ackert AM, Eckel LA. (2003). Development of, and recovery from, activity-based anorexia in female rats. *Physiol Behav*, 80:273–279.

Dragich J, Houwink-Manville I, Schanen C. (2000). Rett syndrome: a surprising result of mutation in MECP2. *Hum Mol Genet*, 9:2365–2375.

Eckel LA, Houpt TA, Geary N. (2000). Spontaneous meal patterns in female rats with and without access to running wheels. *Physiol Behav*, 70:397–405.

Edwards DA. (1970). Induction of estrus in female mice: estrogen-progesterone interactions. *Horm Behav*, 1:299–304.

Everett JW, Sawyer CH (1950) A 24-hour periodicity in the "LH-release apparatus" of female rats, disclosed by barbituate sedation. *Endocrinology* 47: 198–218.

Finegan J, Bartleman B, Wong PY. (1989). A window for the study of prenatal sex hormone influences on postnatal development. *J Genetic Psychol*, 150:101–112.

Finger FW. (1969). Estrus and general activity in the rat. *J Comp Physiol Psychol*, 68:461–466.

Forest MG, de Peretti E, Bertrand J. (1976). Hypothalamic-pituitary-gonadal relationships in man from birth to puberty. *Clin Endocrinol*, 5:551–569.

Frasor J, Barnett DH, Danes JM, Hess R, Parlow AF, Katzenellenbogen BS. (2003). Response-specific and ligand dose-dependent modulation of estrogen receptor (ER) alpha activity by ER-beta in the uterus. *Endocrinology*, 144: 3159–3166.

Freeman ME. (2006). The neuroendocrine control of the ovarian cycle of the rat. In Neill JD (Ed), *Knobil and Neill's physiology of reproduction*, 3rd edition (pp. 2327–2388). New York: Raven Press, Ltd.

Furukawa T, Manabe S, Watanabe T, Sharyo S, Mori Y. (1999). Sex difference in the daily rhythm of hepatic P450 monooxygenase activities in rats is regulated by growth hormone release. *Toxicol Appl Pharmacol*, 161:219–224.

Gatewood JD, Wills A, Shetty S, Xu J, Arnold AP, Burgoyne PS, Rissman EF. (2006). Sex chromosome complement and gonadal sex influence aggressive and parental behaviors in mice. *J Neurosci*, 26:2335–2342.

Gonzalez AS, Rodriguez Echandia EL, Cabrera R, Foscolo MR. (1994). Neonatal chronic stress induces subsensitivity to chronic stress in adult rats: II. Effects on estrous cycles in females. *Physiol Behav*, 56:591–595.

Gorzalka BB, Whalen RE. (1974). Genetic regulation of hormone action: selective effects of progesterone and dihydroprogesterone (5a-pregnane-3,20-dione) on sexual receptivity in mice. *Steroids*, 23:409–505.

Hagino N, Sako T, Nakamoto O, Kunz Y, Saito H. (1983). Prevention of continuous light-induced anovulation in rats by early exposure to continuous light. *Biol Reprod*, 29:355–361.

Harris HA, Katzenellenbogen JA, Katzenellenbogen BS. (2002). Characterization of the biological roles of the estrogen receptors, ERalpha and ERbeta, in estrogen target tissues in vivo through use of an ERalpha-selective ligand. *Endocrinology*, 143:4172–4177.

Herbst AL, Ulfelder H, Poskanzer DC. (1971). Adenocarcinoma of the vagina: Association of maternal stilbestrol therapy with tumor appearance in young women. *New England J Med*, 284:878–881.

Hines M, Sandberg EC. (1996). Sexual differentiation of cognitive abilities in women exposed to diethylstilbestrol (DES) prenatally. *Horm Behav*, 30:354–363.

Hoffman JC. (1969). Light and reproduction in the rat: effect of lighting schedule on ovulation blockade. *Biol Reprod*, 1:185–188.

Huang HH, Marshall S, Meites J. (1976). Capacity of old versus young female rats to secrete LH, FSH, and prolactin. *Biol Reprod*, 14:538–543.

Huang HH, Meites J. (1975). Reproductive capacity of aging female rats. *Neuropsychopharmacology*, 17: 289–295.

Isles AR, Davies W, Burrmann D, Burgoyne PS, Wilkinson LS. (2004). Effects on fear reactivity in XO mice are due to haploinsufficiency of a non-PAR X gene: implications for emotional function in Turner's syndrome. *Hum Mol Genet*, 13:1849–1855.

Jameson KA, Highnote SM, Wasserman LM. (2001). Richer color experience in observers with multiple photopigment opsin genes. *Psychon Bull Rev*, 8:244–261.

Kagabu S, Mamba K, Makita T. (1997). No effect of voluntary exercise on ovarian follicle in rats. *Exp Anim*, 46:247–250.

Konkle AT, Baker SL, Kentner AC, Barbagallo LS, Merali Z, Bielajew C. (2003). Evaluation of the effects of chronic mild stressors on hedonic and physiological responses: sex and strain compared. *Brain Res*, 992:227–238.

Korach KS. (1994). Insights from the study of animals lacking functional estrogen receptor. *Science*, 266: 1524–1527.

Kornstein SG, Kirkwood CK. (2003). Antidepressant drugs. In Steiner M, Koren G (Eds.), *Handbook of female pharmacology* (pp. 1–18). London: Martin Dunitz.

Kraichely DM, Sun J, Katzenellenbogen JA, Katzenellenbogen BS. (2000). Conformational changes and coactivator recruitment by novel ligands for estrogen receptor-alpha and estrogen receptor-beta: correlations with biological character and distinct differences among SRC coactivator family members. *Endocrinology*, 141:3534–3545.

Kudwa AE, Rissman EF. (2003). Double oestrogen receptor alpha and beta knockout mice reveal differences in neural oestrogen-mediated progestin receptor induction and female sexual behaviour. *J Neuroendocrinol*, 15:978–983.

Labrie F. (1993). Mechanism of action and pure anti-androgenic properties of flutamide. *Cancer*, 72: 3816–3827.

LeFevre J, McClintock MK. (1988). Reproductive senescence in female rats: a longitudinal study of individual differences in estrous cycles and behavior. *Biol Reprod*, 38:780–789.

Lehmann ML, Erskine MS. (2004). Induction of pseudopregnancy using artificial VCS: importance of lordosis intensity and prestimulus estrous cycle length. *Horm Behav*, 45:75–83.

Long JA, Evans HM. (1922). The oestrous cycle in the rat and its associated phenomenon. In Leuschner AO (Ed.), *Memoirs of the University of California* (pp. 1–148). University of California Press.

Mani SK, Blaustein JD, O'Malley BW. (1997). Progesterone receptor function from a behavioral perspective. *Horm Behav*, 31:244–255.

Martucci CP, Fishman J. (1979). Impact of continuously administered catechol estrogens on uterine growth and luteinizing hormone secretion. *Eur J Pharmacol*, 105:1288–1292.

Matysek M. (1989). Studies on the effect of stress on the estrus cycle in rats. *Ann Univ Mariae Curie Sklodowska*, 44:143–149.

Maxson SC, Didier-Erickson A, Ogawa S. (1989). The Y chromosome, social signals, and offense in mice. *Behav Neural Biol*, 52:251–259.

Mazeyrat S, Saut N, Grigoriev V, Mahadevaiah SK, Ojarikre OA, et al. (2001). A Y-encoded subunit of the translation initiation factor Eif2 is essential for mouse spermatogenesis. *Nat Genet*, 29:49–53.

McGill TE. (1961). Sexual behavior in three inbred strains of mice. *Behaviour*, 19:341–350.

McFadden D. (1993). A masculinizing effect on the auditory systems of human females having male co-twins. *Proc Natl Acad Sci USA*, 90:11900–11904.

Moradpour F, Naghdi N, Fathollahi Y. (2006). Anastrozole improved testosterone-induced impairment acquisition of spatial learning and memory in the hippocampal CA1 region in adult male rats. *Behav Brain Res*, 175:223–232.

Moriarty K, Kim KH, Bender JR. (2006). Minireview: estrogen receptor-mediated rapid signaling. *Endocrinology*, 147:5557–5563.

Munck A, Guyre PM, Holbrook NJ. (1984). Physiological functions of glucocorticoids in stress and their relation to pharmacological actions. *Endocr Rev*, 5:25–44.

Nakanishi Y, Mori J, Nagasawa H. (1976). Recovery of pituitary secretion of gonadotrophins and prolactin during refeeding after chronic restricted feeding in female rats. *J Endocrinol*, 69:329–339.

Nequin LG, Alvarez J, Schwartz NB. (1979). Measurement of serum steroid and gonadotropin levels and uterine and ovarian variables throughout 4 day and 5 day estrous cycles in the rat. *Biol Reprod*, 20:658–670.

Nguyen DK, Disteche CM. (2006). Dosage compensation of the active X chromosome in mammals. *Nat Genet*, 38:47–53.

Ogawa S, Chester AE, Hewitt SC, Walker VR, Gustafsson JA, Smithies O, et al. (2000). Abolition of male sexual behaviors in mice lacking estrogen receptors alpha and beta (alpha beta ERKO). *Proc Natl Acad Sci USA*, 97:14737–14741.

Palaszynski KM, Smith DL, Kamrava S, Burgoyne PS, Arnold AP, Voskuhl RR. (2005). A yin-yang effect between sex chromosome complement and sex hormones on the immune response. *Endocrinology*, 146:3280–3285.

Panzica G, Viglietti-Panzica C, Balthazart J. (2001). Sexual dimorphism in the neuronal circuits of the quail preoptic and limbic regions. *Microsc Res Tech*, 54:364–374.

Parker KL, Schimmer BP, Schedl A. (1999). Genes essential for early events in gonadal development. *Cell Mol Life Sci*, 55:831–838.

Pfaff DW, Lewis C. (1974). Film analyses of lordosis in female rats. *Horm Behav*, 5:317–335.

Phoenix CH, Goy RW, Gerall AA, Young WC. (1959). Organizing action of prenatally administered testosterone propionate on the tissues mediating mating behavior in the female guinea pig. *Endocrinology*, 65:369–382.

Powers JB. (1970). Hormonal control of sexual receptivity during the estrous cycle of the rat. *Physiol Behav*, 5:831–835.

Reisert I, Karolczak M, Beyer C, Just W, Maxson SC, Ehret G. (2002). Sry does not fully sex-reverse female into male behavior towards pups. *Behav Genet*, 32:103–111.

Richter CP. (1922). A behavioral study of the activity of the rat. *Comp Psychol Monog*, 1.

Ring JR. (1944). The estrogen-progesterone induction of sexual receptivity in the spayed female mouse. *Endocrinology*, 34:269–275.

Rivera HM, Eckel LA (2005) The anorectic effect of fenfluramine is increased by estradiol treatment in ovariectomized rats. *Physiol Behav* 86: 331–337.

Robinson A. (1990). Demography and prevalence of Turner syndrome. In Rosenfeld RG, Grumbach MM (Eds.), *Turner syndrome* (pp. 93–99). New York, NY: Marcel Dekker Inc.

Roozendaal MM, Swartz HJ, Wiegant VM, Mattheij JA. (1995). Effect of restraint stress on the preovulatory luteinizing hormone profile and ovulation in the rat. *Eur J Endocrinol*, 133:347–353.

Roselli CE, Resko JA. (1993). Aromatase activity in the rat brain: hormonal regulation and sex differences. *J Steroid Biochem Mol Biol*, 44:499–508.

Roselli CE, Cross E, Poonyagariyagorn HK, Stadelman HL. (2003). Role of aromatization in anticipatory and consummatory aspects of sexual behavior in male rats. *Horm Behav*, 44:146–151.

Schwartz NB, McCormack CE. (1972). Reproduction: gonadal function and its regulation. *Ann Rev Physiol*, 34:425–472.

Schwartz SM, Blaustein JD, Wade GN. (1979). Inhibition of estrous behavior by progesterone in rats: role of neural estrogen and progestin receptors. *Endocrinology*, 105:1078–1082.

Shetty G, Wilson G, Hardy MP, Niu E, Huhtaniemi I, Meistrich ML. (2002). Inhibition of recovery of spermatogenesis in irradiated rats by different androgens. *Endocrinology*, 143:3385–3396.

Singh RP, Carr DH. (1966). The anatomy and histology of XO human embryos and fetuses. *Anatomical Rec*, 155:369–384.

Singletary SJ, Kirsch AJ, Watson J, Karim BO, Huso DL, Hurn PD, Murphy SJ. (2005). Lack of correlation of vaginal impedance measurements with hormone levels in the rat. *Contemp Top Lab Anim Sci*,44:37–42.

Smith MS, Freeman ME, Neill JD. (1975). The control of progesterone secretion during the estrous cycle and early pseudopregnancy in the rat: prolactin, gonadotropin and steroid levels associated with rescue of the corpus luteum of pseudopregnancy. *Endocrinology*, 96:219–226.

Smith PE. (1926). Ablation and transplantation of the hypophyses in the rat. *Anat Rec*, 32:221.

Stavnezer AJ, McDowell CS, Hyde LA, Bimonte HA, Balogh SA, Denenberg VH. (2000). Spatial ability of XY sex-reversed female mice. *Behav Brain Res*, 112:135–143.

Sun J, Meyers MJ, Fink BE, Rajendran R, Katzenellenbogen JA, Katzenellenbogen BS. (1999). Novel ligands that function as selective estrogens or antiestrogens for estrogen receptor-alpha or estrogen receptor-beta. *Endocrinology*, 140:800–804.

Takeo Y. (1984). Influence of continuous illumination on estrous cycles of rats: time course of changes in levels of gonadotropins and ovarian steroids until occurrence of persistent estrus. *Neuropsychopharmacology*, 39:97–104.

Tapper CM, Greig F, Brown-Grant K. (1974). Effects of steroid hormones on gonadatrophin secretion in female rats after ovariectomy during the estrous cycle. *J Endocrinol*, 62:511–525.

Tarttelin MF, Gorski RA. (1971). Variations in food and water intake in the normal and acyclic female rat. *Physiol Behav*, 7:847–852.

Thompson ML, Edwards DA. (1971). Experiential and strain determinants of the estrogen-progesterone induction of sexual receptivity in spayed female mice. *Horm Behav*, 2:299–305.

Thornhill AR, Burgoyne PS. (1993). A paternally imprinted X chromosome retards the development of the early mouse embryo. *Development*, 118:171–174.

Tilmann C, Capel B. (2002). Cellular and molecular pathways regulating mammalian sex determination. *Recent Prog Horm Res*, 57:1–18.

Tropp J, Markus EJ. (2001). Effects of mild food deprivation on the estrous cycle of rats gustatory system. *Physiol Behav*, 73:553–559.

Tseng AH, Harding JW, Craft RM. (2004). Pharmacokinetic factors in sex differences in Delta 9-tetrahydrocannabinol-induced behavioral effects in rats. *Behav Brain Res*, 154:77–83.

Viau V, Meaney MJ. (1991). Variations in the hypothalamic-pituitary-adrenal response to stress during the estrous cycle in the rat. *Endocrinology*, 129:2503–2511.

Voskuhl RR. (2002). Gender issues and multiple sclerosis. *Curr Neurol Neurosci Rep*, 2:277–286.

Walf AA, Frye CA. (2005). ER-beta selective estrogen receptor modulators produce antianxiety behavior when administered systemically to ovariectomized rats. *Neuropsychopharmacology*, 30:1598–1609.

Walker QD, Nelson CJ, Smith DK, Cynthia M. (2002). Vaginal lavage attenuates cocaine-stimulated activity and establishes place preference in rats. *Pharm Biochem Behav*, 73:743–752.

Weber AL, Adler NT. (1979). Delay of constant light-induced persistent vaginal estrus by 24-hour time cues in rats. *Science*, 204:323–325.

Whalen RE. (1968). Differentiation of the neural mechanisms which control gonadotrophin secretion and sexual behavior. In Diamond M (Ed.), *Reproduction and sexual behavior* (pp 303–340). Bloomington, IN: Indiana University Press.

van Roijen JH, Ooms MP, Weber RF, Brinkmann AO, Grootegoed JA, Vreeburg JT. (1997). Comparison of the response of rat testis and accessory sex organs to treatment with testosterone and the synthetic androgen methyltrienolone (R1881). *J Androl*, 18:51–61.

Xiao L, Becker JB. (1997). Hormonal activation of the striatum and the nucleus accumbens modulates paced mating behavior in the female rat. *Horm Behav*, 32:114–124.

Xu J, Burgoyne PS, Arnold AP. (2002). Sex differences in sex chromosome gene expression in mouse brain. *Hum Mol Genet*, 11:1409–1419.

Xu J, Taya S, Kaibuchi K, Arnold AP. (2005). Sexually dimorphic expression of Usp9x is related to sex chromosome complement in adult mouse brain. *Eur J Neurosci*, 11:3017–3022.

Chapter 4

Methodological Issues in the Study of Hormone-Behavior Relations in Humans: Understanding and Monitoring the Menstrual Cycle

Elizabeth Hampson and Elizabeth A. Young

The ovarian cycle is often a significant variable in studies of hormone-behavior relations in primates, including humans. The two major ovarian steroids, 17β estradiol and progesterone, have been shown to have regulatory effects on a host of brain-related and somatic variables, ranging from the availability of neurotransmitters in certain parts of the brain to the metabolism of drugs in the gut. To the novice researcher, understanding the ovarian cycle and how it can be monitored through assays or other indices of hormonal status can seem bewildering.

In this chapter, we provide a basic overview of the menstrual cycle, including a review of several factors than can influence hormone concentrations or the timing of the cycle. We also briefly describe the advantages and use of conventional serum assays versus saliva for menstrual cycle monitoring, and the indirect methods available. An excellent review of the menstrual cycle can be found in Chabbert Buffet et al. (1998). Our emphasis here will be on practical dimensions of the ovarian cycle that are of greatest relevance to researchers.

IMPORTANCE OF THE MENSTRUAL CYCLE FOR THE STUDY OF SEX DIFFERENCES

Not so long ago researchers believed ovarian hormones were not active in the brain outside the hypothalamic-pituitary region. In the last 25 years, however, it has become clear that receptors for estrogens and progesterone are expressed in many other brain regions as well, including areas considered to be important in the control of behavior, mood, and cognition, such as parts of the cerebral cortex and limbic system. This provides an avenue for ovarian hormones to influence the functioning of these areas, and to exert effects that can be observed at the level of overt behavior and performance. Because there is a difference in the concentrations of estrogen and progesterone produced by the two sexes, at least in adulthood, and because there is variation in ovarian hormones associated with the menstrual cycle, no researcher interested in behavioral sex differences can afford to ignore the potential influence of the ovarian cycle. And, likewise, the menstrual cycle is a significant variable for those interested in the emerging field of sex-based medicine.

ESSENTIAL CHARACTERISTICS OF THE HUMAN MENSTRUAL CYCLE

Among primates who have a menstrual cycle (humans, apes, and old-world monkeys), spontaneous ovulation is the norm. That is, ovulation occurs in the absence of any immediate sensory stimulus. This is different from many species of laboratory animals (e.g., rabbits, cats, ferrets) that are reflex ovulators. Ovulation in primates is controlled by an intricate sequence of hormonal events, mainly controlled by the ovary itself and its cascade of hormonal signals which bathe the hypothalamus and, in turn, actively modify hypothalamic-pituitary control over the menstrual cycle.

Changes in the Ovary

At the ovarian level, the menstrual cycle represents the life cycle of a dominant follicle. By convention, the first day of menses (menstrual bleeding) is denoted Day 1 of the cycle and marks the beginning of the follicular (or proliferative) phase. During the early follicular phase, the growth of one follicle from a larger pool of antral follicles becomes dominant and forms the preovulatory follicle, secreting increasing amounts of estradiol as it matures. Ovulation is the release of the mature oocyte by the ovary and occurs 24–36 hours following a burst in luteinizing hormone (LH) secretion that is triggered by the rapid rise in the concentration of estradiol being secreted by the mature follicle. The LH surge is the event that triggers ovulation. Following ovulation, the residual cells left by the ovulatory follicle are called the corpus luteum, a secretory body that is the source of progesterone, estradiol, and inhibin A. Ovulation, and the formation of the corpus luteum, marks the beginning of the luteal (or secretory) phase of the cycle, which lasts about 13–15 days. Epithelial cells in the endometrium proliferate during the follicular phase of the

cycle under the influence of estradiol; during the luteal phase the epithelial cells differentiate under the influence of progesterone and become secretory. As the luteal phase comes to a close, the corpus luteum regresses, and the production of estradiol, progesterone, and inhibin A drops. The endometrium sheds, marking the beginning of menses and the start of a new cycle.

Pattern of Endocrine Changes

From the standpoint of behavioral research, the most important feature of the menstrual cycle is not the changes in the ovary, but the complex patterns of endocrine changes in several different hormones associated with the ovarian events (Fig. 4.1).

Near the beginning of menses, serum concentrations of the two gonadotropins, follicle-stimulating hormone (FSH) and luteinizing hormone (LH), begin to rise as the anterior pituitary increases production under the stimulus of gonadotropin-releasing hormone (GnRH) released by the hypothalamus. The drop in estradiol as the corpus luteum regresses from the previous cycle is the key signal that initiates the rise. All of these hormones are released in a pulsatile fashion. For example, LH is secreted every 90 minutes during the follicular phase, slowing to one pulse every 4 hours during the mid-luteal phase. The early stages of follicular growth and maturation in the ovary are largely independent of gonadotropins, but FSH is vital in the terminal maturation of the primary follicle. The last ~15 days of follicular growth depend on a cyclical rise in FSH. LH facilitates estradiol production by the follicle, is important for luteinization to occur, and controls the secretion of hormones by the corpus luteum but is inhibited by progesterone (Chabbert Buffet et al., 1998). Concentrations of FSH and LH reach peak levels just before ovulation, with concentrations of around 10–20 mIU/mL and 50–100 mIU/mL, respectively (Abraham, 1978; Thorneycroft et al., 1971). The peak in LH is the event that triggers the release of the mature oocyte. The LH peak is generated under positive feedback control from the high levels of estradiol produced by the mature follicle.

Estradiol levels are minimal during the earliest days of the follicular phase, but increasing concentrations are released into the general circulation as the follicle matures. The highest levels are reached about 24 to 48 hours before the LH peak. In fact, the preovulatory peak in estradiol represents its highest con-

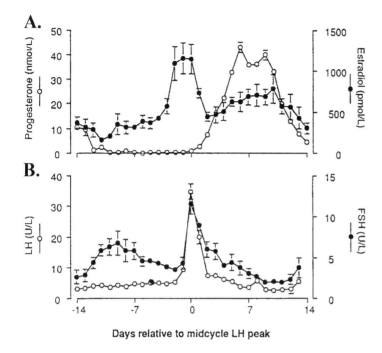

Figure 4.1. Plasma concentrations of: (A) estradiol and progesterone, (B) LH and FSH, during the human menstrual cycle. Data are aligned relative to the day of the midcycle LH peak. Mean concentrations ± SE are shown. Adapted with permission from Chabbert Buffet N, Djakoure C, Maitre, SC, & Bouchard P (1998). Regulation of the human menstrual cycle. *Frontiers in Neuroendocrinology*, 19:151–186.

centration during the entire menstrual cycle. Serum concentrations at this time are typically about 130–200 pg/mL, but concentrations as high as 300–400 pg/mL can be achieved in some women. Following a transient fall in association with ovulation, estradiol secretion is restored by production from the corpus luteum during the luteal phase. Plateau levels of around 100–150 pg/mL (Abraham, 1978; Thorneycroft et al., 1971) are most often seen during the period from −10 to −5 days before the onset of menses. With the regression of the corpus luteum, estradiol levels fall, gradually in some women and precipitously in others, during the last few days of the luteal phase. This ushers in the onset of menses, the sloughing of the endometrium. Serum estradiol during menses is approximately 30–50 pg/mL.

There is insignificant production of progesterone by the ovaries until the formation of the corpus luteum, though a small but discernible increase is evident just prior to ovulation. Peak production of progesterone during the luteal phase typically coincides with the sustained peak in estradiol, from about Day −10 to −5 prior to menses, though the two hormones do not necessarily fall in synchrony at the close of the luteal phase. Maximum progesterone concentration is about 10–20 ng/mL in most women (Abraham, 1978; Thorneycroft et al., 1971). Menstrual bleeding is

triggered by the decrease in progesterone as its trophic effects on the endometrium are lost. Lowest levels of progesterone are found during the follicular phase of the cycle, with nearly undetectable concentrations.

Because estradiol and progesterone have widespread effects on brain function, they are of the greatest relevance to most behavioral researchers. It is less clear whether FSH and LH, being large peptides, are capable of crossing the blood-brain barrier in appreciable quantities from the general circulation (Nicolini et al., 1984; Lei & Rao, 2001).

INDIVIDUAL DIFFERENCES IN THE TIMING OR AMPLITUDE OF HORMONAL EVENTS

We have described the basic pattern of changes in the ovary, gonadotropin, and ovarian steroid secretion that characterize the normal menstrual cycle. However, there are substantial individual differences among women in the exact timing or amplitude of these hormonal events, as well as intra-individual variations in timing and amplitude from one menstrual cycle to the next. At the population level, the average length of the entire cycle, measured from Day 1 of menses, is 29.5 days. This masks significant variation across women in the typical length of the cycle. Normal cycles range in length from about 24 to 35 days, in re-productively healthy adult women during their prime reproductive years (Vollman, 1977). Only a minority of women have the prototypical 28-day cycle. Cycles shorter than 24 days are mostly anovulatory, since it takes at least 12 days for the follicle to develop and the length of the luteal phase is relatively fixed at 13 to 15 days. Some very long cycles are infertile because they reflect subnormal endocrine function, but there are women with long cycles who do not have subnormal function and simply have fewer fertile days per year.

Knowing a woman's typical menstrual cycle length is essential for accurate prospective targeting of men-strual cycle stages. Some women track their own men-strual cycles and can give accurate information about typical length of cycle and its degree of variability from one ovarian cycle to another. However, for many women, self-reports of cycle length are not accurate and sizable disparities can occur between professed cycle length and objective measures. When in doubt, researchers may need to track several ovarian cycles in advance of having the woman participate in research, in order to verify an individual woman's typical length of cycle. This can be accomplished either through keeping menstrual diaries or simply recording the exact date of onset of menses over several successive cycles.

Awareness of the length of a woman's cycle is a basic prerequisite to competent research on the men-strual cycle, because the timing of several endocrine events differs according to cycle length. The length of the luteal phase is relatively fixed at 13 to 15 days. Therefore, most of the variation in cycle length from woman to woman is attributable to differences in the length of the follicular phase. One implication is that the timing of ovulation will be different. A woman with a 35-day cycle will ovulate on about Day 21, whereas a woman with a 24-day cycle will ovulate about Day 10. The timing of research sessions might need to be tai-lored accordingly. Note that neither of these days is 'midcycle,' although ovulation would indeed be ex-pected at or around the middle of the cycle in a woman with the prototypical 28 to 29 day ovarian cycle. Note, also, that these differences in timing have implications for other menstrual cycle events, too. Suppose that a researcher wishes to test research participants at basal hormone concentrations to contrast with testing at a stage associated with high levels of circulating steroids. In a woman with a 24-day cycle, it would be inadvis-able to test on Day 6 of the cycle (where Day 1 is onset of menses), as the timing of ovulation in such a short cycle means that estradiol levels would already be raised in anticipation of ovulation.

To further complicate the life of researchers, there are *intra*-individual differences in the length of the cycle as well as *inter*-individual differences. Women vary in how predictable their cycles are: some women have cycles so regular that they can be predicted with great accuracy. More typically, the onset of menses varies from one cycle to another by 2 to 4 days. Tre-loar's data from more than 25,000 person-years of menstrual history showed that 75% of all cycles among women ages 20 to 40 varied by less than 6 days (Treloar, 1973). This is normal variation; in the situ-ation where a woman fails to ovulate in a particular cycle, departure from the average cycle length may be more substantial. An implication for researchers is that research assessments that are prospectively targeted at particular days of the cycle are unlikely to be com-pletely accurate. Retrospectively, the day of assessment can be confirmed by tracking backward from the onset of the next menses; however, retrospective ver-ification is not practical in all studies. Monitoring hormones by direct measurement is still the best method for confirming hormonal status.

In describing the physiology of the menstrual cycle earlier in this chapter, ranges were provided for typical hormone concentrations at various stages of the cycle. A range of values is required because the amplitude of the hormonal peaks and valleys varies from woman to woman and from cycle to cycle. This reflects a variety of influences including diet, physical or psychological stressors, and factors innate to an individual's metab-olism, among other factors. During the early follicular phase, when steroid production is lowest, estradiol can range from 20 to 50 pg/mL or, at the ovulatory peak, from 100 to as high as 400 pg/mL. With such great variability, it can be difficult to tell with certainty the exact phase of a woman's cycle even when direct measures of hormones are employed. Strategies to help researchers deal effectively with this problem are discussed later in the chapter.

HOW THE MENSTRUAL CYCLE CHANGES OVER THE LIFESPAN

Age has a significant impact on the regularity of the menstrual cycle, its variability, the likelihood of anovulatory cycles, and the concentrations of ovarian hormones observed.

Menarche and the Early Post-Menarcheal Years

Anovulatory cycles are most common in the first and last few years of reproductive life, when hormone levels are less stable. In the first years after menarche, anovulatory cycles are in fact the norm. Attainment of menarche has been hypothesized to require a threshold percentage of body fat of around 17% (Frisch, 1988; Frisch & McArthur, 1974) and in North America, the average age at menarche is about 12.5 years (Bullough, 1981). The advent of menstrual cycling does not imply full ovulatory competence and cycles in the first few years tend to be irregular.

Cycle length ranges from about 21 to 42 days. Regularization is progressively established over the 5 years following menarche, i.e., by gynecologic age 5 (Treloar et al., 1967). Steroid output, even in cycles that appear regular, is comparatively low. Average progesterone levels obtained in ovulatory cycles in a group of 75 post-menarcheal adolescent females were found to be less than half of those attained by women in their mid-20's (Read et al., 1984). Changing patterns of variability with increasing gynecologic age are paralleled by an increase in the incidence of ovulatory cycles. By 5 years after menarche, the number of anovulatory cycles has decreased to about 25%.

Reproductive Maturity

Full reproductive maturity is not reached in many women until the mid-20's. Detailed monitoring of ovarian steroids has shown full ovulatory and luteal phase sufficiency during the years between the mid-20's to about age 35 (Lipson & Ellison, 1992; Fig. 4.2), consistent with suggestions from earlier studies that used basal body temperature recording (Döring, 1969).

It seems that ovarian function peaks later and begins to decline earlier than would be suggested by patterns of menstrual regularity alone. Once full reproductive maturity is achieved the menstrual cycle remains fairly constant, but progressively shortens with age until roughly gynecologic age 25 years. Shortening reflects a modest decrease in the length of the follicular phase (Sherman, West, & Korenman, 1976).

In the last 40 to 50 cycles of a woman's reproductive life, variability in the length of the cycles re-appears, with unusually short and long cycles interspersed (Vollman, 1974).

Full reproductive maturity is accompanied by a very high proportion of ovulatory cycles. Metcalf and Mackenzie (1980) studied ovulation in 254 women over 3 months. Ovulation took place in every cycle in 62% of the women aged 20–24 years, in 88% of women aged 25–29 years, and 91% of women over 30. For research where full ovulatory competence is important, women from their mid-20's to mid-30's constitute the ideal subjects.

Perimenopause and Menopause

During her reproductive life, the average woman ovulates about 350 times. Menopause, defined as a period of one year of amenorrhea (lack of menses) accompanied by increased FSH and LH levels and low estradiol, occurs when the follicular stock in the ovary nears exhaustion. This may sound improbable, given the approximately 7 million germ cells present *in utero*, but nearly all of the germ cells undergo atresia (apoptosis); only about 350–400 ever progress to the stage of a mature follicle. Follicular loss accelerates in women over 36 years of age. Onset of full menopause is reached at a median age of 51.

The term *perimenopause* is sometimes used to describe the menopausal transition in the 2 to 8 years leading up to menopause, when changes in the menstrual cycle begin to occur. In the early part of the transition, menstrual cycles are regular and women may superficially appear to have normal cycles, even while anovulatory cycles become more prevalent. Eventually, in the later part of the transition, the length of the cycle becomes increasingly irregular and menstrual periods may be skipped. It was formerly believed that estrogen production progressively declined throughout perimenopause, but recent evidence suggests that in the early stages of the transition elevated FSH levels can lead to *increased* estradiol production greater than that seen in women under age 35 (e.g., Santoro et al., 1996; Burger, 1996). FSH concentrations in both ovulatory and anovulatory cycles from midlife women are sufficient to produce ovarian hyper-stimulation (Prior, 2005). Eventually, estrogen levels do decrease but this is a late transitional event.

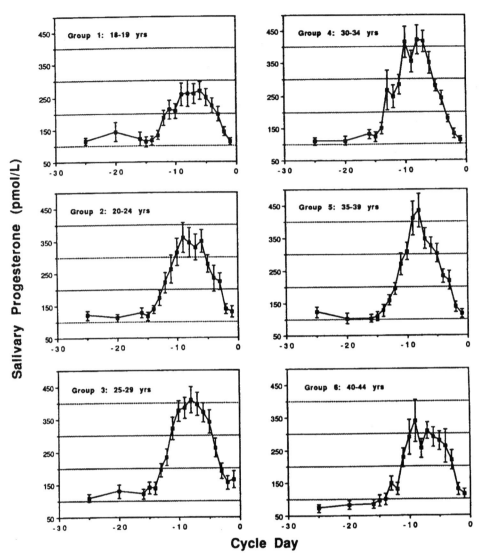

Figure 4.2. Average profiles of salivary progesterone (± SE) attained during the luteal phase of the menstrual cycle, in 6 groups of healthy regularly cycling women ages 18–44. The lowest levels of progesterone were found in the 18–19 year old and the 40–44 year old groups, and highest values in the 25–34 year olds ($n = 20$–22 per group). Data are aligned retrospectively by day of next menstrual onset. Reprinted with permission from Lipson SF, Ellison PT (1992). Normative study of age variation in salivary progesterone profiles. *J Biosoc Sci*, 24:233–244.

Progesterone production tends to be insufficient during perimenopause and there is a shorter luteal phase (Santoro et al., 1996). There may also be changes during perimenopause in the expression of target tissue estradiol receptors, though this is not well-documented (Prior, 2005). It is important for behavioral researchers to recognize that not only do cycles become less predictable in perimenopause,

but also there are significant changes in the endocrine profile compared to earlier stages of reproductive life.

A history of tobacco use is associated with earlier onset of the menopausal transition and menopause by about 2 years (McKinlay et al., 1985). There are also ethnic differences, but prior use of oral contraceptives is not predictive of age at menopause (Gold et al., 2001). The best single predictor of age at menopause is family history; heritability is close to 87% (de Bruin et al., 2001). On an individual basis, the timing of menopause cannot be predicted prospectively.

CONDITIONS THAT CAN INFLUENCE THE ENDOCRINOLOGY OF THE MENSTRUAL CYCLE

Exercise

Interest in associations between energy balance and reproductive function has blossomed in the last two decades (e.g., Cumming, 1990; Frisch & McArthur, 1974; Warren, 1990). In female athletes, interference with the menstrual cycle is well known. Major changes include oligo- or amenorrhea, anovulation, shortened luteal phases (duration of <14 days), and delayed menarche (no occurrence of menses before age 16 years), all of which are accompanied by low levels of estradiol and progesterone (Burrows & Bird, 2000).

Apart from participation in sports requiring sustained high energy demands, however, research suggests that even fairly modest levels of exercise can lead to diminished ovarian steroid output. For example, Ellison and Lager (1985) found progesterone profiles were significantly lower among female recreational runners who averaged only 12.5 miles per week than among age-matched sedentary controls matched on weight, weight-for-height, and menstrual patterns. Progesterone profiles have also been found to be lower in women with moderate weight loss due to dieting in the absence of exercise and lower in women in subsistence ecologies whose endocrine profiles parallel changes in body weight associated with seasonal patterns of food abundance and scarcity (e.g., Ellison et al., 1989). Energy balance may have a significant impact on ovarian function in females.

Exercise is believed to alter the pulsatile pattern of GnRH release from the hypothalamus, leading to the changes in LH and ovarian steroid production (Burrows & Bird, 2000). Exactly how these changes come about, however, is not well understood. Changes in body composition (percentage of body fat) may be involved, but physical stress could conceivably also produce changes in menstrual cyclicity through alterations in the HPA axis.

Stress and Environmental Stimuli

As we have seen, under normal conditions, follicular rupture in the ovary is controlled by a sequence of endogenous hormonal events that unfolds naturally under the control of the ovary, hypothalamus, and pituitary. The ovulatory cycle can be seen as endogenously driven, but subject to exogenous influences which can alter the intrinsic rhythm via changes in hormones. Notably, environmental events that constitute physical or psychological stressors influence the menstrual cycle and the probability of ovulation.

Observations of stress effects on the menstrual cycle go back to ancient times. Stress triggers an endocrine cascade starting in the brain with the release of corticotropin-releasing hormone (CRH) which triggers the release of ACTH from the pituitary which subsequently triggers synthesis and release of cortisol from the adrenal gland. The isolation and sequencing of CRH provided new avenues for exploring stress effects. The majority of studies have been carried out in experimental animals including non-human primates, rodents, and sheep. These studies have shown that injection of CRH into the brain results in inhibition of LH secretion (Jaffee et al., 1990; Petraglia et al., 1987; Gambacciani et al., 1986; Nikolarakis et al., 1986; Olster & Ferin, 1987). CRH is widely distributed in the brain and appears to mediate a number of the behavioral effects of stress, including anorexia and anxiety. The effects of CRH on GnRH secretion may be both direct and indirect: CRH neurons can synapse with GnRH neurons (MacLusky et al., 1988), and CRH can release ß-endorphin from the arcuate ß-endorphin system, an endogenous opioid peptide that is inhibitory to GnRH (Nikolarakis et al., 1986). Inhibitory effects of estrogens, ß-endorphin and CRH all appear to result from actions of these hormones in the brain.

In addition to the inhibitory effects of CRH, older studies suggest that other hormones of the HPA axis can affect LH secretion. Several studies have demonstrated that ACTH administration reduces the increase in serum LH concentrations following removal of the ovaries (Schwartz & Justo, 1977; Mann et al., 1982). This effect is dependent upon the presence of the adrenal and may involve adrenal production of gonadal steroids, which is regulated by ACTH (Putnam et al., 1991). Glucocorticoids may also exert inhibitory effects on GnRH secretion or on LH responsiveness to GnRH, including direct effects of cortisol at the pituitary (Sutter & Schwartz, 1985). A diminished LH response to GnRH challenge has been found in women following long-term predniso- lone treatment (Sakakura et al., 1975). Recent studies in ewes found a clear inhibition of LH secretion by stress levels of cortisol which can be blocked by in- hibiting cortisol synthesis with metyrapone or by giv- ing mifepristone, a cortisol antagonist (Breen et al., 2004; Debus et al., 2002).

Several disorders of menstrual cyclicity have been described which demonstrate HPA axis activation, i.e., increased basal cortisol (Casanueva et al., 1987; Suh et al., 1988; Berga et al., 1989; Hohtari et al., 1988; Villanueva et al., 1986; Loucks et al., 1989; Biller et al., 1990). These include: exercise-induced amenorrhea, anorexia nervosa, and hypothalamic amenorrhea. In all three syndromes, amenorrhea is a primary presenting problem. In anorexia nervosa the hormonal abnormalities in both the HPA and HPG axes are believed to be secondary to weight loss. Weight restriction and low body weight are also ob- served in exercise-induced amenorrhea, and low body weight has been reported in hypothalamic amenor- rhea. Even relatively mild degrees of weight loss in normal weight or obese subjects can lead to distur- bances in both axes as manifested by resistance to dexamethasone and by disturbances in menstrual reg- ularity or amenorrhea (Berger et al., 1983; Edelstein et al., 1983; Pirke et al., 1985; Russel et al., 1970). Consequently, all three of these amenorrheic syn- dromes present with evidence of weight loss, increased HPA axis activation, disrupted HPG functioning and amenorrhea. A recent study on exercise-induced re- productive abnormalities in adolescent girls concluded "in active adolescents, increased cortisol concentra- tion may precede gonadotropin changes seen with higher levels of fitness" (Kasa-Vubu et al., 2004). Consequently, it would appear that similar mecha- nisms may be at work in all three syndromes, by which hormones of the HPA axis contribute to the produc- tion of menstrual cycle irregularities and amenorrhea.

Medical Conditions and Prescription Drugs

A number of pathological conditions can influence the menstrual cycle. To do menstrual cycle research effectively, researchers often need to evaluate whether participants have medical conditions or are taking any drugs that might alter either the temporal patterning or the endocrine profile of the menstrual cycle. In research studies where it is important for the men- strual cycle to be healthy and natural, these factors might constitute exclusionary criteria. In other stud- ies, the conditions themselves might be the subject of study (e.g., Do women with amenorrhea still show cyclic changes in mood and affect?). A full discussion of medical factors is beyond the scope of this chapter. But medications known to alter characteristics of the menstrual cycle include anti-psychotics, psychotropic drugs used as mood stabilizers, and anticonvulsants. Even antibiotics can produce changes in steroid me- tabolism; a back-up method of contraception is re- commended during antibiotic treatment in women who take oral contraceptives.

Failure to ovulate can occur at the extremes of body weight, both over- and underweight, leading to amenorrhea (loss of menstrual cycling). Polycystic ovary syndrome (PCOS) is the single most common cause of irregular and infrequent menses and failure of ovulation in young women. Other conditions that cause irregular menses or amenorrhea include uterine fibroids or polyps, thyroid abnormalities, hyperpro- lactinemia, premature ovarian failure, late-onset congenital adrenal hyperplasia, eating disorders, and stress-induced oligo- or amenorrhea, among others (Adams-Hillard & Deitch, 2005). Menstrual irregu- larities can also be seen in women with diabetes.

Breakthrough bleeding may be observed in anovu- latory cycles, i.e., in the absence of progesterone se- cretion, and can mimic menstruation. However, re- searchers must be wary as this is not menstruation in the usual sense and the normal sequence of hormonal events does not underlie the surface phenomenon of bleeding. Breakthrough bleeding may result from pro- gesterone insufficiency and is also seen in women on oral contraceptives that do not contain enough pro- gesterone (or estradiol) to sustain the endometrium (Ellsworth & Leversee, 1990).

Oral Contraceptives

Apart from pregnancy and lactation, oral contracep- tives (OCs) have perhaps the largest effects on a woman's menstrual cycle. Many women use OCs on only a short-term or intermittent basis; only 50%–75% of women are still using them after 1 year (Ellsworth & Leversee, 1990). OCs sold in the U.S. and Canada contain either ethinyl estradiol or mestranol, in small amounts, combined with one of at least 12 different progestins. Predicting the relative estrogenic and pro-gestogenic potencies of different OC formulations is complex, depending not only on the type and dosage of the estrogens and progestins individually but on the estrogenic, anti-estrogenic, and androgenic effects of each combination. It is important to recognize that not all OCs are alike. Therefore, in experimental de-signs where the physiological effects of OCs are rele-vant, it may be inadvisable to lump OC users together as a single group. Individual differences in metabolism are another important variable: although the dosage administered is fixed, person-to-person variation in the blood levels of ethinyl estradiol and progestin achieved while on OCs is substantial (Goldzieher, 1989).

Oral contraceptives prevent ovulation through neg-ative feedback inhibition at the hypothalamus. In the 1960s, when oral contraceptives first became widely available on the market, they contained a high estro-gen content (~150 μg) and 1 to 10 μg of progestin. They were associated with side effects: water reten-tion, nausea, fatigue, headaches, thrombosis, hyper-tension, and altered blood glucose/lipid metabolism. This gave rise to the idea that oral contraceptive use produces a high estrogen state. The dosage of hor-mone contained in OC pills has progressively been decreased, while retaining contraceptive efficacy. Today's OCs are a different story—they typically contain about 20 to 35 μg of ethinyl estradiol and a correspondingly lower progestin content. One indica-tion of the low hormone content of contemporary OCs is recent reports of decreased bone density, rela-tive to girls not taking OCs, in girls using OCs over a sustained period during their teen to young adult years when peak bone deposition is normally occurring (Teegarden et al., 2005).

Most OC pills are used for 21 consecutive days followed by a pill-free week (or in some cases, a week of inert pills), when menses occurs. Some OC brands contain a fixed daily dosage (monophasic pills), in others (biphasic or triphasic pills) the relative content of the estrogen and progestin components are varied over the 21-day contraceptive cycle to simulate the changes in ovarian hormones that would naturally oc-cur. The simulation is incomplete, producing hor-monal conditions that are still different from an un-assisted menstrual cycle (otherwise the contraceptive effectiveness would be lost). Although the pharma-cological properties of contraceptive steroids are not the same as the naturally occurring hormones, ethinyl

estradiol has been shown to bind to estrogen receptors with affinity similar to 17β estradiol (Briggs & Briggs, 1983). And there is some evidence that ethinyl estra-diol may penetrate into the CNS more readily than estradiol itself (Fishman & Norton, 1977).

A practical problem facing behavioral researchers is how to quantify the effective level of hormone ex-posure in women taking OCs. Tables are available that rank the relative estrogen and progestational po-tencies of various OC pills based on bioassays (e.g., effects on the mouse endometrium), but these tables don't take into account individual differences in me-tabolism from one woman to another. On the surface, an easy solution is to measure the serum concentra-tions of hormones that are achieved using radioim-munoassay (RIA) or enzyme immunoassay (EIA) techniques. Because they have a different molecular structure, however, contraceptive steroids show lim-ited cross-reactivity with the antiserum used in stan-dard assays designed to measure the naturally occur-ring forms of estradiol or progesterone. In one widely used commercial assay kit, the cross-reactivity of the antiserum with ethinyl estradiol is only 1.8% (Diag-nostic Products Corporation, Los Angeles, CA). Therefore, simply measuring the quantities of hor-mones present in OC users with the standard assays used routinely in hospitals or clinical laboratories is not an accurate method to detect the OC steroids. Antiserum with a high specificity for ethinyl estradiol does exist, but is not widely available (e.g., Dibbelt et al., 1991).

Measuring *endogenous* estradiol in OC users typ-ically reveals serum concentrations as low or lower than those found at the menstrual phase of the cycle in OC non-users (De Leo et al., 1991), reflecting the suppressant effects of the OCs on ovarian production. "The secretion of ovarian hormones practically ceases in women taking oestrogen-progestogen mixtures" (Klopper, 1970).

Though combination OCs are the most wide-spread method of hormonal contraception, other methods are available, also involving use of hormones to alter the natural menstrual cycle (e.g., progestin-only contraceptive pills or depot medroxyprogester-one acetate). Because any hormone-based contra-ceptive will affect the endocrine milieu, it is impor-tant for researchers to establish in advance what type of contraception their study participants are using and to ascertain what effects, if any, the contraceptive might have on endocrine profiles.

METHODS FOR MEASURING HORMONE CONCENTRATIONS AND MENSTRUAL CYCLE MONITORING

Most behavioral researchers observe the menstrual cycle with one of two objectives in mind: either passive monitoring of the cycle as it unfolds, or actively targeting particular stages at which behavioral testing will then occur. Often, for the latter type of research, the aim is to use the menstrual cycle to naturalistically 'manipulate' hormones, e.g., to evaluate the impact of high versus low levels of circulating estrogen on some behavioral variable of interest. For both types of research, accurate documentation of the menstrual cycle is essential. Excluding the use of ultrasound to directly visualize the ovaries, which is impractical for most investigations, several techniques are available that can be used for menstrual cycle monitoring. These include the direct quantification of hormones through the use of assays, or the indirect monitoring of the cycle through changes in peripheral physiology.

Radioimmunoassay and Enzyme Immunoassay

In the 1970s and 1980s, the hormonal signature characteristic of the ovulatory menstrual cycle was described, made possible by the development of sensitive and specific immunoassay methods for quantifying steroid and peptide hormones.

a. **Serum or plasma.** Assays suitable for serum or plasma are the most widely available in hospital and laboratory settings. A wide range of analysis methods is supported commercially and the choice of which method is optimal for a given research application depends on variables such as the detection threshold of a particular method, specificity of the antibody, type of subject population to be assessed, volume of specimen available, as well as practical considerations such as cost and the instrumentation available in the laboratory. Commercial availability does not by itself guarantee that a method will be useful: a recent review of widely used kits for testosterone found that only two met reasonable validity criteria for measuring testosterone in women (Taieb et al., 2003). An experienced lab can provide well-informed advice on suitable methods.

Assuming the assay has satisfactory reliability, validity, sensitivity, and precision, how frequently does sampling need to be done, and of which hormones? The answer depends on the research questions being asked. Daily monitoring is generally infeasible due to the prohibitive costs involved and the unwillingness of research participants to have blood taken on a daily basis. Intermittent sampling is one solution. However, often the goal of blood sampling in the first place is not to monitor the whole cycle, but to identify a particular stage or simply quantify the hormone concentrations present during a defined period of time. If the goal is to identify a particular stage, a single serum specimen is usually inadequate. This is because of interpretive ambiguities caused by the large range in hormone concentrations possible at each stage.

There are exceptions, however, where even a single specimen can be useful. If the objective is simply to verify if ovulation has occurred in a particular cycle, then a single well-timed serum sample, obtained during the middle of a woman's luteal phase, might be sufficient to make this judgment if the progesterone concentration falls above a threshold value. A strong correlation has been shown between progesterone and ovulation if values exceed 25 nmol/L, but one can never be sure whether *peak* values are being measured if daily samples are not taken (Abdulla et al., 1983; Israel et al., 1972). Another situation where single time-point sampling might be sufficient is where researchers are concerned with quantifying hormone concentrations at the time that behavioral testing occurs, but are not concerned with defining the exact stage of the menstrual cycle *per se*.

In practice, researchers adopt a wide range of solutions in the trade-off between cost and precision. Obtaining multiple samples is best wherever practically and economically feasible. Serum monitoring can be limited to particular points in the cycle to contain costs; assays can be used jointly with day of cycle tracked by calendar methods or with other indirect methods of monitoring; or two or more hormones can be tracked together to assist in accurately identifying stages of the cycle (e.g., LH as well as estradiol can help to forecast ovulation).

b. **Saliva.** In the last 10 years, saliva has become a practical alternative to serum for the measurement of steroid hormones. Reliable and accurate methods are now available for cortisol and progesterone, and are on the horizon for estradiol with the advent of high-sensitivity chemiluminescent or fluorescence techniques. At present, saliva estradiol assays are available only in a small number of research labs (Table 4.1). Not all hormones pass into the saliva, however. FSH and LH are not represented in saliva to any significant extent (Vining & McGinley, 1986).

Saliva offers practical and theoretical advantages over serum. Daily monitoring becomes feasible because specimen collection is easy, fast, and non-invasive, and can be done by research participants in their own homes. Saliva is stable at room temperature for long periods, or can be frozen. However, its major advantage is a theoretical one: saliva unlike serum provides a direct estimate of the bioavailable fraction of the hormone (Quissell, 1993), i.e., the fraction of the total hormone in the circulation that is biologically active, consisting of free (unbound) and weakly-bound hormone (hormone that readily detaches from weak-affinity carrier proteins and therefore can enter into the saliva). This is the component of interest for behavioral studies, but there is no easy way to measure this important fraction in blood. Existing methods for identifying the 'free' component in serum are inexact (Vining & McGinley, 1986).

As with serum, multiple sampling of hormone concentrations is advisable for improved reliability. Importantly, ovarian secretion of estradiol and progesterone is pulsatile, producing changes in the concentration of the hormone visible in both serum and saliva. Averaging across several samples can help to reduce 'noise' in the measurements caused by pulsatile secretion patterns. For a useful introduction to saliva hormone monitoring, see Hofman (2001) or Vining and McGinley (1986).

Indirect Indicators of Hormonal Status

The hormones associated with the menstrual cycle exert peripheral effects on physiology as well as central nervous system effects, and therefore produce secondary changes in several tissues that constitute useful biomarkers of hormonal activity. These biomarkers can be used by researchers to help monitor the menstrual cycle. Because they are indirect and their effective use depends on women's accurate self-observations, they are less reliable than direct quantification of hormones, in practice. Even when used optimally they provide little indication of the actual levels of hormones attained.

a. **Basal body temperature (BBT).** Body temperature shows a circadian rhythm, rising slowly

Table 4.1. Salivary Estradiol (E$_2$) Concentrations at Different Stages of the Menstrual Cycle in Healthy Women Ages 20 to 38

	n	Median E$_2$ (pg/mL)*
Periovulatory	13	9.54
Midluteal	118	5.79
Day −10[#]	13	5.10
Day −9	19	4.87
Day −8	20	5.84
Day −7	17	6.88
Day −6	28	5.85
Day −5	21	4.83
Premenstrual	7	3.09
Menses	132	4.03
Day +1	2	2.98
Day +2	5	3.08
Day +3	33	4.74
Day +4	43	3.94
Day +5	49	3.97

*Measured by tritium radioimmunoassay, as described in Mead and Hampson (1996).
[#]Days are denoted relative to day of menstrual onset. For example, Day -10 is 10 days before the day of menstrual onset.

from a minimum in the early hours of the morning to an early evening peak. In women, basal temperature is also influenced by the menstrual cycle. There is typically a lower BBT from the beginning of the cycle up to ovulation and a rise thereafter (Fig.4.3). BBT is highest during the luteal phase and begins to drop a few days before menses.

The post-ovulatory rise is thought to be due to the anabolic effects of progesterone, and therefore is considered a sign that ovulation has occurred. No monthly variation in temperature is observed before menarche or after menopause or bilateral oophorectomy. The temperature rise occurs only *after* ovulation (up to several days after), making it impossible to identify the day of ovulation prospectively using the BBT method. Temperature must be taken at the same time every day, which requires a high degree of subject cooperation, and a special expanded scale (or digital) thermometer is required. The shift in BBT is on the order of 0.2°C to 0.6°C. A sustained temperature rise after ovulation is not evident in all women, however, even in cycles that are ovulatory (Moghissi, 1976).

b. **Day count methods—when do they work?** It is generally agreed that forward day count methods for prospectively predicting the day of the menstrual cycle are inaccurate. This partly reflects variability in the length of the cycle. On average, the length varies within-person by 2 to 4 days, or even greater in some women, which is significant for advance prediction of hormonal conditions. However, since the duration of the luteal phase is relatively constant at 13 to 15 days in most women, once the onset of menstruation occurs, it allows the date of ovulation to be estimated retrospectively, and can yield accurate day of cycle information for the just completed luteal phase. This is the reverse day count method of verifying day of cycle.

The accuracy of day count methods also depends on the accuracy of women's estimates of their day of menstrual onset. Reports of menstrual onset based on memory are less accurate than those based on record-keeping (Presser, 1974). Charting of menstrual flow on a menstrual calendar can assist in establishing the length and variability of a woman's cycle; data suggest that recollection of age at menarche, age at menopause, and age at first use of oral contraceptives are 75%–90% accurate by self-report within a confidence interval of one year, but that recollection of menstrual cycle length and variability by interview is not reliable in many women (Bean et al., 1979).

c. **Ovulation detection kits.** Kits for home measurement of urine LH are commercially available. They identify the urine LH surge that occurs on average 18 to 24 hr before ovulation. However, this average disguises a range of variability, as the LH surge can occur from as little as 16 hr to as much as 48 hr before ovulation. These kits may still be useful, because the urine LH surge is considered to be an accurate prospective marker for ovulation. LH detection kits do not help to target the estrogen surge, of interest in many behavioral studies, because estradiol is returning or has returned to basal levels by the time the peak concentration of LH is detected (Harris & Naftolin, 1970). However, as an advance signal of impending ovulation, the urine LH test can be an effective tool. It can also be used to help predict the timing of future

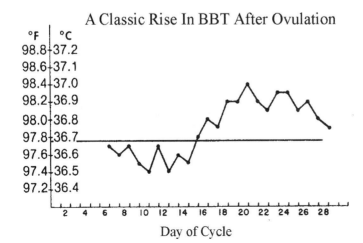

A Classic Rise In BBT After Ovulation

Day of Cycle

Figure 4.3. An example of a basal body temperature (BBT) graph, showing a classic rise in BBT after ovulation.

events, such as the luteal peak in progesterone, that are contingent on the timing of ovulation. In behavioral studies, this may be useful when it is important that women be tested during the luteal phase or to avoid devoting research resources to cycles likely to be anovulatory.

The ClearPlan method (ClearBlue Fertility Monitor) is another type of home monitoring system that utilizes an enzyme immunoassay for the estrogen metabolite estrone-3-glucuronide and LH in first morning urine. Based on a threshold value, the electronic device identifies a time of 'high fertility' that begins with the rise in estrogen prior to ovulation. It is easy to use but expensive, and identifies the rise in estrogen followed by the LH surge. In a validation study of 150 cycles, the measurement of urinary hormones was well-correlated with serum levels (Behre et al., 2000).

d. **Vaginal discharge.** Starting about 5 days before ovulation, estradiol is secreted in increasing amounts from the maturing follicle, stimulating the cervix to secrete type E mucus. Type E mucus is clear, elastic, and slippery and is secreted in increasing abundance as ovulation approaches. The peak day can be identified one day later as the last day of vaginal discharge that has type E features. It identifies the timing of ovulation with a degree of accuracy of ±2 to 3 days (Stanford et al., 2002). After ovulation, there is a rapid change in the quantity and physical properties of the cervical mucus. Progesterone stimulates the cervix to produce a different type of mucus, type G mucus, which is visibly distinct. Type G mucus is associated with minimal or no vaginal discharge. The Billings ovulation method (and its recent successors) detect the fertile period by an increase in "ferning" during the week leading up to ovulation. This method can take 1 month for women to acquire and learn to use proficiently. The monitoring of ferning in dried saliva as an index of rising estrogen levels has been attempted but these devices have undemonstrated validity.

For an up-to-date review of indirect methods of menstrual cycle monitoring, see Stanford et al. (2002).

CONCLUSIONS

The ovarian cycle is a significant source of variability in many brain-related and somatic variables. Some of these, such as variations in neurotransmitter activity, have a clear and direct relevance to understanding hormone-behavior relations. Equipped with a clear understanding of the menstrual cycle, researchers can use it to scientific advantage, leading to potential new insights—the menstrual cycle is far more than a 'nuisance variable' to be controlled. While direct measurement of estradiol and progesterone is often considered the gold standard, it should be emphasized that the effects of steroid hormones can persist for hours or days. Thus, the prior endocrine context is important, not just the current or immediate state of the organism. Times of falling hormone concentrations, such as the late luteal phase, may represent a different endocrine milieu than the early follicular phase although hormone levels may superficially appear similar. Likewise the early luteal phase may not show significant progesterone increases but the brain has still "seen," and responded to, the high estradiol signal driving the LH surge. For these reasons, optimal characterization of the hormonal environment will include some indication of cycle day in addition to direct hormone measures.

References

Abdulla U, Diver MJ, Hipkin L, Davis JC. (1983). Plasma progesterone levels as an index of ovulation. *Br J Obstet Gynaecol.* 90:543–548.

Adams-Hillard PJ, Deitch HR. (2005). Menstrual disorders in the college age female. *Pediatr Clin North Am,* 52:179–197.

Asso D. (1983). *The real menstrual cycle.* New York, NY: Wiley.

Bean JA, Leeper JD, Wallace RB, Sherman BM, Jagger H. (1979). Variations in the reporting of menstrual histories. *Am J Epidemiol,* 109:181–185.

Behre HM, Kuhlage J, Gassner C, Sonntag B, Schem C, Schneider HP, et al. (2000). Prediction of ovulation by urinary hormone measurements with the home use ClearPlan℗ Fertility Monitor: Comparison with transvaginal ultrasound scans and serum hormone measurements. *Hum Reprod,* 15:2478–2482.

Berga SL, Mortola JF, Girton L, Suh B, Laughlin G, Pham P, et al. (1989). Neuroendocrine aberrations in women with functional amenorrhea. *J Clin Endo Metab,* 68:301–308.

Berger M, Pirke K, Doerr P, Krieg C, von Zerssen D. (1983). Influence of weight loss on the dexamethasone suppression test. *Arch Gen Psychiatry,* 40: 585–586.

Biller BM, Federoff HJ, Koenig JI, Klibanski A. (1990). Abnormal cortisol secretion and responses to corticotropin-releasing hormone in women with hypothalamic amenorrhea. *J Clin Endocrinol Metab*, 70:311–317.

Breen KM, Stackpole CA, Clarke IJ, Pytiak AV, Tilbrook AJ, Wagenmaker ER, et al. (2004). Does the type II glucocorticoid receptor mediate cortisol-induced suppression in pituitary responsiveness to gonadotropin-releasing hormone? *Endocrinology*, 145: 2739–2746.

Briggs M, Briggs M. (1983). Oral contraceptives containing estrogen plus progestogen. In Benagiano G., & Diczfalusy E. (Eds.), *Endocrine mechanisms in fertility regulation* (pp.17–48). New York: Raven Press.

Bullough VL. (1981). Age at menarche: a misunderstanding. *Science*, 213:365–366.

Burrows M, Bird S, (2000). The physiology of the highly trained female endurance runner. *Sports Med*, 30: 281–300.

Burger HG. (1996). The endocrinology of the menopause. *Maturitas*, 23:129–136.

Casanueva FF, Borras CG, Burguera B, Muruais C, Fernandez M, Devesa J. (1987). Steroids and neuroendocrine function in anorexia nervosa. *J Steroid Biochem*, 27:635–640.

Chabbert Buffet N, Djakoure C, Christin Maitre S, Bouchard P. (1998). Regulation of the human menstrual cycle. *Front Neuroendocrinol*, 19:151–186.

Cumming DC. (1990). Physical activity and control of the hypothalamic-pituitary-gonadal axis. *Semin Reprod Endocrinol*, 8:15–23.

de Bruin JP, Bovenhuis H, van Noord PA, Pearson PL, van Arendonk JA, te Velde ER, et al. (2001). The role of genetic factors in age at natural menopause. *Hum Reprod*, 16:2014–2018.

Debus N, Barrell GK, Billings HJ, Breen KM, Brown M, Young EA, et al. (2002). Does cortisol mediate endotoxin-induced inhibition of pulsatile LH and GnRH secretion? *Endocrinology*, 143:3748–3755.

De Leo V, Lanzetta D, Vanni AL, D'Antona D, Serveri FM. (1991). Low estrogen oral contraceptives and the hypothalamo-pituitary axis. *Contraception*, 44: 155–161.

Dibbelt L, Knuppen R, Jütting G, Heimann S, Klipping CO, Parikka-Olexik H. (1991). Group comparison of serum ethinyl estradiol, SHBG and CBG levels in 83 women using two low-dose combination oral contraceptives for three months. *Contraception*, 43: 1–21.

Döring GK. (1969). The incidence of anovular cycles in women. *J Reprod Fertil*, Suppl 6:77–81.

Edelstein CK, Roy-Byrne P, Fawzy FI, Dornfeld L. (1983). Effects of weight loss on the dexamethasone suppression test. *Am J Psychiatry*, 140:338–341.

Ellison PT, Lager C. (1985). Exercise-induced menstrual disorders. *N Engl J Med*, 313:825–826.

Ellison PT, Peacock NR, Lager C. (1989). Ecology and ovarian function among Lese women of the Ituri Forest, Zaire. *Am J Phys Anthropol*, 78:519–526.

Ellsworth AJ, Leversee JH. (1990). Oral contraceptives. *Prim Care* 17:603–622.

Ferin M, Vande Wiele R. (1984). Endogenous opioid peptides and the control of the menstrual cycle. *Eur J Obstet Gynecol Reprod Biol*, 18:365–373.

Fishman J, Norton B. (1977). Relative transport of estrogens into the central nervous system. In Garattini S., & Berendes H.W., (Eds.) *Pharmacology of steroid contraceptive drugs* (pp. 37–41). New York: Raven Press.

Frisch RE. (1988). Fatness and fertility. *Sci Am*, 258: 88–95.

Frisch RE, McArthur JW. (1974). Menstrual cycles: fatness as a determinant of minimum weight for height necessary for their maintenance or onset. *Science*, 185:949–951.

Gambacciani M, Yen SS, Rasmussen DD. (1986). GnRH release from the mediobasal hypothalamus: in vitro inhibition by corticotropin-releasing factor. *Neuroendocrinology*, 43:533–536.

Gold EB, Bromberger J, Crawford S, Samuels S, Greendale GA, Harlow SD, et al. (2001). Factors associated with the age of natural menopause in a multiethnic sample of midlife women. *Am J Epidemiol*, 153:865–874.

Goldzieher JW. (1989). Pharmacology of contraceptive steroids: a brief review. *Am J Obstet Gynecol*, 160:1260–1264.

Harris GW, Naftolin F. (1970). The hypothalamus and control of ovulation. *Br Med Bull* 26:3–9.

Hofman L. (2001). Human saliva as a diagnostic specimen. *J Nutr*, 131:1621S-1625S.

Hohtari H, Elovainio R, Salminen K, Laatikainen T. (1988). Plasma corticotropin-releasing hormone, corticotropin, and endorphins at rest and during exercise in eumenorrheic and amenorrheic athletes. *Fertil Steril*, 50:233–238.

Israel R, Mishell DR, Stone SC, Thorneycroft IH, Moyer DL. (1972). Single luteal phase serum progesterone assay as an indicator of ovulation. *Am J Obstet Gynecol*, 112:1043–1046.

Jaffe RB, Plosker S, Marshall L, Martin MC. (1990). Neuromodulatory regulation of gonadotropin-releasing hormone pulsatile discharge in women. *Am J Obstet Gynecol*, 163:1727–1731.

Kasa-Vubu JZ, Sowers M, Ye W, Carlson NE, Meckmongkol T. (2004). Differences in endocrine function with varying fitness capacity in postpubertal females across the weight spectrum. *Arch Pediatr Adolesc Med*, 158:333–340.

Kirschbaum C, Schommer N, Federenko I, Gaab J, Neumann O, Oellers M, et al. (1996). Short-term estradiol treatment enhances pituitary-adrenal axis and sympathetic responses to psychosocial stress in healthy young men. *J Clin Endocrinol Metab*, 81: 3639–3643.

Klopper A. (1970). Developments in steroidal hormonal contraception. *Br Med Bull*, 26:39–44.

Lei ZM, Rao CV. (2001). Neural actions of luteinizing hormone and human chorionic gonadotropin. *Sem Reprod Med*, 19:103–109.

Lipson SF, Ellison PT. (1992). Normative study of age variation in salivary progesterone profiles. *J Biosoc Sci*, 24:233–244.

Loucks AB, Mortola JF, Girton L, Yen SSC. (1989). Alterations in the hypothalamic-pituitary-ovarian and the hypothalamic-pituitary-adrenal axes in athletic women. *J Clin Endocrinol Metab*, 68:402–411.

MacLusky NJ, Naftolin F, Leranth C. (1988). Immunocytochemical evidence for direct synaptic connections between corticotrophin-releasing factor (CRF) and gonadotrophin-releasing hormone (GnRH)-containing neurons in the preoptic area of the rat. *Brain Res*, 439:391–395.

Mann D, Jackson G, Bland M. (1982). Influence of adrenocorticotropin and adrenalectomy on gonadotropin secretion in immature rats. *Neuroendocrinology*, 34:20–26.

McKinlay SM, Bifano NL, McKinlay JB. (1985). Smoking and age at menopause in women. *Ann Intern Med*, 103:350–356.

McNeely MJ, Soules MR. (1988). The diagnosis of luteal phase deficiency: a critical review. *Fertil Steril*, 50:1–15.

Metcalf MG, Mackenzie JA. (1980). Incidence of ovulation in young women. *J Biosoc Sci*, 12:345–352.

Moghissi KS. (1976). Accuracy of basal body temperature for ovulation detection. *Fertil Steril*, 27:1415–1421.

Nicolini A, Buonaguidi R, Ferdeghini M, Carpi A. (1984). Relationship between the circulating levels of adenohypophyseal hormones in blood and in cerebrospinal fluid. *J Neurol Neurosurg Psychiat*, 47:710–714.

Nikolarakis KE, Almeida OF, Herz A. (1986). Corticotropin-releasing factor (CRF) inhibits gonadotropin-releasing hormone (GnRH) release from superfused rat hypothalami in vitro. *Brain Res*, 377:388–390.

Nikolarakis KE, Almeida OF, Herz A. (1986). Inhibition of LH release by CRF may be partially mediated through hypothalamic beta-endorphin release. *NIDA Res Monogr*, 75:403–405.

Olster DH, Ferin M. (1987). Corticotropin-releasing hormone inhibits gonadotropin secretion in the ovariectomized rhesus monkey. *J Clin Endocrinol Metab*, 65:262–267.

O'Rorke A, Kane MM, Gosling JP, Tallon DF, Fottrell PF. (1994). Development and validation of a monoclonal antibody enzyme immunoassay for measuring progesterone in saliva. *Clin Chem*, 40:454–458.

Presser HB. (1974). Temporal data relating to the human menstrual cycle. In Ferin M., Halberg F., Richart R.M., & Vande Wiele R. (Eds.), *Biorhythms and human reproduction* (pp.145–160). New York: Wiley.

Preston FS, Bateman SC, Short RV, Wilkinson RT. (1974). The effects of flying and of time changes on menstrual cycle length and on performance in airline stewardesses. In Ferin M., Halberg F., Richart R.M., & Vande Wiele R. (Eds.), *Biorhythms and human reproduction* (pp. 501–512). New York: Wiley.

Petraglia F, Sutton S, Vale W, Plotsky P. (1987). Corticotropin-releasing factor decreases plasma luteinizing hormone levels in female rats by inhibiting gonadotropin-releasing hormone release into hypophysial-portal circulation. *Endocrinology*, 120:1083–1088.

Pirke KM, Schweiger U, Lemmel W, Krieg JC, Berger M. (1985). The influence of dieting on the menstrual cycle of young, healthy women. *J Clin Endocrinol Metab*, 60:1174–1179.

Prior JC. (2005). Ovarian aging and the perimenopausal transition. *Endocrine*, 26:297–300.

Putnam CD, Brann DW, Mahesh VB. (1991). Acute activation of the adrenocorticotropin-adrenal axis: effect on gonadotropin and prolactin secretion in the female rat. *Endocrinology*, 128:2558–2566.

Quissell DO. (1993). Steroid hormone analysis in human saliva. *Ann N Y Acad Sci*, 694:143–145.

Read GF, Wilson DW, Hughes IA, Griffiths K. (1984). The use of salivary progesterone assays in the assessment of ovarian function in postmenarcheal girls. *J Endocrinol*, 102:265–268.

Russel GFM, Beardwood CJ. (1970). Amenorrhea in feeding disorders: anorexia nervosa and obesity. *Psychother Psychosom*, 18:359–364.

Sakakura M., Takebe K, Nakagawa S. (1975). Inhibition of luteinizing hormone secretion induced by synthetic LRH by long term treatment with glucocorticoids in human subjects. *J Clin Endocrinol Metab*, 40:774–779.

Santoro N, Brown JR, Adel T, Skurnick JH. (1996). Characterization of reproductive hormonal dynamics in the perimenopause. *J Clin Endocrinol Metab*, 81:1495–1501.

Sherman BM, West JH, Korenman SG. (1976). The menopausal transition: analysis of LH, FSH, estradiol and progesterone concentrations during menstrual cycles of older women. *J Clin Endocrinol Metab*, 42:629–636.

Stanford JB, White Jr, GL, Hatasaka H. (2002). Timing intercourse to achieve pregnancy: current evidence. *Obstet Gynecol*, 100:1333–1341.

Schwartz N, Justo S. (1977). Acute changes in serum gonadotropins and steroids following orchidectomy in the rat: role of the adrenal gland. *Endocrinology*, 100:1550–1556.

Suh BY, Liu JH, Berga SL, Quigley ME, Laughlin GA, Yen SS. (1988). Hypercortisolism in patients with functional hypothalamic-amenorrhea. *J Clin Endocrinol Metab*, 66:733–739.

Sutter DE, Schwartz NB. (1985). Effect of glucocorticoids on secretion of luteinizing hormone and follicle-stimulating hormone by female rat pituitary cells in vitro. *Endocrinology*, 117:849–854.

Taieb J, Mathian B, Millot F, Patricot MC, Mathieu E, Queyrel N, et al. (2003). Testosterone measured by 10 immunoassays and by isotope-dilution gas chromatography-mass spectrometry in sera from 116 men, women, and children. *Clin Chem*, 49:1381–1395.

Teegarden D, Legowski P, Gunther CW, McCabe GP, Peacock M, Lyle RM. (2005). Dietary calcium intake protects women consuming oral contraceptives from spine and hip bone loss. *J Clin Endocrinol Metab*, 90:5127–5133.

Treloar AE, Boynton RE, Behn BG, Brown BW. (1967). Variation of the human menstrual cycle through reproductive life. *Int J Fertil.*, 12:77–126.

Villanueva AL, Schlosser C, Hopper B, Liu JH, Hoffman DI, Rebar RW. (1986). Increased cortisol production in women runners. *J Clin Endocrinol Metab*, 63:133–136.

Vining R, McGinley R. (1986). Hormones in saliva. *Crit Rev Clin Lab Sci*, 23:95–146.

Vollman N. (1977). *The menstrual cycle: major problems in obstetrics and gynaecology*. Vol. 7. Philadelphia, PA: W.B. Saunders.

Vollman RF. (1974). Some conceptual and methodological problems in longitudinal studies on human reproduction. In Ferin M., Halberg F., Richart R.M., & Vande Wiele R. (Eds.), *Biorhythms and human reproduction* (pp.161–170). New York:Wiley.

Warren MP. (1990). Weight control. *Semin Reprod Endocrinol*, 8:25–31.

Webley GE, Edwards R. (1985). Direct assay for progesterone in saliva: comparison with a direct serum assay. *Ann Clin Biochem*, 22:579–585.

Chapter 5

Sex Differences in Pharmacogenomics as a Tool to Study CNS Disorders

Julia Pinsonneault and Wolfgang Sadée

Genomics or genome science is the study of the structure, function, and evolution of the genome—the total DNA present in cellular organisms. Evolution is driven by random mutations in the genome that can affect genetic regulatory regions, the processing and stability of messenger RNA and non-coding RNA, translation, and protein structure and functions. Genetic variations or polymorphisms can be insertions or deletions, inversions, expansions of DNA repeats, or they can be a base-pair change of a single nucleotide. The term polymorphism implies a frequency of at least 1% in human populations, but this lower abundance limit is not always rigorously applied in the literature.

Representing ~80% of all genetic variations, single nucleotide polymorphisms (SNPs) are single base-pair substitutions occurring every 300–1000 base-pairs in the human genome, comprised of 3 billion base-pairs. While on the one hand genetic variations generate a near infinite spectrum of variations between individuals, we need to acknowledge that overall human genetic diversity is relatively limited, owing to the rather recent emergence of hominids, and in particular modern humans. Yet, subtle genetic differences appear to play a significant role in susceptibility to disease and response to therapy.

Genetic contributions to risk factors vary over a broad range between CNS disorders, often accounting for 50% or more of relative risk. Similarly, genetic factors determine a considerable portion of interindividual differences in response to therapies, with relative risk to overall outcome also dependent upon the type of CNS disorder. Moreover, each drug is affected differently by genetic variations in genes encoding drug metabolizing enzymes, transporters, and drug targets/receptors. Therefore, the study of genetic differences affecting disease and therapy is germane to understanding disease etiology and optimizing therapy. However, our current knowledge of the main genetic factors remains fragmentary. Furthermore, male and female patients display marked differences in the prevalence and progression of CNS disorders and treatment outcomes—with the sex chromosomes yielding arguably the largest common chromosomal differences among individuals. Therefore, the genetics of CNS disorders strongly intertwines with the study of sex differences, and yet, this has often been neglected in the past. Here we review current trends in our understanding of the genetics of CNS disorders and how sex differences impinge on outcomes, or can serve to study the underlying causes of disease.

PHARMACOGENOMICS: DEFINITION AND METHODOLOGIES

Pharmacogenomics is the application of genome science to the field of pharmacology—the study of what the body does to a drug and what a drug does to the body (pharmacokinetics and pharmacodynamics, respectively). Pharmacogenomics broadly encompasses genome-wide analysis of genetic variations that contribute to disease susceptibility and drug efficacy or toxicity. Pharmacogenetics on the other hand can be understood as a targeted analysis of specific candidate genes involved in disease susceptibility, drug efficacy or drug toxicity. However, the terms pharmacogenomics and pharmacogenetics are often used interchangeably. In addition to genotype, pharmacogenomics includes other large-scale techniques, such as profiling of the transcriptome (all mRNAs in a cell) and proteomics.

The trend of moving from pharmacogenetics studies dealing with candidate genes to the large-scale approach of pharmacogenomics has arisen from an explosion of new methodologies with ever increasing capabilities. With regard to genotyping, methods for discovery and scoring of genetic variations have proliferated, moving from the analysis of single SNPs with low throughput to measuring hundreds and even thousands of SNPs in parallel with high throughput. Genotyping methods such as DNA sequencing and primer extension methods provide the researcher with the exact base pair identity of the SNP in question.

Other low through-put methods such as restriction fragment length polymorphism (RFLP) rely on the presence of an SNP to disrupt a restriction enzyme recognition site, thus changing the length of a DNA fragment visible on a gel separated by electrophoresis. High through-put methods, which can genotype thousands of SNPs in a single sample at once, include hybridization-based technology embedded into mi-

croarrays or bead technologies. For review of methodologies see (Imle, 2005; Palmisano et al., 2005; Tsongalis & Coleman, 2006). Not surprisingly, the rise of high-throughput assays has profoundly changed the approach taken in genetic studies, with increasing emphasis on genome-wide association and linkage analyses of complex multigenic disorders (Rannala, 2001; Detera-Wadleigh & McMahon, 2004; Camp & Cannon-Albright, 2005; Wright, 2005). Despite these advances, CNS disorders have proven resistant to attempts at dissecting the underlying causes with the use of genetic and genomic means. We argue here that a systematic evaluation of sex differences could prove essential for gaining entry into the inner workings of complex CNS disorders.

Considerable work has already focused on sex differences in the response to drug treatments. Prominent examples include kappa opioid receptor agonists, which in some circumstances are effective analgesics in females but not in males (Barrett et al., 2002; Mogil et al., 2003). Also, drug metabolism-related differences have been reported, as a function of life cycle, particularly in females going through puberty or menopause (Anthony & Berg, 2002; Schwartz, 2003). This article, however, focuses on disease susceptibility genes that are likely to affect treatment outcomes by acting downstream of immediate drug targets.

BIOLOGY AND GENETICS OF SEX DIFFERENCES

Differential distribution of the sex chromosomes causes a broad spectrum of physiological differences between males carrying a single X and a Y chromosome, and females with two X chromosomes. The ensuing morphological differences include the development of sex organs, causing distinct patterns of sex hormones that are thought to be the main drivers of sex differences. However, chromosomal genetic differences other than those caused by sex hormones are likely to contribute to many differences between males and females, but the responsible mechanisms are still poorly understood. One could argue that the genomic differences between males and females are far greater than a current focus on single polymorphisms in candidate genes would seem to indicate. We further need to consider that abnormalities in structure and distribution of sex chromosomes do occur with some frequency (Linden et al., 2002; Ferlin et al., 2005), and can potentially serve to dissect the contribution to CNS disorders.

The main cause for sex differences is the biology of the X and Y chromosomes. Because the X chromosome exists in only one copy in males, X-linked mutations are fully expressed in males, and are the cause of genetic diseases such as hemophilia or muscular dystrophy that mostly affect males. In females, the presence of two X chromosomes protects against the effects of recessive mutations but could potentially cause a more harmful gene dosage effect if both copies of a gene were expressed at the same levels as in males. This over-expression is avoided by a mechanism of dosage compensation known as X *inactivation*, a process of random silencing of either one of the two X chromosomes in every cell by extensive CpG island methylation (Gartler & Riggs, 1983). This involves cytosine methylation at CpG islands—phosphodiester-linked pairs of cytosine and guanine, usually in or near the promoter of mammalian genes.

As a result, gene expression may be mosaic at the cellular level: those heterozygous for mutations in X-linked genes express the defect in some cells and not in others. While one commonly assumes that in each cell one X chromosome is randomly inactivated in females, unequal X inactivation or selection of one active X chromosome over the other in somatic cells has been observed (Sharp et al., 2000; Van den Veyver, 2001; Sandovici et al., 2004). On the other hand, a recent survey of X inactivation patterns found that 15% of X-linked genes escape inactivation (Carrel & Willard, 2005). For example, MAOA resides in a region of the X chromosomes known to escape X inactivation, potentially causing higher expression of MAOA in females compared to males, with implications for behavior and mental disorders (discussed further). These results reveal the potential for a broad range of expected phenotypic effects in females caused by mutations in X-linked genes.

The silencing of one X chromosome during X inactivation is one example of epigenetic regulation. Epigenetic modifications are reversible but heritable changes in gene function, without a change in the DNA sequence. These modifications can involve histone alteration and methylation at CpG islands, usually in or near the promoter of mammalian genes. For review see (Jiang et al., 2004; Fuks, 2005). Genomic imprinting—the selective expression or repression of a gene allele based on its parent of origin—also involves epigenetic mechanisms. An additional genetic difference between males and females is the transfer of mitochondrial genes, which is largely restricted to mitochondria from the mother. A number of mitochondrial mutations lead to disease or are known to affect drug response or toxicity. For a review see (Chinnery & Turnbull, 2000).

Here we address the question of how genetic factors contribute to disease susceptibility and drug response in complex disorders that are known to vary considerably in male and female patients. This is done with the intention that integration of currently known genetic factors with sex differences could lead to new insights about disease etiology and response to therapy, but we acknowledge that such integration is still in its infancy. We have selected four CNS disorders—depression, schizophrenia, anorexia, and attention-deficit disorder—as a primary focus for this review, because a rich literature already exists on sex differences. Moreover, drugs used in their treatment comprise nearly half of the ten top-selling drugs, with considerable health implications and economic impact.

Each of these diseases is thought to have a genetic component, and specifically, to involve numerous candidate genes as susceptibility factors. The most likely scenario for such common diseases involves combinations of genetic variations in multiple genes that cooperate to increase the risk of disease. Each of these relatively common genetic variations alone appears to have little impact, but combinations that may vary among individual patients can lead to symptoms, likely with somewhat different clinical outcomes for each combination.

Since these disorders present with different clinical manifestations and at different ages in males and females, we ask whether genetic variations underlying the disease process differ among male and female patients. With respect to drug treatment, both efficacy and toxicity play a role in clinical outcome, and again females and males are likely to differ by genetic determinants. These genetic differences are the subject of pharmacogenomics. Yet, in focusing on genetic factors involved in pharmacodynamic drug effects, we cannot readily separate genetic factors contributing to treatment response and disease susceptibility or progression. Failure or success of a specific drug treatment may indeed reveal differences in disease etiology, assuming that complex CNS disorders derive from different pathophysiology and genetics despite similar phenotypes. Therefore, the pursuit of pharmacogenomic principles in CNS drug response may

Table 5.1. Sex Differences in 4 CNS Disorders

Disorder	Female	Male
Depression	Higher prevalence (2:1)	Lower prevalence
Schizophrenia	Less severe Later onset (Age 25)	More severe Earlier onset (Age 21)
Anorexia nervosa	High prevalence	Rare
ADHD	Lower prevalence	Higher prevalence (4:1)

well lead to a better understanding of the treated disease.

Many disorders of the central nervous system display distinct sex differences. Anxiety, depression, eating disorders and Alzheimer's disease are more common in women. Men, on the other hand, are more likely to be afflicted with alcohol and drug abuse problems, antisocial personality, attention deficit disorders, and Tourette's syndrome. We focus on four distinct disorders: depression, schizophrenia, anorexia nervosa and attention deficit hyperactivity disorder (ADHD). Schizophrenia displays sex differences in the development of the disorder and affects men earlier in life and more severely, even though men and women are affected in equal numbers. Depression and anorexia, by contrast, affect women more than men; while ADHD occurs more frequently in males (see Table 5.1). All these mental disorders share some overlapping candidate genes.

SEX DIFFERENCES AND PHARMACOGENOMICS IN DRUG THERAPIES OF CNS DISEASE: EXAMPLES

Depression

Depression is a relatively common condition that affects approximately 19 million Americans in any year. It can strike individuals equally across educational, economic and ethnic boundaries. There are three frequent types of depression that vary in severity of symptoms and persistence: *major depression* (also called unipolar depression) where symptoms interfere with ability to eat, sleep, work and enjoy life; *dysthymia*, which is long-term or chronic but non-disabling; and *bipolar disorder*, which is characterized by wide mood swings ranging from deep lows to manic highs.

Epidemiological and clinical studies have consistently observed significant sex-specific differences among patients with depression, with females outnumbering males 2:1 (Kessler et al., 1993). There is not a significant sex difference between the rates of depression in children, but differences become evident after onset of puberty (Angold et al., 1999; Steiner et al., 2003). In fact, the increase in the rate of depression of adolescent girls is correlated not with age, but with the physical changes that occur during puberty (Angold et al., 1999). Premenstrual syndrome (PMS) and postpartum depression (PPD) are additional conditions involving depression that specifically affect women and are suggestive of hormonal involvement in the pathogenesis of mood disorders.

Depression is often treated with a combination of psychotherapy and medication. The most common antidepressants used in the treatment of depression are selective serotonin reuptake inhibitors (SSRIs), tricyclics, and monoamine oxidase inhibitors (MAOIs). Tricyclics work by inhibiting norepinephrine and serotonin reuptake. They also antagonize many neurotransmitter receptors, which may be the cause of numerous side effects. SSRIs were developed to specifically target the serotonin transporter, and MAOIs function by selectively inhibiting MAO enzymes. Most antidepressants are also effective in treating some anxiety disorders. There is variation in the response of an individual to any particular drug. Drug response rates vary from 85% for MAOIs to as low as 55% for SSRIs (Quitkin et al., 2002).

Candidate genes currently thought to play a role in susceptibility or drug treatment of schizophrenia, depression, anorexia nervosa and/or ADHD are listed in Table 5.2.

Various candidate genes have been studied for variations that are correlated with antidepressant response (Lerer & Macciardi, 2002). The promoter region of serotonin transporter gene, SERT, which exists in two variants: long and short (HTTLPR l and s), has been examined by a number of groups. For example, patients who are homozygous for the short variant were found to respond better to fluoxetine

Table 5.2. Candidate genes thought to be involved in the susceptibility to or pharmacotherapy of schizophrenia (schiz), major depressive disorder (MDD), anorexia nervosa (AN) and/or attention deficit hyperactivity disorder (ADHD).

Gene Name	Symbol	Chr	Schiz	MDD	AN	ADHD
Agouti-related protein precursor (Vink et al., 2001)	AGRP	16			+	
Apolipoprotein-L1 (Mimmack et al., 2002)	APOL1	22	+			
Apolipoprotein-L2 (Mimmack et al., 2002)	APOL2	22	+			
Apolipoprotein-L4 (Mimmack et al., 2002)	APOL4	22	+			
Alpha serine/threonine-protein kinase(Emamian et al., 2004)	AKT1	14	+			
Beta-1-adrenergic receptor (Zill et al., 2003)	ADRB1	10		+		
Brain-derived neurotrophic factor (Ribases et al., 2004; Neves-Pereira et al., 2005)	BDNF	11	+		+	
cAMP response element binding protein (Zubenko et al., 2003)	CREB	2		+		
Catechol-O-methyltransferase (Bray et al., 2003; Qian et al., 2003; Funke et al., 2005)	COMT	22	+	+		+
Calcium-activated potassium channel protein 3 (Koronyo-Hamaoui et al., 2002)	KCNN3	1			+	
Cholinergic receptor, nicotinic, alpha 7 (Freedman et al., 2001)	CHRNA7	15	+			
Corticotropin-releasing hormone receptor-2 (Villafuerte et al., 2002)	CRHR2	7		+		
D-amino acid oxidase (Chumakov et al., 2002)	DAO	12	+			
D-amino acid oxidase activator (G72) (Chumakov et al., 2002)	DAOA	13	+			
Disrupted in schizophrenia (Millar et al., 2002; Hennah et al., 2003)	DISC1	1	+			
Disrupted in schizophrenia 2 (Millar et al., 2002)	DISC2	1	+			
Dopamine beta-hydroxylase (Faraone et al., 2005)	DBH	9				+
Dopamine receptor D2 (Comings et al., 1991; Glatt et al., 2003; Bergen et al., 2005)	DRD2	11	+		+	+
Dopamine receptor D3 (Crocq et al., 1992)	DRD3	3	+			
Dopamine receptor D4 (Seeman et al., 1993; Faraone et al., 2005)	DRD4	11	+			+
Dopamine receptor D5 (Faraone et al., 2005)	DRD5	4				+
Dopamine transporter (DAT) (Faraone et al., 2005)	SLC6A3	5				+
Dysbindin (Straub et al., 2002)	DTNBP1	6	+			
Estrogen receptor alpha (Perlman et al., 2004)	ESR1	6		+		
Estrogen receptor beta (Rosenkranz et al., 1998)	ESR2	14			+	

continued

Table 5.2. *(continued)*

Gene Name	Symbol	Chr	Schiz.	MDD	AN	ADHD
G-protein beta 3 (Lee et al., 2004)	GNB3	12		+		
Methylenetetrahydrofolate reductase (Bjelland et al., 2003)	MTHFR	1		+		
Monoamine oxidase A (Manor et al., 2002; Gutierrez et al., 2004; Urwin and Nunn, 2005)	MAOA	X		+	+	+
Neuregulin 1 (Stefansson et al., 2002)	NRG1	8	+			
Neurotrophin-3 (Hattori et al., 2002)	NTF3	12	+			
Norepinephrine transporter (NET) (Urwin and Nunn, 2005)	SLC6A2	16			+	
Nitric-oxide synthase, neuronal (Yu et al., 2003)	NOS1	12		+		
Opioid receptor, delta (Bergen et al., 2003)	OPRD1	1			+	
Proline dehydrogenase 1 (Jacquet et al., 2002)	PRODH	22	+			
Proline dehydrogenase 2 (Chakravarti, 2002)	PRODH2	19	+			
Reelin (Grayson et al., 2005)	RELN	7	+			
Reticulon 4 receptor (Sinibaldi et al., 2004)	RTN4R	22	+			
Serotonin receptor 1A (Julius, 1998)	HTR1A	5		+		
Serotonin receptor 1B (Moret and Briley, 2000; Faraone et al., 2005)	HTR1B	6		+		+
Serotonin receptor 1D (Bergen et al., 2003)	HTR1D	1			+	
Serotonin receptor 2A (Collier et al., 1997; Arranz et al., 1998; McMahon et al., 2006)	HTR2A	13	+	+	+	
Serotonin receptor 2C (Arranz et al., 1998; Lerer et al., 2001; Westberg et al., 2002)	HTR2C	X	+	+	+	
Serotonin receptor 4 (Suzuki et al., 2003)	HTR4	5	+	+		
Serotonin receptor 5A (Veenstra-VanderWeele et al., 2000)	HTR5A	7	+			
Serotonin transporter (SERT) (Ogilvie et al., 1996; Fan and Sklar, 2005; Faraone et al., 2005; Urwin and Nunn, 2005)	SLC6A4	17	+	+	+	+
Synapsin 2 (Chen et al., 2004)	SYN2	3	+			
Synaptosomal-associated protein 25 (Faraone et al., 2005)	SNAP25	20				+
Tryptophan hydroxylase (Shinkai et al., 2000; Faraone et al., 2005; Gizatullin et al., 2006)	TPH	11	+	+		+
Tryptophan hydroxylase 2 (Zill et al., 2004)	TPH2	12		+		

"+" indicates that a gene is a candidate for the corresponding disorder. "Chr" = chromosome.

(Prozac) than patients with other genotypes (Kim et al., 2000). By contrast, patients homozygous for the short variant responded worse to fluvoxamine (another SSRI) than patients with other genotypes (Smeraldi et al., 1998).

Numerous clinical association studies have supported a role for the LPR polymorphism, but this has not been uniformly confirmed. These studies are predicated on a previous finding that the long and short forms of HTTLPR have different reporter gene activity in a transfected heterologous tissue culture, and in blood lymphocytes (Heils et al., 1996; Lesch et al., 1996). However, we have analyzed the allelic expression activity of the long and short forms in post-mortem tissues derived from pontine nuclei in post-mortem brain samples (pons being the main site of SERT transcription in the brain). The results failed to show a direct relationship between the LPR and allelic expression; moreover, allelic expression in lymphocytes was also unaffected by LPR (Lim et al., 2006).

These results raise doubt as to the validity of clinical association studies, but they do not rule out genetic effects of SERT on disease outcome and drug response. Moreover, we cannot exclude a role of the LPR polymorphism in response to stress or during development, at which time different transcription factors might become active. Any sex-dependent differences also remain to be addressed.

In a study to determine whether men and women respond differently to antidepressants, women were found to have a superior response to MAOIs compared to men but no other differences were noted (Quitkin et al., 2002). Again, our understanding of the genetic factors contributing to depression and drug response in male and female patients is incomplete. We have addressed the issue of genetic and epigenetic variations of the regulation of MAOA, an X-linked gene. Epigenetic processes (CpG island methylation) are thought to decrease gene expression. Previous studies have suggested that a promoter repeat (pVNTR) modulates MAOA expression (Sabol et al., 1998). We find that CpG island methylation also appears to play a role. We have observed variable CpG methylation in females (independent of X inactivation) but not in males, which could represent a kind of dosage compensation but could also contribute to interindividual differences (Pinsonneault et al., 2006). The role of MAOA and B (both adjacent to each other on the X-chromosome) in mental disorders and drug response requires further study, but our results point to distinct differences in the regulation of this important gene in the brain of male and female subjects.

Estrogens have been shown to have antidepressant effects. Women with severe PPD or postpartum psychosis were reported to respond rapidly to oral estradiol treatment (Ahokas et al., 1998; Ahokas et al., 1999; Ahokas et al., 2000). The speed by which therapy becomes effective is important because it may take several weeks for antidepressants to take full effect. Therefore, estrogen-induced accelerated responsiveness is a promising strategy in female patients under special conditions.

High-dose oral estrogens have been used successfully as a prophylactic in women with a history of severe postpartum affective disorder (Sichel et al., 1995). There is some evidence that combining estrogens with traditional antidepressants to treat depression is effective in accelerating the time to response. The effects of estrogen replacement therapy were examined in a randomized, double-blinded trial of fluoxetine versus placebo in elderly depressed women. Women taking estrogens who were treated with fluoxetine improved significantly more than estrogen-treated patients who received a placebo (Schneider et al., 1997). Patients who did not receive estrogens showed no difference in response to fluoxetine versus placebo, suggesting that estrogens may boost the effects of SSRIs, perhaps by interaction with the serotonin system (Schneider et al., 1997).

In such studies, polymorphisms in any of the genes contributing to disease or drug response have yet to be considered systematically. For example, polymorphisms in estrogen receptor alpha (Herrington, 2003) may affect treatment outcome, as could polymorphisms in the serotonin transporter and further genes involved in neurotransmission. However, risk associated with estrogen use must be considered as well.

Schizophrenia

Schizophrenia is a debilitating form of psychosis that affects approximately 1% of the population, showing a strong genetic component. Although the exact mechanism of pathogenesis is unknown, excessive activity at dopaminergic synapses in the brain is thought to play an important role (Carlsson et al., 1999). The onset of schizophrenia coincides with reproductive years and hormonal changes in the brain. Sex differences in schizophrenia have long been observed and established by epidemiological studies (Grigoriadis & Seeman, 2002; Stevens, 2002).

The average age at onset for women (25 years) is significantly later than in men (21 years), and there is a smaller peak of late first-onset seen only in peri- and postmenopausal women after age 44. Male patients generally have more negative symptoms, a history of more maternal obstetric complications and poorer premorbid adjustment (Preston et al., 2002). Even differences in anatomical brain abnormalities have been detected between male and female patients (Cowell et al., 1996).

In males, higher prefrontal lobe volume was associated with mild severity of disorganization, while in females it was associated with more severe disorganization and hostility (Cowell et al., 1996). The greater severity of symptoms in males suggests that estrogens exert a protective effect against schizophrenia (Grigoriadis & Seeman, 2002). A number of susceptibility genes have been proposed to contribute to the etiology of schizophrenia, which is thought to have a strong inheritable component (see Table 5.2). These genes include the serotonin transporter (SLC6A4), the norepinephrine transporter (SLC6A2), and the dopamine D2 receptor (DRD2). However, none of these genes has been unequivocally linked or enables accurate prediction of disease. Lately, several strong candidate genes have been revealed, including COMT (Bray et al., 2003; Wonodi et al., 2003), NRG1 (Stefansson et al., 2002), and DISC1 (Millar et al., 2002) (see above).

Studies directed specifically towards female patients have revealed additional susceptibility genes. Significant differences in the occurrence of polymorphisms in two genes, DRD2 and NTF3, have recently been observed between schizophrenic women and matched female controls (Virgos et al., 2001). Yet, no single gene has emerged as an overriding factor in schizophrenia.

On the one hand, the disease is likely a canopy of different abnormalities with distinct phenotypes, and on the other, there appear to be multiple genes involved each with low penetrance. By penetrance we mean the degree to which an individual with a given genotype manifests an associated phenotype. These complexities make it difficult to resolve the genetic components of schizophrenia, but numerous studies have already demonstrated the need to consider sex differences.

Atypical antipsychotics such as clozapine have become the treatment of choice for patients suffering from psychosis (Arranz & Kerwin, 2000; Larsen et al.,

2001). These medications are approved for acute and chronic management of patients with schizophrenia and are also widely used for other mental disorders with symptoms of psychosis such as schizoaffective, bipolar and depressive disorder (Ichikawa & Meltzer, 1999). While atypical antipsychotics interact with multiple receptor types, the primary mechanism of action is thought to involve serotonin 5-HT-2 and dopamine D2 receptors (Arranz & Kerwin, 2000).

Each atypical antipsychotic has a distinct repertoire of target receptors. Multiple genes may play a role in disease susceptibility and drug response, but the contributions of specific genetic variations to disease remain unclear. The spectrum of genetic variants found in individuals may combine to allow for optimal selection of the antipsychotic drug. Furthermore, males and females may have a different spectrum of genetic variants underlying disease in the same ethnic population, which also could affect treatment outcome. Therefore, it is advisable to design clinical genetic association studies with patient and control cohorts separated by males and females and ethnicity, in anticipation that different genes may play prominent roles between them.

To search for candidate genes, Arranz and colleagues (Arranz et al., 2000b) measured a number of polymorphisms in multiple genes encoding neurotransmitter receptors and transporters, in psychotic patients receiving clozepine, an effective atypical antipsychotic. A combination of 5 polymorphisms, in the serotonin receptors 5HT-2A and 5HT-2C, the histamine receptor H2, and the serotonin transporter SERT, improved the prediction of a positive response to clozepine to 77% accuracy.

In principle, this type of analysis holds promise for predictive genotyping in antipsychotic therapy; however, predictability did not improve sufficiently to have direct impact on therapy because the results could not be replicated or validated in different populations by other groups (Arranz et al., 2000a). The results may not apply to other patient populations, because there are substantial differences among ethnic populations in the prevalence of single nucleotide polymorphisms (SNPs) and varying linkage to polymorphisms that are functional. This is known as population admixture.

Several SNPs often are linked on the same chromosome and interact functionally. Phased SNPs are called *haplotypes*, which are beginning to supersede the use of single indicator SNPs in genetic association studies (Garner & Slatkin, 2003; Zhao et al., 2003). Haplotypes hold promise for improved power of such clinical studies, and leads to the expectation that genetic risk factors will be unraveled in the future.

Anorexia

Anorexia nervosa (AN) is a psychiatric illness that primarily affects females. A severe eating disorder, it is characterized by maintenance of very low body weight through the restriction of food, excessive exercise and purging. It is associated with the highest mortality rate of any mental illness (Sullivan, 1995). Age of onset is usually adolescence, when estrogen levels are high. It has been demonstrated that estrogens can have anorectic effects and that in the brain, estrogen receptors co-localize with corticotrophin releasing hormone (Dagnault & Richard, 1997). This interaction may modulate the hypothalamic pituitary adrenal (HPA) axis, a key component of stress response (Eastwood et al., 2002). Elevated cortisol level caused by HPA axis hyperactivity is well documented in underweight anorexic patients (Licinio et al., 1996). The HPA axis disruption can be partially attributed to the effects of starvation (Licinio et al., 1996), but genetic predisposition is thought to play a role as well. One gene found to have an association with AN is the estrogen receptor ESR2 (Rosenkranz et al., 1998; Eastwood et al., 2002). ESR2 has been shown to be involved in the anorectic action of estrogens (Liang et al., 2002).

There is a substantial contribution of additional genetic factors associated with AN (Bulik et al., 2006). Candidate genes are listed in Table 5.2 and include those associated with monoamine and neuropeptide function, such as DRD2 (Bergen et al., 2005), and MAOA (Urwin et al., 2003; Urwin & Nunn, 2005). No medications have currently been approved by the FDA for this serious, often fatal disease; however, there are numerous pharmacological targets that are promising (Powers & Santana, 2004).

Cyproheptadine for weight restoration, fluoxetine to prevent relapse after weight restoration and atypical antipsychotics, in particular olanzapine, are being utilized in the treatment of anorexia, but efficacy in any of these therapies has not been confirmed. Given the prevalence in females, and the emergence of an estrogen receptor as a candidate gene, sex differences must be considered as important factors in understanding the molecular genetics of AN.

Attention Deficit Hyperactivity Disorder (ADHD)

Attention deficit hyperactivity disorder is a childhood disorder that affects males more than females at a ratio of 4:1. The disorder consists of two distinct underlying types: inattentive and hyperactive, which are moderately correlated, and the combined type (Lahey et al., 1988). Attempts to explain the sex differences in prevalence have resulted in the creation of two competing models: the polygenic multiple threshold (PMT) model (Cloninger et al., 1978) and the constitutional variability (CV) model (Eme, 1992).

The PMT model suggests that the difference in ADHD prevalence between males and females is because females require a greater number of the same causal genetic factors than males to be affected, while the CV model makes the assumption that males and females differ because each sex has different causal factors (Rhee et al., 1999). For example, in girls ADHD is thought to be caused by a distinct pathological event such as brain damage, whereas boys are slower to develop, and those affected with ADHD are at the extreme of a genetic continuum (Rhee et al., 1999).

Another plausible explanation for sex differences is bias: girls with ADHD are less likely to be disruptive and therefore noticed. This bias could affect the number of females that are referred to clinicians, thereby artificially lowering the apparent incidence of ADHD in females (Biederman et al., 2002).

Pharmacological treatment of ADHD is usually by stimulants: methylphenidate (Ritalin) and methamphetamine (Aderall). A non-stimulant alternative is the selective norepinephrine reuptake inhibitor, atomoxetine (Straterra). Stimulant medications used to treat ADHD bind to the dopamine transporter, inhibiting dopamine reuptake and thus increasing its concentration in the synapse. A repeat polymorphism in the dopamine transporter has been associated with methylphenidate dosage response, where youth who are homozygous for a less common 9-repeat allele have a markedly lower response to the drug than those carrying the more common 10-repeat allele (Stein et al., 2005).

While there is no difference between the sexes on the efficacy of stimulants to treat ADHD symptoms (Spencer et al., 2001), treating adolescent and adult female ADHD patients with stimulants brings with it some caveats because of potential interaction of the medication with hormones. In the follicular phase of menstrual cycle (before ovulation), the level of estrogens is high and progesterone levels are low, while in the luteal phase (after ovulation) level of estrogens drop and progesterone rises. Response to stimulants is greater during follicular phase, compared to the luteal phase (Justice & de Wit, 1999; Terner & de Wit, 2006). Cyclical variations of progesterone may decrease effectiveness, while estrogens enhance the effect of stimulants such as amphetamines (Justice & de Wit, 2000; Quinn, 2005).

Candidate genes for ADHD are listed in Table 5.2. Genes that have been consistently associated with ADHD in multiple studies include: DRD4, DRD5, DBH, SLC6A4, HTR1B, and SNAP25 (Faraone et al., 2005). While these candidate genes point to main processes contributing to ADHD, this has yet to be used in therapy of individual patients, or in designing novel treatment strategies. Clearly, we are still at the beginning of a molecular genetic understanding of this disease.

CANDIDATE GENE APPROACH TO PHARMACOGENOMICS: HOW TO EXPLOIT SEX DIFFERENCES FOR UNDERSTANDING THE GENETIC BASIS OF DIFFERENCES IN RESPONSE TO CNS DRUGS

These diseases share putative susceptibility genes and metabolic pathways. However, the pathological significance of most if not all polymorphisms in candidate genes remains to be confirmed. Only recently have several genes definitively been shown to play a significant role in schizophrenia (Millar et al., 2002; Bray et al., 2003; Harrison & Owen, 2003) and depression (Huang et al., 2002; Bjelland et al., 2003; Caspi et al., 2003; Yu et al., 2003; Zill et al., 2003). These include, but are not limited to: COMT (Bray et al., 2003; Wonodi et al., 2003), SERT (Veenstra-Vander-Weele et al., 2000), NRG1 (Stefansson et al., 2002), and DISC1 (Millar et al., 2002) for schizophrenia; and NOS1 (Yu et al., 2003), ADRB1 (Zill et al., 2003), and MTHFR (Bjelland et al., 2003) for depression.

Many of these genes are listed as candidates for both disorders. The overlap between putative susceptibility genes for schizophrenia and depression must be interpreted with caution, as this selection of candidate genes may be biased because investigators tend to focus on well-studied genes. Even though these diseases have opposite sex prevalences, the underlying genetic mechanisms that cause these disorders to be sex specific may be related.

SUMMARY

In the diverse disorders discussed in this chapter, estrogens appear to play a prominent role, primarily as a protective agent in the case of schizophrenia and depression. Even in depression where women are more strongly affected than men, this may be due to a precipitous drop in estrogens, such as happens after delivering a baby or premenstrually. Yet, hormonal levels are but one of the multiple genomic differences between males and females. Our review points out the overriding need to consider sex in understanding the disease and optimizing its therapy, but it also highlights the complexity of genomic factors in multigenic disease and therapy.

We have evidence of genetic variants of some genes that contribute to disease progression and drug response in male patients but not in female patients, while others are more important in women. Yet, this can only be the beginning of a systematic analysis of genetic factors and sex in complex disease. In this review, we have not considered sex differences in drug metabolism and disposition/transport which also affect sex differences in drug response (see example reviews [Gandhi et al., 2004; Chen, 2005; Donovan, 2005]), but rather have focused on drug targets, pharmacodynamic factors, and disease genetics.

We have yet to define the most promising approaches capable of resolving these complexities such that our knowledge can lead to significantly improved drug therapy. With novel genomic technologies emerging at a frantic pace, we must now clearly define the problem in search of the best approach to understanding the genetics of disease and therapy.

Acknowledgments

The authors were supported by a grant from the National Institute of Drug Abuse: R21 DA108744, a grant from the Society for Women's Health Research, and the UCSF Pharmacogenetics of membrane transporters (PMT) project.

References

Ahokas A., Turtiainen S., & Aito M. (1998). Sublingual oestrogen treatment of postnatal depression. *Lancet*, 351:109.

Ahokas A., Kaukoranta J., & Aito M. (1999). Effect of oestradiol on postpartum depression. *Psychopharmacology*, (Berl) 146:108–110.

Ahokas A., Aito M., & Rimon R. (2000). Positive treatment effect of estradiol in postpartum psychosis: a pilot study. *J Clin Psychiatry*, 61:166–169.

Angold A., Costello E., Erkanli A., & Worthman C. (1999). Pubertal changes in hormonal levels and depression in girls. *Psychol Med*, 29:1043–1053.

Anthony M., & Berg M. (2002). Biologic and molecular mechanisms for sex differences in pharmacokinetics, pharmacodynamics, and pharmacogenetics: Part II. *J Womens Health Gend Based Med*, 11:617–629.

Arranz M., Kerwin R. (2000). Neurotransmitter related genes and antipsychotoic response: pharmacogenetics meets psychiatric treatment. *Ann Med*, 32:128–133.

Arranz M., Munro J., Osborne S., Collier D., & Kerwin R. (2000a). Difficulties in replication of results. *Lancet*, 356:1359–1360.

Arranz M., Munro J., Owen M., Spurlock G., Sham PC., Zhao J., et al. (1998). Evidence for association between polymorphisms in the promoter and coding regions of the 5-HT2A receptor gene and response to clozapine. *Mol Psychiatry*, 3:61–68.

Arranz M., Munro J., Birkett J., Bolonna A., Mancama D., Sodhi M., et al. (2000b). Pharmacogenetic prediction of clozapine response. *Lancet*, 355:1615–1616.

Barrett A., Smith E., & Picker M. (2002). Sex-related differences in mechanical nociception and antinociception produced by mu- and kappa-opioid receptor agonists in rats. *Eur J Pharmacol*, 452:163–173.

Bergen A., van den Bree M., Yeager M., Welch R., Ganjei J., Haque K., et al. (2003). Candidate genes for anorexia nervosa in the 1p33–36 linkage region: serotonin 1D and delta opioid receptor loci exhibit significant association to anorexia nervosa. *Mol Psychiatry*, 8:397–406.

Bergen A., Yeager M., Welch R., Haque K., Ganjei J., van den Bree M., et al. (2005). Association of multiple DRD2 polymorphisms with anorexia nervosa. *Neuropsychopharmacology*, 30:1703–1710.

Biederman J., Mick E., Faraone S., Braaten E., Doyle A., Spencer T., et al. (2002). Influence of gender on attention deficit hyperactivity disorder in children referred to a psychiatric clinic. *Am J Psychiatry*, 159:36–42.

Bjelland I., Tell G., Vollset S., Refsum H., & Ueland P. (2003). Folate, vitamin B12, homocysteine, and the MTHFR 677C->T polymorphism in anxiety and depression: the Hordaland Homocysteine Study. *Arch Gen Psychiatry*, 60:618–626.

Bray N., Buckland P., Williams N., Williams H., Norton N., Owen M., et al. (2003). A haplotype implicated in schizophrenia susceptibility is associated with reduced COMT expression in human brain. *Am J Hum Genet*,73:152–161.

Bulik C., Sullivan P., Tozzi F., Furberg H., Lichtenstein P., & Pedersen N. (2006). Prevalence, heritability, and prospective risk factors for anorexia nervosa. *Arch Gen Psychiatry*, 63:305–312.

Camp N., & Cannon-Albright L. (2005). Dissecting the genetic etiology of major depressive disorder using linkage analysis. *Trends Mol Med*, 11:138–144.

Carlsson A., Waters N., & Carlsson M. (1999). Neurotransmitter interactions in schizophrenia-therapeutic implications. *Eur Arch Psychiatry Clin Neurosci*, 249:S37–S43.

Carrel L., & Willard H. (2005). X-inactivation profile reveals extensive variability in X-linked gene expression in females. *Nature*, 434:400–404.

Caspi A., Sugden K., Moffitt T., Taylor A., Craig I., Harrington H., et al. (2003). Influence of life stress on depression: moderation by a polymorphism in the 5-HTT gene. *Science*, 301:386–389.

Chakravarti A. (2002). A compelling genetic hypothesis for a complex disease: PRODH2/DGCR6 variation leads to schizophrenia susceptibility. *Proc Natl Acad Sci U S A*, 99:4755–4756.

Chen M. (2005). Confounding factors for sex differences in pharmacokinetics and pharmacodynamics: focus on dosing regimen, dosage form, and formulation. *Clin Pharmacol Ther*, 78:322–329.

Chen Q., He G., Wang X., Chen Q., Liu X., Gu Z., et al. (2004). Positive association between synapsin II and schizophrenia. *Bio Psychiat*, 56:177–181.

Chinnery P., & Turnbull D. (2000). Mitochondrial DNA mutations in the pathogenesis of human disease. *Mol Med Today*, 6:425–432.

Chumakov I., Blumenfeld M., Guerassimenko O., Cavarec L., Palicio M., Abderrahim H., et al. (2002). Genetic and physiological data implicating the new human gene G72 and the gene for D-amino acid oxidase in schizophrenia. *Proc Natl Acad Sci U S A*, 99:13675–13680.

Cloninger C., Christiansen K., Reich T., & Gottesman II. (1978). Implications of sex differences in the prevalences of antisocial personality, alcoholism, and criminality for familial transmission. *Arch Gen Psychiatry*, 35:941–951.

Collier D., Arranz M., Li T., Mupita D., Brown N., & Treasure J. (1997). Association between 5-HT2A gene promoter polymorphism and anorexia nervosa. *Lancet*, 350:412.

Comings D., Comings B., Muhleman D., Dietz G., Shahbahrami B., Tast D., et al. (1991). The dopamine D2 receptor locus as a modifying gene in neuropsychiatric disorders. *JAMA*, 266:1793–1800.

Cowell P., Kostianovsky D., Gur R., Turetsky B., & Gur R. (1996). Sex differences in neuroanatomical and clinical correlations in schizophrenia. *Am J Psychiatry*, 153:799–805.

Crocq M., Mant R., Asherson P., Williams J., Hode Y., Mayerova A., et al. (1992). Association between schizophrenia and homozygosity at the dopamine D3 receptor gene. *J Med Genet*, 29:858–860.

Dagnault A., & Richard D. (1997). Involvement of the medial preoptic area in the anorectic action of estrogens. *Am J Physiol*, 272:R311-R317.

Detera-Wadleigh S., & McMahon F. (2004). Genetic association studies in mood disorders: issues and promise. *Int Rev Psychiatry*, 16:301–310.

Donovan M. (2005). Sex and racial differences in pharmacological response: effect of route of administration and drug delivery system on pharmacokinetics. *J Womens Health*, (Larchmt) 14:30–37.

Eastwood H., Brown KMO., Markovic D., & Pieri LF. (2002). Variation in the ESR1 and ESR2 genes and genetic susceptibility to anorexia nervosa. *Mol Psychiatry*, 7:86–89.

Emamian E., Hall D., Birnbaum M., Karayiorgou M., & Gogos J. (2004). Convergent evidence for impaired AKT1-GSK3beta signaling in schizophrenia. *Nat Genet*, 36:131–137.

Eme R. (1992). Selective female affliction in the developmental disorders of childhood: a literature review. *J Clinical Child Psychology*, 21:354–364.

Fan J, & Sklar P. (2005). Meta-analysis reveals association between serotonin transporter gene STin2 VNTR polymorphism and schizophrenia. *Mol Psychiatry*, 10:928–938.

Faraone S., Perlis R., Doyle A., Smoller J., Goralnick J., Holmgren M., et al. (2005). Molecular genetics of attention-deficit/hyperactivity disorder. *Biol Psychiatry*, 57:1313–1323.

Ferlin A., Garolla A., & Foresta C. (2005). Chromosome abnormalities in sperm of individuals with constitutional sex chromosomal abnormalities. *Cytogenet Genome Res*, 111:310–316.

Freedman R., Leonard S., Gault J., Hopkins J., Cloninger C., Kaufmann C., et al. (2001). Linkage disequilibrium for schizophrenia at the chromosome 15q13–14 locus of the alpha7-nicotinic acetylcholine receptor subunit gene (CHRNA7). *Am J Med Genet*, 105:20–22.

Fuks F. (2005). DNA methylation and histone modifications: teaming up to silence genes. *Curr Opin Genet Dev*, 15:490–495.

Funke B., Malhotra A., Finn C., Plocik A., Lake S., Lencz T., et al. (2005). COMT genetic variation confers risk for psychotic and affective disorders: a case control study. *Behav Brain Funct*, 1:19.

Gandhi M., Aweeka F., Greenblatt R., & Blaschke T. (2004). Sex differences in pharmacokinetics and pharmacodynamics. *Annu Rev Pharmacol Toxicol*, 44:499–523.

Garner C., & Slatkin M. (2003) On selecting markers for association studies: patterns of linkage disequilibrium between two and three diallelic loci. *Genet Epidemiol*, 24:57–67.

Gartler S.M., & Riggs A. (1983) Mammalian X-chromosome inactivation. *Annu Rev Genet*, 17:155–190.

Gizatullin R., Zaboli G., Jonsson E., Asberg M., & Leopardi R. (2006). Haplotype analysis reveals tryptophan hydroxylase (TPH) 1 gene variants associated with major depression. *Biol Psychiatry*, 59:295–300.

Glatt S., Faraone S., & Tsuang M.T. (2003). Meta-analysis identifies an association between the dopamine D2 receptor gene and schizophrenia. *Mol Psychiatry*, 8(11):911–915.

Grayson D., Jia X., Chen Y., Sharma R., Mitchell C., Guidotti A., et al. (2005). Reelin• promoter hypermethylation in schizophrenia. *Proc Natl Acad Sci U S A*, 102:9341–9346.

Grigoriadis S., & Seeman M. (2002). The role of estrogen in schizophrenia: implications for schizophrenia practice guidelines for women. *Can J Psychiatry*, 47:437–442.

Gutierrez B., Arias B., Gasto C., Catalan R., Papiol S., Pintor L., et al. (2004). Association analysis between a functional polymorphism in the monoamine oxidase A gene promoter and severe mood disorders. *Psychiatr Genet*, 14:203–208.

Harrison P., & Owen M. (2003). Genes for schizophrenia? Recent findings and their pathophysiological implications. *Lancet*, 361:417–419.

Hattori M., Kunugi H., Akahane A., Tanaka H., Ishida S., Hirose T., et al. (2002). Novel polymorphisms in the promoter region of the neurotrophin-3 gene and their associations with schizophrenia. *Am J Med Genet*, 114:304–309.

Heils A., Teufel A., Petri S., Stober G., Riederer P., Bengel D., et al. (1996). Allelic variation of human serotonin transporter gene expression. *J Neurochem*, 66:2621–2624.

Hennah W., Varilo T., Kestila M., Paunio T., Arajarvi R., Haukka J., et al. (2003). Haplotype transmission analysis provides evidence of association for DISC1 to schizophrenia and suggests sex-dependent effects. *Hum Mol Genet*, 12:3151–3159.

Herrington D. (2003). Role of estrogen receptor-alpha in pharmacogenetics of estrogen action. *Curr Opin Lipidol*, 14:145–150.

Huang Y., Oquendo M., Friedman J., Greenhill L., Brodsky B., Malone K., et al. (2002). Substance abuse disorder and major depression are associated with the human 5-HT1B receptor gene (HTR1B) G861C polymorphism. *Neuropsychopharmacology*, 28:163–169.

Ichikawa J., & Meltzer H. (1999). Relationship between dopaminergic and seratonergic neuronal activity in the frontal cortex and the action of typical and atypical antipsychotic drugs. *Eur Arch Psychiatry Clin Neurosci*, 249(Suppl 4):90–98.

Imle P. (2005). Aspects influencing genotyping method selection. *Methods Mol Biol*, 311:63–72.

Jacquet H., Raux G., Thibaut F., Hecketsweiler B., Houy E., Demilly C., et al. (2002). PRODH mutations and hyperprolinemia in a subset of schizophrenic patients. *Hum Mol Genet*, 11:2243–2249.

Jiang Y., Bressler J., & Beaudet A. (2004). Epigenetics and human disease. *Annu Rev Genomics Hum Genet*, 5:479–510.

Julius D. (1998). Serotonin receptor knockouts: a moody subject. *Proc Natl Acad Sci U S A*, 95: 15153–15154.

Justice A., de Wit H. (1999). Acute effects of d-amphetamine during the follicular and luteal phases of the menstrual cycle in women. *Psychopharmacology*, 145:67–75.

Justice A., de Wit H. (2000). Acute effects of estradiol pretreatment on the response to D-amphetamine in women. *Neuroendocrinology*, 71:51–59.

Kessler R., McGonagle K., Swartz M., Blazer D., & Nelson C. (1993). Sex and depression in the National Comorbidity Survey. I: Lifetime prevalence, chronicity and recurrence. *J Affect Disord*, 29:85–96.

Kim K., Lim S., Lee S., En Sohn S., Kim S., Gyu Hahn C., et al. (2000). Serotonin transporter gene and antidepressant response. *NeuroReport*, 11:215–219.

Koronyo-Hamaoui M., Danziger Y., Frisch A., Stein D., Leor S., Laufer N., et al. (2002). Association between anorexia nervosa and the hsKCa3 gene: a family-based and case control study. *Mol Psychiatry*, 7:82–85.

Lahey B., Pelham W., Schaughency E., Atkins M., Murphy H., Hynd G., et al. (1988). Dimensions and types of attention deficit disorder. *J Am Acad Child Adolesc Psychiatry*, 27:330–335.

Larsen T., Friis S., Haahr U., Joa I., Johannessen J., Melle I., et al. (2001). Early detection and intervention in first-episode schizophrenia: a critical review. *Acta Psychiatr Scand*, 103:323–324.

Lee H., Cha J., Ham B., Han C., Kim Y., Lee S., et al. (2004). Association between a G-protein beta 3 subunit gene polymorphism and the symptomatology and treatment responses of major depressive disorders. *Pharmacogenomics*, 4:29–33.

Lerer B., & Macciardi F. (2002). Pharmacogenetics of antidepressant and mood-stabilizing drugs: a review of candidate-gene studies and future research directions. *Neuropsychopharmacol*, 5:255–275.

Lerer B., Macciardi F., Segman R., Adolfsson R., Blackwood D., Blairy S., et al. (2001). Variability of 5-HT2C receptor cys23ser polymorphism among European populations and vulnerability to affective disorder. *Mol Psychiatry*,6:579–585.

Lesch K., Bengel D., Heils A., Sabol S., Greenberg B., Petri S., et al. (1996). Association of anxiety-related traits with a polymorphism in the serotonin transporter gene regulatory region. *Science*, 274:1527–1531.

Liang Y., Akishita M., Kim S., Ako J., Hashimoto M., Iijima K., et al. (2002). Estrogen receptor beta is involved in the anorectic action of estrogen. *Int J Obes Relat Metab Disord*, 26:1103–1109.

Licinio J., Wong M., & Gold P. (1996). The hypothalamic-pituitary-adrenal axis in anorexia nervosa. *Psychiatry Res*, 62:75–83.

Lim J., Papp A., Pinsonneault J., Sadee W., & Saffen D. (2006). Allelic expression of serotonin transporter (SERT) mRNA in human pons: lack of correlation with the polymorphism SERTLPR. *Mol Psychiatry*, 11:649–662.

Linden M., Bender B., & Robinson A. (2002). Genetic counseling for sex chromosome abnormalities. *Am J Med Genet*, 110:3–10.

Manor I., Tyano S., Mel E., Eisenberg J., Bachner-Melman R., Kotler M., et al. (2002). Family-based and association studies of monoamine oxidase A and attention deficit hyperactivity disorder (ADHD): preferential transmission of the long promoter-region repeat and its association with impaired performance on a continuous performance test (TOVA). *Mol Psychiatry*, 7:626–632.

McMahon F., Buervenich S., Charney D., Lipsky R., Rush A., Wilson A., et al. (2006). Variation in the gene encoding the serotonin 2A receptor is associated with outcome of antidepressant treatment. *Am J Hum Gen*, 78:804–814.

Millar JK., Wilson-Annan J., Anderson S., Christie S., Taylor M., Semple C., et al. (2002). Disruption of two novel genes by a translocation co-segregating with schizophrenia. *Hum Molec Genet*, 9:1415–1423.

Mimmack M., Ryan M., Baba H., Navarro-Ruiz J., Iritani S., Faull R., et al. (2002). Gene expression analysis in schizophrenia: reproducible up-regulation of several members of the apolipoprotein L family located in a high-susceptibility locus for schizophrenia on chromosome 22. *Proc Natl Acad Sci U S A*, 99:4680–4685.

Mogil J., Wilson S., Chesler E., Rankin A., Nemmani K., Lariviere W., et al. (2003). The melanocortin-1 receptor gene mediates female-specific mechanisms of analgesia in mice and humans. *Proc Natl Acad Sci U S A*, 100:4867–4872.

Moret C., & Briley M. (2000). The possible role of 5-HT(1B/D) receptors in psychiatric disorders and their potential as a target for therapy. *Eur J Pharmacol*, 404:1–12.

Neves-Pereira M., Cheung J., Pasdar A., Zhang F., Breen G., Yates P., et al. (2005). BDNF gene is a risk factor for schizophrenia in a Scottish population. *Mol Psychiatry*, 10:208–212.

Ogilvie A., Battersby S., Bubb V., Fink G., Harmar A., Goodwin G., et al. (1996). Polymorphism in serotonin transporter gene associated with susceptibility to major depression. *Lancet*, 347:731–733.

Palmisano G., Delfino L., Fiore M., Longo A., & Ferrara G. (2005). Single nucleotide polymorphisms detection based on DNA microarray technology: HLA as a model. *Autoimmun Rev*, 4:510–514.

Perlman W., Webster M., Kleinman J., & Weickert C. (2004). Reduced glucocorticoid and estrogen receptor alpha messenger ribonucleic acid levels in the amygdala of patients with major mental illness. *Biol Psychiatry*, 56:844–852.

Pinsonneault J., Papp A., & Sadee W. (2006). Allelic mRNA expression of X-linked monoamine oxidase A (MAOA) in human brain: dissection of epigenetic and genetic factors. *Hum Molec Genet*, 15(17): 2636–2649.

Powers P., & Santana C. (2004). Available pharmacological treatments for anorexia nervosa. *Expert Opin Pharmacother*, 5:2287–2292.

Preston N., Orr K., Date R., Nolan L., & Castle D. (2002). Gender differences in premorbid adjustment of patients with first episode psychosis. *Schizophr Res*, 55:285–290.

Qian Q., Wang Y., Zhou R., Li J., Wang B., Glatt S., et al. (2003). Family-based and case-control association studies of catechol-O-methyltransferase in attention deficit hyperactivity disorder suggest genetic sexual dimorphism. *Am J Med Genet B Neuropsychiatr Genet*, 118:103–109.

Quinn P. (2005). Treating adolescent girls and women with ADHD: gender-specific issues. *J Clin Psychol*, 61:579–587.

Quitkin F., Stewart J., McGrath P., Taylor B., Tisminetsky M., Petkova E., et al. (2002). Are there differences between women's and men's antidepressant responses? *Am J Psychiatry*, 159:1848–1854.

Rannala B. (2001). Finding genes influencing susceptibility to complex diseases in the post-genome era. *Am J Pharmacogenomics*, 1:203–221.

Rhee S., Waldman I., Hay D., & Levy F. (1999). Sex differences in genetic and environmental influences on DSM-III-R attention-deficit/hyperactivity disorder. *J Abnorm Psychol*, 108:24–41.

Ribases M., Gratacos M., Fernandez-Aranda F., Bellodi L., Boni C., Anderluh M., et al. (2004). Association of BDNF with anorexia, bulimia and age of onset of weight loss in six European populations. *Hum Mol Genet*, 13:1205–1212.

Rosenkranz K., Hinney A., Ziegler A., Hermann H., Fichter M., Mayer H., et al. (1998). Systematic mutation screening of the estrogen receptor beta gene in probands of different weight extremes: identification of several genetic variants. *J Clin Endocrinol Metab*, 83:4524–4527.

Sabol S., Hu S., & Hamer D. (1998). A functional polymorphism in the monoamine oxidase A gene promoter. *Hum Genet*, 103:273–279.

Sandovici I., Naumova A., Leppert M., Linares Y., & Sapienza C. (2004). A longitudinal study of X-inactivation ratio in human females. *Hum Genet*, 115:387–392.

Schneider L., Small G., Hamilton S., Bystritsky A., Nemeroff C., & Meyers B. (1997). Estrogen replacement and response to fluoxetine in a multicenter geriatric depression trial. *Am J Geriatr Psychiatry*, 5:97–106.

Schwartz J. (2003). The influence of sex on pharmacokinetics. *Clin Pharmacokinet*, 42:107–121.

Seeman P., Guan H., & Van Tol H. (1993). Dopamine D4 receptors elevated in schizophrenia. *Nature*, 365:441–445.

Sharp A., Robinson D., & Jacobs P. (2000). Age- and tissue-specific variation of X chromosome inactivation ratios in normal women. *Hum Genet*, 107:343–349.

Shinkai T., Ohmori O., Suzuki T., Kojima H., Hori H., Terao T., et al. (2000). Polymorphisms of tryptophan hydroxylase gene and the symptomatology of schizophrenia: an association study. *Psychiatr Genet*, 10: 165–171.

Sichel D., Cohen L., Robertson L., Ruttenberg A., & Rosenbaum J. (1995). Prophylactic estrogen in recurrent postpartum affective disorder. *Biol Psychiatry*, 38:814–818.

Sinibaldi L., De Luca A., Bellacchio E., Conti E., Pasini A., Paloscia C., et al. (2004). Mutations of the Nogo-66 receptor (RTN4R) gene in schizophrenia. *Hum Mutat*, 24:534–535.

Smeraldi E., Zanardi R., Benedetti F., Di Bella D., Perez J., & Catalano M. (1998). Polymorphism within the serotonin transporter and antidepressant efficacy of fluvoxamine. *Mol Psychiatry*, 3:508–511.

Spencer T., Biederman J., Wilens T., Faraone S., Prince J., Gerard K., et al. (2001). Efficacy of a mixed amphetamine salts compound in adults with attention-deficit/hyperactivity disorder. *Arch Gen Psychiatry*, 58:775–782.

Stefansson H., Sigurdsson E., Steinthorsdottir V., Bjornsdottir S., Sigmundsson T., Ghosh S., (2002). Neuregulin 1 and susceptibility to schizophrenia. *Am J Hum Genet*, 71:877–892.

Stein M., Waldman I., Sarampote C., Seymour K., Robb A., Conlon C., et al. (2005). Dopamine transporter genotype and methylphenidate dose response in children with ADHD. *Neuropsychopharmacol*, 30: 1374–1382.

Steiner M., Dunn E., & Born L. (2003). Hormones and mood: from menarche to menopause and beyond. *J Affect Disord*, 74:67–83.

Stevens J. (2002). Schizophrenia: reproductive hormones and the brain. *Am J Psychiatry*, 159:713–719.

Straub R., Jiang Y., MacLean C., Ma Y., Webb B., Myakishev M., et al. (2002). Genetic variation in the 6p22.3 gene DTNBP1, the human ortholog of the mouse dysbindin gene, is associated with schizophrenia. *Am J Hum Gen*, 71:337–348.

Sullivan P. (1995). Mortality in anorexia nervosa. *Am J Psychiatry*, 152:1073–1074.

Suzuki T., Iwata N., Kitamura Y., Kitajima T., Yamanouchi Y., Ikeda M., et al. (2003). Association of a haplotype in the serotonin 5-HT4 receptor gene (HTR4) with Japanese schizophrenia. *Am J Med Genet B Neuropsychiatr Genet*, 121: 7–13.

Terner J., & de Wit H. (2006). Menstrual cycle phase and responses to drugs of abuse in humans. *Drug Alcohol Depend*, 84(1):1–13.

Tsongalis G., & Coleman W. (2006). Clinical genotyping: the need for interrogation of single nucleotide polymorphisms and mutations in the clinical laboratory. *Clin Chim Acta*, 363:127–137.

Urwin R., & Nunn K. (2005) Epistatic interaction between the monoamine oxidase A and serotonin transporter genes in anorexia nervosa. *Eur J Hum Genet*, 13:370–3755.

Urwin R., Bennetts B., Wilcken B., Lampropoulos B., Beumont P., Russell J., et al. (2003). Gene-gene interaction between the monoamine oxidase A gene and solute carrier family 6 (neurotransmitter transporter, noradrenalin) member 2 gene in anorexia nervosa (restrictive subtype). *Eur J Hum Genet*, 11:945–950.

Van den Veyver I. (2001). Skewed X inactivation in X-linked disorders. *Semin Reprod Med*, 19:183–191.

Veenstra-VanderWeele J., Anderson G., & Cook E. (2000). Pharmacogenetics and the serotonin system: initial studies and future directions. *European J Pharmacology*, 410:165–181.

Villafuerte S., Del-Favero J., Adolfsson R., Souery D., Massat I., Mendlewicz J., et al. (2002). Gene-based SNP genetic association study of the corticotropin-releasing hormone receptor-2 (CRHR2) in major depression. *Am J Med Gen*, 114:222–226.

Vink T., Hinney A., van Elburg A., van Goozen S., Sandkuijl L., Sinke R., et al. (2001). Association between an agouti-related protein gene polymorphism and anorexia nervosa. *Mol Psychiatry*, 6:325–328.

Virgos C., Martorell L., Valero J., Figuera L., Civeira F., Joven J., et al. (2001). Association study of schizophrenia with polymorphisms at six candidate genes. *Schizophrenia Research*, 49:65–71.

Westberg L., Bah J., Rastam M., Gillberg C., Wentz E., Melke J., et al. (2002). Association between a polymorphism of the 5-HT2C receptor and weight loss in teenage girls. *Neuropsychopharmacol*, 26: 789–793.

Wonodi I., Stine O., Mitchell B., Buchanan R., & Thaker G. (2003). Association between Val108/158 Met polymorphism of the COMT gene and schizophrenia. *Am J Med Genet*, 120B:47–50.

Wright A. (2005). Neurogenetics II: complex disorders. *J Neurol Neurosurg Psychiatry*, 76:623–631.

Yu Y., Chen T., Wang Y., Liou Y., Hong C., & Tsai S. (2003). Association analysis for neuronal nitric oxide synthase gene polymorphism with major depression and fluoxetine response. *Neuropsychobiology*, 47: 137–140.

Zhao H., Pfeiffer R., & Gail M. (2003). Haplotype analysis in population genetics and association studies. *Pharmacogenomics*, 4:171–178.

Zill P., Baghai T., Zwanzger P., Schule C., Eser D., Rupprecht R., et al. (2004). SNP and haplotype analysis of a novel tryptophan hydroxylase isoform (TPH2) gene provide evidence for association with major depression. *Mol Psychiatry*, 9:1030–1036.

Zill P., Baghai T., Engel R., Zwanzger P., Schule C., Minov C., et al. (2003). Beta-1-adrenergic receptor gene in major depression: influence on antidepressant treatment response. *Am J Med Genet*, 120B:85–89.

Zubenko G., Hughes H., III, Stiffler J., Brechbiel A., Zubenko W., & Maher B., (2003). Sequence variations in CREB1 cosegregate with depressive disorders in women. *Mol Psychiatry*, 8:611–618.

Chapter 6

Sex Differences in HPA
Axis Regulation

Elizabeth A. Young, Ania Korszun,
Helmer F. Figueiredo, Matia Banks-Solomon,
and James P. Herman

Living organisms survive by maintaining a complex dynamic equilibrium or homeostasis. Internal stressors (e.g., infection, blood glucose changes, hemodynamic changes) and external stressors (e.g., threat, danger, pain) occur constantly. Stressors set in motion responses aimed at preserving homeostasis, including activation of the hypothalamic-pituitary-adrenal (HPA) axis. HPA activation is a hormonal cascade that is initiated with the activation of neurons in the hypothalamic paraventricular nucleus and subsequent release of corticotropin-releasing hormone (CRH), which stimulates the release of adrenocorticotropic hormone (ACTH) from the anterior pituitary corticotrope. ACTH, in turn, triggers the release of adrenal glucocorticoids into systemic circulation. The stress response is turned off by glucocorticoid negative feedback at brain and pituitary sites (Fig. 6.1).

There is evidence in both rats and humans that stress response is sexually dimorphic, and our studies in rats and humans have suggested that gonadal steroids play an important role in modulating the HPA axis (Young et al., 1993). Gonadal steroids may influence the HPA axis regulatory mechanisms through effects on glucocorticoid receptors, on brain CRH systems, on pituitary responsiveness to CRH, and on adrenal responsiveness to ACTH (Figueiredo et al., 2007).

HPA AXIS REGULATION

Glucocorticoids act via multiple mechanisms and at several sites to inhibit their own release. At the pituitary level, glucocorticoids exert direct effects on the ACTH precursor prohormone, proopiomelanocortocotropin (POMC) gene transcription, POMC mRNA levels, and subsequent ACTH peptide stores in primary pituitary cell cultures *in vitro* (Birnberg et al., 1982; Roberts et al., 1979; Schacter et al., 1982). These effects involve the classic glucocorticoid receptor (GR, Type II), which binds glucocorticoids, is translocated to the nucleus, and binds to sites on the

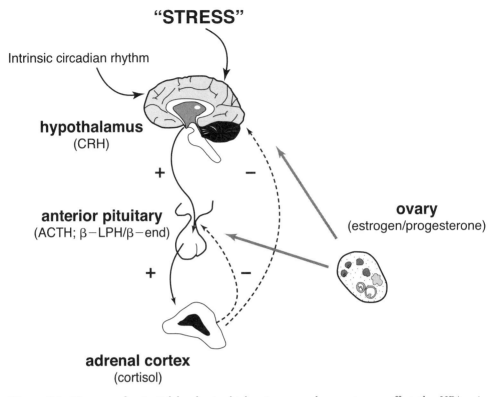

Figure 6.1. Diagram of potential levels at which estrogen and progesterone affect the HPA axis. Studies to date indicate that estradiol can regulate stress responsiveness at the brain, including effects on CRH regulation in the hypothalamus. Data also suggest direct effects of estradiol on pituitary responsiveness in rodents. In humans, progesterone has been found to increase stress responsiveness to exercise stress in normal women in a hypogonadal state. Finally, estradiol affects levels of corticosteroid binding globulin (CBG), which can lead to greater activation of the stress axis since levels of free glucocorticoids are regulated by the amount of CBG.

DNA (Schacter et al., 1982). Studies have demonstrated that glucocorticoids interact with the CRH receptors in the anterior pituitary, acutely inhibiting the binding of CRH to its receptor and chronically decreasing CRH receptor number (Childs et al., 1986; Schwartz et al., 1986). Such direct effects of glucocorticoids on CRH receptors may account for some of the inhibitory action of glucocorticoids on ACTH release *in vitro*.

In addition to pituitary sites of action, glucocorticoids act at brain sites to modulate HPA axis activity. Early work by McEwen and colleagues (1968) demonstrated a very high-affinity uptake of corticosterone in the hippocampus of adrenalectomized rats injected *in vivo* with radiolabeled steroids. These receptors were difficult to demonstrate in non-adrenalectomized rats, presumably because these sites were saturated under resting conditions (McEwen et al., 1970). The receptors were not labeled by [^{3}H]dexamethasone, suggesting multiple types of glucocorticoid receptors (deKloet et al., 1975).

The observation of receptor heterogeneity has been expanded upon by deKloet and colleagues, who subsequently demonstrated two glucocorticoid receptor types: the mineralocorticoid receptor (MR) which has particularly high affinity for the glucocorticoid corticosterone (rats) or cortisol (humans) and the glucocorticoid receptor (GR), which preferentially binds dexamethasone (Reul & deKloet, 1985). Like other steroid receptors, both MR and GR function as transcription factors to regulate gene activation. GRs are widely distributed throughout multiple stress-regulatory sites in the brain, whereas MRs exist predominantly in the hippocampus, amygdala and septum. In addition to action at the pituitary and hypothalamus, there is evidence from animal experiments that forebrain "limbic" sites, including the hippocampus and medial prefrontal cortex, are prominent glucocorticoid feedback sites in the brain.

SEX DIFFERENCES IN HPA AXIS REGULATION – ANIMAL STUDIES

Studies in rodents reveal sex differences in several elements of the HPA axis. Female rats appear to have a more robust HPA axis response to stress than do male rats, and estradiol appears at least partly responsible for this sexual difference. For example, compared with male rats, female rats secrete corticosterone sooner after stress and display higher rates of increase in plasma corticosterone concentration (Jones et al., 1972). This increased corticosterone response is accompanied by a greatly increased ACTH response (Young, 1996). HPA axis hyper-responsiveness to acute stressful stimuli is especially pronounced during proestrus (Ogle & Kitay, 1977; Viau & Meaney, 1991), when circulating estrogens and progesterone peak, and is abolished by ovariectomy (Critchlow et al., 1963; Seale et al., 2004b), suggesting that activational hormonal effects mediate the sex difference. In addition, exogenous estradiol replacement in ovariectomized rats enhances basal ACTH secretion (Carey et al., 1995) (but see (Viau & Meaney, 1991). Compared to gonadally intact males, ovaeriectomized females still demonstrate stress hyper-responsiveness (Young, 1996) although the difference may be due to inhibitory effects of testosterone on stress responsiveness (Viau & Meaney, 1996).

Hormone replacement studies have yielded a complicated picture of the role of gonadal hormones as positive regulators of the HPA axis. Early investigations demonstrated that exogenous administration of estradiol to ovariectomized rats increases plasma ACTH and plasma corticosterone concentrations in response to restraint, footshock, or novelty stress (Viau & Meaney, 1991; Burgess & Handa, 1992; Carey et al., 1995). However, some of these studies used either supra-physiological doses or prolonged time periods (21 days) of estradiol replacement.

In contrast, data from our group (Young et al., 2001; Figueiredo et al., 2004) and others (Redei et al., 1994; Dayas et al., 2000) indicate that when ovariectomized rats are given estradiol at physiologically-relevant concentrations, the ACTH response to acute stress is decreased, suggesting that short-term exposure to estradiol inhibits rather than stimulates plasma ACTH responses to stress and that the effects of higher doses and/or longer periods of estradiol exposure are likely to be pharmacological rather than physiological (Young et al., 2001).

There are further interesting complications. Recently, we found that estradiol enhances plasma corticosterone response to restraint, despite dampening the ACTH response (Figueiredo et al., 2004). This surprising finding suggests that estradiol acts at least peripherally to stimulate adrenal gland sensitivity to ACTH. Indeed, emerging findings from our laboratory indicate that exogenous estradiol administration dramatically enhances adrenal sensitivity to ACTH in dexamethasone-treated ovariectomized rats.

This finding indicates that the increased sensitivity to ACTH in estradiol-treated females potentially overcomes estradiol-mediated reduction in central drive of the HPA axis, resulting in a net increase in glucocorticoid release in these animals' response (Figueiredo et al., 2004). Finally, corticosteroid-binding globulin (CBG), which reduces free corticosterone concentration, is positively regulated by estradiol and thus higher in female rats. Therefore, at least part of the elevated corticosterone levels seen in females is negated by elevated CBG levels.

It is likely that estradiol also acts centrally to regulate hypothalamic CRH response to stress. Interestingly, a partial estrogen response element is found on the CRH gene, which confers estradiol enhancement of CRH expression in CV-1 transfected cells (Vamvakopoulos & Chrousos, 1993); and thus, provides a plausible mechanism by which estradiol may modulate stress responsiveness in females. Systemic administration of estradiol increases CRH mRNA expression in the PVN (Patchev & Almeida, 1996; Li et al., 2003). Together, these data suggest that estradiol can drive transcription of the CRH gene, which may then affect subsequent response capacity. Some reports, however, in which estradiol either decreased PVN CRH peptide/mRNA (Haas & George, 1988; Paulmyer-Lacroix et al., 1996) or had no effect on PVN CRH transcription (Redei et al., 1994) appear contradictory. In short, consensus has not yet emerged regarding the impact of estrogens on PVN CRH transcription *in vivo*. It is important to note that estrogen receptor ERα expression is quite sparse in the PVN (Shughrue et al., 1997; Laflamme et al., 1998);

and while ERβ colocalization with CRH PVN neurons is very limited, it is richly expressed in the magnocellular oxytocin and AVP neurons of the PVN (Alves et al., 1998; Hrabovszky et al., 1998; Isgor et al., 2003). Thus, estradiol's effects on CRH-secreting parvocellular neurons likely occur indirectly, perhaps via transsynaptic inputs. It remains possible that chronic stress may change ER expression in the PVN as noted by Gerritis et al. (2005).

Another mechanism by which estradiol might pharmacologically increase the HPA stress response is through inhibition of glucocorticoid feedback mechanisms. A steeper rate of rise of corticosterone is necessary to elicit glucocorticoid fast feedback in female rats than male rats (Jones et al., 1972). Two studies (Burgess & Handa, 1992; Viau & Meaney, 1991) demonstrate that estradiol treatment delays the ACTH and glucocorticoid shut-off following stress in estradiol-treated female rats, compared with ovariectomized female rats. In addition, estradiol treatment blocks down regulation of hippocampal glucocorticoid receptors following chronic administration of RU 28362, a glucocorticoid agonist in rats. Following long-term (21 days) estradiol treatment, the potent and selective glucocorticoid RU 28362 was ineffective in blocking ether-stress-induced ACTH secretion (Burgess & Handa, 1992). Given the doses and timing of estradiol used in this study, these may be pharmacological effects of estradiol.

Progesterone, like estradiol, may dampen feedback mechanisms in the HPA axis. Progesterone infusions into ewes diminished the effectiveness of cortisol feedback on stress responsiveness *in vivo* (Keller-Wood et al., 1988). Similar effects were observed in pregnant ewes, which have naturally elevated progesterone levels (Keller-Wood et al., 1988). In addition, progesterone promotes anti-glucocorticoid effects on feedback in intact rats *in vivo* and *in vitro* (Svec 1988, Duncan & Duncan, 1979).

Progesterone binds avidly to GR, but at a different site than do glucocorticoids (Svec, 1988). Progesterone can also increase the rate of dissociation of glucocorticoids from the GR (Rousseau et al., 1972). In addition, in cultured rat hepatoma cells, dexamethasone and progesterone bind to the same receptor, and progesterone is a clear competitive antagonist of dexamethasone binding. In expressed human MR, progesterone and dexamethasone displayed similar affinity for MR (Arriza et al., 1987). Furthermore, in female rats, progesterone treatment increased MR

binding as measured with dexamethasone (Carey et al., 1995). Finally, progesterone upregulated glucocorticoid receptor number in the hippocampus (Ahima et al., 1992), which may account for greater glucocorticoid receptor number in the hippocampus of female rats relative to males (Turner & Weaver, 1985).

We examined sex differences in sensitivity to glucocorticoid-negative feedback, and the extent to which removal of estrogens and progesterone by ovariectomy affects glucocorticoid-negative feedback in rats. The designs exploited our finding that both corticosterone pellets and corticosterone injections lead to clear suppressions of circadian-driven ACTH and corticosterone secretion, as well as profound inhibition of the stress response in male rats (Young & Vasquez, 1996).

We used these two treatments to block stress responsiveness in the morning and evening in male, intact female, and ovariectomized female rats (Young, 1996). Both treatments produced similar effects, including: failure of exogenous cortisol to block the stress response of intact female rats; and increased sensitivity to corticosterone in ovariectomized female rats, generating a response similar to that of male rats. However, there remained a difference between ovariectomized female rats and male rats, suggesting that in addition to activational effects of ovarian steroid hormones present at the time of study, organizational effects dependent upon prenatal effects of steroid hormones on the organization of brain systems accounted for some of the sex differences (Young, 1996).

Furthermore, we found dexamethasone to inhibit stress responsiveness in male and female rats similarly, suggesting that resistance to corticosterone may involve mechanisms not invoked by dexamethasone, such as MR. Estradiol may inhibit glucocorticoid feedback mechanisms by altering GR (Burgess & Handa, 1992) or by increasing CRH mRNA levels and thus increasing CRH stores (Vamvakopoulos & Chrousos, 1993). However, it is unlikely that sex differences in resistance to glucocorticoid suppression can be accounted for by sex differences in the number of glucocorticoid receptors (Turner & Weaver, 1985), as females have higher numbers of receptors than males.

Although relevant to human health, the roles of sex differences and ovarian steroids in chronic stress responses have received little attention. To address this issue, our group used a chronic variable stress (CVS) model to investigate male-female differences in long-term stress (Figueiredo & Herman, 2005). The

CVS model circumvents habituation of the stress response by using several stressors, including vibration, hypoxia, cold room, cold swim and warm swim, presented twice daily and unpredictably (one stressor in the morning and another in the afternoon).

Exposure to a 15-d CVS significantly reduced weight gain in both sexes. Adrenal gland weights were significantly greater in control females than males, and CVS increased adrenal weight only in males. Thus, thymus weight (an immune tissue sensitive to mean glucocorticoid exposure) normalized to body weight was significantly decreased only in females, suggesting that chronic stress increases the vulnerability of immune function in females. Importantly, while CVS significantly enhanced plasma corticosterone response to novel restraint stress in both sexes, this response was dramatically exacerbated in CVS females (Fig. 6.2).

In keeping with this finding, glucocorticoid hypersecretion in chronically stressed female rats has also been reported during chronic restraint stress (Galea et al., 1997) and after chronic mild stress (Duncko et al., 2001). Taken together, these findings indicate that female rats are particularly sensitive to chronic stress and to the deleterious effects of corticosterone hypersecretion.

Again, it is likely that the sexual dimorphism in the HPA responses to chronic stress is mediated at least in part by activational effects of ovarian steroids at multiple levels of the HPA axis. Thus, high doses of es-

tradiol potentiated plasma corticosterone secretion and AVP mRNA expression in the PVN of ovariectomized female rats submitted to repeated restraint stress (Lunga & Herbert, 2004). Interestingly, however, while estradiol decreased basal CRH mRNA in the PVN of ovariectomized rats compared to vehicle-treated animals, it had no effect on that of acute or repeated stressed rats (Lunga & Herbert, 2004), suggesting the presence of additional mechanisms in the stress response of females. It is clear that future animal studies examining the precise interplay between ovarian steroids and chronic stress will be of valuable importance for understanding the pathophysiology of HPA axis dysregulation that occurs in stress-related disorders that predominate in women, such as major depression and anorexia nervosa.

In contrast to the stimulatory actions of estrogens and progesterone, several studies demonstrate that testosterone inhibits basal and stress-induced HPA axis activity in male rats (for review, see Viau, 2002). Under basal conditions, gonadectomized male rats have higher plasma ACTH, higher plasma corticosterone levels and increased corticosterone pulsatility relative to intact controls (Seale et al., 2004). Similarly, gonadectomized males display increased corticosterone and ACTH responses to a variety of stressors, including footshock, novel open field, restraint, noise, or lipopolysaccharide administration (Handa et al., 1994; Viau & Meaney, 1996; Seale et al., 2004). This

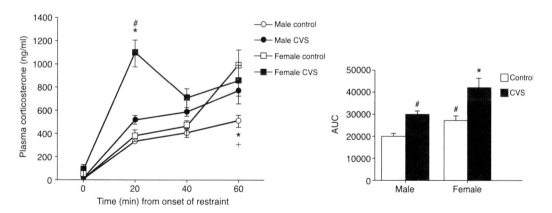

Figure 6.2. Plasma corticosterone responses to a novel 40-min restraint stress one day after a 15-day CVS exposure. Note the robust response in the female rats, notably CVS females, compared to their male counterpart. *P<.05 vs. CVS male and control female; #P<.05 vs. control male; +P<.05 vs. CVS female. Reprinted with permission from Young EA, Korszun A (1999). Women stress and depression: sex differences in hypothalamic-pituitary-adrenal axis. In Leibenluft E. (Ed.), *Gender differences in mood and anxiety disorders: from bench to bedside*. Washington DC: American Psychiatric Press, Inc.

orchiectomy-induced enhancement of HPA axis responses to acute stressors can be reversed with replacement of testosterone or with the non-aromatizable androgen dihydrotestosterone proprionate (Handa et al., 1994; Viau & Meaney, 1996; Seale et al., 2004), suggesting a role of androgen receptors in mediating the inhibitory effect of androgens on the HPA axis.

Orchiectomy also increases AVP, CRH, and GR mRNA expression in the PVN in unstressed male rats. Furthermore, in males, the activity of the HPA axis is apparently regulated by corticosterone-dependent effects on CRH and testosterone-dependent effects on AVP in the PVN (Viau et al., 1999). For example, castration blocked stress enhancement of AVP mRNA, but not CRH mRNA expression in the PVN following adrenalectomy in male rats (Viau et al., 1999). In contrast, stress-induced PVN activity is modulated by interactions between testosterone and corticosterone (Viau, 2002).

Like ERα and ERβ expression, androgen receptor expression is present within the PVN, but is absent in the medial parvocellular neurosecretory neurons (Zhou et al., 1994). In addition, anterior pituitary corticotrophs express few, if any, androgen receptors (Thieulant & Duval, 1985). Thus, if testosterone acts via the androgen receptor, it is likely doing so above the level of the PVN. However, testosterone is aromatized to estradiol in the brain (Martini et al., 1996; Celotti et al., 1997), and thus may act through estrogen receptors as well.

Several sites outside the PVN have been identified where gonadal hormones may modulate HPA axis activity. The medial preoptic area (MPOA) is a region rich in ER, ERβ and androgen receptor, and MPOA implants of testosterone or corticosterone reduce plasma ACTH and corticosterone responses to restraint and decrease AVP (but not CRH) content in the median eminence (Viau & Meaney, 1996). Furthermore, lesions of the MPOA block inhibitory actions of testosterone on ACTH and corticosterone responses to restraint (Viau & Meaney, 1996). In addition, systemic testosterone stimulated CRH expression in the anterior fusiform cortex and AVP mRNA expression in the posterior bed nucleus of the stria terminalis: two regions that are intimately involved in regulation of HPA function (Viau et al., 2001).

Social stress studies indicate that plasma testosterone correlates with dominant behavior whereas reduced testosterone levels are related to submission. For example, in the visible burrow system model of rodent social stress (Blanchard et al., 1995), subordinate males rats are characterized by severe weight loss, decreased plasma testosterone levels, and increased basal levels of corticosterone compared to dominant males (Monder et al., 1994). The neural mechanisms relating plasma testosterone levels with social stress remain to be determined.

SEX DIFFERENCES IN HPA AXIS REGULATION—STUDIES IN HUMANS

The data reviewed thus far in this chapter indicate that sexual dimorphism in HPA axis regulation exists in rats and other animal models. But do similar dimorphisms exist in humans? Until recently, the lack of a reliable stress test has limited the studies on sex differences in stress response in humans.

In the Trier Social Stress Test (TSST), in which subjects undergo a mock job interview in front of a panel of interviewers who are instructed not to provide any verbal or non-verbal feedback, is a reliable and robust stressor in normal subjects (Kirschbaum et al., 1995).

It has been shown that oral contraceptives decrease the free cortisol response to this social stressor in women (Kirschbaum et al., 1995), whereas 48-h treatment of gonadally intact men with estradiol hours increased ACTH and cortisol responses to it (Kirschbaum et al., 1996). These effects of estradiol treatment in men are consistent with results of studies in rats (Burgess & Handa, 1992; Viau & Meaney, 1991) while the effects of oral contraceptives in women are not consistent with the animal literature.

The results from studies of oral contraceptives are harder to interpret, however, because they are synthetic steroids that may differ from endogenous steroids in their effects. Furthermore, since the effect of estradiol was tested in gonadally-intact men, the enhanced responsiveness to stress could have resulted from decreased testosterone levels (see section on testosterone effect on the HPA axis). This finding is confirmed in postmenopausal women by the lack of effect of estradiol replacement on stress response to the TSST (Kudielka et al., 1999). Komesaroff et al., (1999) also showed decreased ACTH and cortisol response to mental arithmetic following estradiol replacement in post-menopausal women. Length of estradiol treatment, type of stressor, and pre-existing hormonal milieu may all affect the results of estradiol administration in humans.

In addition to these studies on HPA responses to social stress, there are sex differences in the response of the HPA axis to pharmacologic challenges. For example, we found a 40% greater cortisol response to oCRH in women than in men, again consistent with animal studies. As oCRH acts in the pituitary, this result suggests that the sex difference arises at the level of the pituitary or adrenal rather than the brain. In a study of the cortisol response to dexamethasone-CRH challenge in premenopausal and postmenopausal women before and after 2 weeks of estradiol treatment, Kudielka et al. (1999) found that estradiol inhibited the cortisol response to this challenge in postmenopausal women only.

Many studies that were conducted before assays could measure ACTH reliably in humans were available measured another product derived from proopiomelanocortin, the ACTH precursor, beta-lipotropin / beta-endorphin. In one study, we found that infusion of cortisol turns off corticotroph secretion within 15 minutes of the onset of a rise in cortisol in both premenopausal females and age-matched male control subjects (Young et al., 1995). However, following the termination of the infusion, men exhibited continued inhibition of corticotroph secretion for 60 min, whereas women began to secrete ß-lipotropin / ß-endorphin within this hour. This difference may be dependent upon progesterone.

Women in the follicular phase with low plasma progesterone concentrations exhibited patterns of suppression of ß-lipotropin / ß-endorphin secretion similar to the men (Young et al., 1995). In contrast, women with progesterone concentrations typical of the luteal phase showed rebound ß-lipotropin/ ß-endorphin secretion following termination of cortisol infusion. Thus, these data suggest that progesterone antagonizes the feedback effects of cortisol in humans, consistent with the Keller-Wood (1988) demonstration of an antagonistic effect of progesterone on the feedback effects of cortisol infusion in ewes. Combined with the *in vitro* evidence for antagonistic effects of progesterone at the GR described above, the data suggest that progesterone is an important modulator of HPA axis function in humans.

The interactions between gonadal steroids and the HPA axis activity have also been examined in pregnancy and in the menstrual cycle. In pregnancy, increases in both estrogens and progesterone occur.

Increases in plasma CBG and cortisol during pregnancy are also well documented, and dexamethasone challenge studies indicate resistance to glucocorticoid negative feedback during pregnancy (Carr et al., 1981; Demey-Ponsart et al., 1982; Nolten & Rueckert, 1981).

However, the degree to which post-dexamethasone hypercortisolism is simply an artifact of increased CBG levels (leading to higher levels of plasma cortisol following dexamethasone administration) is not completely known. Although dexamethasone itself is not bound by CBG, pregnancy could alter the metabolism of dexamethasone so as to result in less dexamethasone bioavailability. At least one study (Nolten & Rueckert, 1981) demonstrated higher free cortisol, higher free cortisol production following an ACTH infusion, decreased suppression of free cortisol by dexamethasone, and a normal circadian rhythm of cortisol during pregnancy, taken together suggesting a change in cortisol set-point during pregnancy. Again, these data are compatible with both animal and human studies showing that both estradiol and progesterone can antagonize the effects of glucocorticoids on negative feedback.

With respect to the menstrual cycle, Altemus and her colleagues (1997) reported increased resistance to dexamethasone suppression during the luteal phase of the menstrual cycle, as compared to the follicular phase, a change that may again be related to either increased estradiol or progesterone during the luteal phase. We, however, found no menstrual cycle variations in basal ACTH or cortisol levels across 24 h (Young et al., 2001). We also found no difference in the ACTH response to glucocorticoid blockade with metyrapone between the follicular and luteal phases (Altemus & Young, unpublished data). Together, these data suggest that basal drive is unchanged by the menstrual cycle, but that negative feedback may be altered across the menstrual cycle. Consistent with this, Kirschbaum et al. (1999) found that ACTH and free (saliva) cortisol responses to the TSST were greater in the luteal phase than the follicular phase, although total (plasma) cortisol showed no menstrual cycle difference, and Altemus et al. (2001) found a greater ACTH response to exercise stress in the mid-luteal compared to the follicular phase in normal women.

An alternative to the classic ovariectomy and replacement hormone studies that can be done in animals is short-term suppression of gonadal steroids with gonadotrophin-releasing hormone (GnRH) agonists, such as Lupron, which causes suppression of both estradiol and progesterone secretion. Roca et al. (2003) first treated normal women with Lupron and then gave them sequential estradiol and progesterone replacement. They found that the exercise stress response was increased and that the response to dexamethasone feedback was decreased during the progesterone "add back" phase, but not during the estradiol "add back" phase, thus providing further evidence that that progesterone acts as a glucocorticoid antagonist.

More recently, the researchers compared leuprolide-induced hypogonadal hormone conditions in normal men and women and found a greater response to exercise stress in men than women, suggesting that sex differences in stress response may be organizational effects of gonadal hormones (Roca et al., 2005). Thus, the data from human studies suggest that ovarian steroids influence the HPA axis response to stress by modulating sensitivity to negative feedback and in addition that there are overall sex differences in stress responsiveness that persist in hypogonadal states.

SUMMARY AND CONCLUSIONS

This review focuses on the interactions between gonadal steroids and the HPA axis, especially the ability of gonadal steroids to modulate glucocorticoid-negative feedback during stress. It is clear that gonadal steroids play a modulatory role in HPA axis regulation in both animals and humans. Although the precise mechanisms mediating ovarian hormone actions remain largely unclear, it is likely that both estrogens and progestins act at multiple sites of the HPA axis. Substantial experimental evidence supports an anti-glucocorticoid effect of progesterone, mediated in part by a modulatory site for progesterone on GR, it is also likely that estradiol plays a role in females' increased resistance to HPA feedback inhibition. Studies in rodents demonstrate that exogenous estradiol treatment enhances or diminishes stress responsiveness depending on the dose and/or exposure time periods of steroid exposure. Finally, it is important to bear in mind that estradiol can increase adrenal gland sensitivity to circulating ACTH, thus offering an additional peripheral mechanism for glucocorticoid hypersecretion in females.

It is possible that gonadal steroid antagonism of glucocorticoid feedback mechanisms and the consequent increased stress responsiveness of females contribute to the increased prevalence of anxiety disorders and autonomic hyper-arousal in women compared with men. In addition, as noted above, organizational differences between male and female brains are caused by exposure to high levels of gonadal steroids in the pre- and perinatal periods. The interactions of these organizational effects in females with cyclical gonadal steroid hormone changes following puberty, followed then by menopause and the loss of these same steroids, suggest that stress responsiveness and susceptibility to stress-related disorders could vary substantially over the lifetime of women. Women's increased vulnerability to depression arises at puberty, when gonadal steroids could further enhance stress responsiveness (Kessler et al., 1993). Further research is needed into the interaction of stress, cyclic hormone changes, and menopause.

References

Ahima RS, Lawson ANL, Osei SYS and Harlan RE. (1992). Sexual dimorphism in regulation of type II corticosteroid receptor immunoreactivity in the rat hippocampus *Endocrinology*, 131:1409–1416.

Altemus M, Redwine L, Yung-Mei L, Yoshikawa T, Yehuda R, Detera-Wadleigh S, Murphy D. (1997). Reduced sensitivity to glucocorticoid feedback and reduced glucocorticoid receptor mRNA expression in the luteal phase of the menstrual cycle. *Neurosychopharmacology*, 17(2):100–109.

Altemus M, Roca C, Galliven E, Romanos C, Deuster P. (2001). Increased vasopressin and adrenocorticotropin responses to stress in the midluteal phase of the menstrual cycle. *J Clin Endocrinol Metab*, 86(6):2525–2530.

Alves SE, Lopez V, McEwen BS, Weiland NG. (1998). Differential colocalization of estrogen receptor beta (ERbeta) with oxytocin and vasopressin in the paraventricular and supraoptic nuclei of the female rat brain: an immunocytochemical study. *Proc Natl Acad Sci USA*, 17;95(6):3281–3286.

Arriza JL, Weinberger C, Cerelli G, Glaser TM, Handelin BL, Housman DE, Evans, RM. (1987). Cloning of human mineralocorticoid receptor complementary DNA: structural and functional kinship with the glucocorticoid receptor. *Science*, 237:268–275.

Birnberg NC, Civelli O, Lissitzski JC, Hinman M, Herbert E. (1979). Regulation of pro-opiomelanocortin gene expression in the pituitary and central nervous system. *Endocrinology*, 110:134A.

Blanchard DC, Spencer RL, Weiss SM, Blanchard RJ, McEwen B, Sakai RR. (1995). Visible burrow system as a model of chronic social stress: behavioral and neuroendocrine correlates. *Psychoneuroendocrinology*, 20:117–134.

Burgess LH, Handa RJ. (1992). Chronic estrogen-induced alterations in adrenocorticotropin and corticosterone secretion, and glucocorticoid receptor-mediated functions in female rats. *Endocrinology*, 131:1261–1269.

Carey MP, Deterd CH, de Koning J, Helmerhorst F, de Kloet ER. (1995). The influence of ovarian steroids on hypothalamic-pituitary-adrenal regulation in the female rat. *J Endocrinol*, 144:311–321.

Carr BR, Parker CR Jr, Madden, JD, MacDonald PC, Porter JC. (1981). Maternal plasma adrenocorticotropin and cortisol relationships throughout human pregnancy. *Am J Obstet Gynecol*, 139:416–422.

Celotti F, Negri-Cesi P, Poletti A. (1997). Steroid metabolism in the mammalian brain: 5alpha-reduction and aromatization. *Brain Res Bull*, 44:365–375.

Childs GV, Morell JL, Niendorf A, Aguilera G. (1986). Cytochemical studies of corticotropin releasing factor receptors in anterior lobe corticotrophs: binding, glucocorticoid regulation and endocytosis of [Biotinyl-Ser1] CRF. *Endocrinology*, 119:2129.

Critchlow V, Liebelt RA, Bar-Sela M, Mountcastle W, Lipscomb HS. (1963). Sex difference in resting pituitary-adrenal function in the rat. *Am J Physiol*, 205: 807–815.

Dayas CV, Xu Y, Buller KM, Day TA. (2000). Effects of chronic oestrogen replacement on stress-induced activation of hypothalamic-pituitary-adrenal axis control pathways. *J Neuroendocrinol*, 12:784–794.

deKloet R. Wallach G, McEwen BS. (1975). Differences in corticosterone and dexamethasone binding to rat brain and pituitary. *Endocrinology*, 96:598.

Demey-Ponsart E, Foidart JM, Sulon J, Sodoyez JC. (1982). Serum CBG, free and total cortisol and circadian patterns of adrenal function in normal pregnancy. *J Steroid Biochem*, 16:165–169.

Duncan MR, Duncan GR. (1979). An in vivo study of the action of antiglucocorticoids on thymus weight ratio, antibody titre and the adrenal-pituitary-hypothalamus axis. *J Steroid Biochem*, 10:245–259.

Duncko R, Kiss A, Skultetyova I, Rusnak M, Jezova D. (2001). Corticotropin-releasing hormone mRNA levels in response to chronic mild stress rise in male but not in female rats while tyrosine hydroxylase mRNA levels decrease in both sexes. *Psychoneuroendocrinology*, 26:77–89.

Figueiredo HF, Herman JP. (2005). Chronic stress-induced facilitation is exacerbated in female rats. In: *Society for Neuroscience*. Washington, DC: Society for Neuroscience Online.

Figueiredo HF, Ulrich-Lai YM, Herman JP. (2004). Estrogen promotes glucocorticoid hypersecretion in female rats by increasing adrenal gland sensitivity to ACTH. In: *Society for Neuroscience*. Washington, DC: Society for Neuroscience Online.

Figueiredo HF, Ulrich-Lai YM, Choi DC, Herman JP. (2007). Estrogen potentiates adrenocortical responses to stress in female rats. *Am J Physiol Endocrinol Metab*, 292(4):E1173–1182.

Galea LA, McEwen BS, Tanapat P, Deak T, Spencer RL, Dhabhar FS. (1997). Sex differences in dendritic atrophy of CA3 pyramidal neurons in response to chronic restraint stress. *Neuroscience*, 81: 689–697.

Gerrits M, Grootkarijn A, Bekkering BF, Bruinsma M, Den Boer JA, Ter Horst GJ. (2005). Cyclic estradiol replacement attenuates stress-induced c-Fos expression in the PVN of ovariectomized rats. *Brain Res Bull*, 67:147–155.

Haas DA, George SR. (1988). Gonadal regulation of corticotropin-releasing factor immunoreactivity in hypothalamus. *Brain Res Bull*, 20: 361–367.

Handa RJ, Burgess LH, Kerr JE, O'Keefe JA. (1994a). Gonadal steroid hormone receptors and sex differences in the hypothalamo-pituitary-adrenal axis. *Horm Behav*, 28:464–476.

Hrabovszky E, Kallo I, Hajszan T, Shughrue PJ, Merchenthaler I, Liposits Z. (1998). Expression of estrogen receptor-beta messenger ribonucleic acid in oxytocin and vasopressin neurons of the rat supraoptic and paraventricular nuclei. *Endocrinology*, 139:2600–2604.

Isgor C, Shieh KR, Akil H, Watson SJ. (2003). Colocalization of estrogen beta-receptor messenger RNA with orphanin FQ, vasopressin and oxytocin in the rat hypothalamic paraventricular and supraoptic nuclei. *Anat Embryol* (Berl), 206:461–469.

Jones MT, Brush FR, Neame RLB. (1972). Characteristics of fast feedback control of corticotrophin release by corticosteroids. *J Endocrinol*, 55:489.

Keller-Wood M, Silbiger J, Wood CE. (1988). Progesterone attenuates the inhibition of adrenocorticotropin responses by cortisol in nonpregnant ewes. *Endocrinology*, 123:647–651.

Kessler RC, McGonagle KA, Swartz M, Blazer DG, Nelson CB. (1993). Sex and depression in the National Comorbidity Survey I: lifetime prevalence, chronicity and recurrence. *J Affect Dis*, 29:85–96.

Kirschbaum C, Kudielka BM, Gaab J, Schommer NC, Hellhammer DH. (1999). Impact of gender, menstrual cycle phase, and oral contraceptives on the activity of the hypothalamus-pituitary-adrenal axis. *Psychosom Med*, 61(2):154–162.

Kirschbaum C, Pirke K-M, Hellhammer DH. (1995). Preliminary evidence for reduced cortisol responsivity to psychological stress in women using oral contraceptive medication. *Psychoneuroendocrinology*, 20:509–514.

Kirschbaum C, Schommer N, Federenko I, Gaab J, Neumann O, Oellers M, et al. (1996). Short-term estradiol treatment enhances pituitary-adrenal axis and sympathetic responses to psychosocial stress in healthy young men. *JCEM*, 81:3639–3643.

Komesaroff PA, Esler MD, Sudhir K. (1999). Estrogen supplementation attenuates glucocorticoid and catecholamine responses to mental stress in perimenopausal women. *J Clin Endocrinol Metab*, 84(2):606–610.

Kudielka BM, Schmidt-Reinwald AK, Hellhammer DH, Kirschbaum C. (1999). Psychological and endocrine responses to psychosocial stress and dexamethasone/corticotropin-releasing hormone in healthy postmenopausal women and young controls: the impact of age and a two-week estradiol treatment. *Neuroendocrinology*, 70(6):422–430.

Laflamme N, Nappi RE, Drolet G, Labrie C, Rivest S. (1998). Expression and neuropeptidergic characterization of estrogen receptors (ERalpha and ERbeta) throughout the rat brain: anatomical evidence of distinct roles of each subtype. *J Neurobiol*, 36:357–378.

Li XF, Mitchell JC, Wood S, Coen CW, Lightman SL, O'Byrne KT. (2003). The effect of oestradiol and progesterone on hypoglycaemic stress-induced suppression of pulsatile luteinizing hormone release and on corticotropin-releasing hormone mRNA expression in the rat. *J Neuroendocrinol*, 15:468–476.

Lunga P, Herbert J. (2004). 17Beta-oestradiol modulates glucocorticoid, neural and behavioural adaptations to repeated restraint stress in female rats. *J Neuroendocrinol*, 6:776–785.

McCormick CM, Smythe JW, Sharma S, Meaney MJ. (1995). Sex-specific effects of prenatal stress on hypothalamic-pituitary-adrenal responses to stress and brain glucocorticoid receptor density in adult rats. *Brain Res Dev Brain Res*, 84:55–61.

McEwen BS, Weiss JM, Schwartz LS. (1968). Selective retention of corticosterone by limbic structures in the rat brain. *Nature*, 220:911–913.

Monder C, Sakai RR, Miroff Y, Blanchard DC, Blanchard RJ. (1994). Reciprocal changes in plasma corticosterone and testosterone in stressed male rats maintained in a visible burrow system: evidence for a mediating role of testicular 11 beta-hydroxysteroid dehydrogenase. *Endocrinology*, 134:1193–1198.

Nolten WE, Rueckert PA. (1981). Elevated free cortisol index in pregnancy: possible regulatory mechanisms. *Am J Obstet Gynecol*, 139:492–498.

Ogle TF, Kitay JI. (1977). Ovarian and adrenal steroids during pregnancy and the oestrous cycle in the rat. *J Endocrinol*, 74:89–98.

Patchev VK, Almeida OF. (1996). Gonadal steroids exert facilitating and "buffering" effects on glucocorticoid-mediated transcriptional regulation of corticotropin- releasing hormone and corticosteroid receptor genes in rat brain. *J Neurosci*, 16:7077–7084.

Paulmyer-Lacroix O, Hery M, Pugeat M, Grino M. (1996). The modulatory role of estrogens on corticotropin-releasing factor gene expression in the hypothalamic paraventricular nucleus of ovariectomized rats: role of the adrenal gland. *J Neuroendocrinol*, 8:515–519.

Redei E, Li L, Halasz I, McGivern RF, Aird F. (1994a). Fast glucocorticoid feedback inhibition of ACTH secretion in the ovariectomized rat: effect of chronic estrogen and progesterone. *Neuroendocrinology*, 60: 113–123.

Redei E, Li L, Halasz I, McGivern RF, Aird F. (1994b). Fast glucocorticoid feedback inhibition of ACTH secretion in the ovariectomized rat: effect of chronic estrogen and progesterone. *Neuroendocrinology*, 60: 113–123.

Reul JMH, deKloet ER. (1985). Two receptor systems for corticosterone in rat brain: microdistribution and differential occupation. *Endocrinology*, 117: 2505–2511.

Roberts JL, Johnson LK, Baxter JD, Budarf ML, Allen RG, Herbert E. (1979). Effect of glucocorticoids on the synthesis and processing of the common precursor to adrenocorticotropin and endorphin in mouse pituitary tumor cells. In Sato GH and Ross R (Eds.), *Hormones and cell culture, Book B*. Cold Spring Harbor Laboratory.

Roca CA, Schmidt PJ, Altemus M, Deuster P, Danaceau MA, Putnam K, Rubinow DR. (2003). Differential menstrual cycle regulation of hypothalamic-pituitary-adrenal axis in women with premenstrual syndrome and controls. *J Clin Endocrinol Metab*, 88: 3057–3063.

Roca CA, Schmidt PJ, Deuster PA, Danaceau MA, Altemus M, Putnam K, et al. (2005). Sex-related differences in stimulated hypothalamic-pituitary-adrenal axis during induced gonadal suppression. *J Clin Endocrinol Metab*, 90:4224–4231.

Rousseau GG, Baxter JD, Tomkins GM. (1972). Glucocorticoid receptors: relations between steroid binding and biological effects. *Mol Biol*, 67: 99–115.

Schacter BS, Johnson LK, Baxter JD, Roberts JL. (1982). Differential regulation by glucocorticoids of proopiomelanocortin mRNA levels in the anterior and intermediate lobes of the rat pituitary. *Endocrinology*, 110:1142.

Schwartz J, Billestrup N, Perrin M, Rivier J, Vale W. (1986). Identification of corticotropin releasing factor target cells and effects of dexamethasone on binding in anterior pituitary using a flourescent analog of CRF. *Endocrinology*, 119:2376.

Seale JV, Wood SA, Atkinson HC, Bate E, Lightman SL, Ingram CD, et al. (2004b). Gonadectomy reverses the sexually diergic patterns of circadian and stress-induced hypothalamic-pituitary-adrenal axis activity in male and female rats. *J Neuroendocrinol*, 16:516–524.

Seale JV, Wood SA, Atkinson HC, Harbuz MS, Lightman SL. (2004a). Gonadal steroid replacement reverses gonadectomy-induced changes in the corticosterone pulse profile and stress-induced hypothalamic-pituitary-adrenal axis activity of male and female rats. *J Neuroendocrinol*, 16:989–998.

Shughrue PJ, Lane MV, Merchenthaler I. (1997). Comparative distribution of estrogen receptor-alpha and -beta mRNA in the rat central nervous system *J Comp Neurol*, 388:507–525.

Svec F. (1988). Differences in the interaction of RU 486 and ketoconazole with the second binding site of the glucocorticoid receptor. *Endocrinology*, 123:1902–1906.

Thieulant ML, Duval J. (1985). Differential distribution of androgen and estrogen receptors in rat pituitary cell populations separated by centrifugal elutriation. *Endocrinology*, 116:1299–1303.

Turner BB, Weaver DA. (1985). Sexual dimorphism of glucocorticoid binding in rat brain. *Brain Res*, 343:16–23.

Vamvakopoulos NC, Chrousos GP. (1993). Evidence of direct estrogenic regulation of human corticotropin-releasing hormone gene expression. Potential implications for the sexual dimophism of the stress response and immune/inflammatory reaction. *J Clin Invest*, 92:1896–1902.

Viau V, Meaney MJ. (1991). Variations in the hypothalamic-pituitary-adrenal response to stress during the estrous cycle in the rat. *Endocrinology*, 129:2503–2511.

Viau V, Meaney MJ. (1996). The inhibitory effect of testosterone on hypothalamic-pituitary-adrenal responses to stress is mediated by the medial preoptic area. *J Neurosci*, 16:1866–1876.

Viau V, Chu A, Soriano L, Dallman MF. (1999). Independent and overlapping effects of corticosterone and testosterone on corticotropin-releasing hormone and arginine vasopressin mRNA expression in the paraventricular nucleus of the hypothalamus and stress-induced adrenocorticotropic hormone release. *J Neurosci*, 19:6684–6693.

Viau V, Soriano L, Dallman MF. (2001). Androgens alter corticotropin releasing hormone and arginine vasopressin mRNA within forebrain sites known to regulate activity in the hypothalamic-pituitary-adrenal axis. *J Neuroendocrinol*, 13:442–452.

Viau V. (2002). Functional cross-talk between the hypothalamic-pituitary-gonadal and -adrenal axes. *J Neuroendocrinol*, 14:506–513.

Young EA. (1995). Glucocorticoid cascade hypothesis revisited: role of gonadal steroids. *Depression*, 3:20–27.

Young EA. (1996). Sex differences in response to exogenous corticosterone. *Molecular Psychiatry*, 1:313–319.

Young EA, Korszun A. (1999). Women stress and depression: sex differences in hypothalamic-pituitary-adrenal axis. In Leibenluft E, (Ed.), *Gender differences in mood and anxiety disorders: from bench to bedside*. Washington DC: American Psychiatric Press, Inc.

Young EA, Altemus M, Parkison V, Shastry S. (2001). Effects of estrogen antagonists and agonists on the ACTH response to restraint stress in female rats. *Neuropsychopharmacology*, 25:881–891.

Young EA, Vazquez D. (1996). Hypercortisolemia, hippocampal glucocorticoid receptors and fast feedback. *Molecular Psychiatry*, 1:149–159.

Zhou L, Blaustein JD, De Vries GJ. (1994). Distribution of androgen receptor immunoreactivity in vasopressin- and oxytocin-immunoreactive neurons in the male rat brain. *Endocrinology*, 134:2622–2627.

Part II

Sex Differences in Neurobiology and Behavior

Chapter 7

Steroid Hormone Receptors and Sex Differences in Behavior

Toni R. Pak and Robert J. Handa

Animal and human behaviors can be dramatically influenced by the presence of the gonads. Early humans learned that castration of a male animal reduced its dominant and aggressive behavior, and removed its unpredictable behavior while in rut. Such observations allowed humans to harness animals as beasts of burden.

As reported by the Greek historian, Herodotus, at about 500 BC, behavioral effects of castration were also seen in men. Even at that time, castration of slaves was a long-standing practice; and as such, docile eunuch slaves were readily sold by Greek traders. From many sources, we know that eunuchs were commonplace in African, Assyrian, Chinese, Egyptian, Greek, and Roman civilizations. The lack of dominant and aggressive behaviors in these individuals made them appealing to rulers; and throughout history, eunuchs often sat at the highest levels of the court, administering justice in the name of the emperors.

Morphological effects of castration have also been observed over the years. In his treatise, *History of*

Animals, written at about 350 BC, Aristotle described the differential effects of prepubertal and postpubertal castration on secondary sex characteristics (Aristotle, 1910). However, it wasn't until studies performed by Arnold Berthold in 1849, while curator of the Gottingen Zoo, showed that substances secreted from the gonad can permanently affect the developing brain (Burrows, 1949). In his pioneering studies, Berthold demonstrated that castration of roosters shortly after hatching modified their adult appearance as well as their behaviors. Grafts of testicular tissue to these neonatally castrated males reversed the effects of castration, resulting in normal adult behaviors (Burrows, 1949). Nonetheless, the isolation and synthesis of some gonadal steroid hormones was not accomplished until the 1930s and the importance of metabolic pathways in the synthesis of steroid hormones was not recognized as important, particularly in studies of behavior, for many years to come.

Similarly, investigations into steroid hormone action made their initial appearance in the late 1950s and early 1960s with Elwood Jensen demonstrating *estrophillin* (later termed *estrogen receptor*), and Gerald Müeller showing estrogen induction of uterine protein synthesis (Jensen et al., 1982).

ACTIONS OF HORMONES ON THE DEVELOPING BRAIN

In 1959, a pioneering study by Phoenix and colleagues (Phoenix et al., 1959), determined that, in guinea pigs, the effects of neonatal castration in the male was to reduce the incidence of adult male behavior and increase female-typical reproductive behaviors. Moreover, administration of testosterone to neonatally castrated males or females abolished adult female behavior, but male-typical behaviors were retained.

This study introduced the concept of *organizational* and *activational* effects of gonadal steroids. Organizational effects were permanent effects that occurred when the developing brain was exposed to gonadal steroids, whereas activational effects were transient effects seen after steroids were given in adulthood. Numerous studies examining the organizational actions of gonadal steroid hormones on reproductive behaviors have followed and remarkably, this concept has been maintained largely intact over the years (see McCarthy & Konkle, 2005 for review).

The concept of organizational actions of gonadal steroid hormones was extended to brain morphology in the 1970s with reports of sex differences in synapses (Raisman & Field, 1973) and dendritic arrays of neurons (Greenough et al., 1977) in the preoptic area, and brain nuclear volume (Gorski et al., 1978). In particular, the studies of the Gorski laboratory later demonstrated that the sex differences in the size of the sexually dimorphic nucleus of the preoptic area (SDN-POA) are established early by exposure to perinatal gonadal steroid hormones. Given that the size of the male SDN-POA was much larger than that of the female and that this volume difference can be sex reversed by perinatal testosterone treatment (Jacobson et al., 1981), these observations fit perfectly with the concept of organizational actions of steroid hormones.

In the developing rodent brain, testosterone acts to prevent the development of female-typical characteristics (*defeminization*) and this has been shown to be estrogen-receptor dependent. For example, estrogen treatment of neonatal females or neonatally castrated males will mimic the actions of testosterone in re-

ducing female-typical reproductive behaviors and hormone secretory patterns, whereas treatment with non-aromatizable androgens have little effect in this regard (Luttge & Whalen, 1970; Gorski, 1971). Moreover, treatment of neonatal male rats with aromatase inhibitors effectively blocks the actions of testosterone on the defeminization of adult reproductive behaviors (McEwen et al., 1977).

Such observations led to the development of the aromatization hypothesis which postulates that the organizational effects of testosterone on male brain morphology and function are predominantly due to the intracellular conversion of testis-derived testosterone to estrogen by the aromatase enzyme (Naftolin et al., 1975; McEwen et al., 1977).

Accordingly, females are protected from estrogen-induced masculinization and defeminization of the brain by two factors: a) the relative lack of androgen as a substrate for intraneuronal estrogen production, and b) the presence in early development of liver-derived estrogen binding proteins (alpha-fetoprotein or sex hormone binding globulin) in the circulation, which prevents estrogen from crossing the blood-brain barrier and effectively sequesters the brain from the actions of peripheral-derived estrogen. In males, testosterone can freely access the brain and, once inside neurons, can be metabolized to estrogen which is now free to bind the intracellular estrogen receptor. This hypothesis has been strongly supported by animal studies over the past 30 years; however, the role of testosterone aromatization in human brain organization is arguably of less importance (Swaab, 2004).

NUCLEAR FAMILY OF STEROID HORMONE RECEPTORS

Nuclear Receptors Are Classified as Ligand-Activated Transcription Factors

Gonadal steroid hormones exert their downstream effects primarily through the binding and subsequent activation of steroid hormone receptors. These receptors belong to a large family of ligand-activated proteins called the *nuclear receptor superfamily*. Steroid hormones such as progestins, androgens, estrogens, glucocorticoids, mineralocorticoids, and thyroid hormones are among some of the cognate ligands for the receptor proteins included in this family.

Since the first successful isolation and complete cloning of a nuclear steroid receptor (human gluco-corticoid receptor; GR) in 1985, the number of identified nuclear receptors has grown at a remarkable pace. In 1999, the Nuclear Receptors Nomenclature Committee proposed a formal classification scheme based on the phylogenetic similarities of the well-conserved DNA binding domain. Hence, this large family of receptors has been subdivided into six classes; most of which include an ever growing number of orphan receptors whose endogenous ligands remain to be determined. In addition, two public databases, the Nuclear Receptor Database (NuReBase; http://www.ens-lyon.fr/LBMC/laudet/nurebase.html) and the Nuclear Receptor Signaling Atlas (NURSA; http://www.nursa.org) have been created as internet-based resources for disseminating and cataloging the rapidly changing knowledge in this field.

Members of the Nuclear Receptor Superfamily Have Distinct Functional Domains

All members of the nuclear receptor superfamily exhibit a similar structure comprised of five functional domains (Fig. 7.1A). Although each of these domains serves distinct functional roles which are consistent across receptor types, the inter-receptor homology of the domains is highly variable and likely explains some of the observed specificity that steroid hormones have in various tissue types.

A/B domain. At the -NH$_3$ terminus of the protein is the A/B domain which contains an activation function (AF-1) region. The AF-1 region of most steroid receptors confers constitutive transcriptional activity of the receptor in the absence of hormone binding. Researchers identified this property of steroid receptors by mutating the C-terminus ligand-binding domain (LBD) and then measuring basal levels of transcription using reporter gene assays (Warnmark et al., 2003). For most steroid hormone receptors, mutations within the LBD resulted in increased basal transcriptional activity of a hormone-sensitive gene. The exception is the AR, where mutation of the LBD resulted in a protein that was transcriptionally weak, leading to the conclusion that the LDB of AR is more important than the AF-1 region for transcriptional activation (Doesburg et al., 1997; Brinkmann, 2001). In addition to the AF-1 region, the A/B domain consists of several threonine, tyrosine, and serine residues

which are important sites of phosphorylation. The A/B domain is the most divergent among the groups of nuclear receptors and can vary in length up to 600 bases.

C domain. Immediately adjacent to the A/B domain is the C domain (DNA binding domain; DBD) which contains a cysteine-rich segment that is highly conserved among species. Within this region, eight cysteine residues serve to harness two zinc ions which fold the protein into two parallel loops referred to as zinc fingers (Fig. 7.1B). These two zinc ions, and hence the two zinc fingers, are critical for normal receptor functioning as studies have demonstrated by the fact that DNA binding is obstructed in the absence of zinc (Cano-Gauci and Sarkar, 1996; Low et al., 2002).

The first (upstream) zinc finger contains a short amino acid segment called the P-box which determines where the receptor binds to DNA. Typically, steroid hormone receptors bind to specific DNA sequences termed hormone response elements (HRE). HREs are comprised of two short, inverted palindromic DNA sequences that are separated by three variable nucleotides (n). The canonical HRE sequence specific for AR, PR, and GR is AGAACAnnnTGTTCT and AGGTCAnnnTGACCT for ER.

The second (downstream) zinc finger is responsible for directing the correct spacing of receptor binding to the DNA as well as the specification of receptor dimerization. Most steroid hormone receptors function as a dimer: a homodimer occurs when two receptors of the same type form a link, such as ERα with ERα, and a heterodimer occurs when two different receptor types link, such as ERα with ERβ. Specific amino acid sequences in the second zinc finger determine whether the receptor will form a homodimer or heterodimer.

D domain. The D domain consists of a flexible hinge region between the C and E domains which allows for conformational changes of the receptor upon ligand binding. In addition, the D domain contains the nuclear localization signal (NLS): an area of positively charged amino acids which maintains the receptor inside the cell nucleus (Guiochon-Mantel, 1994). The D domain is one of the least conserved regions among nuclear receptors and the crystal structure has not been fully characterized.

E domain. The E domain (ligand binding domain; LBD) is the largest segment for all the nuclear receptors. The secondary structure of the LBD is ar-

A

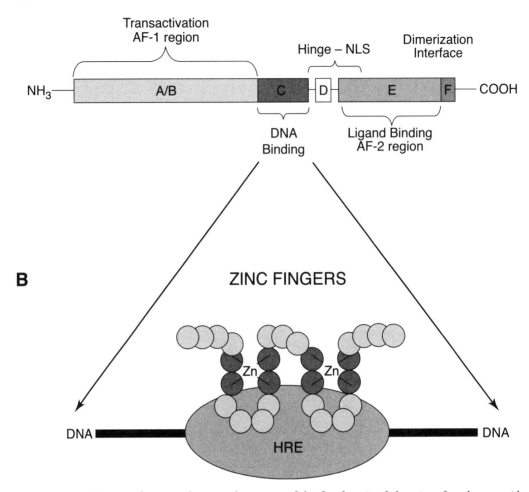

Figure 7.1(A). Diagram depicting the general structure of the five functional domains of nuclear steroid receptors. Domains include: A/B = transactivation region; C = DNA binding domain; D = hinge region (NLS = nuclear local signal); E = ligand binding domain; F = variable domain. (B). Enlarged view of the DNA binding domain showing zinc finger structure. Dark circles represent cysteine residues. HRE = hormone response element.

ranged as 12 α helices. These helices are important for subsequent binding of ligand and coregulatory proteins. For instance, helices 3, 4, and 12 are arranged in a pattern that forms a "hydrophobic pocket" called the activation function-2 (AF-2) region. Upon ligand binding, the LBD undergoes a conformational change that often results in helix 12 shifting to close the opening of the pocket. Interestingly, recent studies detailing the crystal structure of the LBD have shown that the conformational change of the helices differs depending on whether the ligand acts as an antagonist or an agonist (Hillisch et al., 2004; Hurth et al., 2004).

In addition to ligand binding, the E domain also contains the interface for receptor dimerization and regions important for the binding of coregulatory proteins. Recent advances in our understanding of nuclear steroid receptor signaling have revealed a host of proteins that serve to enhance or repress the transcriptional activity of the receptor; hence they are called nuclear receptor coactivators or corepressors. These proteins usually form large multiprotein complexes with the receptor and have a wide variety of functions including modification of histones, chromatin remodeling, and receptor stabilization.

An important component of the LBD is its ability to interact with nuclear receptor interacting sites (NR box) located on coregulatory proteins. The NR-box consists of the amino acid motif leu-x-x-leu-leu (LXXLL, where X is any amino acid). Upon ligand binding, the receptor undergoes a conformational change allowing accessibility for the LXXLL motif. The AR is an important exception to this paradigm. Studies have shown that AR preferentially binds coregulators in the AF-1 region at a phe-x-x-leu-phe (FXXLF) motif which facilitates interaction of the N-terminus with the C-terminus.

F domain. Of the gonadal steroid hormone receptors, only ERs contain an F domain which consists of approximately 50 amino acids at the extreme end of the C-terminus. Mutations of this region do not alter the ability of the cognate ligand, 17β-estradiol (E_2), to induce transcriptional activity nor does it alter DNA binding. Thus, the function of the F domain remains the least understood of all regions in the nuclear receptor superfamily. However, recent studies suggest that the F domain might be important for inhibiting dimerization because of its proximity to the dimerization interface of the E domain. In addition, some studies have shown that specific amino acid sequences in this region might alter the affinity of the ER for binding E_2 and could alter the transactivational activity of the receptor in response to a typical ER antagonist, such as tamoxifen.

Nuclear Receptors Activate Transcription in a Ligand-Dependent and a Ligand-Independent Manner

Ligand-dependent. The classic model of hormone action as described by Elwood Jensen in 1968 portrayed a "two-step" process with nuclear steroid receptors functioning solely as ligand-inducible transcription factors (Jensen, 1968). It was postulated that gonadal steroid hormones, synthesized in peripheral reproductive tissues such as the testes and ovaries, were secreted into the circulation and then transported to various target tissues. Upon entering the target cell, the hormone would then bind its appropriate nuclear

steroid receptor and initiate transcription of a steroid-sensitive gene. (Fig. 7.2A). Over the years, this model of steroid hormone action has proven to be remarkably accurate; however research from the past three decades has shown that it describes only one of the many mechanisms by which steroid hormones exert their effects.

Within the target cell, the unliganded nuclear steroid receptor (apo-receptor) resides as part of a larger complex attached to heat shock proteins. This term was originally coined due to the fact that heat shock proteins are upregulated under conditions of extreme cellular heat stress. Studies suggest that heat shock proteins serve to ensure proper folding of the newly synthesized receptor, prevent DNA binding and receptor dimerization, and shuttle receptors between the cytoplasm and nucleus (Elbi, 2004; Pratt et al., 2004). Ligand binding induces a conformational change in the receptor that dissociates it from the heat shock protein complex allowing the formation a dimer, binding to HREs, and activation of transcription.

Historically, apo-receptors were thought to reside exclusively in the cytoplasm and then translocate to the nucleus upon ligand binding (Gorski & Gannon, 1976). Evidence now suggests that nuclear steroid receptors occupy a variety of subcellular locations, including the plasma membrane and cytoplasmic organelles (Razandi, 2004; Pawlak, 2005) (Fig. 2B).

Further, ligand binding can alter the intranuclear localization of steroid receptors. Recent studies have used receptors that are fused to selected fluorophores, such as green fluorescent protein (GFP), which permits the monitoring of nuclear receptor trafficking within a living cell. For instance, Price and colleagues (Price et al., 2001) showed that ER apo-receptor was diffusely spread throughout the nucleus and then aggregated into punctuate clusters upon E_2 binding. Thus, changes in the C and D regions could alter the trafficking of the receptor within the nucleus, or its location within a cell. Similarly, the PR-A and PR-B isoforms are distributed distinctly from each other; with PR-A predominantly found in the nucleus and PR-B mainly found in the cytoplasm (Lim, 1999). Collectively, studies such as these have radically altered our view of nuclear steroid receptor action.

Another component of the classical model suggested that direct binding of the receptor to DNA was required for transcriptional regulation. However, early studies in the 1990s demonstrated that nuclear steroid

A CLASSICAL MODEL

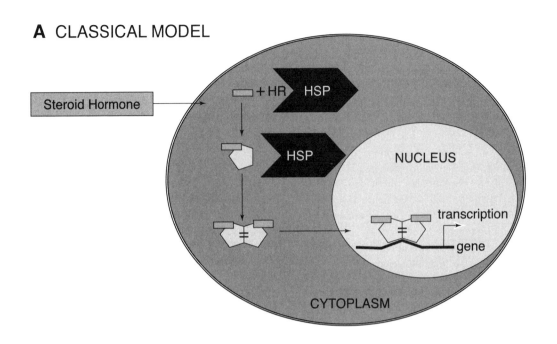

B CURRENT MODEL

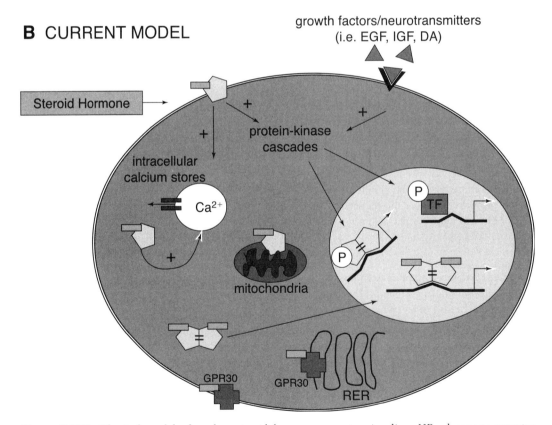

Figure 7.2(A). Classical model of nuclear steroid hormone receptor signaling. HR = hormone receptor; HSP = heat shock protein. (B) Current model of nuclear steroid hormone receptor signaling. EGF = epidermal growth factor; IGF = insulin-like growth factor; DA = dopamine; TF = transcription factor; RER = rough endoplasmic reticulum.

receptors could activate transcription by interacting with other proteins that bind DNA. Furthermore, these protein:protein interactions conveyed a large degree of specificity to the receptors. For example, activator protein-1 (AP-1) is a heterodimer consisting of two protooncogene proteins c-jun and c-fos. This protein complex acts as a transcription factor that binds specific DNA sequences.

Diamond and colleagues (Diamond et al., 1990) first coined the term *GRE composite* site through an observation that GR could form a complex with c-jun and c-fos while bound to a GRE *in vitro*. Their study demonstrated that the arrangement of whether the GRE was bound preferentially to GR, c-jun, or c-fos dictated the transcriptional response of the mouse proliferin gene. Similarly, Yang-Yen and colleagues (Yang-Yen HF, 1990) showed glucocorticoid repression of AP-1 activity was a direct result of glucocorticoid receptor interaction with c-jun and did not require binding to a GRE.

These studies were quickly followed by Gaub and colleagues (Gaub MP, 1990) who showed that ER-induced transcription of the chicken ovalbumin gene was unaffected by a mutation of the ER-DBD; lending further support for the hypothesis that DNA binding was not an absolute requirement for nuclear steroid receptor transcriptional activation. Moreover, they showed that the chicken ovalbumin gene promoter contained a canonical AP-1 site that was activated by ER. Since those early studies, researchers have identified numerous proteins that can interact with nuclear steroid receptors and activate transcription in the absence of direct receptor:DNA binding (see Gottlicher et al., 1998 for review).

It is important to note that nuclear steroid receptors can also mediate a variety of cell functions without directly modulating transcription of a given gene. For example, E_2 has been shown to mobilize intracellular calcium stores and activate second messenger signaling pathways within 5 minutes of hormone treatment (Aronica et al., 1994; Improta-Brears et al., 1999). The general consensus is that such responses are too rapid to be mediated by the transcriptional machinery of the cell and are therefore commonly referred to as the non-genomic actions of steroid hormones.

Ligand-independent. Most nuclear steroid receptors regulate gene transcription even in the absence of ligand binding. There are two possible molecular mechanisms for ligand-independent regulation of transcriptional activity by nuclear steroid receptors. First, compounds such as growth factors, neuropeptides, plasma membrane-associated proteins, and catecholamines can activate protein-kinase cascades which, in turn activate steroid receptors, usually through phosphorylation events. Second, the expression of the receptor stimulates or represses transcription in a concentration-dependent fashion independent of an interaction with any known outside factor (Fig. 7.3). This second mechanism is referred to as *constitutive* regulation and has been described only in reporter gene assays. Constitutive regulation will be discussed in more detail in the following section.

Peptide growth factors such as epidermal growth factor (EGF) and insulin-like growth factor 1 (IGF-1) have been shown to activate ERs through second messenger signaling pathways in cell culture model systems (Ignar-Trowbridge et al., 1992; Ignar-Trowbridge et al., 1993). Epidermal growth factor also elicited sexual behavior in ovariectomized female rats which demonstrated a possible physiological role for ligand-independent activation of steroid hormone receptors (Apostolakis et al., 2000). The EGF-induced sexual behavior was abolished when the animal was given an ER antagonist or ER anti-sense oligonucleotide indicating that the response was mediated through EGF activation of ER (Apostolakis et al., 2000). Similarly, the catecholamine, dopamine (DA), has been shown to activate PR and facilitate female sexual behavior in the absence of progesterone (see Auger, 2001; Blaustein, 2003; Mani, 2005 for review).

Constitutive. The constitutive regulation of target genes by gonadal steroid hormone receptors has not been well described. Most of the observed constitutive activation by gonadal steroid receptors has been demonstrated in studies using reporter gene assays. Although the wild-type ERα has not been shown to display constitutive activity, an ER with a point mutation at position tyr537 has been shown to activate ERE-mediated transcription in an E_2-free culture system (Zhang et al., 1997). By contrast, ERβ has been shown to constitutively regulate a number of estrogen-responsive neuropeptide genes including the gonadotropin-releasing hormone (GnRH) (Pak et al., 2006), corticotropin-releasing hormone (CRH) (Miller et al., 2004), and arginine vasopressin (AVP) (Shapiro et al., 2000) gene promoters. These data suggest that ERα and ERβ serve different physiological functions and potentially regulate gene networks through very different intracellular mechanisms.

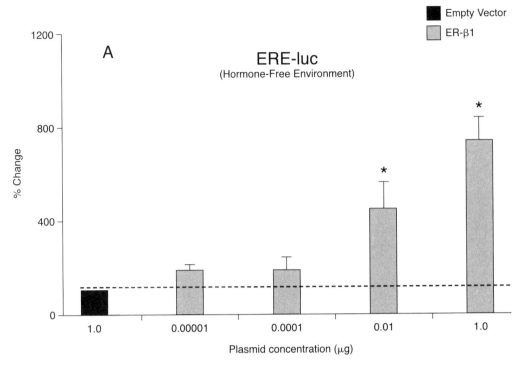

Figure 7.3. Constitutive regulation of ERE-mediated gene transcription by ERβ1 in a hormone-free environment. A hippocampal-derived cell line (HT-22) was co-transfected with an ERE-tk-luciferase reporter construct and varying concentrations of an expression vector containing full length rat ERβ1. Following transfection, cells were treated with 0.01% DMSO (vehicle) in DMEM supplemented with 10% dextran-charcoal stripped fetal bovine serum for 15 hours. Data are represented as percent change in RLU from vehicle-treated empty vector control ± SEM. The presence of a symbol denotes a significant difference from empty vector controls.

The AR has also been shown to activate promoter activity in the absence of ligand (Pak et al., 2005). An important question, however, is whether steroid hormone receptors can bind an HRE without first binding a hormone. This is especially significant for AR because it is predominantly localized in the cytoplasm and translocates to the nucleus as a consequence of ligand-binding. Studies using recombinant steroid receptor protein as well as cellular nuclear extracts have clearly demonstrated that ERs and ARs bind to an HRE in the absence of hormone (Huang et al., 2002; Pak et al., 2005). It is likely that many of the same signaling mechanisms regulating growth factor and neuropeptide activation of steroid hormone receptors, such as receptor phosphorylation, also regulate the constitutive activity of these receptors; however, the precise factors involved have yet to be determined. In addition, because constitutive activation of gene transcription has only been demonstrated

in vitro the physiological consequences of constitutively active receptors remain to be elucidated.

Co-Regulatory Proteins Are Important Mediators of Nuclear Receptor Action

The activation or repression of gene transcription mediated by steroid hormone receptors depends upon their interaction with various co-regulatory proteins. These proteins form a scaffold for the assembly of enzymes which modify chromatin and also serve to stabilize the RNA polymerase-containing preinitiation complex required for basal transcription. In general, they are grouped into one of two categories: coactivators or corepressors. However, recent evidence suggests that these broad designations do not always reflect the action of the protein.

Coactivators. Proteins that enhance the ability of steroid hormone receptors to increase gene tran-

P160/SRC FAMILY OF COACTIVATOR PROTEINS

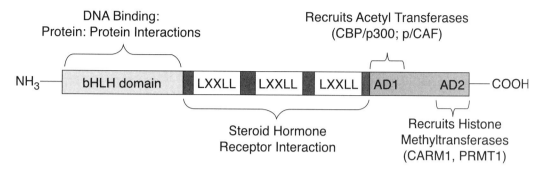

Figure 7.4. Diagram depicting the general structure of the p160 family of coactivator proteins. bHLH = basic helix-loop-helix domain; LXXLL = NR box.

scription are coactivators. Ligand-binding induces a conformational change in the receptor thereby exposing a region that recognizes the amino acid motif (LXXLL) located on the coactivator protein (Fig. 7.4).

This motif, called the NR box, has been shown to be essential for coactivator binding to nuclear steroid receptors. Most coactivator proteins belong to a large group called the SRC/p160 family. Functionally, all members of the SRC family have intrinsic histone acetyltransferase (HAT) activity which modifies the chromatin thus allowing for the interaction of chromatin with the basal transcriptional machinery of the cell. The first cloned member, steroid receptor coactivator 1 (SRC-1), was shown to interact with and

enhance the ligand-dependent activation of PR, ER, and GR demonstrating its ability to act as a general cofactor for all steroid hormone nuclear receptors (Onate et al., 1995). Importantly, SRC-1 had no effect on receptor-mediated transcriptional activation in the absence of ligand. Following the identification of SRC-1, several other coactivator proteins were identified that associate specifically with steroid hormone receptors (see Table 7.1).

Corepressors. Unlike coactivators which are recruited to the receptor-ligand complex upon ligand binding, corepressors appear to be associated with the receptor in its inactive state. They are functionally opposite of coactivators in that they possess intrinsic

Table 7.1. Nuclear Steroid Receptor Coactivator Proteins

SRC Family of Coactivators	*Steroid Hormone Receptor*	*Steroid Hormone Receptor Interaction Domain*
SRC-1	PR, ER, TR, RXR, GR, PPAR	AF-2
SRC-2 (GRIP1, TIF2, NCoA2)	GR, ER	AF-2
SRC-3 (RAC3, pCIP, ACTR, TRAM1, AIB1)	GR, AR, ER, TR, RXR	AF-2

Coactivators (non-SRC family)	*Steroid Hormone Receptor*	*Steroid Hormone Receptor Interaction Domain*
TRAP/DRIP	ER, VDR	AF-2
SRA/SRAP	AR, GR, PR, ER	AF-1
PIAS1	AR, GR, ER	DBD
SNURF	AR, GR, PR, ER	DBD
E6-AP	AR, GR, PR, ER	Amino terminus

histone deacetylase (HDAC) activity thereby blocking RNA polymerase interaction with chromatin. Further, whereas coactivator proteins tend to associate with the LBD of the receptor, corepressors associate with the transactivational AF-1 domain. To date, there are three well-described nuclear receptor corepressor proteins: nuclear receptor corepressor (N-Cor) (Horlein et al., 1995); silencing mediator of retinoid and thyroid receptors (SMRT) (Chen and Evans, 1995); and repressor of estrogen receptor activity (REA) (Montano et al., 1999).

Gonadal Steroid Hormone Receptors Are Located in the Plasma Membrane

Classical receptors. The classical model of steroid hormone action predicted that unbound receptors were localized in the cytoplasm and then translocated to the nucleus upon ligand-binding (Jensen, 1968). A substantial body of evidence taken from studies that manipulated the biochemical properties of the cell, such as changing salt and temperature gradients, supported that hypothesis (Gorski & Gannon, 1976). Moreover, in a sucrose gradient the unbound ER appears as a 4S form (equivalent to 76 Kd) in the cytosolic fraction and the ligand-bound ER is converted to a 5S form which is found in the nuclear fraction.

Two landmark papers, published back-to-back in 1984, caused a major divergence from this classical model and radically altered the field of endocrinology. First, King and Greene (King & Greene, 1984) used monoclonal antibodies to visualize ER in frozen tissue and revealed that the protein was confined to the nucleus. This study was the first to use immunocytochemistry to determine the subcellular localization of ER.

Next, Welshons and colleagues (Welshons et al., 1984) showed that when the nucleus was removed from the cell there was no E_2-binding activity in the remaining cytoplasm of the cell. These data suggested that for ER the unbound and bound forms of the receptor reside exclusively in the nucleus, and that the early data obtained through biochemical studies were perhaps artifacts of the methodology. Together, these studies prompted a re-evaluation of the classical model and further investigations into the subcellular localization of steroid hormone receptors.

Several studies have demonstrated that E_2 can have rapid effects, within seconds to several minutes, on many intracellular events that govern cell function. These effects included the mobilization of intracellular calcium stores (Kelly & Levin, 2001); activation of the MAPK and PI3 second messenger signaling pathways (Watters et al., 1997; Simoncini et al., 2000); and phosphorylation of intracellular transcription factors (Abraham et al., 2003). In addition, many of these rapid effects persisted when E_2 was physically prevented from entering the cell; such as by conjugation to large proteins like bovine serum albumin (BSA). Because these effects occur faster than what would be theoretically possible to be mediated by classical gene transcription mechanisms, these data raised the possibility that steroid receptors might be localized within the plasma membrane.

Indeed, early studies by Pietras and Szego (Pietras & Szego, 1977) demonstrated that in isolated liver and endometrial cells E_2 binding was associated with the plasma membrane. More recently, the cloning of ER, PR, and AR have allowed for the visualization of plasma membrane receptors using specific antibodies (Luconi et al., 1998; Li et al., 2003; Benten et al., 2004). Despite these functional data however, controversy as to the nature of these membrane receptors continues largely because they have not yet been isolated and cloned. Hence, the general consensus is that membrane steroid receptors are products of the same genes that encode the nuclear steroid receptors with some noteworthy exceptions (see Bjornstrom & Sjoberg, 2005; Levin, 2005 for reviews).

Novel receptors. Novel membrane receptors are characterized by their ability to bind hormone with a high affinity, yet are not encoded by the same gene that encodes the classical receptor for that hormone. For instance, in recent years two receptors have been identified that appear to functionally mediate the actions of E_2 and also bind E_2 with high affinity.

The first, termed *ER-X*, was identified as a putative membrane ER that differs from ERα and ERβ (Toran-Allerand et al., 2002). Although the receptor has not yet been isolated and cloned, considerable evidence exists pointing to its unique properties as a functionally distinct ER (Toran-Allerand, 2004). The second, GPR30, is a G protein-coupled receptor that bears no structural similarity to classical steroid hormone receptors. GPR30 was originally identified as an orphan membrane receptor, yet recent evidence indicates that it binds E_2 with modest affinity (Thomas et al., 2005). Subsequent studies revealed that GPR30 can be located in the endoplasmic reticulum membrane and mediates the E_2-induced mobilization of intracellular calcium (Revankar et al., 2005).

Similar membrane-associated G protein-coupled receptors, termed PRα, PRβ and PRγ, have also been proposed as mediating the rapid effects of progesterone (Karteris et al., 2006). An important consideration is whether these membrane receptors interact with the receptors confined to the nucleus. The physiological implications of this "cross-talk" are an exciting new area of research that is just beginning to be elucidated.

STEROID HORMONE RECEPTORS
IN THE BRAIN

Gonadal steroid hormone receptors are anatomically distributed throughout the body and are especially concentrated in the organs associated with reproduction. Here, we will focus only on where steroid hormone receptors are found in the brain with particular emphasis on those regions of the brain that are known to mediate adult sexual behaviors. Our current knowledge of centrally mediated sex behaviors comes mainly from studies using a rat model; consequently, the discussion on the neuroanatomical distribution of gonadal steroid receptors will concentrate on the rat brain.

The development of two important techniques, *in situ* hybridization (ISH) and immunocytochemistry (ICC) has led to the detailed mapping of the neural localization of steroid receptors in the brain. *In situ* hybridization uses a labeled DNA or RNA probe targeted to a specific mRNA sequence of the receptor. The radioactive probe is incubated with thin sections of brain tissue which permits its hybridization with native mRNA in the cells. A number of techniques have been developed to visualize hybridization either at the level of a single cell or at the level of brain regions or nuclei. Based on the detection method, this technique can be highly sensitive and specific; however, because it targets mRNA only, it does not allow for detection of the translated protein. By contrast, in ICC, brain sections are incubated with specific antibodies generated against an antigenic site in the steroid receptor protein. Although this approach might be considered more physiologically relevant since the protein of interest is being examined, a recurring caveat in the steroid hormone receptor field is that highly specific antibodies are not always readily available or easy to generate, leading to inconsistent and sometimes conflicting results.

Androgen Receptors Are Widely
Distributed in the Brain

Androgen receptors are widely distributed throughout most regions of the forebrain including the isocortex (ISO), olfactory cortex (O), and hippocampal formation (HF) (Simerly et al., 1990; Kerr et al., 1995; Nunez et al., 2003). Dense clusters of AR-expressing cells are also observed in the septum, amygdala (AMY) and bed nucleus of the stria terminalis (BST) which are components of the limbic system (Zhou et al., 1994). Male sexual behavior relies heavily on the coordination of sensory cues that are detected by neurons in the olfactory cortex which project to the AMY and BST. Within the preoptic-hypothalamic region, AR-expressing cells are predominant in the preoptic area (POA), paraventricular nucleus (PVN), arcuate nucleus (ARC), and ventromedial nucleus (VMH) (Simerly et al., 1990; Handa et al., 1996). The POA receives input from the BST and is an integral part of the olfactory circuit mediating sex behavior. In general, all AR-expressing cells in the rat brain appear to be neurons; however, there is some evidence for AR expression in astrocytes (Doncarlos et al., 2006).

Neurochemical Phenotypes of
Androgen Receptor-Expressing Cells

The majority of cells expressing high levels of AR are located in brain regions that mediate various aspects of reproduction. As such, we would expect to find AR co-expressed with neuropeptides that are regulated by androgens and known to modulate reproductive function. Nonetheless, data describing AR co-localization with any of these peptides remains limited.

Dopamine has been shown to facilitate sexual motivation in regions that also contain AR, such as the POA. Castration of male rats abolished the mating-induced release of DA in the POA (Dominguez & Hull, 2005), suggesting that AR might mediate the gonadal steroid hormone requirement for DA release. Furthermore, co-expression of AR with neurons containing tyrosine hydroxylase (TH), the rate limiting enzyme for DA synthesis, has been demonstrated in the ventral tegmental area (VTA), substantia nigra (SN) and retrorubral field (RRF), with virtually all AR containing cells in the VTA being positive for TH (Kritzer, 1997).

Some of these areas project to the nucleus accumbens where significant amounts of DA are also released in response to a mating stimulus. Although AR is virtually absent in the n. accumbens, because it is a region associated with the reward component of many pleasurable behaviors, it is likely that the observed increase in DA release following copulation is not specific to reproductive behavior but may be modulated by AR found in afferent projection neurons.

Oxytocin is a neuropeptide that has been shown to be very important for stimulating the female-typical sexual behavior, lordosis, but its role in male-typical sexual behavior is less defined. Oxytocin is synthesized in the PVN and SON and high levels are released in response to mating. The fibers transporting oxytocin from the PVN and SON to the bloodstream have the capacity to interact with neurons in the VMH; the brain region central in the control of the lordosis reflex. However, there is no evidence that androgens regulate oxytocin synthesis or release in females. In males, androgens appear to regulate oxytocin receptor mRNA levels in the VMH (Bale & Dorsa, 1995) but the physiological significance of this is unclear. Moreover, oxytocin receptors and AR are not co-expressed in neurons in the septum, amygdala, cortex, hippocampus, or hypothalamus of adult male rats (Bingaman et al., 1994).

Finally, most studies point to an indirect effect of androgens on the inhibitory neuropeptides or neurotransmitters that modulate reproductive behavior, such as serotonin, prolactin and endorphins due to the general lack of evidence for co-expression in AR neurons (Fodor et al., 2001; Sheng et al., 2004).

The expression of AR in the rat brain is primarily governed by circulating levels of testosterone (T), in a fashion that is somewhat different from other steroid hormone receptors. Autologous upregulation of receptor expression in response to reduced circulating androgen levels has been noted in some brain regions, under some conditions (Burgess & Handa, 1993; Handa et al., 1996). However, AR expression is also reported to decrease when T levels are low (Kerr et al., 1995; Handa et al., 1996; McAbee & DonCarlos, 1999b).

For instance, AR mRNA in the hypothalamus and hippocampus was reduced following castration (Kerr et al., 1995; McAbee & DonCarlos, 1999b) and restored to intact levels after T replacement (McAbee & DonCarlos, 1999b), suggesting the possibility that AR activation drives AR expression. Testosterone is converted intracellulary to 5α-dihydrotestosterone (DHT), which binds exclusively to AR, and E_2 which binds

ER. Surprisingly, both E and DHT have been reported to regulate AR expression in the brain (Handa et al., 1996; McAbee & DonCarlos, 1999a) depending on age, brain region and time following castration.

Anatomical Sex Differences in Androgen Receptor Expression

In adult rats, there are no sex differences in the general distribution of AR- expressing cells in the brain. However, in brain regions that are normally sexually dimorphic in size, such as the medial POA which is larger in males than females, there are more AR-expressing cells (Simerly et al., 1990). Contrary to the equivalent levels of AR expression in adults of both sexes, significantly higher levels of AR-expressing cells are observed in the BST and mPOA of males during early postnatal development (McAbee & DonCarlos, 1998). Interestingly, this sex difference occurs between postnatal days 4 and 10 when there are no appreciable sex differences in circulating levels of T, raising the possibility that this is in response to increased aromatase activity in the male brain during this point in development.

Two Main Forms of Progestin Receptors Are Expressed in the Brain

The PR gene contains two promoters resulting in distinct transcripts that encode two functional PR proteins, designated PR-A and PR-B (Kastner et al., 1990a). The PR-B isoform, referred to as the long form, contains an additional 164 amino acids in the A/B domain that are lacking in the PR-A isoform. Functionally, PR-A and PR-B have been shown to activate transcription of PR responsive genes with different potency; PR-B showing several-fold greater efficacy than PR-A. (Tora et al., 1988; Kastner et al., 1990b; Kastner et al., 1990a; Mulac-Jericevic et al., 2000).

Similar to the distribution of AR, PR-expressing cells are located in many regions of the rat brain that are important for mediating adult female sexual behavior. Specifically, very high levels of PR expression have been demonstrated in the POA and VMH with more moderately expressing cell populations in the BST, ARC, and AMY (Auger et al., 1996; Shughrue et al., 1997b; Greco et al., 2001; Mills et al., 2002). In most of these areas both PR-A and PR-B exist; however, their expression is regulated in a hormone-, region- and sex-dependent manner. For instance, in the hypothalamus adult females reportedly have higher levels of PR-B than males (Scott et al., 2002).

Estrogen Is Required for Progestin Receptor Expression

The primary regulator of PR expression is E_2, and transcriptional activation of the PR gene is strongly induced by E_2, however, elevated progesterone levels can act as a molecular brake to this system to decrease PR through an autoregulatory mechanism (Brown & Blaustein, 1984; Romano et al., 1989; Camacho-Arroyo et al., 1998). A good example of the ability of E_2 to induce PR expression can be seen during early postnatal development of the rat brain. Progestin receptor expression is abundant in the neonatal male POA, yet it is virtually absent in the female. Female rats, as neonates, have low to undetectable levels of circulating T. Moreover, most circulating E_2 is hidden from the brain by the presence of the liver-derived serum binding protein, α-feto protein, which binds E_2 with high affinity and sequesters it from its receptor. Therefore, this dramatic sexual dimorphism is a direct result of E_2 derived from the intracellular metabolism of T in specific regions of the male brain (McEwen et al., 1977; MacLusky & Naftolin, 1981).

In adult female rats, the lordosis reflex is most easily induced when an increase in circulating E_2 is closely followed by an increase in progesterone. During the estrous cycle, PR is transiently expressed in the POA and VMH and the timing of expression correlates well with the cyclic pattern of circulating E_2. Numerous studies have shown that the precisely timed increases in PR-expression in these brain regions are regulated by increases in E_2 and it appears that such a mechanism is designed to facilitate gonadal steroid hormone modulation of reproductive behavior.

In addition to E_2, many plant-derived estrogens (phytoestrogens) and selective estrogen receptor modulators (SERM) can regulate the expression of PR by acting as ER agonists or antagonists (Etgen & Shamamian, 1986; Shughrue et al., 1997b; Funabashi et al., 2001; Jacob et al., 2001; Schreihofer, 2005). For example, the administration of the phytoestrogen, coumestrol partially prevented the E_2-induced increase in PR in the POA and VMH (Jacob et al., 2001). By contrast, the phytoestrogen, genistein, significantly increased PR expression in a neuronal cell line (Schreihofer, 2005). Phytoestrogens, therefore, can behave as ER agonists or antagonists on E_2-re-

sponsive genes in neural tissues. SERMs, such as tamoxifen, specifically designed to act as ER antagonists, tend to prevent estrogen induction of PR expression as would be expected (Etgen & Shamamian, 1986; Shughrue et al., 1997b).

During neonatal rat development, E_2-induced PR expression is mediated by ERα and not ERβ (Chung et al., 2006). In rats treated with agonists specific for each ER subtype, the ERα-specific agonist induced PR levels equivalent to that of E_2-treated animals whereas the ERβ-specific agonist had no effect. In mice, however, there does appear to be some involvement of ERβ. For instance, E_2 treatment induced PR expression in the ERα null mouse model (Moffatt et al., 1998; Kudwa & Rissman, 2003) suggesting the possibility of important species differences in this system.

The molecular mechanism through which E_2 acts to regulate PR expression is unclear because the PR promoter does not contain a canonical ERE. One possibility is that ERs interact with the PR promoter through protein:protein interactions instead of direct DNA binding. Indeed, several studies have demonstrated the presence of multiple AP-1 and SP-1 sites on the PR promoter (Petz & Nardulli, 2000; Petz et al., 2002; Petz et al., 2004). Functionally, the AP-1 sites appear to be involved in the inhibition of ER-induced PR expression; whereas the SP-1 site, in conjunction with an ERE half-site, might contribute to PR promoter activation (Petz & Nardulli, 2000; Petz et al., 2004).

In contrast, PR expression is not induced by estrogen in some brain regions. These areas include the cortex, the oval nucleus of the BST, and the central AMY (Olesen et al., 2005). The molecular mechanisms governing PR expression in cells that are responsive to gonadal steroid hormones versus those that are not responsive have not been determined. One possibility is that the lack of estrogen responsiveness is due in part to a lack of ER expression in these same regions. Interestingly, activation of the DA receptor (D1) increased PR expression in brain regions devoid of ER but did not have any effect in regions that contained ER. These data suggest that DA can act as a compensatory mechanism for the regulation of PR expression in brain areas that are not targets for gonadal steroid hormones.

Another possibility is that a different suite of intracellular coregulatory proteins are expressed, or recruited by the PR promoter, in estrogen-responsive brain regions compared with those regions that do not respond to estrogen. For instance, the long isoform PR-B contains an AF3 region that is not present on the PR-A isoform. This AF3 region is an efficient recruiter of the coactivators GRIP and SRC-1 which leads to differential transcriptional activity between the two isoforms (Giangrande et al., 2000). Further, selective knock-down of SRC-1 expression significantly reduced the E_2-induced expression of PR in the VMH (Molenda et al., 2002) suggesting that SRC-1 is required for the E_2 regulation of PR expression.

Neurochemical Phenotypes of Progestin Receptor-Expressing Cells

For E_2 to have a direct effect of PR gene transcription, it would require that ER and PR be expressed in the same cells. Using *in situ* hybridization, Lauber and colleagues (Lauber et al., 1991) first showed that PR and ER are expressed in overlapping regions of the POA. Definitive co-localization was later confirmed in a study which demonstrated that 30%–50% of PR-expressing cells in the POA, BST, and AMY also contained ER (Greco et al., 2001). Together these anatomical data, along with the functional promoter studies mentioned earlier, strongly suggest that E_2 activates transcription of PR in the rat brain by directly acting in PR-expressing neurons.

Dopamine has been well characterized as a ligand-independent modulator of PR and is important for facilitating PR-mediated sexual behavior. In female rats, the DA-synthesizing enzyme, tyrosine hydroxylase, is co-expressed with PR in many hypothalamic regions (Lonstein & Blaustein, 2004). However, this neuroanatomical relationship does not support the ability of DA to activate PR as DA receptors must be also be found on PR-containing neurons. Receptors mediating DA action (D1/D5) are located throughout the hypothalamus, particularly in regions that are critical for sexual behavior (Zhou et al., 1999; Ciliax et al., 2000) indicating the latter is a possibility.

Progestin Receptor Expression in the Brain Is Highly Sexually Dimorphic

The expression of PR in the rat brain is a very well-described system in which there are striking sex differences. During ontogeny, PR expression is very high in the male BST, POA, VMH, AMY, and ARC (Quadros et al., 2002; Chung et al., 2006). Progestin receptors in the POA and ARC are highly sensitive to gonadal steroid hormone regulation; therefore these regions are sexually dimorphic with females exhibiting few to no PR-containing cells (Kato et al., 1993). On the other hand, PR in the BST and AMY are not responsive to regulation by gonadal steroid hormones during development resulting in equal levels of PR expression in both sexes (Olesen et al., 2005; Chung et al., 2006). Importantly, this marked sexual dimorphism in the POA and ARC has been used as a model system to study how gonadal steroid hormones participate in the masculinization or feminization of the brain during development. Unfortunately, the function of the elevated levels of PR in the male neonate has not been determined to date.

Two Estrogen Receptors: ERα and ERβ

Despite many lines of evidence pointing to the existence of multiple ERs, only two have been isolated and fully sequenced. The first, now referred to as ERα, has been the most extensively characterized to date. The second, ERβ, was isolated 10 years after ERα and its physiological function remains to be fully understood. Estrogen receptor α and ERβ are encoded by separate genes and are functionally distinct (Kuiper et al., 1996; Mosselman et al., 1996; Tremblay et al., 1997). They share approximately a 97% homology in their DBD and a 60% homology in their LBD, whereas the N-terminal region is highly variable (Kuiper et al., 1997). In addition to the original full-length ERs, several functional splice variants have also been identified for both ERα and ERβ (Petersen et al., 1998; Hanstein et al., 1999; Price et al., 2001; Swope et al., 2002; Wang et al., 2005. (Fig. 7.5))

Ligand binding affinities of most naturally-occurring and synthetic estrogens are equivalent for both forms of ER (Kuiper et al., 1997) making it difficult to discern the specific role each receptor has in mediating various physiological processes that are estrogen dependent. Transgenic mouse models designed with targeted disruption of one or both receptors (ERαKO; βERKO) is one tool that has been commonly used to address this issue (Couse et al., 1995; Krege et al., 1998). Another very important tool has been the implementation of numerous tumorogenic cell lines for reporter gene assays. While these models have their inherent limitations, they have proved invaluable for broadening our understanding of steroid hormone receptor function.

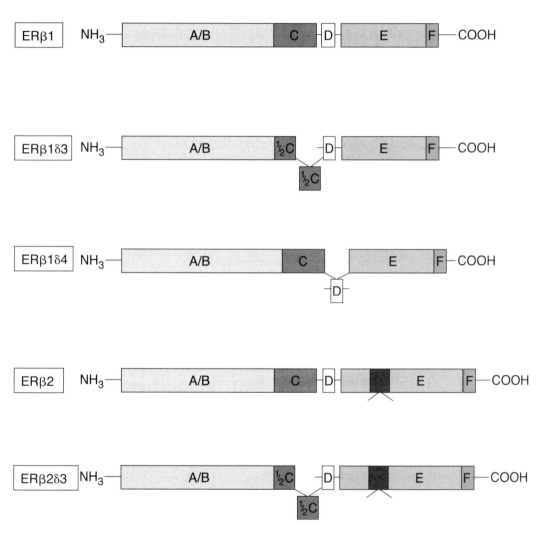

Figure 7.5. Diagram of the ERβ splice variants. Domains include: A/B = transactivation region; C = DNA binding domain; D = hinge region (NLS = nuclear local signal); E = ligand binding domain; F = variable domain. Variants designated with a δ3 are missing exon 3 which codes for the second zinc finger located in the DNA binding domain. Variants designated with a δ4 are missing exon 4 which codes for the hinge region. ERβ2 variants contain an 18 amino acid insert located in the ligand binding domain. A ⌃ symbol denotes an insertion and v symbol represents a deletion.

ERα and ERβ Have Distinct Patterns of Expression in the Brain

In the rat neonate, ERα and ERβ are widely distributed throughout the forebrain and expression overlaps in many areas. However, the number of neurons and degree of receptor expression per neuron differs for each ER subtype. Specifically, ERα is expressed in fairly high levels throughout the neonatal cortex while ERβ expression is limited to a few cells (Perez et al., 2003). Notably, the entorhinal cortex, an important integrator of cortical inputs, contains only ERβ-expressing cells. Both ERα and ERβ are also expressed throughout many regions that are critical for reproductive behavior in the adult including the hypothalamus, BST, and AMY.

In some brain regions like the BST, ERβ and ERα are equally represented; yet in others such as the PVN, AVPv, and AMY there is considerable variability. For example, in the neonatal PVN, a nucleus of the hypothalamus with important neuroendocrine functions, ERα expression is found in only a few cells although it contains high levels of ERβ. In contrast, the AVPv, a nucleus in the rostral preoptic area that is important for reproductive hormone secretion, contains only ERα-expressing cells. Similarly, in the AMY, ERβ is notably absent in the lateral and cortical subdivisions whereas ERα is highly expressed throughout.

In general, this distribution pattern is similar in the adult rat hypothalamus but some interesting developmental differences are found in extra-hypothalamic tissues. First, in the neonate there is no ERβ in the cortical region of the AMY whereas it is highly abundant in the adult (Shughrue et al., 1997a). Second, in the hippocampus there is a reversal of ERβ and ERα expression. Within the infantile rat hippocampus, only ERα-containing cells are observed (Perez et al., 2003) whereas predominantly ERβ-containing cells are found in the adult (Shughrue et al., 1997a). According to Solum and Handa (Solum & Handa, 2001), ERα expression in the hippocampus is virtually absent on the day of birth, peaks at postnatal day 10, and then declines to very few ERα-expressing cells in the adult.

Although not directly involved in mediating sexual behavior, the hippocampus is a very important region for learning and memory and social recognition. A similar switch in ERα and ERβ expression occurs in the cortex. Estrogen receptor alpha is highest during development, with levels peaking on PND 10–12, whereas ERβ is low. This pattern is reversed in adulthood where ERβ is the predominant receptor form, and ERα is found in only scattered cells. Finally, ERβ is the predominant form of estrogen receptor in the cerebellum, both in neonates and adults. The factors responsible for these developmental switches in receptor expression have not been determined although earlier studies examining the transient expression of ER in hippocampus and cortex showed that their development profile seem to be programmed very early in development. Hippocampal and cortical transplants, taken at E13 and placed into the cortex of neonates, expressed the same developmental ontogeny regardless of the age of the host (O'Keefe et al., 1993).

Neurochemical Phenotypes of Estrogen Receptor-Expressing Cells

Estrogen receptors are coexpressed with many neuromodulators/neurotransmitters and their associated receptors. This list includes, but is not restricted to: the serotonin, dopamine, norepinephrine, vasopressin, oxytocin, CRH, galanin, GnRH and proenkephalin systems. Of particular interest for adult female sexual behavior is the neuropeptide oxytocin and the monoamine, DA. As will be discussed in subsequent sections, oxytocin is an important modulator of the lordosis response in females. Infusion of oxytocin into the CNS has been shown to increase the frequency of the female-typical sex behavior, lordosis (Caldwell et al., 1986; Caldwell et al., 1989). Oxytocin is produced primarily in neurons of the PVN and SON whose axonal projections extend toward and innervate the VMH; an essential region for the stimulatory control of female sexual behaviors. Approximately 84% of oxytocin-containing neurons in the PVN express ERβ, yet few SON neurons co-express ERβ and oxytocin (Suzuki & Handa, 2005). By contrast, ERα was not co-expressed with oxytocin in either the PVN or SON.

Dopamine-producing neurons are identified by the immunochemical detection of its rate-limiting enzyme, TH. Dopamine has been shown to enhance all parameters of both female- and male-typical sexual behavior, presumably through the disinhibition of neurons providing tonic inhibitory stimuli. In the AVPv, ERα and TH are co-expressed in a sexually dimorphic manner with females having a higher number of co-expressed cells than males (Patisaul et al., 2006). Projections from the AVPv extend to a number of brain regions, such as the POA, BST, AMY, and periaqueductal gray (PAG), that are critical for the display of sexual behavior (Gu & Simerly, 1997).

Further, TH promoter activity has been shown to be regulated by E_2 and is mediated differentially by ERα and ERβ (Maharjan et al., 2005). For example, E_2 increased TH promoter activity when mediated by ERα but decreased promoter activity through ERβ. These data provide a potential molecular mechanism for some of the diverse cyclical, seasonal, and age-dependent actions of E_2 in the central nervous system.

In addition to ER co-expression with neuropeptides and neurotransmitters there is considerable overlap between ER containing cells and other gonadal steroid hormone receptors, such as PR and AR. As mentioned previously, PR and ER are co-expressed in some cells of the BST, POA and AMY. These same regions also have neurons that co-express AR and ER (Greco et al., 1998). Together, these data provide neuroanatomical evidence that gonadal steroid hormones might work in a coordinated fashion to regulate adult sexual behaviors.

SEXUAL BEHAVIOR

The rat is a particularly good model for the study of sexual behavior. When presented with a mating stimulus rats display consistent, well-stereotyped behaviors that occur in a predictable sequence. This has allowed investigators to quantify the behaviors and correlate them temporally with circulating hormone levels, neural expression of steroid hormone receptors, and external sensory cues. In general, female-specific behaviors are only displayed by females and male-specific behaviors are only displayed by males. This seemingly obvious fact is dictated not by sex chromosomes, but by morphological and biochemical differences in specific brain nuclei that are organized perinatally under the guidance of the gonadal steroid hormone mileu.

As such, if the female brain is *masculinized* perinatally with exogenous testosterone treatment, she will display male typical sexual behaviors as an adult. The presence of this same hormone will also *defeminize* the brain and thus, she is no longer able to exhibit female typical behaviors in adulthood. The reverse is true for the male brain. Elimination of circulating testosterone causes the brain to presumably develop along the default conditions which is to show female typical behaviors in adulthood.

Phoenix and Goy first categorized the effects of gonadal steroid hormones on adult sexual behavior as organizational or activational (Phoenix et al., 1959). Organizational effects refer to the permanent consequences hormones have on directing the differentiation of neural structures towards a male- or female-typical function. An example of this is the dramatic anatomical sex differences observed in certain regions of the rat brain. For instance, the sexually dimorphic nucleus (SDN) of the POA (later termed MPNc) is approximately four times larger in males than in females. The organizational effects of gonadal steroid hormones are reflected in the fact that the female SDN can be made morphologically larger with the administration of a single dose of TP and/or E_2 on the day of birth (Gorski et al., 1978; Jacobson et al., 1981).

Dohler and colleagues (Dohler et al., 1982) went on to demonstrate that the critical period for the development of the SDN occurs during the pre- and perinatal period and that it is regulated entirely by circulating gonadal steroid hormones. In their study, pregnant dams were administered daily TP injections beginning on gestation day 16. Following birth, the pups were treated with daily injections of TP for 10 days. This regimen of TP treatment was sufficient to completely sex-reverse the female SDN making it morphologically identical to that of the male.

Although the POA is a critical mediator of adult male sexual behavior, and SDN volume size correlates with the appearance of male behaviors, the sex difference in the SDN does not seem to play a role in regulating male behavior. Lesion studies have been unable to identify a role for the SDN in most reproductive behaviors. By contrast, activational effects of gonadal steroid hormones are transient changes in behavior and function that occur throughout life, but are present only when the hormone is present. Activational effects of gonadal steroid hormones on sexual behavior will be discussed in greater detail in the following sections.

Female Sexual Behavior

Female-Specific Sex Behaviors Are Well-Characterized

A sexually receptive female will display solicitory behaviors when she first encounters a male. These proceptive behaviors, ear wiggling, hopping and darting abruptly about the cage, and allowing the male to investigate her anogenital region, are designed to attract the male and also convey her sexually receptive state. When the male attempts to mount the receptive female, flank stimulation elicits a lordosis reflex in which the female assumes a characteristic posture with her back arched and her tail moved to one side exposing her elevated perineum. This posture facilitates the insertion of the male penis into her vaginal opening; a behavioral endpoint termed *intromission.*

Quantification of the lordosis response is used as a common denominator for assessing the degree of female sexual receptivity. The lordosis quotient (LQ) is calculated as the number of lordotic responses divided by the number of male mounts multiplied by 100. Thus, a high LQ is assigned when a female assumes the lordosis posture with nearly every mounting attempt (i.e. 80–90); whereas unsuccessful mounting attempts, (e.g. due to the failure of a lordosis response), would result in a low LQ. This standardized method of quantifying female sexual behavior makes it possible to critically compare behavioral results from one experimental paradigm to another.

Following a successful intromission by the male, the female rat will engage in pacing behavior. In a behavior testing situation, if a barrier is placed in the cage the female will actively retreat behind the barrier to avoid further contact with the male. The consequence of pacing is that the female delays subsequent intromission attempts by the male. Physiologically, this escape behavior allows time for the activation of the progestational reflex; a neural activation of prolactin secretion from the anterior pituitary that ultimately serves to prime the uterus for embryo implantation. Hence, pacing behavior increases the probability that each mating attempt results in a successful pregnancy.

Gonadal Steroid Hormones
Are Required for Female
Sexual Behavior

Circulating gonadal steroid hormones in females fluctuate over the course of a single reproductive cycle. In the rat, the length of the reproductive, or "estrous" cycle is 4–5 days, whereas in women the menstrual cycle is approximately 28 days in length. Each reproductive cycle is initiated by a surge of GnRH from the hypothalamus, which in turn stimulates the synthesis and release of two gonadotropic hormones from the anterior pituitary gland: follicle stimulating hormone (FSH) and luteinizing hormone (LH). The rat estrous

cycle is divided into four distinct segments based primarily on follicular morphology and circulating hormone levels: diestrus (II), proestrus, estrus, and metestrus (or diestrus I).

Diestrus is characterized by the growth and maturation of the ovarian follicles. Follicular development is controlled by FSH, whereas LH stimulates the synthesis and secretion of E_2 from the growing follicle. The rapid growth of the follicle on diestrus evening and proestrus, correlates with the rise in circulating estradiol levels which peak late in the morning of *proestrus*, approximately 12 hours prior to ovulation. At this time mature eggs are ready for release into the oviducts. Circulating P levels begin to rise on the afternoon of proestrus, several hours after the E_2 peak. As mentioned earlier, E_2 induces PR expression in the brain, thereby priming the brain for the subsequent increase in circulating progesterone.

Behaviorally, P synergizes with the high levels of circulating E_2 to induce the lordosis reflex. It is possible to induce a lordosis reflex in the absence of P, but doses of E_2 much higher than what is considered physiologically relevant are required. As rodents are nocturnal animals, the beginning of the dark phase on the afternoon of proestrus marks the start of behavioral *estrus.* Estrus is the day of ovulation and, in reproductively mature rodents, coincides precisely with sexual receptivity and behavioral exhibition of the lordosis reflex. Following ovulation the remnants of the ruptured follicles degenerate marking the start of *metestrus.* The day of metestrus marks a time when circulating gonadal steroid hormone levels are at their nadir and follicular development begins anew.

In addition to the absolute requirements of E_2 and P for initiating lordosis behavior, several other neuropeptides and neurotransmitters play a facilitatory role in modulating the intensity, duration, and frequency of the response. One important neuropeptide is oxytocin which is synthesized by neurons in the PVN and SON. Oxytocin is released from the anterior pituitary into the circulation following a mating stimulus. Additionally, oxytocin-containing neuronal fibers originating from the PVN interact with oxytocin receptors that are highly expressed in the VMH. This neural activation of oxytocin receptors is thought to play an important role in mediating the lordosis response. Studies have shown that central administration of oxytocin receptor agonists enhance the duration and frequency of lordosis behavior in response to male mounting attempts (Arletti & Bertolini, 1985;

Caldwell et al., 1986; Caldwell et al., 1989; Schulze & Gorzalka, 1991). This effect is attenuated by infusion of an oxytocin receptor antagonist or an antisense oligonucleotide directed at oxytocin mRNA (Witt & Insel, 1991; Caldwell et al., 1994; McCarthy et al., 1994). Interestingly, oxytocin has been shown to also facilitate some of the solicitory female sexual behaviors such as hopping and darting (Pedersen & Boccia, 2002).

Dopamine is also an important modulator of female sex behavior. Dopamine is a catecholamine that functions in the brain as both a neurotransmitter and a neurohormone. The results of early studies that suggested DA might be involved in mediating female sexual behavior demonstrated that administration of apomorphine, a non-selective DA receptor agonist, induced a lordosis response in ovariectomized rats treated with E_2 alone (Hamburger-Bar & Rigter, 1975). Surprisingly, the degree of the lordosis response was equivalent to that in rats treated with both E_2 and P suggesting that DA could also synergize with E_2 and act as a substitute for P. Since that early experiment a considerable amount of evidence has been collected that conclusively shows DA activates PR in a ligand-independent fashion resulting in modulation of female sexual behavior (see Mani, 2005 for review).

Gonadotropin-releasing hormone is another neuropeptide that has been implicated in modulating female sex behavior. Gonadotropin-releasing hormone is the most upstream regulator of reproduction in mammals and failure to produce GnRH results in sterility. Most importantly, GnRH controls the preovulatory surge in LH that occurs on the afternoon of proestrus. Because GnRH has been shown to facilitate both solicitory behaviors and lordosis (Moss & McCann, 1975; Dudley et al., 1981; Wu et al., 2006), this raises the possibility that GnRH is important for the temporal coordination of ovulation and subsequent behavioral responses. It is important to note that oxytocin, DA, and GnRH are incapable of inducing a lordosis response in the absence of E_2, highlighting the absolute requirement of gonadal steroid hormones for the display of female sexual behavior.

In nature, most mammals exhibit some degree of seasonality in their reproductive strategies; they do not show ovulatory cycles year-round as is found in the laboratory rat raised in constant conditions. From a species population standpoint this strategy is extremely useful because it provides a biological mechanism to impede reproduction during times that are not optimal for offspring survival. As expected, in seasonal breeders there are considerable species variations in the duration of the reproductive cycle and in the timing of behavioral receptivity. For an excellent review on reproduction in seasonal breeders see Bronson, 1985.

Sexual Maturation and the Onset of Female Sex Behaviors

The attainment of sexual maturity requires a temporal coordination of the physiological and behavioral events necessary for reproductive success. In female rats, the most common indicator for puberty onset is the first day of vaginal introitus. Vaginal introitus occurs as the result of rising levels of circulating estrogen, which is coincident with the first day of estrus and the occurrence of ovulation. Södersten (Södersten, 1975) thoroughly characterized the age at which female sexual behaviors emerge. Interestingly, behavioral estrus and vaginal introitus were not temporally coordinated in the peripubertal female rat. In some cases, lordosis behavior preceded vaginal introitus and in others, the behavior occurred several days after vaginal introitus. Further, they noted that the first two behavioral cycles tended to be longer than subsequent behavioral cycles, reflecting an attainment of the mature phenotype. These data suggest that the timing mechanisms controlling centrally-mediated behaviors are shaped by the stimulus of cyclical, circulating hormones.

The onset of female sexual behaviors can be induced precociously with hormone treatments, however there is a minimum age before which time hormones are ineffective. This indicates that a neural maturation of the brain must occur before it is able to respond to a subsequent temporal coordination induced by cyclical circulating steroid hormones. Immature rats treated daily with 10 μg estradiol-benzoate displayed the solicitory behavior of ear wiggling as early as 11 days of age; however a lordosis response could not be evoked in a majority of animals (94%) until 19 days of age (Södersten, 1975). At this time it is unclear what additional factors mediate solicitory behaviors and why these types of behaviors can be hormonally induced at a much earlier age than lordosis. Moreover, a lordosis response could not be elicited in adult rats ovariectomized at 15 days of age when given the same dose of estradiol-benzoate that elicited the response in rats ovariectomized at 20 days of age. Overall, these data point to a critical window of time for neural maturation occurring between 15 and 20 days of age. Indeed, gross morphological and neurochemical changes have been shown to occur in the brain during the pubertal transition in rodents (Sisk & Zehr, 2005).

The Ventromedial Nucleus of the Hypothalamus and the Preoptic Area Are the Primary Brain Regions Directing Lordosis Behavior

The VMH, located in the caudal portion of the hypothalamus, is of central importance for mediating lordosis behavior. The VMH contains high concentrations of ER, PR, and oxytocin receptors thereby being anatomically positioned as a prime integrator of multiple signaling inputs. Studies have shown that local infusion of E_2 into the VMH is sufficient to induce a lordosis response even in the absence of all other hormones. Similarly, disruption of this region by pharmacological or mechanical lesions abolishes the lordosis response. Estrogen signaling in the VMH is relayed through efferent projections that target the PAG in the midbrain; an important brain area responsible for mediating information from the spinal cord.

In contrast to the VMH, which is considered to be the most critical brain region for stimulating lordosis, the POA is widely regarded as the most critical region for inhibiting lordosis. The POA, located rostral to the optic chiasm near the anterior portion of the hypothalamus, has direct axonal projections to the VMH thereby providing an anatomical conduit for the regulation of lordosis behavior. Pharmacological lesions of the POA increased the LQ in female rats, whereas a decreased LQ was observed following electrical stimulation of the POA (Hoshina et al., 1994). Further, Kato and Sakuma (Kato & Sakuma, 2000) demonstrated that during a mating test specific populations of neurons in the POA decreased their firing rate, suggesting a decrease in inhibitory neurotransmitter signaling. Moreover, the underlying mechanism for lordosis inhibition has been shown to be mediated by opioid receptors located in the medial portion of the POA (Sinchak et al., 2004).

While these data strongly implicate the POA as the primary center governing lordosis inhibition, it is important to mention that other brain regions are also involved. For instance, it has been demonstrated that axonal projections to the POA, especially those coming from the septum, might be equally important (Yamanouchi & Arai, 1990; Tsukahara & Yamanouchi, 2001).

Efferent projections from the VMH target the midbrain central gray, specifically the PAG, which immediately surrounds the cerebral aqueduct connecting the 3rd and 4th ventricles. The PAG acts as central relay in the midbrain for many basic physiological functions such as anxiety, pain, and heart rate. As such, the PAG innervates midbrain and brainstem regions that target motor neurons in the spinal cord (Kow & Pfaff, 1998; Daniels et al., 1999). Projections to the PAG arise from the POA and the VMH separately suggesting that both inhibitory and facilitatory signals are integrated at the level of the PAG. An important question is whether the projections from the VMH and/or POA to the PAG express gonadal hormone steroid receptors. Morrell and Pfaff (Morrell & Pfaff, 1982) demonstrated that up to 30% of E_2-concentrating neurons in the VMH send projections to the PAG, however only 12% of those neurons were activated in response to a mating stimulus as measured by expression of the immediate early gene product Fos (Calizo & Flanagan-Cato, 2003).

Similarly, only a small percentage of VMH-projecting cells co-expressed PR and Fos during a mating test (Flanagan-Cato et al., 2006). Importantly, E_2 has been shown to produce a general increase in VMH neuronal activity that primes the region to respond to other neuromodulatory peptides known to facilitate lordosis behavior (Kow & Pfaff, 1998). Taken together, these data suggest that the important steroid-responsive region is the VMH but that other factors are involved in modulating lordosis behavior at the level of the PAG.

Male Sexual Behavior

Sexual Behavior in the Male Is Stereotypical and Sequential

Male sexual behaviors are easily recognized, precisely quantifiable, and occur in a predictable order. Upon presentation of a sexually-receptive female the sexually-experienced male begins to investigate her anogenital region to confirm her reproductive status. Initially, the female will repeatedly run away compelling the male to aggressively pursue her. This behavior provides important olfactory cues to brain regions that mediate subsequent sexual behaviors in the male. With every successful encounter the male will palpate the female flanks with his forepaws and attempt to mount the female. As the male mounts the female, he will rapidly thrust his pelvis back and forth which leads to intromission.

Typically, the male must make several mounting and intromission attempts before he is able to achieve ejaculation. Determination of whether the male has a successful intromission or an ejaculation can be ascertained by observing specific postural and behavioral parameters. For instance, a mount without a successful intromission results in the male simply backing away from the female. When the male ejaculates his posture becomes rigid, he stands upright on his hindlegs, and then moves quickly backward away from the female. The male will immediately begin to groom his genitalia and is unable to display subsequent sexual behaviors without a rest period. The duration of time in which subsequent sexual behavior is impeded is referred to as the refractory period.

Male sexual behavior in the rodent is easily quantified and has been standardized between the laboratories of various investigators. Quantification commonly consists of counting the number of mounts, intromissions, and ejaculations that occur in a given time period. Additional parameters can also be measured that reflect the sexually receptive state of the male, such as latency to mount, latency to intromission, and time (or number of intromissions) to ejaculation.

Sexual Maturation and the Onset of Male Sex Behaviors

Unlike females, in which puberty is defined as the first day of vaginal introitus, males do not have one specific physiological benchmark that defines pubertal onset. A spontaneous increase in GnRH pulsatility is one clear initiator of sexual maturation in both males and females, although the exact mechanism responsible for GnRH secretory activation remains controversial. GnRH drives the pulsatile release of FSH and LH from the anterior pituitary gland and in turn, this stimulates spermatogenesis and steroidogenesis in the male, respectively. Plasma FSH levels are moderately high just after birth and then decline to nearly undetectable levels between 5 and 15 days of age (Ketelslegers et al., 1978).

Beginning on day 15, FSH levels gradually increase and reach concentrations approximating those during the early postnatal period by day 25. On day 30, plasma FSH levels rapidly increase and reach peak values by day 40 that is followed by an equally rapid return to 25-day-old levels by day 60. This pubertal peak in FSH is critical for the initiation of sperm production by sertoli cells in the testes. On the other hand, plasma LH levels remain relatively stable from birth through sexual maturation. Leydig cells in the testes synthesize and release T in response to LH stimulation and as the testes enlarge, testicular LH receptors reach adult values by 50 days of age. Therefore, increased T production during puberty is not due to a change in plasma LH levels, but rather due to a heightened testicular responsiveness to LH stimulation. Together, these data suggest that sexual maturation in the rat begins at 25–30 days of age and is complete by 50–60 days of age.

Physiologically, the culmination of sexual maturity in the male is defined as the point in which mature sperm are present in the epididymis. However, the presence of mature sperm precedes the display of sexual behavior by several days raising the question of how sexual behaviors and physical maturation become temporally coordinated in the male. It has been well established that T, E_2 and DHT, acting on both central and peripheral targets, are required for the expression of male sexual behavior. Moreover, the levels of expression of AR and ERα in the brain are similar in juvenile and adult males (Weiland et al., 1997; Romeo et al., 1999; Romeo et al., 2001) indicating that the juvenile brain is capable of responding to steroid hormones. Yet, juvenile males given exogenous T do not display copulatory behaviors in the presence of a stimulus female (Sodersten et al., 1977; Meek et al., 1997). These data suggest that the pubertal transition encompasses a critical period for the remodeling of neural processes that govern adult sexual behaviors.

Gonadal Steroid Hormones Are Required for Male Sexual Behavior

Activational actions of gonadal steroid hormones are important for the display of male sexual behaviors. In general castration in adulthood abolishes, and T treatment restores, all types of mating behavior as well as accessory sex organ responsiveness, such as penile erection, in response to the stimulus of an estrous female. Due to the extensive metabolism of T in target tissues, two primary questions arise as to how hormones regulate male sexual behavior: first, which metabolite of T is most important for initiating and maintaining sexual behaviors and second, what are the critical central sites of hormone action.

When administered separately, neither T's aromatized metabolite E_2, nor its reduced metabolite DHT, were able to restore the entire array of male sexual behaviors in castrated adult male rats (Davidson, 1969; McDonald et al., 1970). These data suggested that DHT and E_2 work synergistically to regulate sex behavior. Baum and Vreeburg (Baum & Vreeburg, 1973) confirmed this hypothesis by demonstrating that co-treatment with E_2 and DHT in castrated animals restored all parameters of male sexual behavior comparable to that of animals treated with T alone. Further, their data suggested that E_2 was important for inducing mounting and thrusting behavior whereas, DHT was primarily acting in motor neurons innervating the penis to facilitate erection and ejaculation.

Several important brain regions associated with sexual behavior are E_2 responsive. Further, these brain regions contain aromatase activity (Naftolin et al., 1975; Selmanoff et al., 1977) indicating that T can be converted to E_2 within these brain regions to regulate male sexual behavior. Direct infusion of aromatase inhibitors into the mPOA significantly inhibited mounting and ejaculatory behaviors in adult male mice (Clancy et al., 1995). Studies using the aromatase null mouse model (ArKO) have provided further evidence for the importance of brain aromatase for male sexual behavior in rodents. The ArKO mouse was created by the targeted mutagenesis of exons 1 and 2 of the aromatase gene resulting in an inability to convert T to E_2 (Honda et al., 1998). Male gonadally intact ArKO mice fail to display any copulatory behaviors in the presence of an estrous female (Matsumoto et al., 2003) yet, subcutaneous treatment with EB restored the display of sexual behaviors to that of wild type mice (Bakker et al., 2004).

Interestingly, aromatase activity in many brain regions is upregulated by androgens (Roselli et al., 1997) which re-emphasizes the synergistic role of androgens and estrogens in mediating the normal display of sexual behaviors. Notably, in some mammalian species like the ferret, E_2 is unable to recapitulate some of the social aspects of mating behavior, such as the initial approach and investigation of an estrous female (Baum, 1990). This suggests that androgens act centrally to regulate motivational behaviors and has led investigators to draw a distinction between the hormonal regulation of sexual motivation versus that of sexual ability.

The Medial Preoptic Area Is the Primary Brain Region that Controls Male Sexual Behavior

Determination of the neuroanatomical sites responsible for mediating male sexual behavior was initially accomplished through lesioning studies or the placement of hormone receptor agonists and/or antagonists in specific brain nuclei. In 1968, Lisk (Lisk, 1968) demonstrated that lesions to the mPOA abolished male sexual behavior as measured by the number of copulatory plugs found beneath the cage following pairing with an estrous female. These data were consistent with a previous study showing that TP implanted directly into the preoptic-anterior hypothalamic area resulted in increased sexual behavior (Lisk, 1967).

Using radiolabeled T, Sar and Stumpf (Sar & Stumpf, 1972) went on to show that the mPOA contains a large population of androgen-concentrating cells. Overall, these data clearly demonstrated that the POA contained hormone responsive cells that were critical for the display of male sexual behavior; however they were not conclusive in determining that the mPOA was the primary neuroanatomical site of regulation for the behavior. For instance, the possibility remained that lesions of the mPOA simply disrupted an important pathway for sexual behavior, perhaps by severing afferent cortical connections.

To address this issue, investigators began looking at which neuronal populations were activated during a mating test by measuring the immediate early gene product Fos. Following a mating test, intact male rats showed a dramatic increase in Fos immunoreactivity in the piriform cortex, mPOA, BST and nucleus accumbens (Robertson et al., 1991; Baum and Everitt, 1992). Further, the BST and mPOA neurons that express mating-induced c-Fos also contained AR and ER (Greco et al., 1998). These studies helped confirm that the POA is not just a component of a particular regulatory pathway, but instead the primary central hormone responsive regulator of male sexual behavior. Moreover, there is now a substantial body of evidence that points to the POA as the primary regulatory site in most vertebrate species studied (Larsson & Ahlenius, 1999).

The mPOA is also an important target for DA innervation. Direct infusion of the DA receptor agonist apomorphine into the mPOA enhanced sexual behavior as measured by an increased number of mounts and intromissions and a decreased ejaculatory latency (Hull et al., 1986). Similarly, DA receptor antagonists reduced, but did not abolish these same parameters (Pehek et al., 1988). These data provoke important questions such as how DA is regulated during sexual behavior and what the molecular mechanisms are for DA-enhanced copulatory behavior. One hypothesis is that dopaminergic innervation of the mPOA disinhibits other brain nuclei responsible for the control of the motor functions associated with sexual behavior. Moreover, because the mPOA is an important target of sensory input from several brain regions there is some evidence that DA disinhibits sensory neurons thereby facilitating integration of relevant sensory cues like odorant stimuli (Hull et al., 2004).

Limbic Structures Integrate and Process Olfactory Cues that Enhance Male Sexual Behavior

Brain regions that are not necessarily critical for the display of male sexual behavior but are associated with facilitation include components of the limbic and olfactory systems. Specifically, the vomeronasal pathway in males is important for the integration of sensory cues that establish partner preference and determination of female sexual receptivity (see Keverne, 2004 for review). As mentioned previously, when a male is paired with an estrous female he first engages in a period of anogenital investigation that involves direct contact with the female genitalia. This behavior provides access to nonvolatile odors which are primarily processed by sensory neurons in the vomeronasal organ (VNO). Processing of volatile odors, such as urinary excretions, is mediated primarily by the main olfactory bulb. Sensory neurons in the vomeronasal organ (VNO) send axonal projections to the accessory olfactory bulb (AOB). Efferents from the AOB project to the BST and AMY which are primary components of the limbic system.

In general, the vomeronasal system is sexually dimorphic with males having a larger AOB and VNO than females (see Guillamon and Segovia, 1997 for review). Ablation of the VNO in sexually-naïve rats severely impairs adult sexual behavior; however, in rats that are sexually experienced ablation of the VNO is of minimal consequence (Saito & Moltz, 1986). These data highlight an interesting aspect of male

sexual behavior that seems to involve learning and memory. Indeed, early studies in the field of sex behavior demonstrated that experienced males far outperformed inexperienced males in the number of mounts, intromissions, and ejaculations (Dewsbury, 1969). Although the precise brain regions required for the learning component have not been defined, they are likely a combination of areas that control both motor reflexes and memory. Overall, the prevailing view is that the vomeronasal system contributes to the overall state of sexual arousal but is not required for sexual performance.

The BST and AMY are integral parts of the limbic system and provide direct anatomical inputs to the POA. As mentioned above, the BST and AMY are also areas that contain gonadal steroid receptors and are targets for the actions of gonadal steroid hormones. Odorant stimuli from an estrous female, either from direct vaginal secretions or soiled bedding, induces the expression of Fos immunoreactivity in these brain nuclei (Bressler & Baum, 1996; Coolen et al., 1997).

Further, the induction of Fos is dependent on the presence of gonadal steroid hormones, as Fos is not induced by odoriferous stimuli in gonadectomized males (Paredes et al., 1998). The importance of the BST for the integration of olfactory cues was nicely illustrated in a report by Claro and colleagues (Claro et al., 1995). In their study, sexual behavior tests were performed in sexually-naïve and sexually-experienced male rats that received bilateral lesions to the BST. They found that although both groups showed copulatory deficiencies, the sexually-naïve rats had significantly increased latencies for all behavioral parameters measured, such as mounts, intromissions, and ejaculations. Further, inexperienced lesioned rats demonstrated indiscriminate sniffing behavior that did not improve with subsequent behavioral tests (i.e. more sexual experiences). The rate of olfactory investigation was not measured in the experienced lesioned rats.

Overall, the authors concluded that the BST was critical for mediating sexual arousal, potentiated by olfactory cues, primarily in sexually-naïve animals; whereas sexually-experienced animals displayed deficiencies primarily in areas related to sexual performance.

SUMMARY

The goal of this chapter was to provide the reader with a general understanding of how gonadal steroid hormones contribute to broad sex differences in the behavior of adult animals and the underlying molecular mechanisms that mediate hormone action. During ontogeny, gonadal steroid hormones organize many sex differences that are not manifested behaviorally until sexual maturity is attained.

Moreover, these hormones act centrally through their specific receptors in discrete brain regions that are critical for integrating external cues, monitoring internal homeostatic conditions, and executing appropriate behavioral responses. Nuclear steroid hormone receptors are widely distributed throughout regions of the brain critical for the normal display of adult sexual behavior in both males and females. These receptors rely on a complex suite of intracellular regulatory proteins that dictate whether the hormone will have an inhibitory or stimulatory effect on subsequent gene transcription. Finally, this chapter highlights how the field of neuroendocrinology has substantially advanced our understanding of how the neonatal steroid hormone environment contributes at the molecular, cellular, and behavioral levels to define gender-specific differences.

References

Abraham IM, Han SK, Todman MG, Korach KS, Herbison AE. (2003). Estrogen receptor beta mediates rapid estrogen actions on gonadotropin-releasing hormone neurons in vivo. *J Neurosci*, 23:5771–5777.

Apostolakis EM, Garai J, Lohmann JE, Clark JH, O'Malley BW. (2000). Epidermal growth factor activates reproductive behavior independent of ovarian steroids in female rodents. *Mol Endocrinol*, 14:1086–1098.

Aristotle (1910). *Historia animalium.* Oxford: Clarendon Press.

Arletti R, Bertolini A. (1985). Oxytocin stimulates lordosis behavior in female rats. *Neuropeptides*, 6:247–253.

Aronica SM, Kraus WL, Katzenellenbogen BS. (1994). Estrogen action via the cAMP signaling pathway: stimulation of adenylate cyclase and cAMP-regulated gene transcription. *Proc Natl Acad Sci U S A*, 91:8517–8521.

Auger AP. (2001). Ligand-independent activation of progestin receptors: relevance for female sexual behaviour. *Reproduction*, 122:847–855.

Auger AP, Moffatt CA, Blaustein JD. (1996). Reproductively-relevant stimuli induce Fos-immunoreactivity within progestin receptor-containing neurons in localized regions of female rat forebrain. *J Neuroendocrinol*, 8:831–838.

Bakker J, Honda S, Harada N, Balthazart J. (2004). Restoration of male sexual behavior by adult exogenous estrogens in male aromatase knockout mice. *Horm Behav*, 46:1–10.

Bale TL, Dorsa DM. (1995). Regulation of oxytocin receptor messenger ribonucleic acid in the ventromedial hypothalamus by testosterone and its metabolites. *Endocrinology*, 136:5135–5138.

Baum MJ, Vreeburg JT. (1973). Copulation in castrated male rats following combined treatment with estradiol and dihydrotestosterone. *Science*, 182:283–285.

Baum MJ, Everitt BJ. (1992). Increased expression of c-fos in the medial preoptic area after mating in male rats: role of afferent inputs from the medial amygdala and midbrain central tegmental field. *Neuroscience*, 50:627–646.

Baum MJ, Carroll RS, Cherry JA, Tobet SA. (1990). Steroidal control of behavioural, neuroendocrine, and brain sexual differentiation: studies in a carnivore, the ferret. *J Neuroendocrinology*, 2:1–18.

Benten WP, Guo Z, Krucken J, Wunderlich F. (2004). Rapid effects of androgens in macrophages. *Steroids*, 69:585–590.

Bingaman EW, Baeckman LM, Yracheta JM, Handa RJ, Gray TS. (1994). Localization of androgen receptor within peptidergic neurons of the rat forebrain. *Brain Res Bull*, 35:379–382.

Bjornstrom L, Sjoberg M. (2005). Mechanisms of estrogen receptor signaling: convergence of genomic and nongenomic actions on target genes. *Mol Endocrinol*, 19:833–842.

Blaustein JD. (2003). Progestin receptors: neuronal integrators of hormonal and environmental stimulation. *Ann N Y Acad Sci*, 1007:238–250.

Bressler SC, Baum MJ. (1996). Sex comparison of neuronal Fos immunoreactivity in the rat vomeronasal projection circuit after chemosensory stimulation. *Neuroscience*, 71:1063–1072.

Brinkmann AO. (2001). Lessons to be learned from the androgen receptor. *Eur J Dermatol*, 11:301–303.

Bronson FH. (1985). Mammalian reproduction: an ecological perspective. *Biol Reprod*, 32:1–26.

Brown TJ, Blaustein JD. (1984). Supplemental progesterone delays heat termination and the loss of progestin receptors from hypothalamic cell nuclei in female guinea pigs. *Neuroendocrinology*, 39:384–391.

Burgess LH, Handa RJ (1993) Hormonal regulation of androgen receptor mRNA in the brain and anterior pituitary gland of the male rat. Brain Res Mol Brain Res 19:31–38.

Burrows H. (1949.) *Biological actions of sex hormones.* London: Cambridge University Press.

Caldwell JD, Prange AJ, Jr., Pedersen CA. (1986). Oxytocin facilitates the sexual receptivity of estrogen-treated female rats. *Neuropeptides*, 7:175–189.

Caldwell JD, Jirikowski GF, Greer ER, Pedersen CA. (1989). Medial preoptic area oxytocin and female sexual receptivity. *Behav Neurosci*, 103:655–662.

Caldwell JD, Johns JM, Faggin BM, Senger MA, Pedersen CA. (1994). Infusion of an oxytocin antagonist into the medial preoptic area prior to progesterone inhibits sexual receptivity and increases rejection in female rats. *Horm Behav*, 28:288–302.

Calizo LH, Flanagan-Cato LM. (2003). Hormonal-neural integration in the female rat ventromedial hypothalamus: triple labeling for estrogen receptor-alpha, retrograde tract tracing from the periaqueductal gray, and mating-induced Fos expression. *Endocrinology*, 144:5430–5440.

Camacho-Arroyo I, Guerra-Araiza C, Cerbon MA. (1998). Progesterone receptor isoforms are differentially regulated by sex steroids in the rat forebrain. *Neuroreport*, 9:3993–3996.

Cano-Gauci DF, Sarkar B. (1996). Reversible zinc exchange between metallothionein and the estrogen receptor zinc finger. *FEBS Lett*, 386:1–4.

Chen JD, Evans RM. (1995). A transcriptional co-repressor that interacts with nuclear hormone receptors. *Nature*, 377:454–457.

Chung WC, Pak TR, Weiser MJ, Hinds LR, Andersen ME, Handa RJ. (2006). Progestin receptor expression in the developing rat brain depends upon activation of estrogen receptor alpha and not estrogen receptor beta. *Brain Res*, 1082(1):50–60.

Ciliax BJ, Nash N, Heilman C, Sunahara R, Hartney A, Tiberi M, et al. (2000). Dopamine D(5) receptor immunolocalization in rat and monkey brain. *Synapse*, 37:125–145.

Clancy AN, Zumpe D, Michael RP. (1995). Intracerebral infusion of an aromatase inhibitor, sexual behavior and brain estrogen receptor-like immunoreactivity in intact male rats. *Neuroendocrinology*, 61:98–111.

Claro F, Segovia S, Guilamon A, Del Abril A. (1995). Lesions in the medial posterior region of the BST impair sexual behavior in sexually experienced and inexperienced male rats. *Brain Res Bull*, 36:1–10.

Coolen LM, Peters HJ, Veening JG. (1997). Distribution of Fos immunoreactivity following mating versus anogenital investigation in the male rat brain. *Neuroscience*, 77:1151–1161.

Couse JF, Curtis SW, Washburn TF, Eddy EM, Schomberg DW, Korach KS. (1995). Disruption of the mouse oestrogen receptor gene: resulting phenotypes and experimental findings. *Biochem Soc Trans*, 23:929–935.

Daniels D, Miselis RR, Flanagan-Cato LM. (1999). Central neuronal circuit innervating the lordosis-producing muscles defined by transneuronal transport of pseudorabies virus. *J Neurosci*, 19:2823–2833.

Davidson JM. (1969). Effects of estrogen on the sexual behavior of male rats. *Endocrinology*, 84:1365–1372.

Dewsbury DA. (1969). Copulatory behaviour of rats (*Rattus norvegicus*) as a function of prior copulatory experience. *Anim Behav*, 17:217–223.

Diamond MI, Miner JN, Yoshinaga SK, Yamamoto KR. (1990). Transcription factor interactions: selectors of positive or negative regulation from a single DNA element. *Science*, 249:1266–1272.

Doesburg P, Kuil CW, Berrevoets CA, Steketee K, Faber PW, Mulder E, et al. (1997). Functional in vivo interaction between the amino-terminal, transactivation domain and the ligand binding domain of the androgen receptor. *Biochemistry*, 36:1052–1064.

Dohler KD, Coquelin A, Davis F, Hines M, Shryne JE, Gorski RA. (1982). Differentiation of the sexually dimorphic nucleus in the preoptic area of the rat brain is determined by the perinatal hormone environment. *Neurosci Lett*, 33:295–298.

Dominguez JM, Hull EM. (2005). Dopamine, the medial preoptic area, and male sexual behavior. *Physiol Behav*, 86:356–368.

Doncarlos LL, Sarkey S, Lorenz B, Azcoitia I, Garcia-Ovejero D, Huppenbauer C, et al. (2006). Novel cellular phenotypes and subcellular sites for androgen action in the forebrain. *Neuroscience*, 138:801–807.

Dudley CA, Vale W, Rivier J, Moss RL. (1981). The effect of LHRH antagonist analogs and an antibody to LHRH on mating behavior in female rats. *Peptides*, 2:393–396.

Elbi C WD, Romero G, Sullivan WP, Toft DO, Hager GL, DeFranco DB. (2004). Molecular chaperones function as steroid receptor nuclear mobility factors. *Proc Natl Acad Sci U S A*, 101:2876–2881.

Etgen AM, Shamamian P. (1986). Regulation of estrogen-stimulated lordosis behavior and hypothalamic progestin receptor induction by antiestrogens in female rats. *Horm Behav*, 20:166–180.

Flanagan-Cato LM, Lee BJ, Calizo LH. (2006). Co-localization of midbrain projections, progestin receptors, and mating-induced fos in the hypothalamic ventromedial nucleus of the female rat. *Horm Behav*, 50(1):52–60.

Fodor M, Oudejans CB, Delemarre-van de Waal HA. (2001). Absence of androgen receptor in the growth hormone releasing hormone-containing neurones in the rat mediobasal hypothalamus. *J Neuroendocrinol*, 13:724–727.

Funabashi T, Kawaguchi M, Kimura F. (2001). The endocrine disrupters butyl benzyl phthalate and bisphenol A increase the expression of progesterone receptor messenger ribonucleic acid in the preoptic area of adult ovariectomized rats. *Neuroendocrinology*, 74:77–81.

Gaub MP BM, Scheuer I, Chambon P, Sassone-Corsi P. (1990). Activation of the ovalbumin gene by the estrogen receptor involves the fos-jun complex. *Cell*, 63:1267–1276.

Giangrande PH, Kimbrel EA, Edwards DP, McDonnell DP. (2000). The opposing transcriptional activities of the two isoforms of the human progesterone receptor are due to differential cofactor binding. *Mol Cell Biol*, 20:3102–3115.

Gorski J, Gannon F. (1976). Current models of steroid hormone action: a critique. *Annu Rev Physiol*, 38:425–450.

Gorski R. (1971). *Gonadal hormones and the perinatal development of neuroendocrine function.* New York: Oxford University Press.

Gorski RA, Gordon JH, Shryne JE, Southam AM. (1978). Evidence for a morphological sex difference within the medial preoptic area of the rat brain. *Brain Res,* 148:333–346.

Gottlicher M, Heck S, Herrlich P. (1998). Transcriptional cross-talk, the second mode of steroid hormone receptor action. *J Mol Med,* 76:480–489.

Greco B, Edwards DA, Michael RP, Clancy AN. (1998). Androgen receptors and estrogen receptors are colocalized in male rat hypothalamic and limbic neurons that express Fos immunoreactivity induced by mating. *Neuroendocrinology,* 67:18–28.

Greco B, Allegretto EA, Tetel MJ, Blaustein JD. (2001). Coexpression of ER beta with ER alpha and progestin receptor proteins in the female rat forebrain: effects of estradiol treatment. *Endocrinology,* 142:5172–5181.

Greenough WT, Carter CS, Steerman C, DeVoogd TJ. (1977). Sex differences in dentritic patterns in hamster preoptic area. *Brain Res,* 126:63–72.

Gu GB, Simerly RB. (1997). Projections of the sexually dimorphic anteroventral periventricular nucleus in the female rat. *J Comp Neurol,* 384:142–164.

Guillamon A, Segovia S. (1997). Sex differences in the vomeronasal system. *Brain Res Bull,* 44:377–382.

Guiochon-Mantel A, Delabre K, Lescop P, Milgrom E. (1994). Nuclear localization signals also mediate the outward movement of proteins from the nucleus. *Proc Natl Acad Sci U S A,* 91:7179–7183.

Hamburger-Bar R, Rigter H. (1975). Apomorphine: facilitation of sexual behaviour in female rats. *Eur J Pharmacol,* 32:357–360.

Handa RJ, Kerr JE, DonCarlos LL, McGivern RF, Hejna G. (1996). Hormonal regulation of androgen receptor messenger RNA in the medial preoptic area of the male rat. *Brain Res Mol Brain Res,* 39:57–67.

Hanstein B, Liu H, Yancisin MC, Brown M. (1999). Functional analysis of a novel estrogen receptor-beta isoform. *Mol Endocrinol,* 13:129–137.

Hillisch A, Peters O, Kosemund D, Muller G, Walter A, Schneider B, et al. (2004). Dissecting physiological roles of estrogen receptor alpha and beta with potent selective ligands from structure-based design. *Mol Endocrinol,* 18:1599–1609.

Honda S, Harada N, Ito S, Takagi Y, Maeda S. (1998). Disruption of sexual behavior in male aromatase-deficient mice lacking exons 1 and 2 of the cyp19 gene. *Biochem Biophys Res Commun,* 252:445–449.

Horlein AJ, Naar AM, Heinzel T, Torchia J, Gloss B, Kurokawa R, et al. (1995). Ligand-independent repression by the thyroid hormone receptor mediated by a nuclear receptor co-repressor. *Nature,* 377:397–404.

Hoshina Y, Takeo T, Nakano K, Sato T, Sakuma Y. (1994). Axon-sparing lesion of the preoptic area enhances receptivity and diminishes proceptivity

among components of female rat sexual behavior. *Behav Brain Res,* 61:197–204.

Huang ZQ, Li J, Wong J. (2002). AR possesses an intrinsic hormone-independent transcriptional activity. *Mol Endocrinol,* 16:924–937.

Hull EM, Muschamp JW, Sato S. (2004). Dopamine and serotonin: influences on male sexual behavior. *Physiol Behav,* 83:291–307.

Hull EM, Bitran D, Pehek EA, Warner RK, Band LC, Holmes GM. (1986). Dopaminergic control of male sex behavior in rats: effects of an intracerebrally-infused agonist. *Brain Res,* 370:73–81.

Hurth KM, Nilges MJ, Carlson KE, Tamrazi A, Belford RL, Katzenellenbogen JA. (2004). Ligand-induced changes in estrogen receptor conformation as measured by site-directed spin labeling. *Biochemistry,* 43:1891–1907.

Ignar-Trowbridge DM, Teng CT, Ross KA, Parker MG, Korach KS, McLachlan JA. (1993). Peptide growth factors elicit estrogen receptor-dependent transcriptional activation of an estrogen-responsive element. *Mol Endocrinol,* 7:992–998.

Ignar-Trowbridge DM, Nelson KG, Bidwell MC, Curtis SW, Washburn TF, McLachlan JA, et al. (1992). Coupling of dual signaling pathways: epidermal growth factor action involves the estrogen receptor. *Proc Natl Acad Sci U S A,* 89:4658–4662.

Improta-Brears T, Whorton AR, Codazzi F, York JD, Meyer T, McDonnell DP. (1999). Estrogen-induced activation of mitogen-activated protein kinase requires mobilization of intracellular calcium. *Proc Natl Acad Sci U S A,* 96:4686–4691.

Jacob DA, Temple JL, Patisaul HB, Young LJ, Rissman EF. (2001). Coumestrol antagonizes neuroendocrine actions of estrogen via the estrogen receptor alpha. *Exp Biol Med* (Maywood), 226:301–306.

Jacobson CD, Csernus VJ, Shryne JE, Gorski RA. (1981). The influence of gonadectomy, androgen exposure, or a gonadal graft in the neonatal rat on the volume of the sexually dimorphic nucleus of the preoptic area. *J Neurosci,* 1:1142–1147.

Jensen EV. (1968). A two-step mechanism for the interaction of estradiol with rat uterus. *Proc Natl Acad Sci U S A,* 59:632–638.

Jensen EV, Greene GL, Closs LE, DeSombre ER, Nadji M. (1982). Receptors reconsidered: a 20-year perspective. *Recent Prog Horm Res,* 38:1–40.

Karteris E, Zervou S, Pang Y, Dong J, Hillhouse EW, Randeva HS, Thomas P. (2006). Progesterone signaling in human myometrium through two novel membrane G protein coupled receptors: potential role in functional progesterone withdrawal at term. *Mol Endocrinol,* 20(7):1519–1534.

Kastner P, Krust A, Turcotte B, Stropp U, Tora L, Gronemeyer H, Chambon P. (1990a). Two distinct estrogen-regulated promoters generate transcripts encoding the two functionally different human progesterone receptor forms A and B. *Embo J,* 9:1603–1614.

Kastner P, Bocquel MT, Turcotte B, Garnier JM, Horwitz KB, Chambon P, et al. (1990b). Transient expression of human and chicken progesterone receptors does not support alternative translational initiation from a single mRNA as the mechanism generating two receptor isoforms. *J Biol Chem*, 265:12163–12167.

Kato A, Sakuma Y. (2000). Neuronal activity in female rat preoptic area associated with sexually motivated behavior. *Brain Res*, 862:90–102.

Kato J, Hirata S, Nozawa A, Mouri N. (1993). The ontogeny of gene expression of progestin receptors in the female rat brain. *J Steroid Biochem Mol Biol*, 47:173–182.

Kelly MJ, Levin ER. (2001). Rapid actions of plasma membrane estrogen receptors. *Trends Endocrinol Metab*, 12:152–156.

Kerr JE, Allore RJ, Beck SG, Handa RJ. (1995). Distribution and hormonal regulation of androgen receptor (AR) and AR messenger ribonucleic acid in the rat hippocampus. *Endocrinology*, 136:3213–3221.

Ketelslegers JM, Hetzel WD, Sherins RJ, Catt KJ. (1978). Developmental changes in testicular gonadotropin receptors: plasma gonadotropins and plasma testosterone in the rat. *Endocrinology*, 103:212–222.

Keverne EB. (2004). Importance of olfactory and vomeronasal systems for male sexual function. *Physiol Behav*, 83:177–187.

King WJ, Greene GL. (1984). Monoclonal antibodies localize oestrogen receptor in the nuclei of target cells. *Nature*, 307:745–747.

Kow LM, Pfaff DW. (1998). Mapping of neural and signal transduction pathways for lordosis in the search for estrogen actions on the central nervous system. *Behav Brain Res*, 92:169–180.

Krege JH, Hodgin JB, Couse JF, Enmark E, Warner M, Mahler JF, et al. (1998). Generation and reproductive phenotypes of mice lacking estrogen receptor beta. *Proc Natl Acad Sci U S A*, 95:15677–15682.

Kritzer MF. (1997). Selective colocalization of immunoreactivity for intracellular gonadal hormone receptors and tyrosine hydroxylase in the ventral tegmental area, substantia nigra, and retrorubral fields in the rat. *J Comp Neurol*, 379:247–260.

Kudwa AE, Rissman EF. (2003). Double oestrogen receptor alpha and beta knockout mice reveal differences in neural oestrogen-mediated progestin receptor induction and female sexual behaviour. *J Neuroendocrinol*, 15:978–983.

Kuiper GG, Enmark E, Pelto-Huikko M, Nilsson S, Gustafsson JA. (1996). Cloning of a novel receptor expressed in rat prostate and ovary. *Proc Natl Acad Sci U S A*, 93:5925–5930.

Kuiper GG, Carlsson B, Grandien K, Enmark E, Haggblad J, Nilsson S, Gustafsson JA. (1997). Comparison of the ligand binding specificity and transcript tissue distribution of estrogen receptors alpha and beta. *Endocrinology*, 138:863–870.

Larsson K, Ahlenius S. (1999). Brain and sexual behavior. *Ann N Y Acad Sci*, 877:292–308.

Lauber AH, Romano GJ, Pfaff DW. (1991). Gene expression for estrogen and progesterone receptor mRNAs in rat brain and possible relations to sexually dimorphic functions. *J Steroid Biochem Mol Biol*, 40:53–62.

Levin ER. (2005). Integration of the extranuclear and nuclear actions of estrogen. *Mol Endocrinol*, 19:1951–1959.

Li L, Haynes MP, Bender JR. (2003). Plasma membrane localization and function of the estrogen receptor alpha variant (ER46) in human endothelial cells. *Proc Natl Acad Sci U S A*, 100:4807–4812.

Lim CS BC, Htun H, Xian W, Irie M, Smith CL, Hager GL. (1999). Differential localization and activity of the A- and B-forms of the human progesterone receptor using green fluorescent protein chimeras. *Mol Endocrinol*, 13:366–375.

Lisk RD. (1967). Neural localization for androgen activation of copulatory behavior in the male rat. *Endocrinology*, 80:754–761.

Lisk RD. (1968). Copulatory activity of the male rat following placement of preoptic-anterior hypothalamic lesions. *Exp Brain Res*, 5:306–313.

Lonstein JS, Blaustein JD. (2004). Immunocytochemical investigation of nuclear progestin receptor expression within dopaminergic neurones of the female rat brain. *J Neuroendocrinol*, 16:534–543.

Low LY, Hernandez H, Robinson CV, O'Brien R, Grossmann JG, et al. (2002). Metal-dependent folding and stability of nuclear hormone receptor DNA-binding domains. *J Mol Biol*, 319:87–106.

Luconi M, Bonaccorsi L, Maggi M, Pecchioli P, Krausz C, Forti G, Baldi E. (1998). Identification and characterization of functional nongenomic progesterone receptors on human sperm membrane. *J Clin Endocrinol Metab*, 83:877–885.

Luttge W, Whalen R. (1970). Dihydrotestosterone, androstenedione, testosterone: comparative effectiveness in masculinizing and defeminizing reproductive systems in male and female rats. *Horm Behav*, 1:265.

MacLusky NJ, Naftolin F. (1981). Sexual differentiation of the central nervous system. *Science*, 211:1294–1302.

Maharjan S, Serova L, Sabban EL. (2005). Transcriptional regulation of tyrosine hydroxylase by estrogen: opposite effects with estrogen receptors alpha and beta and interactions with cyclic AMP. *J Neurochem*, 93:1502–1514.

Mani SK. (2005). Signaling mechanisms in progesterone-neurotransmitter interactions. *Neuroscience*, 138(3):773–781.

Matsumoto T, Honda S, Harada N. (2003). Alteration in sex-specific behaviors in male mice lacking the aromatase gene. *Neuroendocrinology*, 77:416–424.

McAbee MD, DonCarlos LL. (1998). Ontogeny of region-specific sex differences in androgen receptor messenger ribonucleic acid expression in the rat forebrain. *Endocrinology*, 139:1738–1745.

McAbee MD, Doncarlos LL. (1999a). Estrogen, but not androgens, regulates androgen receptor messenger ribonucleic acid expression in the developing male rat forebrain. *Endocrinology*, 140:3674–3681.

McAbee MD, DonCarlos LL. (1999b). Regulation of androgen receptor messenger ribonucleic acid expression in the developing rat forebrain. *Endocrinology*, 140:1807–1814.

McCarthy MM, Konkle AT. (2005). When is a sex difference not a sex difference? *Front Neuroendocrinol*, 26:85–102.

McCarthy MM, Kleopoulos SP, Mobbs CV, Pfaff DW. (1994). Infusion of antisense oligodeoxynucleotides to the oxytocin receptor in the ventromedial hypothalamus reduces estrogen-induced sexual receptivity and oxytocin receptor binding in the female rat. *Neuroendocrinology*, 59:432–440.

McDonald P, Beyer C, Newton F, Brien B, Baker R, Tan HS, et al. (1970). Failure of 5alpha-dihydrotestosterone to initiate sexual behaviour in the castrated male rat. *Nature*, 227:964–965.

McEwen BS, Lieberburg I, Chaptal C, Krey LC. (1977). Aromatization: important for sexual differentiation of the neonatal rat brain. *Horm Behav*, 9:249–263.

Meek LR, Romeo RD, Novak CM, Sisk CL. (1997). Actions of testosterone in prepubertal and postpubertal male hamsters: dissociation of effects on reproductive behavior and brain androgen receptor immunoreactivity. *Horm Behav*, 31:75–88.

Miller WJ, Suzuki S, Miller LK, Handa R, Uht RM. (2004). Estrogen receptor (ER)beta isoforms rather than ERalpha regulate corticotropin-releasing hormone promoter activity through an alternate pathway. *J Neurosci*, 24:10628–10635.

Mills RH, Romeo HE, Lu JK, Micevych PE. (2002). Site-specific decrease of progesterone receptor mRNA expression in the hypothalamus of middle-aged persistently estrus rats. *Brain Res*, 955:200–206.

Moffatt CA, Rissman EF, Shupnik MA, Blaustein JD. (1998). Induction of progestin receptors by estradiol in the forebrain of estrogen receptor-alpha gene-disrupted mice. *J Neurosci*,18:9556–9563.

Molenda HA, Griffin AL, Auger AP, McCarthy MM, Tetel MJ. (2002). Nuclear receptor coactivators modulate hormone-dependent gene expression in brain and female reproductive behavior in rats. *Endocrinology*, 143:436–444.

Montano MM, Ekena K, Delage-Mourroux R, Chang W, Martini P, Katzenellenbogen BS. (1999). An estrogen receptor-selective coregulator that potentiates the effectiveness of antiestrogens and represses the activity of estrogens. *Proc Natl Acad Sci U S A*, 96:6947–6952.

Morrell JI, Pfaff DW. (1982). Characterization of estrogen-concentrating hypothalamic neurons by their axonal projections. *Science*, 217:1273–1276.

Moss RL, McCann SM. (1975). Action of luteinizing hormone-releasing factor (lrf) in the initiation of lordosis behavior in the estrone-primed ovariectomized female rat. *Neuroendocrinology*, 17:309–318.

Mosselman S, Polman J, Dijkema R. (1996). ER beta: identification and characterization of a novel human estrogen receptor. *FEBS Lett*, 392:49–53.

Mulac-Jericevic B, Mullinax RA, DeMayo FJ, Lydon JP, Conneely OM. (2000). Subgroup of reproductive functions of progesterone mediated by progesterone receptor-B isoform. *Science*, 289:1751–1754.

Naftolin F, Ryan KJ, Davies IJ, Reddy VV, Flores F, Petro Z, et al. (1975). The formation of estrogens by central neuroendocrine tissues. *Recent Prog Horm Res*, 31:295–319.

Nunez JL, Huppenbauer CB, McAbee MD, Juraska JM, DonCarlos LL. (2003). Androgen receptor expression in the developing male and female rat visual and prefrontal cortex. *J Neurobiol*, 56:293–302.

O'Keefe JA, Pedersen EB, Castro AJ, Handa RJ. (1993). The ontogeny of estrogen receptors in heterochronic hippocampal and neocortical transplants demonstrates an intrinsic developmental program. *Brain Res Dev Brain Res*, 75:105–112.

Olesen KM, Jessen HM, Auger CJ, Auger AP. (2005). Dopaminergic activation of estrogen receptors in neonatal brain alters progestin receptor expression and juvenile social play behavior. *Endocrinology*, 146:3705–3712.

Onate SA, Tsai SY, Tsai MJ, O'Malley BW. (1995). Sequence and characterization of a coactivator for the steroid hormone receptor superfamily. *Science*, 270:1354–1357.

Pak TR, Chung WC, Roberts JL, Handa RJ. (2006). Ligand-independent effects of estrogen receptor beta on mouse gonadotropin releasing hormone (GnRH) promoter activity. *Endocrinology*, 147(4): 1924–1931.

Pak TR, Chung WC, Lund TD, Hinds LR, Clay CM, Handa RJ. (2005). The androgen metabolite, 5alpha-androstane-3beta, 17beta-diol, is a potent modulator of estrogen receptor-beta1-mediated gene transcription in neuronal cells. *Endocrinology*, 146:147–155.

Paredes RG, Lopez ME, Baum MJ. (1998). Testosterone augments neuronal Fos responses to estrous odors throughout the vomeronasal projection pathway of gonadectomized male and female rats. *Horm Behav*, 33:48–57.

Patisaul HB, Fortino AE, Polston EK. (2006), Neonatal genistein or bisphenol-A exposure alters sexual differentiation of the AVPV. *Neurotoxicol Teratol*, 28:111–118.

Pawlak JKM, Krust A, Chambon P, Beyer C. (2005). Estrogen receptor-alpha is associated with the plasma membrane of astrocytes and coupled to the MAP/Src-kinase pathway. *Glia*, 50:270–275.

Pedersen CA, Boccia ML. (2002). Oxytocin maintains as well as initiates female sexual behavior: effects of a highly selective oxytocin antagonist. *Horm Behav*, 41:170–177.

Pehek EA, Warner RK, Bazzett TJ, Bitran D, Band LC, Eaton RC, Hull EM. (1988). Microinjection of cis-flupenthixol, a dopamine antagonist, into the medial preoptic area impairs sexual behavior of male rats. *Brain Res*, 443:70–76.

Perez SE, Chen EY, Mufson EJ. (2003).Distribution of estrogen receptor alpha and beta immunoreactive profiles in the postnatal rat brain. *Brain Res Dev Brain Res*, 145:117–139.

Petersen DN, Tkalcevic GT, Koza-Taylor PH, Turi TG, Brown TA. (1998). Identification of estrogen receptor beta2, a functional variant of estrogen receptor beta expressed in normal rat tissues. *Endocrinology*, 139:1082–1092.

Petz LN, Nardulli AM. (2000). Sp1 binding sites and an estrogen response element half-site are involved in regulation of the human progesterone receptor A promoter. *Mol Endocrinol*, 14:972–985.

Petz LN, Ziegler YS, Loven MA, Nardulli AM. (2002). Estrogen receptor alpha and activating protein-1 mediate estrogen responsiveness of the progesterone receptor gene in MCF-7 breast cancer cells. *Endocrinology*, 143:4583–4591.

Petz LN, Ziegler YS, Schultz JR, Nardulli AM. (2004). Fos and Jun inhibit estrogen-induced transcription of the human progesterone receptor gene through an activator protein-1 site. *Mol Endocrinol*, 18:521–532.

Phoenix CH, Goy RW, Gerall AA, Young WC. (1959). Organizing action of prenatally administered testosterone propionate on the tissues mediating mating behavior in the female guinea pig. *Endocrinology*, 65:369–382.

Pietras RJ, Szego CM. (1977). Specific binding sites for oestrogen at the outer surfaces of isolated endometrial cells. *Nature*, 265:69–72.

Pratt WB, Galigniana MD, Morishima Y, Murphy PJ. (2004). Role of molecular chaperones in steroid receptor action. *Essays Biochem*, 40:41–58.

Price RH, Jr., Butler CA, Webb P, Uht R, Kushner P, Handa RJ. (2001). A splice variant of estrogen receptor beta missing exon 3 displays altered subnuclear localization and capacity for transcriptional activation. *Endocrinology*. 142:2039–2049.

Quadros PS, Lopez V, De Vries GJ, Chung WC, Wagner CK. (2002). Progesterone receptors and the sexual differentiation of the medial preoptic nucleus. *J Neurobiol*, 51:24–32.

Raisman G, Field PM. (1973). Sexual dimorphism in the neuropil of the preoptic area of the rat and its dependence on neonatal androgen. *Brain Res*, 54:1–29.

Razandi M PA, Merchenthaler I, Greene GL, Levin ER. (2004). Plasma membrane estrogen receptors exist and functions as dimers. *Mol Endocrinol*, 18:2854–2865.

Revankar CM, Cimino DF, Sklar LA, Arterburn JB, Prossnitz ER. (2005). A transmembrane intracellular estrogen receptor mediates rapid cell signaling. *Science*, 307:1625–1630.

Robertson GS, Pfaus JG, Atkinson LJ, Matsumura H, Phillips AG, Fibiger HC. (1991). Sexual behavior increases c-fos expression in the forebrain of the male rat. *Brain Res*, 564:352–357.

Romano GJ, Krust A, Pfaff DW. (1989). Expression and estrogen regulation of progesterone receptor mRNA in neurons of the mediobasal hypothalamus: an in situ hybridization study. *Mol Endocrinol*, 3:1295–1300.

Romeo RD, Diedrich SL, Sisk CL. (1999). Estrogen receptor immunoreactivity in prepubertal and adult male Syrian hamsters. *Neurosci Lett*, 265:167–170.

Romeo RD, Cook-Wiens E, Richardson HN, Sisk CL. (2001). Dihydrotestosterone activates sexual behavior in adult male hamsters but not in juveniles. *Physiol Behav*, 73:579–584.

Roselli CE, Abdelgadir SE, Resko JA. (1997). Regulation of aromatase gene expression in the adult rat brain. *Brain Res Bull*, 44:351–357.

Saito TR, Moltz H. (1986). Copulatory behavior of sexually-naive and sexually-experienced male rats following removal of the vomeronasal organ. *Physiol Behav*, 37:507–510.

Sar M, Stumpf WE. (1972). Cellular localization of androgen in the brain and pituitary after the injection of tritiated testosterone. *Experientia*, 28:1364–1366.

Schreihofer DA. (2005). Transcriptional regulation by phytoestrogens in neuronal cell lines. *Mol Cell Endocrinol*, 231:13–22.

Schulze HG, Gorzalka BB. (1991). Oxytocin effects on lordosis frequency and lordosis duration following infusion into the medial pre-optic area and ventromedial hypothalamus of female rats. *Neuropeptides*, 18:99–106.

Scott RE, Wu-Peng XS, Pfaff DW. (2002). Regulation and expression of progesterone receptor mRNA isoforms A and B in the male and female rat hypothalamus and pituitary following oestrogen treatment. *J Neuroendocrinol*, 14:175–183.

Selmanoff MK, Brodkin LD, Weiner RI, Siiteri PK. (1977). Aromatization and 5alpha-reduction of androgens in discrete hypothalamic and limbic regions of the male and female rat. *Endocrinology*, 101:841–848.

Shapiro RA, Xu C, Dorsa DM. (2000). Differential transcriptional regulation of rat vasopressin gene expression by estrogen receptor alpha and beta. *Endocrinology*, 141:4056–4064.

Sheng Z, Kawano J, Yanai A, Fujinaga R, Tanaka M, Watanabe Y, Shinoda K. (2004). Expression of estrogen receptors (alpha, beta) and androgen receptor in serotonin neurons of the rat and mouse dorsal raphe nuclei; sex and species differences. *Neurosci Res*, 49:185–196.

Shughrue PJ, Lane MV, Merchenthaler I. (1997a). Comparative distribution of estrogen receptor-alpha and -beta mRNA in the rat central nervous system. *J Comp Neurol*, 388:507–525.

Shughrue PJ, Lane MV, Merchenthaler I. (1997b). Regulation of progesterone receptor messenger ribonucleic acid in the rat medial preoptic nucleus by estrogenic and antiestrogenic compounds: an in situ hybridization study. *Endocrinology*, 138:5476–5484.

Simerly RB, Chang C, Muramatsu M, Swanson LW. (1990). Distribution of androgen and estrogen receptor mRNA-containing cells in the rat brain: an in situ hybridization study. *J Comp Neurol*, 294:76–95.

Simoncini T, Hafezi-Moghadam A, Brazil DP, Ley K, Chin WW, Liao JK. (2000). Interaction of oestrogen receptor with the regulatory subunit of phosphatidylinositol-3-OH kinase. *Nature*. 407:538–541.

Sinchak K, Mills RH, Eckersell CB, Micevych PE. (2004). Medial preoptic area delta-opioid receptors inhibit lordosis. *Behav Brain Res* 155:301–306.

Sisk CL, Zehr JL. (2005). Pubertal hormones organize the adolescent brain and behavior. *Front Neuroendocrinol*, 26:163–174.

Sodersten P. (1975). Receptive behavior in developing female rats. *Horm Behav*, 6:307–317.

Sodersten P, Damassa DA, Smith ER. (1977). Sexual behavior in developing male rats. *Horm Behav*, 8:320–341.

Solum DT, Handa RJ. (2001). Localization of estrogen receptor alpha (ER alpha) in pyramidal neurons of the developing rat hippocampus. *Brain Res Dev Brain Res*, 128:165–175.

Suzuki S, Handa RJ. (2005). Estrogen receptor-beta, but not estrogen receptor-alpha, is expressed in prolactin neurons of the female rat paraventricular and supraoptic nuclei: comparison with other neuropeptides. *J Comp Neurol*, 484:28–42.

Swaab D. (2004). Sexual differentiation of the human brain: relevance for gender identity, transsexualism and sexual orientation. *Gynecol Endocrinol*, 19:301–312.

Swope D, Harrell JC, Mahato D, Korach KS. (2002). Genomic structure and identification of a truncated variant message of the mouse estrogen receptor alpha gene. *Gene*, 294:239–247.

Thomas P, Pang Y, Filardo EJ, Dong J. (2005). Identity of an estrogen membrane receptor coupled to a G protein in human breast cancer cells. *Endocrinology*, 146:624–632.

Tora L, Gronemeyer H, Turcotte B, Gaub MP, Chambon P. (1988). The N-terminal region of the chicken progesterone receptor specifies target gene activation. *Nature*, 333:185–188.

Toran-Allerand CD. (2004). Minireview: a plethora of estrogen receptors in the brain: where will it end? *Endocrinology*, 145:1069–1074.

Toran-Allerand CD, Guan X, MacLusky NJ, Horvath TL, Diano S, Singh M, et al. (2002). ER-X: a novel, plasma membrane-associated, putative estrogen receptor that is regulated during development and after ischemic brain injury. *J Neurosci*, 22:8391–8401.

Tremblay GB, Tremblay A, Copeland NG, Gilbert DJ, Jenkins NA, Labrie F, Giguere V. (1997). Cloning, chromosomal localization, and functional analysis of the murine estrogen receptor beta. *Mol Endocrinol*, 11:353–365.

Tsukahara S, Yamanouchi K. (2001). Neurohistological and behavioral evidence for lordosis-inhibiting tract from lateral septum to periaqueductal gray in male rats. *J Comp Neurol*, 431:293–310.

Wang Z, Zhang X, Shen P, Loggie BW, Chang Y, Deuel TF. (2005). Identification, cloning, and expression of human estrogen receptor-alpha36, a novel variant of human estrogen receptor-alpha66. *Biochem Biophys Res Commun*, 336:1023–1027.

Warnmark A, Treuter E, Wright AP, Gustafsson JA. (2003). Activation functions 1 and 2 of nuclear receptors: molecular strategies for transcriptional activation. *Mol Endocrinol*, 17:1901–1909.

Watters JJ, Campbell JS, Cunningham MJ, Krebs EG, Dorsa DM. (1997). Rapid membrane effects of steroids in neuroblastoma cells: effects of estrogen on mitogen activated protein kinase signalling cascade and c-fos immediate early gene transcription. *Endocrinology*, 138:4030–4033.

Weiland NG, Orikasa C, Hayashi S, McEwen BS. (1997). Distribution and hormone regulation of estrogen receptor immunoreactive cells in the hippocampus of male and female rats. *J Comp Neurol*, 388:603–612.

Welshons WV, Lieberman ME, Gorski J. (1984). Nuclear localization of unoccupied oestrogen receptors. *Nature*, 307:747–749.

Witt DM, Insel TR. (1991). A selective oxytocin antagonist attenuates progesterone facilitation of female sexual behavior. *Endocrinology*, 128:3269–3276.

Wu TJ, Glucksman MJ, Roberts JL, Mani SK. (2006). Facilitation of lordosis in rats by a metabolite of luteinizing hormone releasing hormone (LHRH). *Endocrinology*, 147(5):2544–2549.

Yamanouchi K, Arai Y. (1990). The septum as origin of a lordosis-inhibiting influence in female rats: effect of neural transection. *Physiol Behav*, 48:351–355.

Yang-Yen HF CJ, Sun YL, Smeal T, Schmidt TJ, Drouin J, Karin M. (1990). Transcriptional interference between c-Jun and the glucocorticoid receptor: mutual inhibition of DNA binding due to direct protein-protein interaction. *Cell*, 62:1205–1215.

Zhang QX, Borg A, Wolf DM, Oesterreich S, Fuqua SA. (1997). An estrogen receptor mutant with strong hormone-independent activity from a metastatic breast cancer. *Cancer Res*, 57:1244–1249.

Zhou D, Apostolakis EM, O'Malley BW. (1999). Distribution of D(5) dopamine receptor mRNA in rat ventromedial hypothalamic nucleus. *Biochem Biophys Res Commun*, 266:556–559.

Zhou L, Blaustein JD, De Vries GJ. (1994). Distribution of androgen receptor immunoreactivity in vasopressin- and oxytocin-immunoreactive neurons in the male rat brain. *Endocrinology*, 134:2622–2627.

Chapter 8

Sex Differences in Affiliative Behavior and Social Bonding

Larry J. Young and C. Sue Carter

The normal establishment of social relationships and social bonds is critical for the survival of most mammalian species and is particularly important in our own species. Several social behaviors, such as territorial aggression or parental care are typically sexually dimorphic, but these sex differences are often diminished in monogamous species that form breeding pairs and work together to raise the offspring.

Various psychiatric disorders including autism spectrum disorders (ASD) and schizophrenia are characterized by severe disruption in social engagement, social reciprocity and communication. ASD, which reportedly has a prevalence of approximately 1 in 166, is 4–5 times more common in males than in females (Fombonne, 2003; Chakrabarti & Fombonne, 2005). Therefore, an understanding of sex differences in the underlying neurobiological and molecular mechanisms regulating affiliative behavior and social bond formation may have important implication for human mental health.

The past 15 years have witnessed phenomenal advances in our understanding of mechanisms un-derlying affiliative behaviors in animal models, including social bonding and parental care. In most mammals, parental care is provided exclusively by the mother, with males displaying little interest or antagonistic behavior toward their offspring (Lonstein & De Vries, 2000). However, in monogamous species, both parents contribute to the care of the offspring. Monogamous species also display selective social attachments, or pair bonds, toward their mates. Although the basic behavioral components of parental care and pair bonding are similar between the sexes, separate, yet related molecular and neurobiological mechanisms appear to be regulating these behaviors in males and females. The underlying neurobiological mechanisms regulating affiliative behavior are influenced by both genetic and epigenetic factors. Here we will discuss both the similarities and differences in the regulation of social bonding and parental behavior between the sexes.

Using the monogamous prairie vole (*Microtus ochrogaster*) as a model system we will focus primarily on the neurobiology of affiliative behavior and social bonding in prairie voles. We will also focus mainly on the roles of the neuropeptides oxytocin (OT) and vasopressin (AVP) and the effects of stress on social bonding and parental care. However, it should be recognized that these neuropeptides do not work in a vacuum, but are simply the most well-characterized systems in a complex network of factors and circuits that regulate these complex behaviors. Finally, we will briefly discuss some implications of these findings for translational research on human social behavior.

VOLES AS A MODEL FOR
AFFILIATIVE BEHAVIOR

The development of microtine rodents, or voles, as laboratory rodent models of affiliation has greatly facilitated our understanding of the sexually dimorphic neurobiological mechanisms of affiliative behaviors, including social bonding and parental care. Vole species vary tremendously in terms of their mating and social structures. Prairie voles are highly affiliative, and are characterized as socially monogamous (Getz et al., 1981; Carter et al., 1995). Although extra-pair copulations do occur (Wolff et al., 2002), nesting pairs are stable over time and both male and female prairie voles cooperate in the rearing of the offspring. This socially monogamous mating structure is rare, occurring in approximately 3%–5% of mammalian species (Kleiman, 1977). Thus, prairie voles are an excellent model for investigating social attachment and parental care, but not sexual monogamy per se. In contrast to prairie voles, montane and certain populations of meadow voles are much less social, do not typically form pair bonds, and the males do not participate in the rearing of the offspring (Jannett, 1980). These species provide valuable opportunities for comparative studies that facilitate the elucidation of mechanisms regulating affiliative behavior.

It may seem counterintuitive that prairie voles would be a useful model for exploring the sexually dimorphic regulation of affiliative behavior, since male and female prairie voles exhibit quite similar social behaviors. Unlike most laboratory animal models, both male and female prairie voles exhibit extensive parental care for their offspring. Similarly, male and female prairie voles form enduring social attachments for their mates. Despite these similarities in behavior, the regulatory mechanisms underlying these behaviors are in

some cases distinct. Furthermore, the sensitivity of the underlying neurobiology regulating these behaviors to environmental influences may also be different between males and females. While this socially monogamous species may not be representative of many mammalian species, prairie voles can provide valuable insights into the sexually dimorphic nature of behaviors that are relevant to our own species.

PARTNER PREFERENCE
FORMATION

In order to examine the neurobiology of social bonding, one needs an appropriate laboratory proxy for the behavior. In the laboratory, pair bonding can be assessed in part using a partner preference test. In this test the experimental subject is placed in a 3-chambered arena in which the partner is tethered to restrict its movement to one chamber and a novel animal of equal stimulus value is placed in the opposite chamber (Williams et al., 1992). In the initial phase of the test, a male and female are housed together and at this time experimental manipulations can occur. Following this cohabitation, the experimental animal, either the male or the female, is placed in the center of the chamber and allowed to freely move about the arena. During a 3-hr test, a pair-bonded prairie vole will spend more than twice as much time in contact with the partner than the stranger.

The initial studies examining partner preference formation revealed that mating facilitates partner preference formation in male and female prairie voles, but is apparently not essential. This partner preference has been postulated to be indicative of a pair bond since the partner preference remained for up to 2 weeks of separation from the partner (Insel & Hulihan, 1995).

Recent studies suggest that genetic and epigenetic factors may influence the length and quality of social interactions needed for the development of partner preferences. For this reason, the exact period of cohabitation necessary for a partner preference to form can vary across laboratories and under different rearing conditions (Bales, et al., 2007b). However, in every case in which comparisons were made, we have found that females form preferences for a familiar partner more quickly than males. In addition, in females mating experience hastened the onset of a partner preference (Williams et al., 1992; DeVries et al., 1996). It was the original finding that mating facilitated pair bond formation that led to the hypothesis that oxytocin (OT), known to be released during sexual behavior, might play a role in pair bond formation (Carter, 1992; Williams et al., 1994).

Pair bonding in prairie voles also is characterized by an increase in mate guarding in both sexes. However, the behavioral experiences and physiological underpinnings necessary for mate guarding are sexually dimorphic. In males, mating was followed by a dramatic increase in male-male aggression, apparent within 24 hrs of the onset of a sexual interaction; nonsexual cohabitation did not trigger the onset of mate guarding in males. Subsequent studies revealed that activation of central arginine vasopressin (AVP) receptors was necessary for the postmating induction of male-male aggression (Winslow et al., 1993). However, in female prairie voles a period of several days of cohabitation—with or without mating—was required to induce intrasexual aggression (Bowler et al., 2002). The neuroendocrine correlates of female-female aggression remain to be identified, but preliminary studies did not implicate vasopressin (Carter, unpublished data). These findings support the more general hypothesis that the neural substrates of pair bond formation are sexually dimorphic, and may rely on differential effects of oxytocin and vasopressin (Carter, 2007).

SEX DIFFERENCES IN PARENTAL CARE

Unlike the situation in non-monogamous species, such as rats, in which the mother is the sole caregiver to the offspring, in monogamous mammals, including prairie voles, both males and females exhibit extensive parental care. A careful analysis of the parental care of primiparous lactating females and their male partners revealed a nearly identical repertoire of parental responsiveness between the sexes (Lonstein & De Vries, 1999b). Subtle quantitative differences in parental care behavior were reported, including the observation that males spent less time in contact with pups, but when in contact with the pups, the males spent more time licking and grooming the pups than females. In addition, males spent less time quiescently positioned over the pups, but more time hunched over the pups than females. These results demonstrate that the neural circuitry for parental behavior is present in both sexes.

Despite these remarkable similarities in nurturing, there are also interesting paradoxical sex differences in parental behavior of sexually-naïve prairie voles. While the majority of sexually-naïve male prairie voles display parental responsiveness when exposed to pups, a high percentage of sexually-naïve, adult-female prairie voles either attack or ignore pups (Lonstein & De Vries, 1999a).

In order to determine whether these sex differences were mediated by circulating gonadal steroid hormones, males and females were gonadectomized for 4 weeks prior to testing for parental behavior. Castrated males continued to display high levels of parental care, whereas ovariectomized females continued to display low levels of maternal care (Lonstein & De Vries, 1999a). These data suggest that sex differences in parental care of virgin prairie voles are independent of the activational effects of gonadal steroids.

In order to determine whether these sex differences were established by perinatal steroid exposure, males were castrated at birth and their spontaneous paternal behavior was assessed as adults (Lonstein et al., 2002). Postnatal castration significantly reduced the percentage of males acting parentally. In contrast, pre- and postnatal treatment with androgen did not increase the percentage of females displaying parental care as adults. These data suggest that while gonadal secretions appear to masculinize paternal responsiveness, i.e. increase the frequency of parental care, testosterone may not be the primary factor responsible for this sexual differentiation.

OXYTOCIN, VASOPRESSIN AND AFFILIATIVE BEHAVIOR

The first studies of the neurochemical mechanisms underlying pair-bond formation focused on the roles of the neuropeptides oxytocin (OT) and arginine vasopressin (AVP). In a wide range of taxa, ranging from fish to mammals, both peptides have been widely implicated in the regulation of several sexually dimorphic social behaviors, including parental care, aggression, territorial behaviors and vocal communication (Goodson & Bass, 2001; Burbach et al., 2006). Oxytocin and AVP are nonapeptides synthesized primarily in the paraventricular and supraoptic nuclei of the hypothalamus.

Magnocellular neurosecretory neurons in these regions project to the posterior pituitary where they release OT and AVP into the blood stream (Burbach et al., 2006). Peripherally circulating OT stimulates uterine contraction during parturition and milk ejection during lactation. Peripheral AVP regulates water reabsorption in the kidney as well as vascular tone. In addition, parvocellular OT and AVP neurons send neuropeptidergic projections throughout the brain. The distribution of OT-producing cells and their projections have not been reported to be sexually dimorphic, at least in voles (Fig. 8.1) (Lim et al., 2004a; Yamamoto et al., 2004).

However, certain neuronal populations of vasopressinergic neurons are highly sexually dimorphic across vertebrate taxa. AVP-synthesizing neurons in the bed nucleus of the stria terminalis and medial amygdala produce significantly more AVP mRNA in males than in females. These neurons are believed to result in the dense AVP immunoreactive fiber plexus in the ventral pallidum and lateral septum that have been implicated in pair-bond formation and paternal behavior in male prairie voles (Fig. 8.1) (De Vries & Buijs, 1983; Liu et al., 2001; Lim & Young, 2004; De Vries & Panzica, 2006).

These neurons are sensitive to gonadal steroids, both early in development and in adulthood (De Vries & Panzica, 2006). Castration of males dramatically reduces the AVP mRNA and immunoreactivity in these regions. Androgen replacement restores AVP synthesis. Androgen treatment increases AVP expression in females, however not to the same degree as in males (De Vries et al., 1994). This difference in sensitivity to gonadal steroids appears to be due to early organizational effects of androgens since treating early postnatal females with testosterone abolishes the sex difference in sensitivity to androgen (Wang et al., 1993).

OXYTOCIN AND PAIR BONDING IN FEMALES

Because of the demonstrated role of OT in regulating maternal care and mother-infant bonding (Pedersen & Prange, 1979; Kendrick et al., 1987; Kendrick et al., 1997), and because its release is stimulated by vaginocervical stimulation (Kendrick et al., 1986; Sansone et al., 2002), OT was an excellent candidate for facilitating pair-bond formation in female prairie voles. Intracerebroventricular infusion of OT via osmotic minipumps during a 6-hour cohabitation pe-

riod without mating stimulated the development of a partner preference in female prairie voles. Control females receiving CSF during the same cohabitation failed to display a partner preference (Williams et al., 1994). Furthermore, infusion of an OT receptor antagonist (OTA) prevented the OT-induced partner preference.

A second study replicated this finding, but also reported that equivalent doses of AVP were not sufficient to stimulate pair-bond formation in females (Insel & Hulihan, 1995). That same report found that infusion of an OTA, but not an AVP receptor antagonist prevented partner preference formation in female prairie voles after a 14-hr cohabitation period (Insel & Hulihan, 1995). Although AVP receptor activation does not appear to be necessary for mating-induced pair bonding in female prairie voles, exogenous AVP is capable of inducing partner preferences in females after a short 1-hr cohabitation (Cho et al., 1999). Interestingly, partner preferences in this paradigm could be blocked by either OTA or AVP antagonists, suggesting that exogenous peptide may be acting to promote selective partner preference formation via both OT and AVP receptors. However, access to either OT or AVP may be sufficient to facilitate non-selective social behaviors in both sexes (Cho, et al., 1999). Clues regarding the neural circuitry involved in OT-mediated pair-bond formation in females emerged from comparative neuroanatomical studies examining OT receptor distribution in prairie voles and non-monogamous species, including montane voles (Witt et al., 1991; Insel & Shapiro, 1992). Prairie voles have high densities of OT receptors in the nucleus accumbens and prefrontal cortex, while montane voles have very low densities of OT receptors in the nucleus accumbens (Fig. 8.2). Given their role in reward and reinforcement, these regions are attractive candidates for regulating social attachments. In fact, infusion of an OT receptor antagonist into the prefrontal cortex or the nucleus accumbens, but not the adjacent caudate putamen, prevents mating-induced partner preference formation (Fig. 8.2) (Young et al., 2001). These results suggest that partner preference formation in female prairie voles involves the activation of the mesolimbic dopamine reward circuitry. In fact, dopamine is released within the nucleus accumbens in female prairie voles during mating and dopamine receptor antagonists prevent pair-bond formation in female prairie voles (Gingrich et al., 2000).

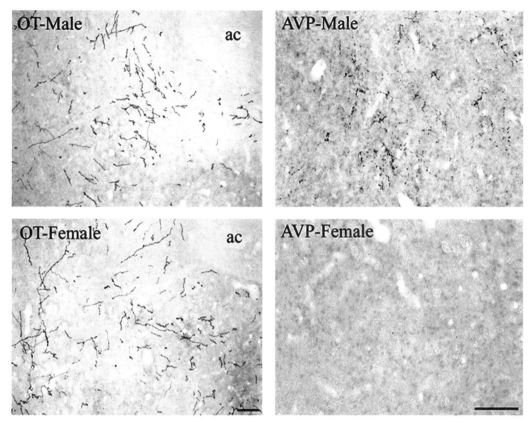

Figure 8.1. OT and AVP immunocytochemistry in males and females. OT-immunoreactive fibers are observed in the nucleus accumbens in both males and females, with no apparent sexual dimorphism (left column). AVP-immunoreactive fibers appear in the ventral pallidum in males but not females (right column). Scale bar = 100 μm. Note that the OT photomicrographs are taken at twice the magnification of the AVP photomicrographs. *Abbreviations:* ac = anterior commissure. Adapted with permission from Lim MM, Murphy AZ, Young LJ. (2004). Ventral striatopallidal oxytocin and vasopressin V1a receptors in the monogamous prairie vole (*Microtus orchorogaster*). *J of Comparative Neurology*, 468:555–570.

VASOPRESSIN AND PAIR BONDING IN MALES

In studies paralleling those discussed for females, AVP has been shown to facilitate partner preference formation in male prairie voles. The actions of AVP in the brain are mediated by V1a and V1b receptor (V1aR and V1bR, respectively) subtypes of AVP receptors, although most of the social behavioral effects of AVP have been attributed to the V1aR subtype.

Intracerebroventricular infusion of a selective V1aR antagonist prevents mating-induced partner preference formation as well as the selective aggression associated with mating in male prairie voles (Winslow et al., 1993). In that same study, infusion of AVP, but not OT, facilitated partner preference formation in the absence of mating. Infusion of an OT receptor antagonist did not block mating-induced partner preference formation. These data suggest that AVP, but not OT, regulates pair-bond formation in male prairie voles. However, a separate study using a different paradigm slightly contradicted these findings by demonstrating that a single infusion of either OT or AVP could stimulate partner preference formation after a 1-hr cohabitation period (Cho et al., 1999). Another study also provides evidence that OT may play a role in pair bonding in males since OT antagonist into the lateral septum prevented partner preference formation (Liu et al., 2001).

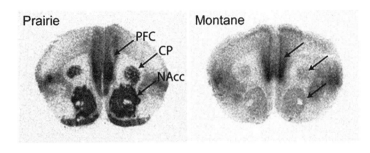

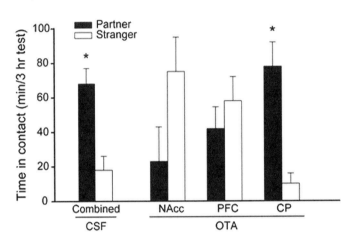

Figure 8.2. Oxytocin regulation of pair bonding in female prairie voles. Top: Receptor autoradiograms illustrating that prairie voles have much higher densities of oxytocin receptor in the nucleus accumbens (NAcc) and caudate putamen (CP) compared to non-monogamous montane voles. Both species have oxytocin receptor in the prefrontal cortex (PFC). Bottom: An OT receptor antagonist (OTA; 1ng/side in 200 nl) infused bilaterally into the NAcc or PFC, but not the (CP) blocks partner preference formation in female prairie voles. Adapted with permission from Young LJ, Wang Z. (2004). The neurobiology of pair bonding. *Nature Neuroscience*, 7(10):1048–1054.

As in females, candidate sites of action of AVP for stimulating partner preference formation in males were identified by comparing the distribution of V1aR binding sites in monogamous prairie voles and non-monogamous montane and meadow voles (Insel et al., 1994; Lim & Young, 2004). Prairie voles have higher levels of receptors in several brain regions including the ventral pallidum, medial dorsal thalamus, and medial amygdala than do montane or meadow voles (Fig. 8.3). When V1aR antagonist was site-specifically infused into each of these regions, only infusions into the vental pallidum prevented partner preference formation (Fig. 8.3) (Lim & Young, 2004).

Furthermore, viral vector mediated up-regulation of V1aR binding in the ventral pallidum of male prairie voles stimulated partner preferences in the absence of mating (Pitkow et al., 2001). Finally, overexpression of the prairie vole V1aR in the ventral pallidum of male meadow voles, which typically do not form partner preferences, resulted in the development of partner preferences (Lim et al., 2004b).

A separate study found that infusing V1aR antagonist into the lateral septum inhibited partner preference (Liu et al., 2001). This is interesting in light of the role of septal V1aR in regulating social recognition in males (Bielsky et al., 2005). The lateral septum projects heavily to the nucleus accumbens and could potentially relay social signals to the reward pathway.

These data suggest that species differences in pair bonding may arise from species differences in expression pattern of the AVP receptors in males. Molecular studies have begun to address the mechanisms that may underlie this species difference. A comparison of the prairie and montane vole V1aR gene revealed two intriguing differences. First, the prairie vole V1aR gene has been duplicated, a process which could have altered the expression pattern of the gene (Young et al., 1999). Second, a highly repetitive microsatellite DNA element found in the promoter of the prairie vole AVP receptor gene promoter is nearly absent in the montane and meadow vole genes. This altered promoter structure may alter expression pattern since it has been demonstrated in cell culture reporter assays that variations in this microsatellite can alter gene expression in a cell-specific manner (Hammock & Young, 2004).

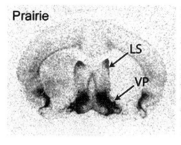
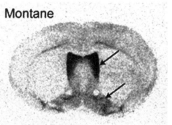
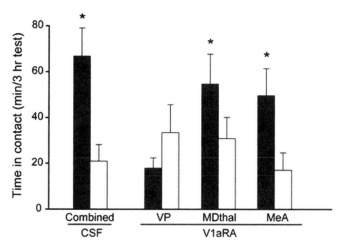

Figure 8.3. Vasopressin regulation of pair bonding in male prairie voles. Top: Receptor autoradiograms illustrating that prairie voles have higher densities of V1a vasopressin receptors (V1aR) in the ventral pallidum (VP) compared to montane voles. Bottom: Infusion of a selective V1aR antagonist (V1aRA, 0.05 ng/side in 1 μl) into the VP, but not into the mediodorsal thalamus (MDthal) or medial amygdala (MeA) prevents mating-induced partner preference formation in male prairie voles. Scale bar = 1mm. Adapted from Young LJ, Wang Z (2004). The neurobiology of pair bonding. *Nature Neuroscience*, 7(10):1048–1054.

However, it should be noted that a recent survey of other non-monogamous vole species suggest that the microsatellite is also present in several other non-monogamous rodent species, suggesting that the presence or absence of the microsatellite alone is not responsible for differences in social organization across other vole species (Fink et al., 2006). This observation does not rule out the possibility that more subtle differences in microsatellite length or composition may contribute to variation in receptor gene expression.

The highly repetitive microsatellite in the V1aR promoter is unstable and there is a significant amount of variability in the length of the microsatellite between individual prairie voles (Hammock & Young, 2002, 2005). There is also an extraordinary amount of individual variation in V1aR binding in specific brain regions of male prairie voles (Phelps & Young, 2003).

In order to determine whether variation in the V1aR promoter was associated with variation in V1aR density in the brain, male and female prairie voles were genotyped and selectively bred to produce a group of breeders and offspring that were homozygous for either short alleles, or long alleles of the microsatellite. Adult male offspring from the two genotypes

were then paired with females and subjected to a partner preference test. Male prairie voles with a long microsatellite had higher levels of V1aR receptor expression in several brain regions, including the olfactory bulb and lateral septum, and were more likely to display partner preferences than males with short microsatellite (Hammock & Young, 2005). This finding demonstrates that variations in promoter of the AVP receptor gene result in variations in social bonding in males. Females were not examined in this study for partner preference formation.

SEX DIFFERENCES IN THE ROLES OF OT AND AVP IN PAIR BONDING

As demonstrated, most of the studies examining pair bonding in females have focused on OT rather than AVP, while studies examining pair bonding in males have focused on AVP. But is the regulation of social bonding in voles really sexually dimorphic?

One study reports that OT antagonist, but not V1aR antagonist prevents mating-induced pair bonding in females (Insel & Hulihan, 1995). A separate study found that a V1aR antagonist, but not an OT antagonist blocks partner preference in males (Winslow et al., 1993). These data suggest a clear sex difference in the relative role of endogenous OT and AVP in pair-bond formation. However, infusions of either OT or AVP are capable of facilitating partner preferences after a brief cohabitation, suggesting that capacity for both peptides to stimulate partner preferences are similar between the sexes (Cho et al., 1999).

Furthermore, one study reported that infusion of an OT antagonist into the lateral septum blocked partner preference formation in male prairie voles, suggesting that both OTR and V1aR activation may be necessary in partner preference formation in male prairie voles (Liu et al., 2001). This would be consistent with the known role of both OT and AVP in regulating social recognition in males (Popik & Ree, 1991; Popik et al., 1992; Bielsky & Young, 2004; Bielsky et al., 2005), a process that undoubtedly is critical for the development of a pair bond.

Most studies have failed to report sex differences in OT or V1aR binding in the prairie vole brain (Insel & Shapiro, 1992; Wang et al., 1996). A recent study reporting a sex difference in OTR binding in the prefrontal cortex is the exception (Smeltzer et al., 2006), but other studies have not reported this difference. One potential explanation for the sex difference in the roles of OT and AVP lies in the sexually dimorphic release of the peptides during cohabitation and mating. AVP is clearly sexually dimorphic and is likely what is responsible for the male-specific role of this peptide; not only in pair bonding, but a host of other male-typical social behaviors (Goodson & Bass, 2001).

Oxytocin synthesis in the brain is not typically sexually dimorphic (Yamamoto et al., 2004). However, it is possible that OT is preferentially released in the female (Kramer et al., 2004), which might be especially relevant during the vaginocervical stimulation associated with copulation (Fig. 8.4). In addition, OT is essential for social recognition (Ferguson et al., 2000; Ferguson et al., 2001), a process that is implicit in pair bonding in both sexes.

OXYTOCIN, VASOPRESSIN, AND PARENTING

While there have been no studies examining the regulation of maternal care in lactating female prairie voles, studies have examined the potential role of neu-

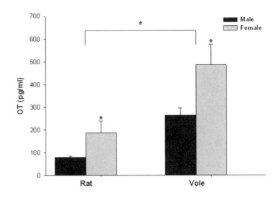

Figure 8.4. Plasma levels of OT are higher in females than in males, and also higher in prairie voles than in rats. Adapted with permission from Kramer KM, Cushing BS, Carter CS, Wu J, Ottinger MA (2004). Sex and species differences in plasma oxitocin using an enzyme immunoassay. *Can J Zoology*, 82: 1194–1200.

ropeptides in the regulation of spontaneous maternal care, or alloparental care, in juvenile and adult virgin female prairie voles. In contrast to virgin adult female prairie voles, juvenile females display high levels of alloparental care (Fig. 8.5) (Olazabal & Young, 2006a).

Among juvenile females, individual variation in alloparental care is positively correlated with OT receptor density in the nucleus accumbens (Olazabal & Young, 2006a). This relationship also holds across species. Meadow voles and mice have little or no OT receptor in the nucleus accumbens and juveniles of these species do not display alloparental care. Rats have intermediate levels of OT receptors in the striatum and display more alloparental behavior than do meadow voles or mice.

As mentioned previously, the majority of adult female prairie voles are not maternal. Spontaneously maternal individuals have higher densities of OT receptor in the nucleus accumbens than non-maternal females (Olazabal & Young, 2006b). Furthermore, infusion of an OT receptor antagonist into the nucleus accumbens blocks spontaneous maternal care. These data suggest that OT acting in the nucleus accumbens plays a role in facilitating maternal care in female prairie voles. Comparable studies in male prairie voles are needed to determine whether similar relationships hold for male parental care. Furthermore, there have been no studies examining the potential role of AVP in regulating maternal care in female prairie voles.

The initial studies of the regulation of paternal care in males focused again on the role of AVP. A sexually dimorphic plexus of AVP-immunoreactive fibers is concentrated in the lateral septum of the male prairie vole. Prairie vole fathers, or males that had been paired with a female for 3 days, have decreased levels of AVP-immunoreactivity in the septum compared to sexually-naïve males (Bamshad et al., 1993; Bamshad et al., 1994). The decrease in septal AVP after cohabitation with a female was coincident with an increase in paternal behavior as well as in increase in AVP mRNA in the cells giving rise to these projections (Wang et al., 1994b). These data were interpreted as being consistent with AVP being released from the immunoreactive plexus and an associated increase in AVP synthesis to replenish stores. Subsequent studies found that infusion of AVP into the lateral septum of sexually-naïve male prairie voles facilitated paternal care, while a selective V1aR antagonist inhibited paternal care (Wang et al., 1994a).

Variations in V1aR expression patterns in the brain have also been associated with individual variation in paternal care in prairie voles. Male prairie voles with shorter alleles of the microsatellite sequence in the 5′ flanking region of the V1aR gene have lower levels V1aR binding in the lateral septum and olfactory bulb compared to males with longer alleles of the same microsatellite (Hammock & Young, 2005). When tested for paternal behaviors with their own pups, short allele males displayed slightly less licking and grooming than did long allele males. Interestingly, there were no differences in licking and grooming of pups between long allele and short allele females, consistent with the sexually dimorphic regulation of parental behavior. It is not known whether these differences in paternal behavior are due to the variations in septal V1aR density, but this finding is consistent with the pharmacological studies demonstrating the role of septal AVP in regulating paternal care.

Despite these observations, the role of AVP in regulating paternal care is not as simple as it may seem. As mentioned, castration of males for up to 8 weeks did not significantly decrease the percentage of male prairie voles that displayed paternal care even though it resulted in a nearly complete loss of AVP immunoreactivity in the septum (Lonstein & De Vries, 1999a). The authors attributed this contradictory result potentially to differences in genetic background in the colony over time, although it is possible that AVP from other sources may have compensated for the decrease in septal AVP.

In addition, even small differences in animal husbandry can affect alloparental behavior in this species (Bates, et al., 2007b). Another study found that both OT and AVP may be contributing to the regulation of paternal care. While a central infusion of a V1aR antagonist or an OT receptor antagonist alone did not inhibit alloparental behavior, a cocktail of both inhibitors did reduce parental care and increased the number of attacks, suggesting that activation of either the V1aR or the OT receptor may be sufficient to facilitate paternal behavior (Bales et al., 2004b).

SEXUALLY DIMORPHIC DEVELOPMENTAL EFFECTS OF OT AND AVP

Exposure to peptides and steroids, especially during development, can reprogram the nervous system, altering thresholds for sociality, emotionality and aggression (Carter, 2003). Among the likely targets of developmentally-induced variations in behavior are OT and AVP and their receptors. For example, in rats enhanced maternal stimulation is capable of increasing expression of the OTR in females and the V1aR in males (Champagne et al., 2001; Francis et al., 2002; Champagne et al., 2003). In prairie voles exposure to AVP in the first week of life increased the tendency toward aggression in adulthood; these effects also were most obvious in males (Stribley & Carter, 1999).

The literature on effects of either hormonal manipulations or handling in early life support the general hypothesis that males are especially sensitive to developmental perturbations in part because the AVP system, including AVP synthesis (Yamamoto et al., 2004) and expression of V1aRs (Bales et al., 2007a), may be more easily disrupted in males and also of greater importance in male behavior (Carter, 2003; 2007). The OT system also is sensitive to early experience (Yamamoto et al., 2004), probably capable of affecting both females and males.

One study examined the effects of neonatal disruption of OT neurotransmission by treating pups with either saline, OT or an OT antagonist. The OT antagonist resulted in a decrease in alloparental care in 21 day old males, but did not significantly affect this behavior in females (Fig. 8.5) (Bales et al., 2004a). Interestingly, OT treatment in neonatal males

5a.

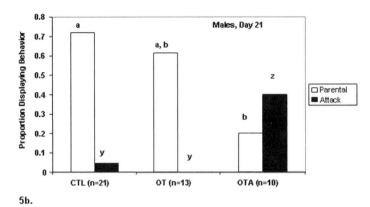

5b.

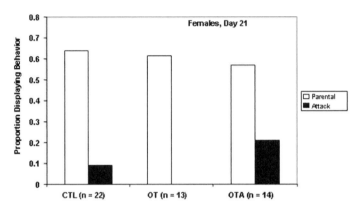

Figure 8.5. The effects of neonatal manipulations are often sexually dimorphic. (A). Effects of neonatal exposure to oxytocin (OT), an OT antagonist (OTA), or control (CTL) treatment on male parental and attack behavior, day 21 (Fisher's exact test, P=.021). Different letters indicate groups that are different at P<.05.* (B). Effects of neonatal exposure to OT, OTA, or CTL treatments on female parental and attack behavior, day 21. Adapted with permission from Bales KL, Pfeifer LA, Carter CS (2004). Sex differences and developmental effects of manipulations of oxytocin on alloparenting and anxiety in prairie voles. *Develomental Psychobiology*, 44:123–131.

also resulted in an increased likelihood of developing a partner preference after a brief cohabitation (Bales & Carter, 2003). Deficits in the OT system may yield increased sensitivity to stress and a corresponding change in the capacity to manage stressful experiences (Ragnauth et al., 2005).

SEX DIFFERENCES IN THE EFFECTS OF STRESS ON SOCIAL BEHAVIORS

Sexually-dimorphic neuropeptides, including AVP and OT, may be of particular relevance to sex differences in emotional reactivity to social stimuli and other forms of stressors. With references to both social behaviors and the management of related challenges or stress, males seem to be more dependent on AVP than females. Thus, male behavior may be especially sensitive to changes in this system. Females might be less reliant on AVP in part because they have lower central levels of this peptide in critical brain regions,

such as the bed nucleus of the stria terminalis, medial amygdala, lateral septum, all of which have been implicated in stress and coping. Alternatively, females may be insensitive to AVP, or even show directionally different effects when exposed to AVP (Winslow et al., 1993; Thompson et al., 2006).

Several of the functions normally served by AVP in males may rely on OT in females; a lack of dependence on AVP also could serve to protect females from over reacting to stimuli, such as those encountered during social interactions.

Sex differences in reproductive strategies may be mirrored by sex differences in reactivity to stressors, including those associated with social interactions. In general, male reproductive strategies are associated with increased mobilization, while more passive strategies are found in females. In male prairie voles, pair-bond formation is facilitated by either exposure to a stressor or increases in corticosterone and possibly an associated increase in AVP. Females in contrast, responded to stressors or corticosterone treatments by showing a decreased tendency to form a heterosexual pair bond, possibly because stress inhibits OT, upon which they are more dependent than males (DeVries et al., 1995; DeVries et al., 1996).

Reactions to stimuli from infants may be physiological related to the responses to other forms of stressors, and thus might be expected to be sexually dimorphic and possibly regulated differently in males and females. Data from prairie voles also support this hypothesis. Exposure to a stressor, such as swimming, has sexually dimorphic effects on parental behavior, tending to increase parental behavior in males, but not in females (Bales et al., 2006). Parental behavior in male prairie voles also appears to require AVP (Wang et al., 1994a) and perhaps OT as well (Bales et al., 2004b); preliminary data suggest that parental behavior in female prairie voles, as in other species, may be primarily reliant on OT (Bales & Carter, 2002; Olazabal & Young, 2006b). Adding AVP to the endogenous hormonal cocktail for parental behavior may allow males to overcome fear or anxiety and attend to infants even under stressful conditions.

The absence of social interactions can be a stressor for highly social mammals, such as prairie voles. Females may be generally more vulnerable to the effects of social isolation, again possibly in part due to sex differences in the functions of OT and AVP. In nature, female prairie voles rarely remain in social isolation, although males may live alone. In adult female prairie vole social isolation, followed by a social stressor, was associated with increased OT as well as AVP, CRF, ACTH and corticosterone (Grippo et al., 2007). OT was also elevated in isolated males, but AVP, ACTH and corticosterone did not differ in males living with a sibling versus alone, once more suggesting a sex difference in reactivity to stress. In general, the effects of isolation on stress hormones are more pronounced in females than in males (Ruscio et al., 2007; Grippo et al., 2007). In males versus females the actions of AVP might be protective against the negative consequences of living alone.

TRANSLATIONAL IMPLICATIONS FOR SEXUALLY DIMORPHIC REGULATION OF AFFILIATIVE BEHAVIORS

Sex differences in psychiatric disorders are common. A better understanding of the role of sexually dimorphic neuropeptides will inform our understanding of

such differences or may suggest biologically-based interventions. Particularly striking is the sex difference in autism spectrum disorders (ASD), which are usually characterized by atypical social behaviors as well as anxiety. ASD is 4–5 times more prevalent in males than females. It has been hypothesized that high levels of testosterone during early development, may create a predisposition to ASD, producing phenotypic changes associated with "extreme" maleness (Baron-Cohen & Belmonte, 2005). Neural mechanisms through which testosterone or related steroids might potentiate ASD have not been fully elaborated. Alternatively, variations in OT or AVP activity may contribute to the social behavioral phenotype of ASD.

Blood levels of OT are low in certain forms of ASD (Modahl et al., 1998). An extended form of OT (termed OT-X), considered a precursor for OT, was measured at higher than normal levels in blood from children described as autistic (Green et al., 2001). The extended form of OT may be less active than regular OT and indicates altered processing of the OT precursor. Whether differences in OT might play a causal role in the features of ASD remains to be determined, however there is some evidence that OT infusions may reduce some of the behavioral symptoms in ASD (Hollander et al., 2003; Bartz & Hollander, 2006).

Recent pharmacological and imaging studies in humans suggest that OT may in fact alter social cognition, including interpersonal trust (Heinrichs et al., 2003; Kirsch et al., 2005; Kosfeld et al., 2005). The OT receptor also has been a target for several linkage and linkage disequilibrium studies in families containing family members diagnosed with ASD (Ylisaukko-Oja et al., 2005). Single nucleotide polymorphisms (SNPs) in the OTR have been associated with ASD in the Chinese Han population (Wu et al., 2005) and in a Caucasian population within the United States (Jacob, et al., 2007). Measurements of the AVP peptide as a function of ASD have not been reported. However, linkage and linkage disequilibrium for the gene for the AVP V1a receptor have been described in a subset of families including members diagnosed with ASD (Kim et al., 2001; Wassink et al., 2004; Yirmiya et al., 2006).

Research to date supports the general hypothesis that males are especially sensitive to developmental perturbations in part because the AVP system, including AVP synthesis, and expression of V1aRs, are more easily disrupted in males and also of greater importance in male behavior (Carter, 2007). In humans, elevations in central AVP, experimentally induced by intranasal infusion of this peptide, can have behavioral consequences, possibly by increasing behavioral or emotional reactivity to normally irrelevant stimuli or non-threatening social stimuli. The behavioral effects of exogenous AVP also are sexually dimorphic. Men given additional AVP showed increases in activity in corregator muscles, a component of frowning, and also rated neutral facial expression as more "unfriendly." In contrast, females given AVP smiled more and reported more positive, affiliative responses to unfamiliar neutral faces (Thompson et al., 2006). In males (but possibly less so in females), AVP-facilitated hypersensitivity to or misinterpretation of social stimuli might exacerbate the features of ASD.

We are only in the earliest stages of understanding the sexually dimorphic nature of the brain mechanisms that regulate affiliative behavior and social bonding. Animal models such as the prairie vole are essential for an understanding of how males and females differentially regulate social behaviors. These studies will provide valuable insights that may be useful for understanding sexually dimorphic pathologies in social behaviors such as that found in autism.

Acknowledgments

We express gratitude to our many colleagues, hopefully all appropriately credited below, who contributed the research upon which this review is based. Research described here was supported by NIH (HD 38490; MH 073022; MH 072935), and the National Alliance for Autism Research (CSC) and NIH (MH056538, MH56897 and MH64692), NSF STC IBN-9876754 and the Yerkes Center Grant RR00165 (LJY).

References

Bales KL, Carter CS. (2003). Developmental exposure to oxytocin facilitates partner preferences in male prairie voles (*Microtus ochrogaster*). *Behav Neurosci*, 117:854–859.

Bales KL, Carter CS. (2002). Oxytocin facilitates parental care in female prairie voles (but not in males). *Soc Neurosci* Abstr, 89.3.

Bales KL, Pfeifer LA, Carter CS. (2004a). Sex differences and developmental effects of manipulations of oxytocin on alloparenting and anxiety in prairie voles. *Dev Psychobiol*, 44:123–131.

Bales KL, Kim AJ, Lewis-Reese AD, Sue Carter C. (2004b). Both oxytocin and vasopressin may influ-

ence alloparental behavior in male prairie voles. *Horm Behav*, 45:354–361.

Bales KL, Kramer KM, Lewis-Reese AD, Carter CS. (2006). Effects of stress on parental care are sexually dimorphic in prairie voles. *Physiol Behav*, 87:424–429.

Bales KL, Plotsky PM, Young LJ, Lim MM, Grotte N, Ferrer E, Carter CS. (2007a). Neonatal oxytocin manipulations have long-lasting, sexually dimorphic effects on vasopressin receptors. *Neuroscience* 144: 38–45.

Bales KL, Lewis-Reese AD, Pfeifer LA, Kramer KM, Carter CS. (2007b). Early experience affects the traits of monogamy in a sexually dimorphic manner. *Dev Psychobiology* 49:335–342.

Bamshad M, Novak MA, DeVries GJ. (1993). Sex and species differences in the vasopressin innervation of sexually naive and parental prairie voles, *Microtus ochrogaster* and meadow voles, *M. pennsylvanicus.J Neuroendocrinol*, 5:247–255.

Bamshad M, Novak M, de Vries G. (1994). Cohabitation alters vasopressin innervation and paternal behavior in prairie voles (*Microtus ochrogaster*). *Physiol and Behav*, 56:751–758.

Baron-Cohen S, Belmonte MK. (2005). Autism: a window onto the development of the social and the analytic brain. *Annu Rev Neurosci*, 28:109–126.

Bartz J, Hollander E. (2006). The neuroscience of affiliation: forging links between basic and clinical research on neuropeptides and social behavior. *Horm Behav*, 50(4):518–528.

Bielsky IF, Young LJ (2004) Oxytocin, vasopressin, and social recognition in mammals. *Peptides*, 25:1565–1574.

Bielsky IF, Hu SB, Ren X, Terwilliger EF, Young LJ. (2005). The V1a vasopressin receptor is necessary and sufficient for normal social recognition: a gene replacement study. *Neuron*, 47:503–513.

Bowler, CM, Cushing BS, Carter CS. (2002). Social factors regulate female-female aggression and affiliation in prairie voles. *Physiol Behav* 76: 559–566.

Burbach P, Young LJ, Russell J. (2006). Oxytocin: synthesis, secretion and reproductive functions. In Neill JD, (Ed.), 3rd Edition, *Knobil and Neill's Physiology of Reproduction*, (pp 3055–3127). San Diego: Academic Press.

Carter, CS. 1992. Oxytocin and sexual behavior. *Neurosci Biobehav Rev*, 16: 131–144.

Carter CS. (2003). Developmental consequences of oxytocin. *Physiol Behav*, 79:383–397.

Carter CS. (2007). Sex differences in oxytocin and vasopressin: implications for autism spectrum disorders? *Behav Brain Res*, 176:170–186.

Carter CS, DeVries AC, Getz LL. (1995). Physiological substrates of mammalian monogamy: the prairie vole model. *Neurosci Biobehav Rev*, 19:303–314.

Chakrabarti S, Fombonne E. (2005). Pervasive developmental disorders in preschool children: confirmation of high prevalence. *Am J Psychiatry*, 162:1133–1141.

Champagne F, Diorio J, Sharma S, Meaney MJ. (2001). Naturally occurring variations in maternal behavior in the rat are associated with differences in estrogen-inducible central oxytocin receptors. *Proc Natl Acad Sci U S A*, 98:12736–12741.

Champagne FA, Weaver IC, Diorio J, Sharma S, Meaney MJ. (2003). Natural variations in maternal care are associated with estrogen receptor alpha expression and estrogen sensitivity in the medial preoptic area. *Endocrinology*, 144:4720–4724.

Cho MM, DeVries AC, Williams JR, Carter CS. (1999). The effects of oxytocin and vasopressin on partner preferences in male and female prairie voles (*Microtus ochrogaster*). *Behav Neurosci*, 113:1071–1079.

De Vries G, Buijs R. (1983). The origin of vasopressinergic and oxytocinergic innervation of the rat brain with special reference to the lateral septum. *Brain Res*, 273:307–317.

De Vries GJ, Panzica GC. (2006). Sexual differentiation of central vasopressin and vasotocin systems in vertebrates: different mechanisms, similar endpoints. *Neuroscience*, 138:947–955.

De Vries GJ, Wang Z, Bullock NA, Numan S. (1994). Sex differences in the effects of testosterone and its metabolites on vasopressin messenger RNA levels in the bed nucleus of the stria terminalis of rats. *J Neurosci*, 14:1789–1794.

DeVries AC, DeVries MB, Taymans SE, Carter CS. (1996). The effects of stress on social preferences are sexually dimorphic in prairie voles. *Proc Natl Acad Sci USA*, 93:11980–11984.

DeVries CA, DeVries MB, Taymans S, Carter CS. (1995). Modulation of pair bonding in female prairie voles (*Microtus ochrogaster*) by corticosterone. *Proc Natl Acad Sci USA*, 92:7744–7748.

Ferguson JN, Aldag JM, Insel TR, Young LJ. (2001). Oxytocin in the medial amygdala is essential for social recognition in the mouse. *J Neuroscience*, 21:8278–8285.

Ferguson JN, Young LJ, Hearn EF, Insel TR, Winslow JT. (2000). Social amnesia in mice lacking the oxytocin gene. *Nature Genetics*, 25:284–288.

Fink S, Excoffier L, Heckel G. (2006). Mammalian monogamy is not controlled by a single gene *Proc Natl Acad Sci USA*, 103:10956–10960.

Fombonne E. (2003). The prevalence of autism. *JAMA*, 289:87–89.

Francis DD, Young LJ, Meaney MJ, Insel TR. (2002). Naturally occurring differences in maternal care are associated with the expression of oxytocin and vasopressin (V1a) receptors: gender differences. *J Neuroendocrinol*, 14:349–353.

Getz LL, Carter CS, Gavish L. (1981). The mating system of the prairie vole *Microtus ochrogaster*: field and laboratory evidence for pair bonding. *Behav Ecol Sociobiol*, 8:189–194.

Gingrich B, Liu Y, Cascio C, Wang Z, Insel TR. (2000). Dopamine D2 receptors in the nucleus accumbens are important for social attachment in female prairie voles (*Microtus ochrogaster*). *Behav Neurosci*, 114:173–183.

Goodson JL, Bass AH. (2001). Social behavior functions and related anatomical characteristics of vasotocin/vasopressin systems in vertebrates. *Brain Res Rev*, 35:246–265.

Green LA, Fein D, Mohahl C, Feinstein C, Waterhouse L, Morris M. (2001). Oxytocin and autistic disorder: alterations in peptide forms. *Biol Psychiatry*, 50:609–613.

Grippo AJ, Lamb DG, Carter CS, Porges SW. (2007) Social isolation disrupts autonomic regulation of the heart and influences negative affective behaviors. *Biol Psychiatry*, in press.

Hammock EAD, Young LJ. (2002). Variation in vasopressin V1a receptor promoter and expression: implications for inter- and intraspecific variation in social behavior. *Eur J Neurosci*, 16:399–402.

Hammock EAD, Young LJ. (2004). Functional microsatellite polymorphisms associated with divergent social structure in vole species. *Mol Biol Evol*, 21:1057–1063.

Hammock EAD, Young LJ. (2005). Microsatellite instability generates diversity in brain and sociobehavioral traits. *Science*, 308:1630–1634.

Heinrichs M, Baumgartner T, Kirschbaum C, Ehlert U. (2003). Social support and oxytocin interact to suppress cortisol and subjective responses to psychosocial stress. *Biol Psychiatry*, 54:1389–1398.

Hollander E, Novotny S, Hanratty M, Yaffe R, DeCaria CM, Aronowitz BR, Mosovich S. (2003). Oxytocin infusion reduces repetitive behaviors in adults with autistic and Asperger's disorders. *Neuropsychopharmacology*, 28:193–198.

Insel TR, Shapiro LE. (1992). Oxytocin receptor distribution reflects social organization in monogamous and polygamous voles. *Proc Natl Acad Sci*, 89:5981–5985.

Insel TR, Hulihan T. (1995). A gender-specific mechanism for pair bonding: oxytocin and partner preference formation in monogamous voles. *Behav Neurosci*, 109:782–789.

Insel TR, Wang Z, Ferris CF. (1994). Patterns of brain vasopressin receptor distribution associated with social organization in microtine rodents. *J Neurosci*, 14:5381–5392.

Insel TR, Preston S, Winslow JT. (1995). Mating in the monogamous male: behavioral consequences. *Physiol Behav*, 57:615–627.

Jannett FJ. (1980). Social dynamics of the montane vole *Microtus montanus*, as a paradigm. *The Biologist*, 62:3–19.

Jacob S, Brune CW, Carter CS, Leventhal B, Lord C, Cook EH, Jr. (2007). Association of the oxytocin receptor gene (*OXTR*) in Caucasian children and adolescents with autism. *Neuroscience Letters*, 417: 6–9.

Kendrick KM, Keverne EB, Baldwin BA. (1987). Intracerebroventricular oxytocin stimulates maternal behaviour in the sheep. *Neuroendocrinol*, 46:56–61.

Kendrick KM, Keverne EB, Baldwin BA, Sharman DF. (1986). Cerebrospinal fluid levels of acetylcholinesterase, monoamines and oxytocin during labor, parturition, vaginocervical stimulation, lamb separation and suckling in sheep. *Neuroendocrinol*, 44: 149–156.

Kendrick KM, Costa APCD, Broad KD, Ohkura S, Guevara R, Levy F, Keverne EB. (1997). Neural control of maternal behavior and olfactory recognition of offspring. *Brain Res Bull*, 44:383–395.

Kim S, Young LJ, Gonen D, Veenstra-VanderWeele J, Courchesne R, Courchesne E, et al. (2001). Transmission disequilibrium testing of arginine vasopressin receptor 1A (AVPR1A) polymorphisms in autism. *Mol Psychiatry*, 7:503–507.

Kirsch P, Esslinger C, Chen Q, Mier D, Lis S, Siddhanti S, et al. (2005). Oxytocin modulates neural circuitry for social cognition and fear in humans. *J Neurosci*, 25:11489–11493.

Kleiman D. (1977). Monogamy in mammals. *Q Rev Biol*, 52:39–69.

Kosfeld M, Heinrichs M, Zak PJ, Fischbacher U, Fehr E. (2005). Oxytocin increases trust in humans. *Nature*, 435:673–676.

Kramer KM, Cushing BS, Carter CS, Wu J, Ottinger M. (2004). Sex and species differences in plasma oxytocin using an enzyme immunoassay. *Canad J Zoology*, 82:1194–1200.

Lim MM, Young LJ. (2004). Vasopressin-dependent neural circuits underlying pair-bond formation in the monogamous prairie vole. *Neurosci*, 125:35–45.

Lim MM, Murphy AZ, Young LJ. (2004a). Ventral striato-pallidal oxytocin and vasopressin V1a receptors in the monogamous prairie vole (*Microtusochrogaster*). *J Comp Neurol*, 468:555–570.

Lim MM, Wang Z, Olazábal DE, Ren X, Terwilliger EF, Young LJ. (2004b). Enhanced partner preference in promiscuous species by manipulating the expression of a single gene. *Nature*, 429:754–757.

Liu Y, Curtis JT, Wang ZX. (2001). Vasopressin in the lateral septum regulates pair-bond formation in male prairie voles (*Microtus ochrogaster*). *Behav Neurosci*, 115:910–919.

Lonstein JS, De Vries GJ. (1999a). Sex differences in the parental behaviour of adult virgin prairie voles: independence from gonadal hormones and vasopressin. *J Neuroendocrinol*, 11:441–449.

Lonstein JS, De Vries GJ. (1999b). Comparison of the parental behavior of pair-bonded female and male prairie voles (*Microtus ochrogaster*). *Physiol and Behav*, 66:33–40.

Lonstein JS, De Vries GJ. (2000). Sex differences in parental behavior of rodents. *Neurosci Biobehav Rev*, 24:669–686.

Lonstein JS, Rood BD, De Vries GJ. (2002). Parental responsiveness is feminized after neonatal castration in virgin male prairie voles, but is not masculinized by perinatal testosterone in virgin females. *Horm Behav*, 41:80–87.

Modahl C, Green LA, Fein D, Morris M, Waterhouse L, Feinstein C, Levin H. (1998). Plasma oxytocin levels in autistic children. *Biol Psychiatry*, 43:270–277.

Olazabal DE, Young LJ. (2006a). Species and individual differences in juvenile female alloparental care are associated with oxytocin receptor density in the striatum and the lateral septum. *Horm Behav*, 49: 681–687.

Olazabal DE, Young LJ. (2006b). Oxytocin receptors in the nucleus accumbens facilitate "spontaneous" maternal behavior in adult female prairie voles. *Neuroscience*, 25;141(2):559–568.

Pedersen CA, Prange AJ, Jr. (1979), Induction of maternal behavior in virgin rats after intracerebroventricular administration of oxytocin. *Proc Natl Acad Sci USA*, 76:6661–6665.

Phelps SM, Young LJ. (2003). Extraordinary diversity in vasopressin (V1a) receptor distributions among wild prairie voles (*Microtusochrogaster*): patterns of variation and covariation. *J Comp Neurol*, 466:564–576.

Pitkow LJ, Sharer CA, Ren X, Insel TR, Terwilliger EF, Young LJ. (2001). Facilitation of affiliation and pair-bond formation by vasopressin receptor gene transfer into the ventral forebrain of a monogamous vole. *J Neurosci*, 21:7392–7396.

Popik P, Ree JMV. (1991). Oxytocin but not vasopressin facilitates social recognition following injection into the medial preoptic area of the rat. *Eur Neuropsychopharm*, 1:555–560.

Popik P, Vos PE, Ree JMV. (1992). Neurohypophyseal hormone receptors in the septum are implicated in social recognition in the rat. *Behav Pharm*, 3:351–358.

Ragnauth AK, Devidze N, Moy V, Finley K, Goodwillie A, Kow LM, et al. (2005). Female oxytocin gene-knockout mice, in a semi-natural environment, display exaggerated aggressive behavior. *Genes, Brain, & Behavior*, 4:229–239.

Ruscio MG, Sweeny T, Hazelton J, Suppatkul P, Carter C S. (2007) Social environment regulates corticotropin releasing factor, corticosterone and vasopressin in juvenile prairie voles. *Horm Behav* 51:54–61.

Sansone GR, Gerdes CA, Steinman JL, Winslow JT, Ottenweller JE, Komisaruk BR, Insel TR. (2002). Vaginocervical stimulation releases oxytocin within the spinal cord in rats. *Neuroendocrinol*, 75:306–315.

Smeltzer MD, Curtis JT, Aragona BJ, Wang Z. (2006). Dopamine, oxytocin, and vasopressin receptor binding in the medial prefrontal cortex of monogamous and promiscuous voles. *Neurosci Lett*, 394:146–151.

Stribley JM, Carter CS. (1999). Developmental exposure to vasopressin increases aggression in adult prairie voles. *Proc Natl Acad Sci U S A*, 96:12601–12604.

Thompson RR, George K, Walton JC, Orr SP, Benson J. (2006). Sex-specific influences of vasopressin on human social communication. *Proc Natl Acad Sci USA*, 103:7889–7894.

Wang Z, Bullock NA, De Vries GJ. (1993). Sexual differentiation of vasopressin projections of the bed nucleus of the stria terminalis and medial amygdaloid nucleus in rats. *Endocrinol,* 132:2299–2306.

Wang Z, Ferris CF, De Vries GJ. (1994a). Role of septal vasopressin innervation in paternal behavior in prairie voles (*Microtusochrogaster*). *Proc Natl Acad Sci USA,* 91:400–404.

Wang Z, Smith W, Major DE, DeVries GJ. (1994b). Sex and species differences in the effects of cohabitation on vasopressin messenger RNA expression in the bed nucleus and stria terminalis in prairie voles (*Microtusorchogaster*) and meadow voles (*Microtuspennsylvanicus*). *Brain Res,* 650:212–218.

Wang Z, Young LJ, Liu Y, Insel TR. (1996). Species differences in vasopressin receptor binding are evident early in development: comparative anatomic studies in prairie and montane voles. *J Comp Neurol,* 378:535–546.

Wassink TH, Piven J, Vieland VJ, Pietila J, Goedken RJ, Folstein SE, Sheffield VC. (2004). Examination of AVPR1a as an autism susceptibility gene. *Mol Psychiatry,* 9:968–972.

Williams J, Catania K, Carter C. (1992). Development of partner preferences in female prairie voles (*Microtusochrogaster*): the role of social and sexual experience. *Horm Behav,* 26:339–349.

Williams JR, Insel TR, Harbaugh CR, Carter CS. (1994). Oxytocin administered centrally facilitates formation of a partner preference in prairie voles (*Microtus ochrogaster*). *J Neuroendocrin,* 6:247–250.

Winslow J, Hastings N, Carter CS, Harbaugh C, Insel T. (1993). A role for central vasopressin in pair bonding in monogamous prairie voles. *Nature,* 365:545–548.

Witt DM, Carter CS, Insel TR. (1991). Oxytocin receptor binding in female prairie voles: Endogenous and exogenous oestradiol stimulation. *J Neuroendocrinol,* 3:155–161.

Wolff JO, Mech SG, Dunlap AS, Hodges KE. (2002). Multi-male mating by paired and unpaired female prairie voles (*Microtusochrogster*). *Behaviour,* 139: 1147–1160.

Wu S, Jia M, Ruan Y, Liu J, Guo Y, Shuang M, et al. (2005). Positive association of the oxytocin receptor gene (OXTR) with autism in the Chinese Han population. *Biol Psychiatry,* 58:74–77.

Yamamoto Y, Cushing BS, Kramer KM, Epperson PD, Hoffman GE, Carter CS. (2004). Neonatal manipulations of oxytocin alter expression of oxytocin and vasopressin immunoreactive cells in the paraventricular nucleus of the hypothalamus in a gender-specific manner. *Neuroscience,* 125:947–955.

Yirmiya N, Rosenberg C, Levi S, Salomon S, Shulman C, Nemanov L, et al. (2006). Association between the arginine vasopressin 1a receptor (AVPR1a) gene and autism in a family-based study: mediation by socialization skills. *Mol Psychiatry,* 11:488–494.

Ylisaukko-Oja T, Alarcon M, Cantor RM, Auranen M, Vanhala R, Kempas E, et al. (2005). Search for autism loci by combined analysis of Autism Genetic Resource Exchange and Finnish families. *Ann Neurol,* 59(1):145–155.

Young LJ, Wang Z. (2004). The neurobiology of pair bonding. *Nat Neurosci,* 7:1048–1054.

Young LJ, Lim M, Gingrich B, Insel TR. (2001). Cellular mechanisms of social attachment. *Horm Behav,* 40: 133–148.

Young LJ, Nilsen R, Waymire KG, MacGregor GR, Insel TR. (1999). Increased affiliative response to vasopressin in mice expressing the vasopressin receptor from a monogamous vole. *Nature,* 400:766–768.

Chapter 9

Sex Differences in the Organization of Movement

Evelyn F. Field and Ian Q. Whishaw

*It is to be expected that some research workers will
always like to watch animals.*
Barnett, 1963, p. xv

One of the first scientists to record his observations regarding how and why males and females differed was Aristotle. He felt that the scientific study of why we come in two sexes, male and female, would ultimately lead to an understanding of what is "naturally more knowable" regarding life's diversity (Cosans, 1998). His analysis of what made males and females distinct from one another was driven by how males and females differed in external physical form and behavior; that is, by what he could see.

Historically, studies of sex differences in sexual and non-sexual behaviors were restricted to what could be seen in real time with the naked eye. Lordosis and mounting during rat sexual behavior could be discriminated as they occurred. Changes in the performance of males and females as they learned to solve a spatial task could be timed with a stop watch. Also, the number of aggressive or playful bouts that occurred during a social encounter could be recorded as they took place. Many of the initial behaviors that were studied, with regards to sex differences in behavior, were deter-mined by what could be seen and tracked in real time. With advances in technology, however, the details of how behaviors are organized can now be observed and quantified in the time scale of milliseconds.

The detailed analysis of movement organization, in vertebrates, is commonly referred to as the study of functional vertebrate morphology or kinematics (Ashley-Ross & Gillis, 2002). Historically, research in this discipline has focused on how the expression of a behavior, such as locomotion, is generated by the overall morphology and skeletomusculature of the organism being studied. Many kinesiologists and functional morphologists, either implicitly or explicitly, focus on how an animal's peripheral form (i.e. number of limbs) determines its kinematic profile during behaviors such as forward locomotion. Consequently, the common, often unspoken, consensus is that differences in the kinematic organization of a behavior between two organisms or between two sexes are due to differences in an animal's form, not to differences in the central nervous system (CNS) instructions that govern the expression of the behavior being studied (Smith, 1994). It is possible, however, that the organization of movement is not determined entirely by the form of the animal. Thus, the kinematic organization of a pattern of movement may be determined by the CNS, in spite of variations in animal morphology. This may be especially true for differences in how movements are coordinated by males and females.

With regards to sex differences in behavior, males and females differ in their frequency of expression of many reproductive (Ward, 1992), and non-reproductive behaviors (Beatty, 1992). For example, males play at a higher frequency as juveniles (Pellis, 2002), and exhibit different patterns of aggression (Blanchard, Sheperd, Carobrez, & Blanchard, 1991) open-field exploration (Elliot & Grunberg, 2005; Palanza, 2001) as adults, than females. In general, research regarding sex differences in behavior has focused on whether there are differences in the sex-typical frequency of expression of a selected behavior. Rarely, has the question of whether sex differences are present in the kinematic organization of behaviors, that are functionally similar and equally successful, been addressed.

In this chapter, research will be presented that has focused on the question of whether there are sex differences in the kinematic organization of movement. In addition, the relative contributions of gonadal steroids, the CNS, and of body morphology, to the development and subsequent adult expression of sex-typical patterns of movement will be discussed.

The concept that sex differences can exist in the kinematic organization of behavior, and that gonadal steroids can influence the expression of a non-reproductive pattern of movement is not without precedent. Frank Beach has shown that the execution of a movement pattern can differ between male and female dogs and that these differences can be influenced by gonadal hormones. Prior to the onset of sexual maturity, both male and female dogs squat during micturition. After puberty, while females continue to squat, males often raise one hind leg. The sex difference in adult micturition patterns is modifiable by androgen exposure neonatally (Beach, 1974). Males that are castrated shortly after birth no longer express the male typical pattern of micturition in adulthood (Fig. 9.1).

The successful performance of a movement, in rats, can also be influenced by the stage of the estrous cycle at testing. The ability of a female rat to traverse a beam, and accurately place its feet on that beam, is significantly better at behavioral estrus than proestrus or diestrus (Becker, Snyder, Miller, Westgate, & Jenuwine, 1987). This has been linked directly to 17β-estradiol levels in the striatum (Becker et al., 1987). A correlation between sensorimotor performance and whether an animal is in behavioral estrus or diestrus has also been shown for female rats that are placed on a treadmill that undergoes unpredictable changes in speed. Females in diestrus compensate for the changes in speed by varying the swing phase of the step cycle. In contrast, females in estrus compensate for changes in treadmill speed by changing their stride length (Smith, 1998; Smith & Chapin, 1996; Smith et al., 2000).

Research, using humans, has also shown that motoric performance can vary across the menstrual cycle. Females, at the midluteal phase of the menstrual cycle—when estradiol and progesterone levels are highest—display better performance on manual dexterity tasks than at other times of the cycle, such as menstruation, when estradiol and progesterone levels are at their lowest (Hampson & Kimura, 1988). Thus, there is evidence that the organization of movement can be sex-typical and that the execution of a movement can be modified by gonadal steroid exposure.

In rats, it has been shown that males and females differ in how they organize their movements during their execution of numerous non-reproductive behaviors such as locomotion, spontaneous turning, evasion during juvenile play, dodging to protect a food item, contact righting, skilled reaching, and the postural adjustments made during haloperidol-induced catalepsy (Field, Martens, Watson, & Pellis, 2005; Field, Watson, Whishaw, & Pellis, 2005; Field & Whishaw, 2005; Field, Whishaw, Forgie, & Pellis, 2004; Field, Whishaw, & Pellis, 1996; Field, Whishaw, & Pellis, 1997a; Field, Whishaw, & Pellis, 1997b; Field, Whishaw, & Pellis, 2000). In the subsequent sections of this chapter the sexual differentiation of the kinematic organization of behavior during juvenile play, dodging to protect a food item and contact righting, will be discussed.

SEX DIFFERENCES IN THE KINEMATIC ORGANIZATION OF PLAY BEHAVIOR

The initial description of sex differences in the kinematic organization of a non-sexual behavior, in rats,

MALE

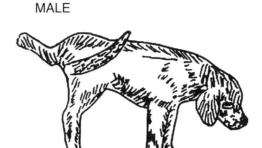

FEMALE

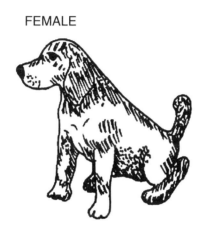

Figure 9.1. The urinary posture of domestic dogs is sexually dimorphic after puberty. Adult females and puppies of both sexes assume a squatting posture (A). During the onset of puberty, however, males switch to the adult male form where one leg is raised (B). Adapted with permission from Beach FA (1974). Effects of gonadal hormones on urinary behavior in dogs. *Physiology & Behavior*, 12:1005–1013.

was conducted for evasion during play. Play-fighting, or rough and tumble play, is an activity common to the juveniles of many mammalian species (Fagen, 1981). The frequency of play fighting in juvenile rats is sexually dimorphic (Pellis, 2002). In general, males initiate more attacks to the nape, the area of preferred contact during social play, than do females (Meaney, 1989; Pellis & Pellis, 1990; Thor & Holloway, 1983).

Males and females also differ in their response to a playful attack. Females are more likely to evade an approaching conspecific than are males. Males, in contrast, are more likely to roll over to a supine position (Pellis & McKenna, 1992; Pellis & Pellis,

1990). While males and females differ in their frequency of play behavior and the type of defense they use in response to a playful attack, they also differ in how they organize their movements during defensive maneuvers such as evasion (Pellis, Field, Smith & Pellis, 1997).

Females, when swerving away laterally from an approaching conspecific pivot around a point close to the pelvis; and thus, their bodies move unidirectionally in a forward, cephalocaudal direction away from the conspecific. Males, in contrast, are more likely to couple evasive tactics with a movement of their pelvis back towards the conspecific that is attempting to make nape contact. Thus, males move their napes away from the attacker and use the lower body to block the approach of the opponent (Pellis et al., 1997; Pellis & Pellis, 1987).

One difficulty, however, with the analysis of sex differences in the organization of movement during play fighting, is that sex differences in the organization of a behavior such as evasion may be due to the males' attempts to enhance their opportunity for counterattack by placing themselves in closer proximity to the attacker after the completion of an evasive maneuver. The motoric behaviors during play fighting are also often composed of movements in multiple directions. The defending animal, while evading an approaching conspecific during a play bout by turning laterally, may also simultaneously leap vertically or incorporate rotation around the longitudinal axis to move the nape away from the conspecific.

Therefore, while the initial study of sex differences in the kinematic organization of behavior was done by analyzing the evasive movements performed during play, the complexity of the movements led to the selection of a different behavioral paradigm. The behavior that was chosen for analysis, to determine whether males and females differed in their organization of lateral evasive maneuvers, was dodging to protect a food item from an approaching conspecific (Whishaw, 1988; Whishaw & Tomie, 1987; Whishaw & Tomie, 1988).

DODGING TO PROTECT A FOOD ITEM

When eating a food item, a rat will typically hold the food in both forepaws and lean backwards onto its hindpaws. If another rat approaches from the side and attempts to grab the food pellet the rat that is eating will dodge laterally away from the approaching conspecific to protect the food item from theft. This behavior was chosen for analysis since the magnitude of the dodge is approximately 180° away from an approaching conspecific, and its beginning and end are easily identified. Males and females are equally successful in the completion of this task (Whishaw, 1988; Whishaw & Gorny, 1994; Whishaw & Tomie, 1987; Whishaw & Tomie, 1988) and it is a behavior that occurs primarily in the horizontal plane (Field et al., 1996). The final advantage is that dodging is a behavior that rats express naturally. It first appears just

after weaning (Bolles & Woods, 1964), and the early onset of this behavior makes it amenable to analysis during development and in adulthood.

A kinematic analysis of dodging in Long-Evans male and female rats revealed that they use different patterns of movement and postural adjustments to complete this behavior even though their overall success in completing the task was equivalent between the sexes (Field et al., 1996). Males make a significantly larger excursion with the pelvis than do females. This difference is due to a larger backwards and sideways movement of the pelvis in the opposite direction to the movement of the snout (Fig. 9.2). The difference in the movement of the pelvis is due, in part, to differences in the stepping patterns of the hindpaws.

The sex-typical hindpaw stepping patterns, used during dodging to protect a food item, are illustrated in Figure 9.3A and 9.3B. After turning laterally, (Aa-b) females make an initial forward and sideways step with the hindpaw ipsilateral to the direction of the dodge (Ab). This step is followed by a forward step by the hindpaw contralateral to the direction of the dodge (Ad) and a final forward step by the hindpaw ipsilateral to the direction of the dodge (Ae). In contrast, males make less lateral movement of the upper body (Ba) before taking a backward step with the hindpaw ipsilateral to the direction of the dodge (Bb). This is often followed by either, or both, a second backward step by the ipsilateral hindpaw (Bd), and a sideways step of the contralateral hindpaw into the approaching conspecific (Bd). The ipsilateral hindpaw then makes a final forward step (Be). Thus, sex differences in hindpaw stepping are present both in the frequency and direction of steps (Fig. 9.3) and these differences contribute to the differences seen in the trajectory traveled by the pelvis during a dodge.

The Role of the Conspecific

It is possible that the sex differences in the kinematic organization of the dodge are due to the influence of the conspecific (in this case, the thief). The initial analysis of sex differences in the organization of dodging movements was conducted using animals that dodged from same-sex conspecifics. While a kinematic analysis of the behavior of male and female robbers revealed no differences in their angle of approach or their proximity to the food item held by the dodging

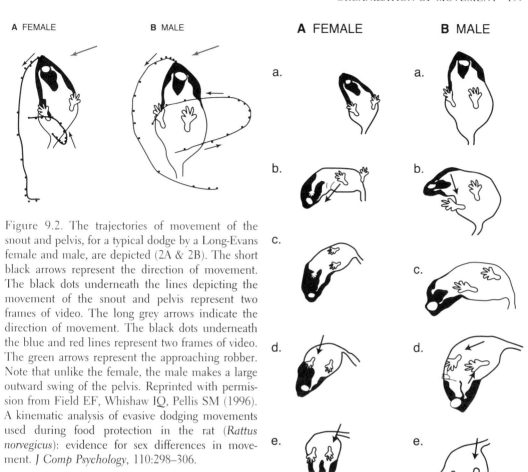

Figure 9.2. The trajectories of movement of the snout and pelvis, for a typical dodge by a Long-Evans female and male, are depicted (2A & 2B). The short black arrows represent the direction of movement. The black dots underneath the lines depicting the movement of the snout and pelvis represent two frames of video. The long grey arrows indicate the direction of movement. The black dots underneath the blue and red lines represent two frames of video. The green arrows represent the approaching robber. Note that unlike the female, the male makes a large outward swing of the pelvis. Reprinted with permission from Field EF, Whishaw IQ, Pellis SM (1996). A kinematic analysis of evasive dodging movements used during food protection in the rat (*Rattus norvegicus*): evidence for sex differences in movement. *J Comp Psychology*, 110:298–306.

Figure 9.3. The number and direction of the steps taken by the hindpaws during a typical female (3A) and male (3B) dodge are shown. Adapted with permission from Field EF, Whishaw IQ, Pellis SM (1996). A kinematic analysis of evasive dodging movements used during food protection in the rat (*Rattus norvegicus*): evidence for sex differences in movement. *J Comp Psychology*, 110:298–306.

animal (Field et al., 1996), it is still possible, that the differences found were a function of being paired with a same-sex partner. Female robbers may be perceived as less threatening than males.

To test this, the dodging patterns of males and females that were paired with opposite sex conspecifics were analyzed. No differences in the sex-typical expression of dodging were found when females or males dodged from a conspecific of the same or opposite sex (Field et al., 1997b). Thus, sex differences in the composition of the dodge are not determined by the behavior or sex of the robber.

The Role of Experience

It is also possible that the expression of sex-typical patterns of movement organization is dependent on the interaction of animals with one another during the juvenile phase. As mentioned previously, dodging is a behavior that begins to be spontaneously expressed just after weaning between postnatal (P) days 21 and 24 (Bolles & Woods, 1964).

In order to determine whether experience during the juvenile period is necessary for the sex-typical kinematic organization of dodging in adulthood, animals were isolated from P21 until P90. Two same-sex animals were housed in cages with a wire mesh partition. This allowed the animals to still see, smell, and huddle beside one another, but they could not engage in physical interaction. As adults, the animals were given free access to one another for three weeks during the training and testing phase. It was found that, as adults, both males and females expressed sex-typical patterns of movement organization that were indistinguishable from controls. This suggests that physical interaction during the juvenile phase is not necessary for the sex-typical expression of dodging in adulthood. One confound, however, is that the three weeks of combined housing may be enough to compensate for the effects of isolation during the juvenile and pubertal phase.

During dodging, males and females are also sexually dimorphic in how they orient their pelvis to the robber at the end of the dodge. Males generally orient their pelvis to the head of the robber whereas females generally orient their pelvis towards the midbody of the robber (Field et al., 2004; Field et al., 1997b) (Fig. 9.4). This sex difference is irrespective of whether the robber is male or female (Field et al., 1997b).

After separation during the juvenile phase males and females no longer orient their pelvis towards the robber in a sex-typical manner. Isolated males and females orient their pelvis, towards the head or midbody, of the robber indiscriminately. This provides evidence that the normal development of at least one aspect of the dodging animal's behavior is dependent on juvenile experience. Thus, while some aspects of the adult-typical interaction of the dodging animal with the conspecific are dependent on juvenile interactions other aspects, such as the sex-typical kinematic organization of dodging, are not.

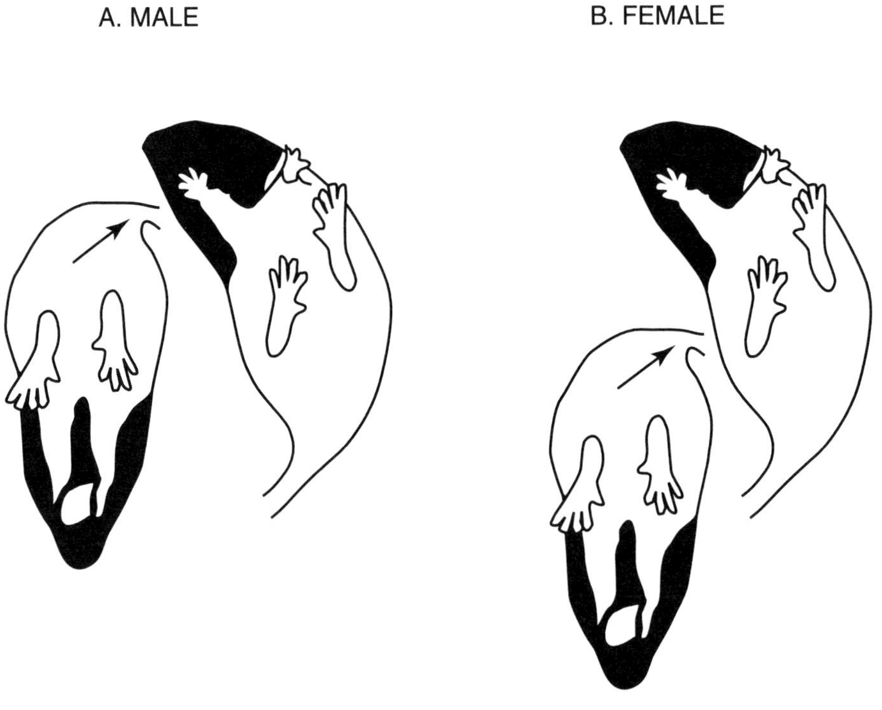

A. MALE   B. FEMALE

Figure 9.4. The final position of the dodger with respect to the robber is shown here. The final, male-typical, position of the dodging rat is shown with its pelvis aligned to the head of the robber (4A). The final, female-typical, position of the dodging rat is shown with its pelvis aligned to the midbody of the robber (4B). Adapted with permission from Field EF, Whishaw IQ, Pellis SM. (1997). Organization of sex-typical patterns of defense during food protection in the rat: the role of the opponent's sex. *Aggressive Behavior*, 23:197–214.

THE ROLE OF GONADAL STEROIDS

Once a sex difference in the organization of a behavior is documented the possible roles that gonadal steroids may play, with regards to the development and sexual differentiation of a behavior, are often investigated (Baum, 2003; Beach, 1975; Beach, 1981; Becker et al., 2005). Traditionally, the model for sexual differentiation of mammals has viewed the female as the default condition (Jost, 1983). Testes are necessary to produce the external genitalia typical of genetic males; ovaries, however, are not needed to produce the external genitalia typical of females (Jost, 1960). Thus, in the absence of testicular hormones, the genetic male develops the female phenotype (Voutilainen, 1992).

The time of exposure to gonadal steroids may also be critical for the expression of sex-typical patterns of behavior. There are periods of time during development when exposure to gonadal steroids may organize the neural circuits that underlie the expression of sex-typical patterns of non-sexual behavior in adulthood. These same neural circuits, in adulthood, may subsequently rely on exposure to gonadal steroids for activation before the sex-typical behavior pattern in question is expressed (Phoenix, Goy, Gerall, & Young, 1959).

Since the seminal work by Phoenix and colleagues (1959), a number of studies have demonstrated the validity of the organizational/activational hypothesis of gonadal steroid effects for sex-typical sexual behavior in mammals (Adkins-Reagan, Mansukhani, Thompson, & Yang, 1997; Baum, 2003), and in non-sexual behaviors such as aggression (Blanchard et al., 1991; Blanchard & Blanchard, 1990), play (Pellis, 2002; Pellis, Field, Smith, & Pellis, 1997; Pellis & Pellis, 1990), spatial behavior (Kanit et al., 2000; Kanit et al., 2000; Roof & Stein, 1999), spontaneous and exploratory behavior (Mead, Hargreaves, & Galea, 1996; Quadagno, Shryne, Anderson, & Gorski, 1972; Swanson, 1966), and anxiety (Beck & Luine, 2002; Papaioannou, Gerozissis, Prokopiou, Bolaris, & Stylianopoulou, 2002).

Thus, it is possible that the kinematic organization of sex-typical patterns of behavior may depend on either or both the organizational and activational effects of gonadal steroids (Baum, 2003). To address the question of whether the sexual differentiation of the organization of the movements used to protect a food item required gonadal steroid exposure, testicular and ovarian hormones were removed at various time points during development, and the subsequent expression of dodging, in adulthood, was analyzed.

Testicular Hormones

The presence or absence of testicular hormones during development can influence the development of male-typical patterns of dodging. Male rats were castrated at three different ages: (a) within the first 24 hours of birth, (b) just prior to puberty, and (c) in adulthood. Females were treated with 200 µl of testosterone propionate (TP) on postnatal days 1 and 2. It was found that males castrated at birth were more similar to intact females than to intact males in the kinematics of their dodging behavior. Castration prior to puberty, or in adulthood, had no effect. TP treated females in contrast, were more like intact males than intact females. Thus, the development and expression of the male-typical pattern of dodging is likely dependent on the organizational, but not activational, effects of testicular hormones (Field et al., 1997a).

Ovarian Hormones

As previously discussed, female-typical patterns of development have often been considered the default condition. Gonadal steroids are often not considered necessary for the development of female-typical form and behavior (Jost, 1983; MacLusky & Naftolin, 1981). There is growing evidence, however, that female-typical patterns of behavior are not simply the default condition, but are actively determined by both genetic (De Vries et al., 2002) and hormonal processes (Collaer & Hines, 1995). Furthermore, a number of behavioral studies have shown that the action of ovarian hormones is necessary for the female-typical development of sexual (Gerall, Dunlap, & Hendricks, 1973; Hendricks & Duffy, 1974) and non-sexual (Field et al., 2000; Forgie & Stewart, 1994; Pellis, 2002; Stewart & Cygan, 1980) behaviors.

In order to determine whether the presence of ovarian steroids is necessary for the development of the female-typical pattern of dodging, the behavior of female rats that were ovariectomized within the first 24 hours after birth, prior to puberty, or as adults was examined. It was found that females ovariectomized just after birth used the same pattern of dodging as intact males. Females ovariectomized prior to puberty exhibited patterns of dodging that qualitatively appeared female-like but incorporated backwards steps of the hindpaw that are typical of males. This suggests that for females, in contrast to males, there is an organizational effect of ovarian steroids during puberty for the development of female-typical patterns of motor behavior in adulthood.

Ovariectomy in adulthood, similar to castration in males, had no effect (Field et al., 2004). Thus, the organization of the female pattern of dodging is dependent on the presence of neonatal and pubertal gonadal steroids (Field et al., 1997a). These data provide evidence that the female-typical pattern of movement organization during dodging is not a default, but is actively feminized and demasculinized (Fitch, Cowell, & Denenberg, 1998; Fitch & Denenberg, 1998; Pellis, 2002) by ovarian steroids.

Further research will need to be conducted to determine the relative contributions of ovarian and testicular steroids, and their associated receptor subtypes to the development of sex-typical patterns of movement and its neural control. For example, the effects of estrogen can be exerted via two intracellular receptor subtypes—ERα and ERβ (McEwen, 2001). Estrogenic effects on behavior can be specific to receptor subtype. For example, the running wheel activity of female mice is dependent on the presence of ERα, not ERβ (Ogawa, Chan, Gustafsson, Korach, & Pfaff, 2003).

It has also been shown that female hormones, most specifically estrogen, can have influences on the biochemical and behavioral output of the dopaminergic system of the basal ganglia (Becker, 1990a; Becker, 1990b; Becker, 1999), a system that is involved in the coordination and selection of motor patterns (Hikosaka, 1998; Mink, 1996). Therefore, it is possible that the effects of androgens and estrogens on the development and the function of the basal ganglia dopaminergic system may be, in part, responsible for the development of sex-typical patterns of movement organization.

THE ROLE OF BODY MORPHOLOGY

One possible confound, or explanatory variable for the sex differences in movement patterns that have been documented for dodging to protect a food item, is the presence of sex differences in overall body mass and morphology. Male Long-Evans rats, as adults, are larger than females; this is due in part to the influence of gonadal steroids during early development (Wade, 1976).

Gonadectomy just after birth influences final adult body mass; males castrated at birth are smaller (Field et al., 1997a), and females ovariectomized at birth are larger, than their intact male and female counterparts (Field et al., 2004). Thus, it is possible that sex differences in the organization of movement and posture may arise from peripheral differences in overall body mass.

Similarly, since there are sex differences in the morphology of the pelvis for a number of species including humans (Coleman, 1969), rats (Bernstein & Crelin, 1967), mice (Shimizu & Awata, 1984), and rabbits (Lowrance, 1968), as well as in muscle and organ weights (Stewart & German, 1999), and skeletal mass (DeMoss & Wright, 1998), it is possible that sex differences in movement are a byproduct of the sexual differentiation of body form. Sex differences in the organization of movement, as has been discussed previously, are often interpreted as due to sex differences in body composition or mass. It is also possible, however, that sex differences in the organization of movement are due primarily to differences in the organization of the CNS and its program for movement rather than differences in peripheral form.

To determine whether sex differences in body mass or morphology can be the sole explanatory variable for sex differences in movement organization during dodging to protect a food item, the kinematics of dodging were examined in gravid females which are similar in mass to intact adult males; in juvenile males and females prior to the sexual differentiation of the pelvis (Berstein & Crelin, 1967); and in testicular feminized males which are female-typical in their body morphology, but are thought to have a masculinized CNS due to the masculinizing effects of estrogens aromatized from androgens (McGinnis, Marcelli, & Lamb, 2002; Olsen, 1992; Stanley, Gumbreck, Allison, & Easley, 1973).

Pregnant Females

Gravid females at G19/20 are indistinguishable from normal males with regards to overall mass (Field et al., 2004). If overall body mass contributes to the expression of sex-typical patterns of movement then gravid females should be more similar to intact males than females. The results from this experiment revealed that gravid females were similar to intact females, not to intact males. Thus, differences in body mass cannot be the sole reason for the expression of sex-typical patterns of dodging in Long-Evans male and female rats (Field et al., 2004).

Juvenile Males and Females

While the study of pregnant females shows that a female-typical pattern of movement is used by females irrespective of mass it is still possible that differences in the development of body morphology and putatively the underlying skeletomusculature have contributed to the adult expression of sex-typical patterns of dodging. As mentioned previously, rats begin to exhibit dodging behavior shortly after weaning (Bolles & Woods, 1964), prior to sex differences in the morphology of the pelvis, which in rats, arise around puberty (Bernstein & Crelin, 1967). Both males and females use sex-typical patterns of dodging prior to puberty (Pellis, Field, & Whishaw, 1999); and thus, prior to the sexual differentiation of the pelvis. These findings provide further support for the hypothesis that sex differences in the organization of movement are neurally based and not determined by sex differences in body composition.

The *tfm* Model

The third approach used to determine whether skeletomusculature was relevant to the type of dodge pattern performed was in the study of behavior in the testicular feminized mutation (*tfm*) or *tfm*-affected male rat.

The *tfm* rat (Stanley et al., 1973), as a consequence of a point mutation in the androgen receptor gene (Yarbrough et al., 1990), is insensitive to the direct effect of androgens which are necessary to masculinize the body (Vanderschueren et al., 1994). Thus, *tfm* males express a feminine peripheral phenotype, including a blind-end vagina, a nipple line (Stanley et al., 1973), an unandrogenized skeleton, as determined by a smaller femur length, width, and weight, and a smaller overall body size than intact males (McGinnis et al., 2002; Vanderschueren et al., 1994).

Masculinization of the rodent CNS, in contrast to the periphery however, is thought to be accomplished primarily by the aromatization of testosterone to estrogen (McCarthy, 1994; Olsen, 1992). *tmf* males have functional secretory testes located in the abdomen, male-like levels of circulating testosterone (Purvis, Haug, Clausen, Naess, & Hansson, 1977), and possess a nuclear estrogen binding system that is similar to

control males (Purvis et al., 1977). It has been demonstrated that *tfm* males can exhibit male sexual behavior as adults (Olsen, 1979b; Shapiro, Levine, & Adler, 1980). In addition, it has been shown that castration during the neonatal period, prior to postnatal day 10 (Olsen, 1979a), in contrast to castration after postnatal day 10 (Olsen & Whalen, 1981), is necessary to induce lordosis with estrogen treatment in adulthood. Therefore, it is thought that the CNS of the *tfm* male is largely masculinized and defeminized via the aromatization of testosterone to estrogen during the perinatal period.

The analysis of the behavior of *tfm* males, during dodging to protect a food item, revealed that even though they were smaller and more feminized in their body morphology, which includes a lack of external testes and thus a caudal testicular mass, they were indistinguishable from control wild-type males, but were significantly different from their control wild-type females, in their performance of male-typical patterns of dodging. There is evidence, however, that they do not perform in a male-typical manner in all aspects of their non-reproductive behavior. Males do not express male-typical patterns of play behavior (Field, Whishaw, Pellis, & Watson, 2006); and thus, the masculinization of the organization of movement is dissociable from male-typical patterns of play behavior that have been shown to be androgen dependent (Pellis, 2002).

The results of the experiments previously described provide evidence that sex differences in movement organization are not due solely to differences in overall body mass, are not dependent on the presence of external testicular mass, and are not likely due to sex differences in skeletomusculature. Thus, sex differences in movement organization must be due, in large part, to sex differences in how the CNS orchestrates the organization of sex-typical patterns of movement and how gonadal steroids during the neonatal and pubertal period influence the sex-typical development of the neural circuits that underlie these behaviors.

CONTACT RIGHTING

While evidence that sex differences are present in the kinematic organization of dodging to protect a food item has been presented, sex differences in movement organization are present in a number of behaviors in the rat, and are thus not task specific (Field et al.,

2005; Field & Whishaw, 2005; Field et al., 2000; Pellis et al., 1997). A second behavior where kinematic differences in the organization of movement have been described is contact righting, or the ability of an animal to role over from supine to prone when placed on a solid surface (Field et al., 2005).

Both male and female Long-Evans rats begin rotation to prone with the shoulders; this rotation passively carries the neck and head towards prone. The recruitment of the hindquarters, however, is different between males and females. In females, once their forepaws have established firm contact with the ground, their hindquarters rotate in the same direction, past their forequarters. This leads to a large angular change in the longitudinal axis of the female animals relative to their starting point when supine.

Males, in contrast, exhibit a small rotation of the hindquarters in the opposite direction to that of the forequarters, within a few frames of the initiation of forequarter rotation. It is only after the initial counter rotation of their hindquarters, in the opposite direction to that of their forequarters, that the males rotate their hindquarters in the same direction as the forequarters to complete the righting sequence and achieve a prone position. Thus, from the initial supine position to the final prone position, there is little angular displacement of the longitudinal axis of the body (Fig. 9.5). Comparing the performance of male and female Long-Evans rats to the *tfm*-affected males and their associated wild-type male and female controls again suggests that these sex differences in movement organization are not due to differences in body mass or morphology (Field et al., 2005).

The role of gonadal steroids with regards to the sexual differentiation of sex-typical patterns of contact righting has not been studied. The effects of CNS injury on the expression of sex-typical tactics of dodging to protect a food item and contact righting, however, has begun to be addressed. One system that is commonly associated with the expression and selection of movement patterns is the basal ganglia and in particular the ascending dopaminergic systems.

THE ROLE OF THE CNS

The role of the ascending dopaminergic systems in the control of the organization of movement and the selection of movement patterns has been extensively studied (Metz, Farr, Ballerman, & Whishaw, 2001;

Metz, Piecharka, Kleim, & Whishaw, 2004; Metz, Tse, Ballerman, Smith, & Fouad, 2005; Miklyaeva, Castañeda, & Whishaw, 1994; Miklyaeva, Martens, & Whishaw, 1995; Miklyaeva & Whishaw, 1996; Miklyaeva et al., 1997; Whishaw et al., 1994; Whishaw, O'Connor, & Dunnett, 1986; Whishaw et al., 2002).

Sex differences in the anatomy and function of dopaminergic neurons have been described during early development (Andersen, Rutstein, Benzo, Hostetter, & Teicher, 1997; Andersen, Thompson, Kreznel, & Teicher, 2002; Beyer, Eusterschulte, Pilgrim, & Reisert, 1992; Beyer, Pilgrim, & Reisert, 1991; Pilgrim, Beyer, & Reisert, 1999) after treatment with drugs, such as amphetamine, apomorphine, and cocaine, (Becker, 1999; Becker, Molenda, & Hummer, 2001; Becker, Robinson, & Lorenz, 1982; Robinson, Becker, & Ramirez, 1980; Savageau & Beatty, 1981), and in the substantia nigra before (Dewing et al., 2006; Ravizza, Galanopoulou, Velíšková, & Moshé, 2002; Ravizza, Velíšková, & Moshé, 2003), and after damage (Cass, Peters, & Smith, 2005; Murray et al., 2003; Tamás, Lubics, Szalontay, Lengvári, & Reglödi, 2005). In the following two sections evidence will be presented to support the hypothesis that sex differences in movement organization may be related, in part, to sex differences in the development and adult function of the nigrostriatal and mesolimbocortical dopaminergic systems.

Lesions of the Dopaminergic System in Early Development

Lesions of the dopaminergic system early in development lead to impairments in motor performance in adulthood (Whishaw et al., 1994). Whether early lesions of the dopaminergic system can influence, in a sex-typical manner, the expression of sex-typical patterns of movement organization in adulthood has been addressed using the dodging to protect a food item and contact righting paradigms.

The analysis of sex-typical patterns of dodging behavior revealed that there were no impairments in the kinematic organization of dodging in males or females, given an intraventricular 6-OHDA lesion on postnatal day 5, as compared to controls. While both males and females used sex-typical kinematic patterns of dodging they were impaired in other aspects of their behavior. As previously mentioned, a dodge is a turn of approximate 180 degrees away from an approaching conspecific (Field et al., 1996; Whishaw, 1988).

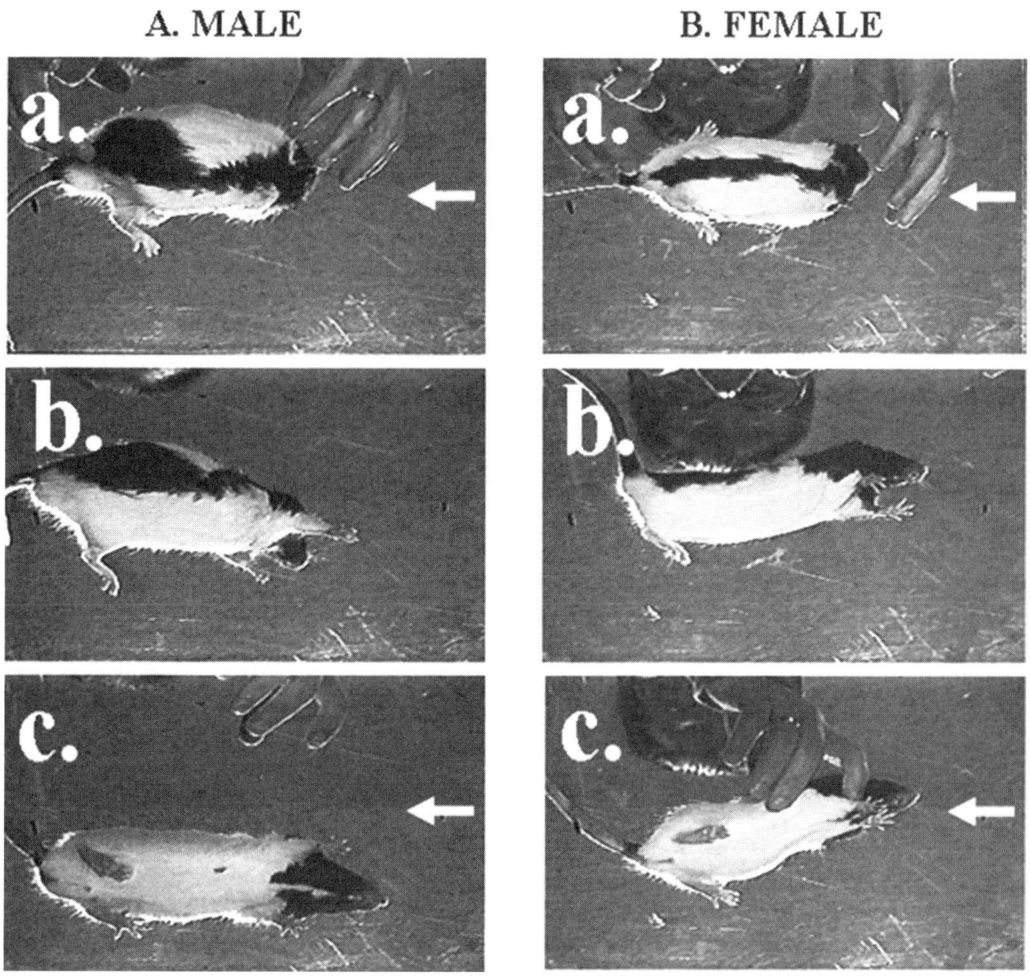

A. MALE

B. FEMALE

Figure 9.5. The pattern of contact righting, from the ventral perspective, is shown for a male (A) and a female (B) Long-Evans rat. Note that the female undergoes a large angular displacement along the longitudinal axis, whereas the male has a large whole body displacement. The white arrow represents the initial supine position for each animal. Adapted with permission from Field EF, Martens DJ, Watson NV, Pellis, SM (2005). Sex differences in righting from supine to prone: a masculinized skeletomusculature is not required. *J Comp Psychology,* 119:238–245.

At the completion of the dodge the animal regains a stationary position and resumes eating. 6-OHDA treated males and females while using normal sex-typical patterns of movement during the dodge are impaired in their ability to resume an immobile position at the end of the dodge. Thus, while the sex-typical kinematic organization of the turn is intact their behavior subsequent to the completion of the dodge is no longer normal (Field, Sherren, Pellis, & Whishaw, 2005).

6-OHDA treated males and females also used, in general, sex-typical patterns of contact righting from supine to prone as determined by the presence or absence of counter rotation by the hindquarters. A deficit was found, however, in the 6-OHDA treated males with regards to the proper timing and placement of the forepaw during contact righting. These males would often place the forepaw, ipsilateral to the direction of the turn, onto the substrate earlier than control males. This corresponded to an overall greater angle of displacement of the longitudinal axis of the 6-OHDA treated males as compared to their male controls (Field et al., 2005).

Given the finding, during contact righting, that the 6-OHDA treated males had greater difficulties in coordinating the movements of the fore- and hindquarters it was predicted that they would also be impaired in other behaviors that required the integration of their forelimb movements with other aspects of movement and/or postural support. This speculation was confirmed by the finding that 6-OHDA treated males were more impaired on a forelimb food handling task than were 6-OHDA treated females (Field et al., 2005). These data suggest that the integration of the movements of the fore- and hindquarters, and their organization by the CNS, may follow different trajectories during the development of males and females. Thus, it should be possible to find sex differences in the kinematic organization of movement and posture early in development.

It has been reported that male and female rats, within the first few days of life, exhibit a difference in how they maintain their posture. Males are more likely to have a tail position bias in the opposite direction to their head position than females (Afonso, Santana, & Rodriguez, 1993; Ross, Glick, & Meibach,

1981) (Fig. 9.6). The analysis of patterns of contact righting and spontaneous turning in rats within the first few days of birth also suggests that males and females differ in how they integrate their movements (Field, unpublished observations). Males again appear to differ in their organization and integration of movements of the fore- and hindquarters. The direction of the movement of the hindquarters is often opposite that of the forequarters; similar to the differences seen in adulthood. A great deal of further study is needed to verify and expand these findings both with regards to the role of gonadal steroids in organizing the sexual differentiation of these behaviors and in turn how these differences are organized within the CNS during development.

Lesions of the Ascending Dopaminergic Systems in Adulthood

Lesions of the dopaminergic systems in adulthood have been shown to alter the selection of sex-typical patterns of movement during contact righting, in adult Long-Evans rats. The basal ganglia, the function of

FEMALE

MALE

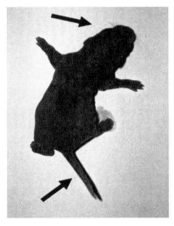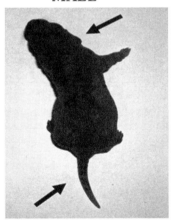

Figure 9.6. Two, 2-day old male and female rats are depicted. In the female the hindpaw ipsilateral to the direction of the turn has just stepped forward in the direction of the forequarters. In the male, the step that occurred subsequent to the photo displayed was with the hindpaw contralateral to the direction of the turn away from the side of the body, thus moving the hindquarters in the direction opposite to that of the forequarters. Note the difference in the direction of the tail in contrast to the head (indicated by arrows). Adapted with permission from Ross DA, Glick SD, Meibach, RC (1981). Sexually dimorphic brain and behavioral asymmetries in the neonatal rat. *Proc Nat Acad Sci U S A*, 78:1958–1961.

which is mediated, in part, by the nigrostriatal dopaminergic pathway, is considered to be important not only for the integration of movement but also for the selection of a pattern of movement (Hikosaka, 1998; Mink, 1996). Thus, it is possible that the choice of a sex-typical pattern of movement can be affected by lesions of the ascending dopaminergic systems. A comparison of the pattern of contact righting, in adult rats with a unilateral 6-OHDA lesion, towards either the affected or non-affected side of the body, has shown that the choice of a sex-typical pattern of movement can be influenced by CNS injury to the nigrostriatal pathway (Field, Metz, Pellis, & Whishaw, 2004).

To test whether males and females used male- or female-typical patterns of contact righting, after a unilateral lesion of the ascending dopaminergic systems, both sham and 6-OHDA treated males and females were filmed during rotation towards the affected, or contralateral side of the body, or the non-affected or ipsilateral side of the body.

Results of this study revealed that the choice of male- or female-typical patterns of righting can be influenced by a unilateral lesion of the ascending dopaminergic systems. Male and female sham-treated animals showed a sex-typical pattern of contact righting irrespective of the side of the body that they rotated towards. In contrast, 6-OHDA treated males and females showed a bias towards the use of a male- or female-typical pattern of rotation that was dependent on the side of the body they rotated towards; irrespective of the sex of the animal. Both 6-OHDA treated males and females had a displacement of the longitudinal axis that was similar to sham-treated males and used a male-typical strategy of hindquarter rotation when rotating towards the side of the body ipsilateral to the lesion.

In contrast, both lesion-treated males and females had an angular displacement of the longitudinal axis and a lack of hindquarter rotation that was more female-typical when rotating towards the side of the body that was contralateral to the lesion (see Fig. 9.7). These differences in the selection of sex-typical patterns of hindquarter movement were not due to differences in the use of the forequarters (Field et al., 2004).

These data provide evidence, for the first time, that the choice of a sex-typical movement pattern is dependent on the function of intact ascending dopaminergic systems. How the choice of a sex-typical motor program is governed by these systems will need further investigation. This study also provides definitive evidence that sex differences in movement organization are not due to differences in body morphology, but are due to sex differences in the selection of movement patterns by the CNS since males, and females, are now exhibiting both sex-typical strategies independent of body morphology.

IMPLICATIONS FOR HUMAN STUDIES

Sex differences in movement organization are also present in humans. Sex differences in sensorimotor behaviors have been reported both pre- and postnatally (Almli, Ball, & Wheeler, 2001; Davies & Rose, 2000; DiPietro et al., 2001; Piek, Gasson, Barrett, & Case, 2002), and with advancing age (Cao, Ashton-Miller, Schultz, & Alexander, 1997; Frandin, Sonn, Svantesson, & Grimby, 1995; Pavol, Owings, Foley, & Grabiner, 1999; Sayers, Guralnik, Thombs, & Fielding, 2005; Schultz, Ashton-Miller, & Alexander, 1997; Wojcik, Thelen, Schultz, Ashton-Miller, & Alexander, 1999).

While the effects of developmental experience (Hall & Kimura, 1995) and the integration of visual information with sex differences in movement organization have been addressed (Tottenham & Saucier, 2004) possible sex differences in movement organization and posture and how they might contribute to sex differences in sensorimotor tasks have not. Thus, it is possible that sex differences in movement during a goal-directed task, such as throwing accuracy, are dependent in part on sex differences in postural support and movement organization within the CNS.

Kinematic analysis, in humans, has primarily focused on how differences in body morphology determine differences in movement. It has recently been argued, however, that this cannot explain the sex differences found in the organization of dynamic movements (Zeller, McCrory, Kibler, & Uhl, 2003).

There are differences in the throwing accuracy of homosexual and heterosexual males who have similar body morphology (Hall & Kimura, 1995; Sanders & Wright, 1997) and the selection of movement patterns can be influenced by an individual's perception of their gender relative to their physical sex (Barlow, Mills, Agras, & Steinman, 1980; Rekers & Morey, 1989). It has also been reported that girls with congenital adrenal hyperplasia (CAH), who are prenatally androgenized are more masculine in their behavior (Collaer & Hines, 1995). Girls with the simple-vir-

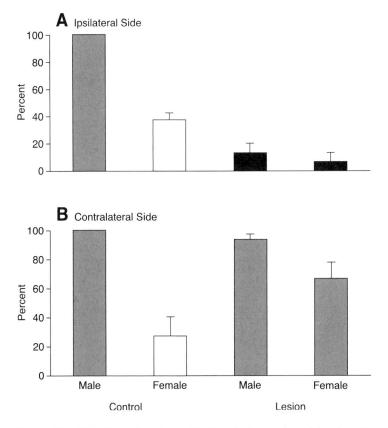

Figure 9.7. This figure depicts the likelihood of contralateral hindquarter rotation during contact righting in males and females that have been either sham treated or given a unilateral 6-OHDA lesion of the ascending dopaminergic systems. Both male and female 6-OHDA animals were more female-like when rotating towards the ipsilateral to the lesion (A) in contrast to being more male-like when rotating towards the side of the body contralateral to the lesion (B).

ilizing variant of CAH, however, who have a more strongly masculinized body morphology, are more feminized in their movements than are CAH girls with the salt-wasting variant, who are more female-like in body morphology, but more masculine in their movements (Dittman, 1992). These findings suggest that sex differences are present in the organization of a number of behaviors in humans; and as has been described for rats, these differences are not due solely to differences in body size or skeletomusculature morphology, and are likely due to the sexual differentiation of the CNS systems that control the production and organization of movement.

Consistent with the sex differences in the organization of lateral maneuvers in rats are preliminary data revealing that when humans turn after walking forward, they do so using a sequence of movement similar to that of rats. Eight female and eight male undergraduates were videotaped, first walking away from the camera and then turning to face the camera. The pattern of shifting body weight and stepping differed between the sexes.

The males shifted their body weight to the leg furthest away from the direction of the turn, whereas the females shifted their body weight to the leg closest to the direction of turning. Because of these different patterns of weight shift, the males ended up making more steps than the females to complete the turn. This cross-species consistency, coupled with further preliminary data demonstrating sex differences in the patterns of spontaneous turning in species such as the laboratory mouse (C57/Black6) (*Mus musculus*), degus (*Octodon degus*), the marsupial cat (*Dasyurus hallacatus*) and two insects, the African field cricket (*Gryllus bimaculatus*) and the giant Madagascan hissing cockroach (*Gromphadorhina portentosa*) further support the argument that sex differences in movement are generated by differences in neural function (Field et al., unpublished obs.).

The differences in body morphology between species are certainly greater than the differences between the sexes within a select species. Sex differences in movement organization, in a diversity of species, suggests that sex differences in movement organization are evolutionarily old and may be highly conserved.

The presence of sex differences in how the nervous system controls movement leads to the prediction that damage to areas of the CNS involved in generating movement, especially in humans, should lead to different behavioral outcomes. There is some evidence that impairments and recovery of function can differ, as a function of sex (Di Carlo et al., 2003; Groswasser, Cohen, & Keren, 1998; Hurn, Vannucci, & Hagberg, 2005; Roof & Hall, 2000; Scivoletto, Morganti, & Molinari, 2004; Sipski, Jackson, Gómez-Marín, Estores, & Stein, 2004), after CNS injury.

There is also some suggestion in the literature that males and females suffering from Parkinson's disease, a disease that is due to the death of dopaminergic neurons within the substantia nigra, may differ in their symptomology (Dunnewold et al., 1998; Lyons, Hubble, Troster, Pahwa, & Koller, 1998; van Hilten et al., 1993). To date, the presence or not of sex differences in the kinematic organization of behavior in Parkinsonian patients, or individuals with CNS injury, have not been well studied. Further study of how movement control develops and is sexually differentiated via genetic and hormonal mechanisms, in humans, and how this relates to CNS dysfunction in adulthood is needed.

The kinematic analysis of movement organization in individuals who have neurodevelopmental disorders, that involve the dysfunction of the CNS, specifically dysfunction of the dopaminergic system, such as autism, schizophrenia, attention deficit hyperactivity disorder, or Tourette's syndrome, have also not been well studied. This is surprising since sex differences in the prevalence and symptomology of these disorders are well known. Furthermore, movement abnormalities are commonly mentioned and are often apparent prior to cognitive and social impairments (Melillo & Leisman, 2004; Teitelbaum et al., 2004). Whether sex differences in movement organization are present in these disorders and how this relates to function in other cognitive and social domains will also require further study.

CONCLUSION

Males and females are different in many aspects of their non-sexual behavior. Sex differences in the organization of non-sexual behaviors likely have evolved due to differences in the advantage of one form of the behavior over the other for males relative to females. The reasons for sex differences in the organization of movement are at present unclear. Future work from a comparative evolutionary perspective is necessary to understand how these differences have evolved and why.

At present, however, irrespective of the evolutionary history of sex differences in movement organization, it is possible that these differences have an adaptive value for a variety of behaviors such as play, aggression, maternal behavior, courtship behaviors and mate selection. Future research directed towards understanding the CNS mechanisms that underlying the motoric expression of these behaviors will need to be done.

In a proximate world the existence of sex differences in the organization of movement in non-reproductive behaviors can be used to understand how a sexually differentiated nervous system develops and how sexually differentiated motor systems are integrated with sexually differentiated sensory, cognitive and social systems to yield a male and female phenotype in both human and non-human species. This can then be used to further our understanding of how events that alter CNS function differentially affect the development and final adult function of both males and females.

Acknowledgments

The authors would like to thank the staff and students, at the Canadian Centre for Behavioural Neuroscience, who have assisted with many of the projects cited in this chapter. They would also like to thank the Alberta Heritage Foundation for Medical Research, National Science and Engineering Research Council of Canada and the Canadian Institutes for Health Research for financial support.

References

Adkins-Reagan E, Mansukhani V, Thompson R, Yang, S. (1997). Organizational actions of sex hormones on sexual partner preference. *Brain Research Bulletin*, 44:497–502.

Afonso, D, Santana, C, Rodriguez M. (1993). Neonatal lateralization of behavior and brain dopaminergic asymmetry. *Brain Research Bulletin*, 32:11–16.

Almli CR, Ball RH, Wheeler ME. (2001). Human fetal and neonatal movement patterns: gender differences and fetal-to-neonatal continuity. *Developmental Psychobiology*, 38:252–273.

Andersen SL, Rutstein M, Benzo JM, Hostetter JC, Teicher MH. (1997). Sex differences in dopamine receptor overproduction and elimination. *Neuroreport*, 8:1495–1498.

Andersen SL, Thompson AP, Kreznel E, Teicher MH. (2002). Pubertal changes in gonadal hormones do not underlie adolescent dopamine receptor overproduction. *Psychoneuroendocrinology*, 27:683–691.

Ashley-Ross MA, Gillis GB. (2002). A brief history of vertebrate functional morphology. *Integrative and Comparative Biology*, 42:183–189.

Barlow DH, Mills JR, Agras WS, Steinman DL. (1980). Comparison of sex-typed motor behavior in male-to-female transsexuals and women. *Archives of Sexual Behavior*, 9:245–253.

Barnett SA. (1963). *The rat: a study in behavior*. Chicago:Aldine Publishing Company.

Baum MJ. (2003). Activational and organizational effects of estradiol on male behavioral neuroendocrine function. *Scandinavian Journal of Psychology*, 44: 213–220.

Beach FA. (1974). Effects of gonadal hormones on urinary behavior in dogs. *Physiology & Behavior*, 12: 1005–1013.

Beach FA. (1975). Behavioral endocrinology: an emerging discipline. *American Scientist*, 63:178–187.

Beach FA. (1981). Historical origins of modern research on hormones and behavior. *Hormones and Behavior*, 15:325–376.

Beatty WW. (1992). Gonadal hormones and sex differences in non-reproductive behaviors. In A. Gerall, H. Moltz, & I. L. Ward (Eds.), *Handbook of behavioral neurobiology: Sexual differentiation* (Vol. 11, pp. 85–128). New York, New York: Plenum Press.

Beck KD, Luine VN. (2002). Sex differences in behavioral and neurochemical profiles after chronic stress: role of housing conditions. *Physiology & Behavior*, 75:661–673.

Becker JB. (1990a). Direct effect of 17β-estradiol on striatum: sex differences in dopamine release. *Synapse*, 5:157–164.

Becker JB. (1990b). Estrogen rapidly potentiates amphetamine-induced striatal dopamine release and rotational behavior during microdialysis. *Neuroscience Letters*, 118:169–171.

Becker JB. (1999). Gender differences in dopaminergic function in striatum and nucleus accumbens. *Pharmacology, Biochemistry and Behavior*, 64:803–812.

Becker JB, Arnold AP, Berkley KJ, Blaustein JD, Eckel LA, Hampson E. et al. (2005). Strategies and methods for research on sex differences in brain and behavior. *Endocrinology*, 146:1650–1673.

Becker JB, Molenda H, Hummer, DL. (2001). Gender differences in the behavioral responses to cocaine and amphetamine: implications for mechanisms mediating gender differences in drug abuse. *Annals of the New York Academy of Sciences*, 937:172–187.

Becker JB, Robinson TE, Lorenz KA. (1982). Sex differences and estrous cycle variations in amphetamine-elicited rotational behavior. *European Journal of Pharmacology*, 80:65–72.

Becker JB, Snyder PJ, Miller MM, Westgate SA, Jenuwine MJ. (1987). The influence of estrous cycle and intrstriatal estradiol on sensorimotor performance in the female rat. *Pharmacology, Biochemistry & Behavior*, 27:53–59.

Bernstein P, Crelin ES. (1967). Bony pelvic sexual dimorphism in the rat. *Anatomical Records*, 157: 517–526.

Beyer C, Eusterschulte B, Pilgrim C, Reisert I. (1992). Sex steroids do not alter sex differences in tyrosine hydroxylase activity of dopaminergic neurons in vitro. *Cell Tissue Research*, 270:547–552.

Beyer C, Pilgrim C, Reisert I. (1991). Dopamine content and metabolism in mesencephalic and diencephalic cell cultures: sex differences and effects of sex steroids. *The Journal of Neuroscience*, 11: 1325–1333.

Blanchard DC, Sheperd JK, Carobrez ADP, Blanchard RJ. (1991). Sex effects in defensive behavior: baseline differences and drug interactions. *Neuroscience & Biobehavioral Reviews*, 15:461–468.

Blanchard RJ, Blanchard CD. (1990). Anti-predator defense as models of animal fear and anxiety. In Brain PF, Parmigiani S, Blanchard RJ, Mainardi D. (Eds.), *Fear and Defense* (pp. 89–108). Chur, Switzerland: Harwood Academic Publishers.

Bolles RC, Woods PJ. (1964). The ontogeny of behavior in the albino rat. *Animal Behavior*, 12:427–441.

Cao C, Ashton-Miller JA, Schultz AB, Alexander NB. (1997). Abilities to turn suddenly while walking: effects of age, gender, and available response time. *The Journals of Gerontology: Series A, Biological Sciences and Medical Sciences*, 52:M88–M93.

Cass WA, Peters LE, Smith MP. (2005). Reductions in spontaneous locomotor activity in aged male, but not female, rats in a model of early Parkinson's disease. *Brain Research*, 1034:153–161.

Coleman WH. (1969). Sex differences in the growth of the human bony pelvis. *American Journal of Physical Anthropology*, 31:125–152.

Collaer ML, Hines M. (1995). Human behavioral sex differences: a role for gonadal hormones during early development? *Psychological Bulletin*, 118:55–107.

Cosans CE. (1998). Aristotle's anatomical philosophy of nature. *Biology and Philosophy*, 13:311–339.

Davies PL, Rose JD. (2000). Motor skills of typically developing adolescents: awkwardness or improvement? *Physical and Occupational Therapy in Pediatrics*, 20:19–42.

De Vries GJ, Rissman EF, Simerly RB, Yang LY, Scordalakes EM, Auger CJ, et al. (2002). A model system for study of sex chromosome effects on sexually dimorphic neural and behavioral traits. *Journal of Neuroscience*, 22:9005–9014.

DeMoss DL, Wright GL. (1998). Sex and strain differences in whole skeletal development in the rat. *Calcified Tissue International*, 62:153–157.

Dewing P, Chiang CW, Sinchak K, Sim H, Fernagut PO, Kelly S, et al. (2006). Direct regulation of adult brain function by the male-specific factor SRY. *Current Biology*, 16:415–420.

Di Carlo A, Lamassa M, Baldereschi M, Pracucci G, Basile AM, Wolfe CDA, et al. (2003). Sex differences in the clinical presentation, resource use, and 3-month outcome of acute stroke in Europe. *Stroke*, 34:1114–1119.

DiPietro JA, Bornstein MH, Costigan KA, Pressman EK, Hahn C-S, Painter K, et al. (2001). What does fetal movement predict about behavior during the first two years of life? *Developmental Psychobiology*, 40:358–371.

Dittman RW (1992). Body positions and movement patterns in female patients with congenital adrenal hyperplasia. *Hormones & Behavior*, 26:441–456.

Dunnewold RJ, Hoff JI, van Pelt HC, Fredrikze PQ, Wagemans EA, van Hilten BJ. (1998). Ambulatory quantitative assessment of body position, bradykinesia, and hypokinesia in Parkinson's disease. *Journal of Clinical Neurophysiology*, 15:235–242.

Elliot BM, Grunberg NE. (2005). Effects of social and physical enrichment on open field activity differ in male and female Sprague Dawley rats. *Behavioral Brain Research*, 165:187–196.

Fagen R. (1981). *Animal play behavior.* New York, New York: Oxford University Press.

Field EF, Martens DJ, Watson NV, Pellis SM. (2005). Sex differences in righting from supine to prone: a masculinized skeletomusculature is not required. *Journal of Comparative Psychology*, 119:238–245.

Field EF, Metz GA, Pellis SM, Whishaw IQ. (2004). Are there sex differences in postural support in a rat model of Parkinson's disease? *Society for Neuroscience*, (2004 Abstract Viewer/Itinerary Planner ed.). Washington DC.

Field EF, Sherren N, Pellis SM, Whishaw IQ. (2005). The neonatal 6-OHDA model of ADHD: do developmental manipulations of the dopaminergic system affect sex-typical patterns of movement organization? *Society for Neuroscience*, (2005 Abstract Viewer/Itinerary Planner ed.). Washington DC.

Field EF, Watson NV, Whishaw IQ, Pellis SM. (2005). A masculinized skeletomusculature is not required for male-typical patterns of food-protective movements. *Hormones and Behavior*, 47:49–55.

Field EF, Whishaw IQ. (2005). Sex differences in postural adjustments during a single pellet skilled reaching task do not affect reaching success. *Behavioural Brain Research*, 163:237–245.

Field EF, Whishaw IQ, Forgie ML, Pellis SM. (2004). Neonatal and pubertal, but not adult, ovarian steroids are necessary for the development of female-typical patterns of dodging to protect a food item. *Behavioral Neuroscience*, 118:1293–1304.

Field EF, Whishaw IQ, Pellis SM. (1996). A kinematic analysis of evasive dodging movements used during food protection in the rat: evidence for sex differences in movement. *Journal of Comparative Psychology*, 110:298–306.

Field EF, Whishaw IQ, Pellis SM. (1997a). A kinematic analysis of sex-typical movement patterns used during evasive dodging to protect a food item: the role of gonadal androgens. *Behavioral Neuroscience*, 111:808–815.

Field EF, Whishaw IQ, Pellis SM. (1997b). The organization of sex-typical patterns of defense during food protection in the rat: the role of the opponent's sex. *Aggressive Behavior*, 23:197–214.

Field EF, Whishaw IQ, Pellis SM. (2000). Sex differences in catalepsy: evidence for hormone-dependent postural mechanisms in haloperidol treated rats. *Behavioural Brain Research*, 109:207–212.

Field EF, Whishaw IQ, Pellis SM, Watson NV. (2006). Play fighting in androgen-insensitive tfm rats: evidence that androgen receptors are necessary for the development of adult playful attack and defense. *Developmental Psychobiology*, 48:111–120.

Fitch RH, Cowell PE, Denenberg VH. (1998). The female phenotype: nature's default? *Developmental Neuropsychology*, 14:213–231.

Fitch RH, Denenberg VH. (1998). A role for ovarian hormones in sexual differentiation of the brain. *The Behavioral and Brain Sciences*, 21:311–327.

Forgie ML, Stewart J. (1994). Effects of prepubertal ovariectomy on amphetamine-induced locomotor activity in adult female rats. *Hormones & Behavior*, 28:241–260.

Frandin K, Sonn U, Svantesson U, Grimby G. (1995). Functional balance tests in 76-year-olds in relation to performance, activities of daily living and platform tests. *Scandinavian Journal of Rehabilitation Medicine*, 27:231–241.

Gerall AA, Dunlap JL, Hendricks SE. (1973). Effect of ovarian secretions on female behavioral potentiality in the rat. *Journal of Comparative Physiology and Psychology*, 82:449–465.

Groswasser Z, Cohen M, Keren O. (1998). Female TBI patients recover better than males. *Brain Injury*, 12:805–808.

Hall JA, Kimura D. (1995). Sexual orientation and performance on sexually dimorphic motor tasks. *Archives of Sexual Behavior*, 24:395–407.

Hampson E, Kimura D. (1988). Reciprocal effects of hormonal fluctuations on human motor and perceptual-spatial skills. *Behavioral Neuroscience*, 102:456–459.

Hendricks SE, Duffy JA. (1974). Ovarian influences on the development of sexual behavior in neonatally androgenized rats. *Developmental Psychobiology*, 7: 297–303.

Hikosaka O. (1998). Neural systems for control of voluntary action: a hypothesis. *Advances in Biophysics*, 35:81–102.

Hurn PD, Vannucci SJ, Hagberg H. (2005). Adult or perinatal injury: does sex matter? *Stroke*, 36:193–195.

Jost A. (1960). Hormonal influences in the sex development of bird and mammalian embryos. *Memoirs of the Society of Endocrinology*, 7:49–62.

Jost A. (1983). Genetic and hormonal factors in sex differentiation of the brain. *Psychoneuroendocrinology*, 8:183–193.

Kanit L, Taskiran D, Yilmaz OA, Balkan B, Demirgoren S, Furedy JJ, et al. (2000). Sexually dimorphic cognitive style in rats emerges after puberty. *Brain Research Bulletin*, 52:243–248.

Kanit L, Yilmaz OA, Taskiran D, Kulali B, Furedy JJ, Demirgoren S, et al. (2000). Sexually dimorphic cognitive style, female sex hormones, and cortical nitric oxide. *Physiology & Behavior*, 71:277–287.

Lowrance EW. (1968). Linear growth and appearance of sex difference in the rabbit pelvis. *Anatomical Records*, 161:413–418.

Lyons KE, Hubble JP, Troster AI, Pahwa R, Koller WC. (1998). Gender differences in Parkinson's disease. *Clinical Neuropharmacology*, 21:118–121.

MacLusky NJ, Naftolin F. (1981). Sexual differentiation of the central nervous system. *Science*, 211:1294–1303.

McCarthy MM. (1994). Molecular aspects of sexual differentiation of the rodent brain. *Psychoneuroendocrinology*, 19:415–427.

McEwen BS. (2001). Invited review: estrogens effects on the brain: multiple sites and molecular mechanisms. *Journal of Applied Physiology*, 91:2785–2801.

McGinnis MY, Marcelli M, Lamb DJ. (2002). Consequences of mutations in androgen receptor genes: molecular biology and behavior. In Pfaff DW, Arnold AP, Etgen AM, Fahrbach SE, Rubin RT (Eds.), *Hormones, brain and behavior* (pp. 347–379). New York, New York: Academic Press.

Mead LA, Hargreaves EL, Galea LAM. (1996). Sex differences in rodent spontaneous activity levels. In Sanberg PR, Ossenkopp KP, Kavaliers M, (Eds.), *Motor activity and movement disorders* (pp. 111–139). Georgetown, Texas: R. G. Landes Company.

Meaney MJ. (1989). The sexual differentiation of social play. *Psychiatric Developments*, 3:347–361.

Melillo R, Leisman G. (2004). *Neurobehavioral disorders of childhood: an evolutionary perspective*. New York, New York: Springer.

Metz GA, Farr T, Ballerman M, Whishaw IQ. (2001). Chronic levodopa therapy does not improve skilled reach accuracy or reach range on a pasta matrix reaching task in 6-OHDA dopamine depleted (hemi-Parkinson analogue) rats. *European Journal of Neuroscience*, 14:27–37.

Metz GA, Piecharka DM, Kleim JA, Whishaw IQ. (2004). Preserved ipsilateral-to-lesion motor map organization in the unilateral 6-OHDA-treated rat model of Parkinson's disease. *Brain Research*, 1026: 126–135.

Metz GA, Tse A, Ballerman M, Smith LK, Fouad K. (2005). The unilateral 6-OHDA rat model of Parkinson's disease revisited: an electromyographic and behavioural analysis. *European Journal of Neuroscience*, 22:735–744.

Miklyaeva EI, Castañeda E, Whishaw IQ. (1994). Skilled reaching deficits in unilateral dopamine-depleted rats: impairments in movement and posture and compensatory adjustments. *Journal of Neuroscience*, 14:7148–7158.

Miklyaeva EI, Martens DJ, Whishaw IQ. (1995). Impairments and compensatory adjustments in spontaneous movement after unilateral dopamine depletion in rats. *Brain Research*, 681:23–40.

Miklyaeva EI, Whishaw IQ. (1996). HemiParkinson analogue rats display active support in good limbs versus passive support in bad limbs on a skilled reaching task of variable height. *Behavioral Neuroscience*, 110:117–125.

Miklyaeva EI, Woodward NC, Nikiforov EG, Tompkins GJ, Klassen F, Ioffe MI, et al. (1997). The ground reaction forces of postural adjustments during skilled reaching in unilateral dopamine-depleted hemiparkinson rats. *Behavioural Brain Research*, 88:143–152.

Mink JW. (1996). The basal ganglia: focused selection and inhibition of competing motor programs. *Progress in Neurobiology*, 50:381–425.

Murray, HE, Pillai AV, McArthur SR, Razvi N, Datla KP, Dexter DT, et al. (2003). Dose- and sex-dependent effects of the neurotoxin 6-hydroxydopamine on the nigrostriatal dopaminergic pathway of adult rats: differential actions of estrogen in males and females. *Neuroscience*, 116:213–222.

Ogawa S, Chan J, Gustafsson JA, Korach KS, Pfaff DW. (2003). Estrogen increases locomotor activity in mice through estrogen receptor alpha: specificity for the type of activity. *Endocrinology*, 144:230–239.

Olsen KL. (1979a). Androgen-insensitive rats are defeminized by their testes. *Nature*, 279:238–239.

Olsen KL. (1979b). Induction if male mating-behavior in androgen-insensitive (*tfm*) rats and normal (King-Holtzman) male rats: effect of testosterone propionate, estradiol benzoate, and dihydrotestosterone. *Hormones and Behavior*, 13:66–84.

Olsen KL. (1992). Genetic influences on sexual behavior differentiation. In Gerall AA, Moltz H, Ward IL (Eds.), *Handbook of behavioral neurobiology: sexual differentiation* (Vol. 11, pp. 1–41). New York, New York: Plenum Press.

Olsen KL, Whalen RE. (1981). Hormonal control of the development of sexual behavior in androgen insensitive (*tfm*) rats. *Experientia*, 38:139–140.

Palanza P. (2001). Animal models of anxiety and depression: how are females different? *Neuroscience & Biobehavioral Reviews*, 25:219–233.

Papaioannou A, Gerozissis K, Prokopiou A, Bolaris S, Stylianopoulou F. (2002). Sex differences in the effects of neonatal handling on the animal's response to stress and the vulnerability for depressive behavior. *Behavioral Brain Research*, 129:131–139.

Pavol MJ, Owings TM, Foley KT, Grabiner MD. (1999). The sex and age of older adults influence the outcome of induced trips. *The Journals of Gerontology: Series A, Biological Sciences and Medical Sciences*, 54:103–108.

Pellis SM. (2002). Sex differences in play fighting revisited: traditional and nontraditional mechanisms of sexual differentiation in rats. *Archives of Sexual Behavior*, 31:17–26.

Pellis SM, Field EF, Smith LK, Pellis VC. (1997). Multiple differences in the play fighting of male and female rats: implications for the causes and functions of play. *Neuroscience and Biobehavioral Reviews*, 21:105–120.

Pellis SM, Field EF, Whishaw IQ. (1999). The development of a sex differentiated defensive motor pattern in rats: a possible role for juvenile experience. *Developmental Psychobiology*, 35:156–164.

Pellis SM, McKenna MM. (1992). Intrinsic and extrinsic influences on play fighting in rats: effects of dominance, partner's playfulness, temperament and neonatal exposure to testosterone propionate. *Behavioural Brain Research*, 50:135–145.

Pellis SM, Pellis VC. (1987). Play-fighting differs from serious fighting in both target of attack and tactics of fighting in the laboratory rat *Rattus norvegicus*. *Aggressive Behavior*, 13:227–242.

Pellis SM, Pellis VC. (1990). Differential rates of attack, defense, and counterattack during the developmental decrease in play fighting by male and female rats. *Developmental Psychobiology*, 23:215–231.

Phoenix CH, Goy RW, Gerall AA, Young WC. (1959). Organizing action of prenatally administered testosterone propionate on the tissues mediating mating behavior in the female guinea pig. *Endocrinology*, 615:369–381.

Piek JP, Gasson N, Barrett N, Case I. (2002). Limb and gender differences in the development of coordination in early infancy. *Human Movement Science*, 21:621–639.

Pilgrim C, Beyer C, Reisert I. (1999). The effects of sex and sex hormones in the development of dopaminergic neurons. In di Porzio U, Pernas-Alonso R, Perrone-Capano C. (Eds.), *Development of dopaminergic neurons* (pp. 75–86). Austin, Texas: R. G. Landes Company.

Purvis K, Haug E, Clausen OPF, Naess O, Hansson V. (1977). Endocrine status of the testicular feminized male (*tfm*) rat. *Molecular and Cellular Endocrinology*, 8:317–334.

Quadagno DM, Shryne JE, Anderson C, Gorski RA. (1972). Influence of gonadal hormones on social, sexual emergence and open field behavior in the rat (Rattus nervegicus). *Animal Behavior*, 20:732–740.

Ravizza T, Galanopoulou AS, Velíšková J, Moshé SL. (2002). Sex differences in androgen and estrogen receptor expression in rat substantia nigra during development: an immunohisotchemical study. *Neuroscience*, 115:685–696.

Ravizza T, Velíšková J, Moshé SL. (2003). Testosterone regulates androgen and estrogen receptor immunoreactivity in rat substantia nigra pars reticulata. *Neuroscience Letters*, 338:57–61.

Rekers GA, Morey SM. (1989). Sex-typed body movements as a function of severity of gender disturbance in boys. *Journal of Psychology and Human Sexuality*, 2:183–195.

Robinson TE, Becker JB, Ramirez VD. (1980). Sex differences in amphetamine-elicited rotational behavior and the lateralization of striatal dopamine in rats. *Brain Research Bulletin*, 5:539–545.

Roof RL, Hall ED. (2000). Gender differences in acute CNS trauma and stroke: neuroprotective effects of estrogen and progesterone. *Journal of Neurotrauma*, 17:367–388.

Roof RL, Stein DG. (1999). Gender differences in Morris water maze performance depend on task parameters. *Physiology & Behavior*, 68:81–86.

Ross DA, Glick SD, Meibach RC. (1981). Sexually dimorphic brain and behavioral assymetries in the neonatal rat. *Proccedings of the National Academy of Sciences U S A*, 78:1958–1961.

Sanders G, Wright M. (1997). Sexual orientation differences in cerebral asymmetry and in the performance of sexually dimorphic cognitive and motor tasks. *Archives of Sexual Behavior*, 26:463–480.

Savageau MM, Beatty WW. (1981). Gonadectomy and sex differences in the behavioral responses to amphetamine and apomorphine of rats. *Pharmacology, Biochemistry & Behavior*, 14:17–21.

Sayers SP, Guralnik JM, Thombs LA, Fielding RA. (2005). Effects of leg muscle contraction velocity on functional performance in older men and women. *Journal of the American Geriatric Society*, 53:467–471.

Schultz AB, Ashton-Miller JA, Alexander NB. (1997). What leads to age and gender differences in balance maintenance and recovery? *Muscle & Nerve*, S5: S60–S64.

Scivoletto G, Morganti B, Molinari M. (2004). Sex-related differences of rehabilitation outcomes of spinal cord lesion patients. *Clinical Rehabilitation*, 18:709–713.

Shapiro BH, Levine DC, Adler NT. (1980). The testicular feminized rat: a naturally occurring model of androgen independent brain masculinization. *Science*, 209:418–420.

Shimizu H, Awata T. (1984). Growth of skeletal bones and their sexual differences in mice. *Jikken Dobutsu (Experimental Animals)*, 33:69–76.

Sipski ML, Jackson AB, Gómez-Marín O, Estores I, Stein A. (2004). Effects of gender on neurologic and functional recovery after spinal cord injury. *Archives of Physical Medicine and Rehabilitation*, 85:1826–1836.

Smith KK. (1994). Are neuromotor systems conserved in evolution? *Brain, Behavior and Evolution*, 43:293–305.

Smith SS. (1998). Estrous hormones enhance coupled, rhythmic olivary discharge in correlation with facilitated limb stepping. *Neuroscience*, 82:83–95.

Smith SS, Chapin JK. (1996). Estrous hormones and the olivo-cerebellar circuit I: contrast enhancement of sensorimotor-correlated Purkinje cell discharge. *Experimental Brain Research*, 1113:371–384.

Smith SS, Hsu F-C, Li X, Frye CA, Faber DS, Markowitz RS. (2000). Oestrogen effects in olivo-cerebellar and hippocampal circuits. *Novartis Foundation Symposium*, 230:155–172.

Stanley AJ, Gumbreck LG, Allison JE, Easley RB. (1973). Part I. Male pseudohermaphroditism in the laboratory Norway rat. *Recent Progress in Hormone Research*, 29:43–64.

Stewart J, Cygan D. (1980). Ovarian hormones act early in development to feminize adult open-field behavior in the rat. *Hormones and Behavior*, 14:20–32.

Stewart SA, German RZ. (1999). Sexual dimorphism and ontogenetic allometry of soft tissues in *Rattus norvegicus*. *Journal of Morphology*, 242:57–66.

Swanson HH. (1966). Sex differences in behavior of hamsters in open field and emergence tests: effects of pre- and post-pubertal gonadectomy. *Animal Behavior*, 14:522–529.

Tamás A, Lubics A, Szalontay L, Lengvári I, Reglödi D. (2005). Age and gender differences in behavioral and morphological outcome after 6-hydroxydopamine-induced lesion of the substantia nigra in rats. *Behavioural Brain Research*, 158:221–229.

Teitelbaum O, Benton T, Shah PK, Prince A, Kelly JL, Teitelbaum P. (2004). Eshkol-Wachman movement notation in diagnosis: the early detection of Asperger's syndrome. *Proceedings of the National Academy of Science*, 101:11909–11914.

Thor DH, Holloway WRJ. (1983). Play-solicitation behavior in juvenile male and female rats. *Animal Learning and Behavior*, 11:173–178.

Tottenham LS, Saucier DM. (2004). Throwing accuracy during prism adaptation: male advantage for throwing accuracy is independent of prism adaptation rate. *Perceptual and Motor Skills*, 98:1449–1455.

van Hilten BJ, Hoogland G, van der Velde EA, van Dijk JG, Kerkhof GA, Roos RA. (1993). Quantitative assessment of parkinsonian patients by continuous wrist activity monitoring. *Clinical Neuropharmacology*, 16:36–45.

Vanderschueren D, Van Herck E, Geusens P, Suiker A, Visser W, Chung K, Bouillon R. (1994). Androgen resistance and deficiency have different effects on the growing skeleton of the rat. *Calcified Tissue International*, 55:198–203.

Voutilainen R. (1992). Differentiation of the fetal gonad. *Hormone Research*, 38:66–71.

Wade GN. (1976). Sex hormones, regulatory behaviors, and body weight. In Rosenblatt JS, Hinde RA, Shaw E, Beer C. (Eds.), *Advances in the study of behavior* (Vol. 6, pp. 201–279). New York, New York: Academic Press.

Ward IL. (1992). Sexual behavior: The product of perinatal hormonal and prepuertal social factors. In Gerall A, Moltz H, Ward IL (Eds.), *Handbook of behavioral neurobiology: sexual differentiation* (Vol. 11, pp. 157–180). New York, New York: Plenum Press.

Whishaw IQ. (1988). Food wrenching and dodging: use of action patterns for the analysis of sensorimotor and social behavior in the rat. *Journal of Neuroscience Methods*, 24:169–178.

Whishaw IQ, Gorny B, Tran-Nguyen LTL, Castañeda E, Miklyaeva EI, Pellis SM. (1994). Making two movements at once: impairments of movement, posture, and their integration underlie the adult skilled reaching deficit of neonatally dopamine-depleted rats. *Behavioural Brain Research*, 61:65–77.

Whishaw IQ, Gorny BP. (1994). Food wrenching and dodging: eating time estimates influence dodge probability and amplitude. *Aggressive Behavior*, 20:35–47.

Whishaw IQ, O'Connor WT, Dunnett SB. (1986). The contributions of motor cortex, nigrostriatal dopamine and caudate putamen to skilled forelimb use in the rat. *Brain*, 109:805–843.

Whishaw IQ, Suchowersky O, Davis L, Sarna J, Metz GA, Pellis SM. (2002). Impairment of pronation, supination, and body co-ordination in reach-to-grasp in human Parkinson's disease (PD) reveals homology to deficits in animal models. *Behavioural Brain Research*, 133:165–176.

Whishaw IQ, Tomie J. (1987). Food wresting and dodging: strategies used by rats (*Rattus norvegicus*) for obtaining and protecting food from conspecifics. *Journal of Comparative Psychology*, 101:202–209.

Whishaw IQ, Tomie J. (1988). Food wrenching and dodging: a neuroethological test of cortical and dopaminergic contributions to sensorimotor behavior in the rat. *Behavioral Neuroscience*, 102:110–123.

Wojcik LA, Thelen DG, Schultz AB, Ashton-Miller JA, Alexander NB. (1999). Age and gender differences in single-step recovery from a forward fall. *The Journals of Gerontology: Series A, Biological Sciences and Medical Sciences*, 54:M44–M50.

Yarbrough WG, Quarmby VE, Simental JA, Joseph DR, Sar M, Lubahn DB, et al. (1990). A single base mutation in the androgen receptor gene causes androgen insensitivity in the testicular feminized rat. *The Journal of Biological Chemistry*, 265:8893–8900.

Zeller BL, McCrory JL, Kibler BW, Uhl TL. (2003). Differences in kinematics and electromygraphic activity between men and women during the single-leg squat. *The American Journal of Sports Medicine*, 31:449–456.

Chapter 10

Sex Differences in Motivation

Jill B. Becker and Jane R. Taylor

This chapter develops the thesis that sexually dimorphic development of the neural systems involved in motivation has evolved due to sex differences in care of young. We proposed that sex differences in the neural systems important for maternal motivation result in sex differences in motivated behaviors in general. In particular, the greater oxytocin projection to the nucleus accumbens (NAcc) in females is hypothesized to play an important role in these sex differences. In addition, there are effects of gonadal hormones that modulate the reward system. Specifically, estradiol enhances the rewarding value of potential targets, while progesterone counteracts the effect of estradiol. Ultimately, research on the neurobiological mechanisms of sex differences in motivation will aid in the treatment and understanding of motivation-related pathologies for females and males.

WHAT IS MOTIVATION?

In psychological terms motivation is the internal state that induces or drives an animal to engage in a specific behavior. There are a number of naturally-occurring motivated behaviors, where it is assumed that an animal engages in these behaviors in order to gain a particular reward i.e., eating, drinking, and engaging in sexual behavior. There are also motivated behaviors that are acquired through experience with reinforcers, such as drugs of abuse. The proximal or immediate motivation to engage in these behaviors is the acquisition of the rewarding item: the food item, a liquid to drink, a sex partner, or a drug of abuse. Sex differences in the motivation to engage in parental behavior, the motivation to engage in sexual behavior, and the motivation to take drugs of abuse exist. In this chapter, we will address sex differences in the neurobiological systems that induce an animal to seek a reward; but first we will examine motivation from an evolutionary perspective, as we believe this view will provide some insight into the neural systems that mediate motivation.

WHY ARE THERE SEX DIFFERENCES IN MOTIVATION?

We have learned a great deal in recent years about the proximal causes for sex differences in motivation. We propose that to make further advances in our knowledge requires an evolutionary approach to how we think about motivation. The fundamental premise of natural selection is that traits are selected that result in an increase in an individual's genes being represented in subsequent offspring, in other words—traits that enhance reproductive success and inclusive fitness. As the behaviors needed to enhance reproductive success are different for males and females, the ultimate (i.e., evolutionary) pressures on the neural systems that mediate motivation have resulted in the evolution of sex differences in motivational systems.

Reproductive success for a male mammal requires insemination of female conspecifics; so the primary reproductive motivation[1] of a male is to gain access to females for the purpose of mating. For non-parental males, which is the majority (90%) of mammalian species, the strategy is to inseminate as many females as possible, thereby increasing the chance that the male's genes will be represented in surviving animals that go on to reproduce. In the male, this is a system that is activated by testosterone and its metabolites, and it is always "on" except in seasonal breeders or when environmental constraints limit testicular function or mating opportunities.

Reproductive success for the female mammal requires a series of related, but distinct behaviors and

---

1. We recognize that there is a distinction between proximate vs. ultimate causes of behavior, with ultimate causes being those contingencies that govern a behavior; and the ultimate causes being the evolutionary constraints that have selected for animals that engage in the behavior— constraints that the animal is unaware of. In a similar fashion, we propose that there are also proximate vs. ultimate motivations to engage in a behavior, with the animal being aware of the proximate motivation of gaining access to the reward (i.e., the female rat), while being unaware of the ultimate motivation (in this case generation of many offspring).

neuroendocrine processes. The female must select the best mate, and then achieve successful fertilization, implantation, pregnancy, parturition, and subsequent maternal behavior to promote survival of her offspring. In other words, the primary reproductive motivation of the female, after she has chosen to mate, is production of and care for her young; in effect, ensuring that her genes will survive in subsequent generations. Each of the functions that contribute to reproductive success in the female is activated by estradiol and progesterone, with contributions from hypothalamic hormones and releasing factors. Different selection pressures operating on female versus male sexual strategies have produced different, but related neural systems to mediate the various components of the behaviors that contribute to reproductive success.

Different areas of the female brain are important for sexual ability (i.e., the ability to exhibit the lordosis reflex) and sexual motivation as well as maternal behavior and maternal motivation. Further on, these roles are discussed in the context of the neural mechanisms of motivation.

As should be apparent from this brief discussion, the neural systems important for motivation and engaging in behaviors essential for reproductive success are different for males and females. The premise that we will be developing in this chapter is that there are sex differences in motivation and that the sexes differ along three dimensions. First, motivation in females varies with reproductive status (i.e., estrous cycle or pregnancy), but is constant in males. Therefore, motivation in females is modulated by gonadal hormones, and the female brain is more vulnerable to be co-opted by exogenous agents that induce constant activation (e.g., drugs of abuse) than are males.

There are neuroanatomical differences in the motivational systems beyond sex itself that are still related to reproduction. In females, neural systems that lead to formation of the mother-infant bond operate in ways that are different than in males, even in males that form paternal attachments where these neural systems may be present, but normally, are inactive. Sex differences in neural circuitry of attachment may spill over into other motivation systems too, including non-reproductive motivations for drugs. The development of strong attachments, and addictions or compulsive behaviors may occur through activation of the neural system that mediates maternal motivation; thus, females can become addicted to drugs more rapidly than males.

Lastly, we emphasize that sex differences in motivation that have been discovered in non-human animals are also likely to be present in humans, since humans have been subject to many of the same evolutionary constraints. In a recent cross-cultural analysis in the behavior of men and women, it was concluded that sex differences in cognitive function present in humans is an evolutionary consequence of specialization of behaviors by the sexes, and in particular behaviors related to female reproductive capacity and maternal behavior (Wood & Eagly, 2002). Even though pregnancy and maternal care of the young may no longer dictate a woman's reproductive success, women retain a brain that evolved under these constraints and understanding the neurobiological factors that underlie these differences should be an emerging area of clinical and preclinical research (Cahill, 2006).

THE NEURAL SYSTEMS THAT MEDIATE MOTIVATION

The areas of the brain that are thought to be especially important for the neurobiology of motivation are illustrated in Figure 10.1 in a generic form. Based primarily on data from males, we see that there is a major role for the ascending dopamine systems that project from the substantia nigra to the dorsal striatum and from the ventral tegmental area (VTA) to the nucleus accumbens (NAcc), amygdala (AMY) and frontal cortex.

The NAcc is composed of the core and shell, which differ in their afferent input and efferent projections. The hippocampus projects to both core and shell, with the dorsal subiculum projecting to the core and the ventral subiculum projecting to the shell (not illustrated). Prelimbic prefrontal cortex projects to the core of the NAcc while infralimbic and piriform cortex project to the shell. (Brog et al., 1993).

Specific subcompartments of the AMY also project to the core versus. shell (Wright et al., 1996). Both core and shell receive input from dopamine neurons in the VTA, and this input is topographically organized. The output from the NAcc core connects to the ventral pallidum, subthalamic nucleus, and substantia nigra, while the shell projects more to the subcortical limbic system, but also projects to the ventral pallidum and substantia nigra. Information from the core and the shell of the NAcc is integrated at the level

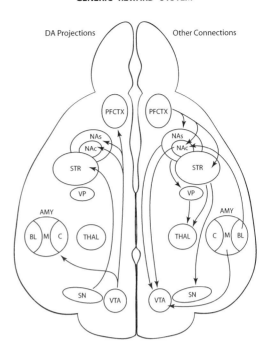

GENERIC "REWARD" SYSTEM

Figure 10.1. The reward system. This is a simplified schematic diagram of the neural systems important for reward. While no brain region is involved in only one aspect of behavior, the brain regions depicted here have been shown to be important for reward in a number of different paradigms. Dopamine (DA) projections are depicted on the left side of the brain. DA cell bodies in the substantia nigra (SN) project to the striatum. DA cell bodies in the ventral tegmental area (VTA) project to all parts of the the amygdala (AMY; BL = basolateral, M = medial, c = central), the nucleus accumbens core (NAc) and shell (NAs), as well as the prefrontal cortex (PFCTX). On the right side of the diagram associations among these various nuclei are illustrated. VP = ventral pallidum, THAL = thalamus.

of the thalamus. Cortical areas (AMY, and orbitofrontal, perhaps the cingulate cortex) are important for learning the association between a conditioned stimulus (CS) and reward (Schoenbaum et al., 2000; Chudasama & Robbins, 2003; Saddoris et al., 2005) as well as mediating changes in the incentive salience of stimuli (Berridge, 2006).

When males and females are compared, variation from the generic version of motivational systems can be seen. There is also variation from this generic scheme for each specific motivated behavior. We know that the brain of males and females are different and that sex differences can be observed in the neurobiological basis of motivation. Research in sexual motivation, paternal behavior, and in the motivation to take drugs of abuse has been done in both male and female rats. These are the behaviors for which we know the most about sex differences in motivation, and the neural systems that underlie these sex differences.

SEX DIFFERENCES IN SEXUAL MOTIVATION

Male Sexual Behavior

Sexual behavior has both appetitive (motivational) and consummatory components (sexual ability) as do many other behaviors (Craig, 1918). This has been elegantly demonstrated in experiments from the Everitt laboratory with male rats (Everitt & Stacey, 1987; Everitt, 1990).

Using a second order schedule of reinforcement, Everitt and collaborators demonstrated that male rats could be trained to bar press for access to a sexually-receptive female rat. Bar pressing was established using a red light as a CS after pairing the red light with odors from a sexually-receptive female rat. Once bar pressing was established on a fixed-interval schedule of 5 minutes, experiments were performed to demonstrate that bar pressing was a measure of sexual motivation and the ability to engage in sexual behavior was measured when the female was delivered into the testing chamber.

These investigators went on to show that castration reduced both bar pressing for the female (i.e., sexual motivation) as well as sexual behavior (i.e., sexual ability). As would be predicted from a large body of research (reviewed in Hull et al, 2006), lesions of the medial preoptic area (POA) resulted in a severe impairment of male copulatory behavior.[2] But, strikingly had little effect on the operant responding for access to the female. On the other hand, lesions of the basolateral amygdala (blAMY) reduced bar pressing for

access to the female rat (i.e., sexual motivation), but failed to affect sexual ability (Everitt & Stacey, 1987; Everitt, 1990).

The results of these experiments clearly demonstrated that there are distinct neural substrates necessary for sexual motivation versus sexual ability. Furthermore, when amphetamine was delivered to the NAcc of male rats with a blAMY lesion, bar pressing for access to the female was reinstated (Everitt, 1990). Since there are projections from the blAMY to the NAcc, dopamine in the NAcc—released by amphetamine—was implicated in sexual motivation. Subsequently, a number of investigators have demonstrated that extracellular dopamine concentrations increase in the NAcc of male rats in anticipation of gaining access to a sexually receptive female as well as during sexual behavior. (Pfaus et al., 1990; Pleim et al., 1990; Pfaus & Phillips, 1991; Damsma et al., 1992).

To summarize, the areas of the brain that are primarily important for the ability to engage in copulatory behavior (i.e., sexual ability) in the male (Fig. 10.2) include the POA, the medial amygdala (mAMY), and the bed nucleus of the stria terminalis (BNST). The blAMY, NAcc, and striatum are more involved in the motivation to engage in sexual behavior (Baum, 2002). The connections among these brain regions involved in sexual motivation and sexual ability are described in more detail in Figure 10.2.

Female Sexual Behavior

While both male and female rats may exhibit an increase in extracellular concentrations of dopamine in the NAcc during sexual behavior (Pfaus et al., 1990; Mermelstein & Becker, 1995; Pfaus et al., 1995), in the female, this increase in NAcc dopamine depends upon the context in which the sexual behavior occurs. This is due to the fact that sexual behavior is rewarding to the female rat only under specific conditions (Oldenberger et al., 1992; Paredes & Alonso, 1997; Paredes & Vazquez, 1999; Martinez & Paredes, 2001; Jenkins & Becker, 2003b). In other words, for the female the context and timing of the sexual encounter is critical to whether sexual behavior is rewarding.

In laboratory experiments on sexual behavior, animals have historically been studied in a small chamber where contacts are initiated by the male who engages in a series of mounts and intromissions that ultimately lead to ejaculation (Bermant, 1961; Ber-

---

2. It should be noted that the POA may also be involved, at least to some extent in sexual motivation, as lesions of the POA decrease partner preferences, pursuit of females, and other indirect measures of sexual motivation (reviewed in Hull et al, 2006).

MALE SEXUAL BEHAVIOR

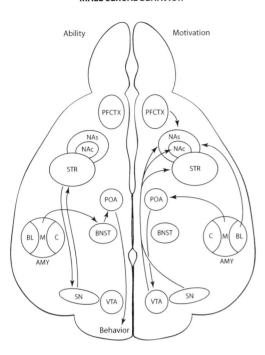

Figure 10.2. The neural systems mediating male sexual behavior. On the left are indicated the neural systems that are most critical for the ability of the male rat to engage in copulatory behaviors. On the right are depicted the neural systems in the male that are involved in the motivation or desire to engage in sexual behavior. The projections from mAMY to BNST and POA are vasopressin containing neurons. BNST = bed nucleus of the stria terminalis, POA = preoptic area.

mant, 1967; Adler, 1969). Under these conditions, the male controls the rate of copulation and will intromit with a female at a relatively rapid rate—approximately once every 30 seconds—until ejaculation occurs after 9 or 10 intromissions.

On the other hand, if sexual behavior takes place in a chamber where the female can escape from the male, she will establish and maintain longer latencies between sexual contacts (Adler, 1969; Adler, 1978; McClintock, 1984; Erskine et al., 1989). For laboratory rodents, the female will remove herself from the presence of the male after an intromission and return to the male about 2 minutes later (Jenkins & Becker, 2003b).

In the wild, rats engage in mating in groups of several females and the dominant male. Under these

conditions the male is able to achieve his preferred rapid rate of intromissions with different females. The females, in turn, achieve their preferred rate of copulation by withdrawing from the male and then returning after the preferred interval (McClintock, 1984). Achieving the preferred rate of copulation is important for the female rodent to optimize the rate of vaginocervical stimulation received from a male which activates a neuroendocrine reflex that is necessary for pregnancy to occur (Adler, 1969; McClintock & Adler, 1977; Adler, 1978; McClintock, 1984; Erskine, 1989).

The female's repeated approach and withdrawal from the male during a sexual encounter is known as *pacing behavior* (Erskine et al., 1989). Pacing behavior allows the female to control both the rate and duration of the copulatory bout. Importantly, sexual behavior is rewarding to the female rat when she achieves her preferred rate of copulation (Paredes & Alonso, 1997; Paredes & Vazquez, 1999; Martinez & Paredes, 2001; Jenkins & Becker, 2003b), whether or not she is actively pacing the rate of copulation (Jenkins & Becker, 2003a).

In support for a role for dopamine in sexual motivation in females, NAcc-dopamine increases only when female rats are receiving copulatory stimulation at their preferred rate of intromissions; *not* when they receive similar numbers of intromissions at a rate that is too fast or too slow. This can be accomplished either by the female actively controlling or "pacing" the rate of copulation or if the experimenter removes the male and then returns him to the female's chamber at appropriate intervals during copulation (Mermelstein & Becker, 1995; Becker et al., 2001). Female hamsters also exhibit an increase of dopamine in dialysate during sexual behavior (Meisel et al., 1993).

It should be noted that female rats engaging in sexual behavior at their preferred pacing interval had greater increases in dopamine in dialysate from the NAcc than did animals in which the male rat was removed and then returned to the female's chamber either too rapidly or much later (Becker et al., 2001). Furthermore, dopamine increases in the NAcc occurred prior to coital stimulation when intromissions were received at the female's preferred pacing interval, but not during the interval when coital stimulation occurred under other conditions (Jenkins & Becker, 2003a). Thus, increases in NAcc dopamine are not induced by coital stimulation or escape from/ removal of the male rat; instead, the NAcc-dopamine increases occur in anticipation of coital stimulation that occurs at a specific interval. These data support the hypothesis that dopamine increases in the NAcc signal the impending receipt of coital stimulation at the female's preferred pacing interval, and that NAcc dopamine plays a role in sexual motivation.

The increase in dopamine in the NAcc is apparently not always necessary for a female to find sexual behavior rewarding. In hamsters, pretreatment of females with the D_2-dopamine receptor antagonist raclopride blocked conditioned place preferences for the place in which mating occurred (Meisel et al., 1996). On the other hand, Paredes et al. found that pretreatment with the dopamine antagonists flupentixol or raclopride did not block conditioned place preference induced by paced mating in female rats (Garcia-Horsman & Paredes, 2004), while the μ-opiate antagonist naloxone prevented establishment of conditioned place preference induced by paced mating (Paredes & Martinez, 2001).

These results suggest that activation of D_2 dopamine receptors may not be necessary for sexual behavior to be rewarding, while μ-opioid receptor mediated activation—with the downstream effects on GABA, dopamine, and glutamate neurotransmission—is important for sexual motivation in the female rat. The study by Garcia-Horseman and Paredes (2004) used a relatively low dose of raclopride, leaving open the possibility that this dose is not sufficient to completely block the rewarding effect of dopamine. Alternatively, it is possible that the way the conditioned place preference test is conducted (animals are placed into the test apparatus for conditioned place preference training immediately after receiving an ejaculation) is particularly sensitive to the effect of opioid antagonists.

To summarize, the brain regions involved in the female rat's lordosis reflex (the behavior that makes it possible for the male to achieve intromission) include the POA, the ventral medial hypothalamus (VMH), the mAMY and the lateral septum (LS) (McCarthy & Becker, 2002). In order to activate a neuroendocrine reflex that promotes implantation and maintains pregnancy as well as for sexual motivation, the NAcc, dorsal striatum, and mAMY have to be involved (Fig. 10.3) (Erskine & Hanrahan, 1997; Becker et al., 2001; Polston et al., 2001; Bradley, 2005).

In particular, dopamine in the NAcc is implicated in the anticipation of sexual behavior that is rewarding. Sexual behavior of the female rat requires new considerations and interpretations of the role of dopamine

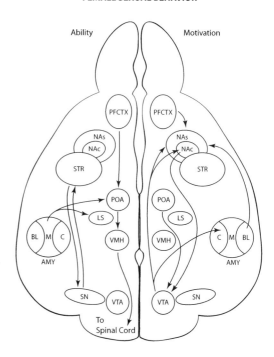

FEMALE SEXUAL BEHAVIOR

Figure 10.3. The neural systems mediating female sexual behavior. On the left are indicated the neural systems that are most critical for the ability of the female rat to engage in copulatory behaviors. On the right are depicted the neural systems in the female that are involved in the motivation or desire to engage in sexual behavior. LS = lateral septal nucleus, VMH = ventromedial nucleus of the hypothalamus.

in reward. Female rats find sexual behavior rewarding and have increased NAcc dopamine when they engage in sex at their preferred interval (Mermelstein & Becker, 1995; Paredes & Alonso, 1997; Becker et al., 2001; Martinez and Paredes, 2001). Sexual experience also plays a role in sexual motivation, with experience enhancing the reinforcing properties of sexual behavior in the female (Meisel & Mullins, 2006).

Sex that is rewarding has been shown to be associated with the triggering of a neuroendocrine reflex necessary for pregnancy (Adler, 1974; Gilman et al., 1979; Erskine et al., 1989). One possibility of this is that the changes in dopamine observed here represent a coupling of the sexual interaction and its physiological consequences, both of which may be necessary for sexual behavior to be rewarding in the female. In other words, increases in dopamine predict the receipt of coital stimulation, but only when the coital stimulation occurs at such a rate that it triggers the neuroendocrine reflex necessary for successful pregnancy to occur. Coital stimulation is known to induce the release of oxytocin in rats and other species (Flanagan et al., 1993). The neuroendocrine reflex that is activated in the female rat also results in the release of prolactin (Erskine, 1995). Since oxytocin is thought to induce the release of prolactin, one possibility is that activation of the intrahypothalamic neurons necessary for coital-induced release of prolactin and oxytocin also enhances dopamine release in the NAcc.

MATERNAL MOTIVATION: A SEXUAL DIMORPHIC BEHAVIOR

The neuroendocrinology and neurochemistry of maternal motivation has recently been reviewed quite thoroughly (Lonstein & Morrell, 2007), and we refer the reader to this excellent review for additional details. The hormones of pregnancy and parturition prime the brain for the onset of maternal behaviors which begin at parturition as a consequence of the exposure to pups. As is true of sexual behavior, there are brain regions important for the ability to engage in the behaviors that comprise maternal behavior and other brain regions important for the motivation to engage in these behaviors.

Maternal behavior consists of a set of behaviors that includes: parturition-related behaviors, nest building, pup retrieval, pup licking, the nursing posture (kyphosis), and maternal aggression. These behaviors are initially dependent on hormones for their rapid establishment at parturition. Once maternal behaviors have been induced, their expression continues to occur without additional hormones, and can be induced more rapidly by exposure to pups, indicating that establishment of maternal behaviors results in long-term changes in the brain.

The hormones necessary for the rapid establishment of maternal behaviors in the rat are estradiol, progesterone, prolactin (and the related hormones decidual luteotrophin and placental lactogens I and II) and oxytocin. During pregnancy, estradiol acts in the POA to prime the brain so that the female rapidly displays maternal behavior at parturition (Rosenblatt, 1992). Progesterone is elevated throughout most of pregnancy, and its withdrawal at the end of pregnancy

is necessary, in most species, for the onset of labor, initiation of lactation, and the estradiol-triggered onset of maternal behavior (Rosenblatt, 1992; Lonstein & Morrell, 2007).

The decline in progesterone is thought to result in an increase in prolactin receptors in the POA, which allows the full expression of maternal behaviors (Bridges & Hay, 2005). Interestingly, in humans progesterone does not decline until after parturition, but there is a shift in the type of progesterone receptors in the myometrium pre-partum that decreases the response to progesterone while enhancing stimulation induced by estradiol which is necessary for parturition (Brown et al., 2004; Fernandes et al., 2005; Karteris et al., 2006; Sheehan, 2006).

Prolactin and related lactogenic hormones are transported into the brain via an active receptor-transport mechanism in the choroid plexus (Lonstein & Morrell, 2007). In the POA, prolactin has been shown to facilitate the onset of maternal behavior in the estradiol primed female rat (Rosenblatt, 1992; Lonstein & Morrell, 2007). Other brain regions where prolactin is thought to influence maternal behavior include the mAMY, lateral septum, anterior hypothalamus.

Finally, oxytocin is thought to act in the POA, NAcc and olfactory-related brain regions to influence maternal behavior (Rosenblatt, 1992; Lonstein & Morrell, 2007). The role of oxytocin in maternal behavior was called into question when it was observed that the oxytocin knock-out (OTKO) mouse had normal reproductive behavior (Nishimori et al., 1996). Recent studies, however, have found that the OTKO mouse has deficits in pup-licking as well as maternal motivational deficits (Pedersen et al., 2006) and social recognition problems (Ferguson et al., 2001). Interestingly, oxytocin is necessary for licking behavior post-partum and is not maintained without oxytocin, as it is reduced by an oxytocin antagonist (Champagne et al., 2001).

To summarize, as illustrated in Figure 10.4, the POA, NAcc, striatum, lateral septum, and paraventricular nucleus (PVN) are thought to be important for maternal behaviors and the rapid formation of the mother-infant bond immediately after parturition (Lonstein et al., 1998; Lonstein et al., 2000; Lonstein et al., 2003; Gatewood et al., 2006; Lonstein and Morrell, 2006). Hormonal regulation of the initiation of maternal behavior converges on the POA, with contributions from the mAMY (which are inhibitory),

MATERNAL BEHAVIOR

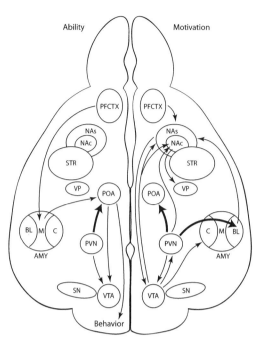

Figure 10.4. The neural systems mediating maternal behavior. On the left are indicated the neural systems that are most critical for the ability of the female rat to engage in maternal behaviors. On the right are depicted the neural systems in the female that are involved in the motivation or desire to engage in maternal behavior. The projections from the PVN (paraventricular nucleus) contain oxytocin.

the paraventricular nucleus (PVN; where oxytocin cell bodies are found), and perhaps the VTA, lateral septum and the anterior hypothalamus.

The neurobiology of maternal motivation has only recently become a topic of research study, although it has been known for some time that female rats will cross electrified grids to gain access to pups (Lonstein & Morrell, 2007). Pup retrieval is the behavior studied most frequently, as recently-parturient female rats will readily learn to bar press for access to pups and will bar press for hours, retrieving hundreds of pups (reviewed in [Lonstein & Morrell, 2007]). Importantly, the withdrawal of progesterone is necessary for dams to bar press for pups, as progesterone treatment prevents responding for pups in pregnancy terminated females (Hauser & Gandelman, 1985). Thus, progesterone appears to dampen maternal motivation.

Operant responding has also been used to identify the areas of the brain that are necessary for bar pressing for access to pups. Lesions of the POA or blAMY reduced bar pressing for access to pups whereas lesions of the NAcc did not (Lee et al., 2000). All lesions disrupted pup retrieval in the home cage (Lee et al., 2000). It is important to note that the operant responding in this experiment was maintained on an FR1 schedule, and that bar-pressing behavior was established with Froot Loops during pregnancy and then parturient dams were given pups when the bar was pressed post-partum. In other paradigms, lesion of the NAcc have been shown to decrease sensitivity to changes in the delivery of reinforcers (Acheson et al., 2006), so it is possible that after NAcc lesions the bar pressing by parturient rats may reflect a learning deficit, rather than lack of involvement of NAcc in maternal motivation. The finding that lesions of the NAcc shell disrupt pup retrieval, but not locomotor activity, argues that the NAcc is involved in some aspect of maternal motivation (Li & Fleming, 2003).

Using c-Fos immunoreactivity to designate brain regions that are active, Morrell and colleagues have shown that cues associated with pups in a conditioned place preference task result in activation of neurons in the POA, prefrontal cortex, NAcc, and the blAMY, but not the dorsal striatum (Mattson et al., 2003; Mattson & Morrell, 2005). Based on their analysis of the neural systems mediating maternal motivation, Lonstein and Morrell (Lonstein & Morrell, 2007) propose that increased dopamine activity in the ascending mesolimbic circuits is necessary for many of active components of maternal behavior. Interestingly, the hedonic impact (i.e., liking) of food and sex may also be regulated by opioid systems within these mesolimbic dopaminergic circuits that control reward motivation (Pecina et al., 2006). Studies of sex differences in these so called "hedonic hot spots" in the NAcc shell and ventral pallidum also would be predicted to reveal a sexually dimorphic pattern of regulation.

It is interesting to note that in biparental species, such as the prairie vole, males display parental behavior in response to vasopressin in the lateral septum (Wang, 1994; Wang et al., 1994a; Wang et al., 1994b) (see Young & Carter, Chapter 8 in this volume). In biparental mice, lesions of the POA reduce parental behavior in both males and females (Gubernick et al., 1993; Lee & Brown, 2002), suggesting that the neural basis of parental behavior is similar in males and females. Male rats can be induced to show parental behaviors by presentation of pups (Rosenblatt et al., 1996); and estradiol given systemically or estradiol implants in the POA enhance the onset of maternal behaviors in male rats (Rosenblatt et al., 1996; Rosenblatt & Ceus, 1998). It takes longer, however, to induce these behaviors in males than in females (Rosenblatt et al., 1996; Rosenblatt & Ceus, 1998). The neural basis of paternal motivation (or maternal motivation in males) is unstudied to date.

SEX DIFFERENCES IN DRUG ABUSE

Once sex differences in motivational circuits had evolved, we postulate that there were unforeseen consequences that resulted in many other motivations systems being sexually dimorphic as well. Nowhere is this so striking as in drug addiction. Sex differences emerge in all phases of the addiction process including initiation and prevalence of use, patterns and levels of use, the progression to addiction, withdrawal, and relapse. We focus our discussion here on cocaine use, but the same patterns of sex differences in addiction are present for all drugs of abuse (Lynch et al., 2002b; Carroll et al., 2004a).

Cocaine addiction is characterized by the transition from casual, recreational use, to habitual or compulsive, including binge patterns. Such changes are hypothesized to be in part due to changes in motivation to use the drug over time. Here we briefly review clinical and pre-clinical evidence for sex/gender differences in addiction, with an emphasis on psychostimulant addiction, and suggest that sex differences in motivation for drug taking, as well as other reinforcers may be due to evolutionary priorities that are the consequence of variations in hormonal status and/or sex-chromosome complement.

Sex Differences in Drug Abuse in Humans

Although the rates of drug abuse are currently lower in women, the number of women using and abusing licit and illicit drugs is on the rise. Adult men are 2 to 3 times more likely than women to have a drug abuse/dependence disorder (SAMHSA, 1996), although some evidence suggests that the gender difference in prevalence of drug use may be due to differences in opportunity, rather than vulnerability to drug use (Van Etten & Anthony, 1999; Van Etten et al., 1999).

Cocaine abuse in particular has increased in the last decade among women so that of the 1.8 million Americans who use cocaine, approximately 30% are now female (Wetherington & Roman, 1995). According to a recent report, 9% of women age 12 and over have used cocaine. The only illicit drug used more by women is marijuana (28% have used marijuana) (Kandel et al., 1995). Among women who have used cocaine, prevalence of lifetime dependence for cocaine is 14.9±2.0% (mean ±S.D.). This is in contrast to alcohol where 79% have used alcohol, but only 9.2±0.8% have developed lifetime dependence (Kandel et al., 1995). The use of all illicit drugs has been increasing among women in the past decade, and stimulant drug use and dependence among women, in particular, is a growing public health concern (Wetherington & Roman, 1995; Lynch et al., 2002b; Carroll et al., 2004a). In particular, recent evidence suggests that women are *more* vulnerable to some aspects of cocaine abuse.

Women begin using cocaine and enter treatment at earlier ages than men (Griffin et al., 1989; Mendelson et al., 1991) and have more severe cocaine use at intake than men (Kosten et al., 1993). Thus, the progression to dependence may differ between men and women, with women progressing through the landmark stages from initial use to dependence at a faster rate (Kosten et al., 1985; Brady & Randall, 1999). This *telescoping* effect reflects a briefer time course for the development of medical consequences and behavioral/psychological factors characteristic of a dependence disorder. An increased vulnerability in women may also account for higher rates of relapse. Although cocaine-addicted women and men typically report similar levels of cocaine use (Evans et al., 1999), abstinent women report higher levels of craving following exposure to cocaine-related cues (Robbins et al., 1999a). Such differences may be due to sociocultural factors or to biological factors. If there are biological factors that impact the rate at which women become addicted, it could be that neural mechanisms that mediate the rapid formation of the mother-infant bond play a role in other types of associations and addiction in particular.

Repeated exposure to addictive drugs may cause sexually dimorphic neuroadaptive alterations in cortico-limbic-striatal circuits that contribute to alterations in motivational function that are critical for craving and relapse (Lynch et al., 2006). Consequently, sex differences in motivation may contribute to, and be a consequence of, addiction. Specifically, neuroadaptations in motivational processes with increased control over behavior by drug-associated cues may be more evident in women than men, which likely contributes to aspects of compulsive drug-seeking and drug-taking behavior. Furthermore, cocaine cues induce more drug craving in female than male addicts (Robbins et al., 1999b). Collectively, these results suggest that women may be more sensitive to the addictive properties of cocaine than men. However, this evidence is based primarily on retrospective reports, and relatively little is known about the neurobiological basis for sex differences in motivational processes in general.

Sex Differences in Animal Models of Drug Use

Basic research on the role of sex and ovarian hormones in the neurochemical and behavioral responses to acute and repeated exposure to drugs of abuse also finds sex differences. The acute behavioral response to psychomotor stimulants that rodents exhibit can reflect both sex differences and be modulated by gonadal hormones in males and females. Research on rodents and humans indicates that the behavioral effects of drugs of abuse, and the psychomotor stimulants in particular, are both sexually dimorphic and modulated by the gonadal steroid hormones (e.g., (Gordon, 1980; Hruska & Silbergeld, 1980; Becker & Ramirez, 1981; Di Paolo et al., 1981; Joyce et al., 1982; Dluzen & Ramirez, 1984; Becker & Beer, 1986; Di Paolo et al., 1986; Hruska, 1988; Van Hartesveldt et al., 1989; Dluzen & Ramirez, 1990; Bazzett et al., 2000; Lynch et al., 2002b; Sell et al., 2002; Carroll et al., 2004a).

With repeated exposure to psychomotor stimulants there is an increase in the psychomotor activating effects of the drug, known as *behavioral sensitization.* Behavioral sensitization can be different in males and females, and can be differentially affected by gonadal steroid hormones.

If one considers sensitization of amphetamine or cocaine-induced psychomotor behavior to be the absolute increase in the behavioral response exhibited when two tests are compared, females exhibit more robust sensitization than do intact males (Robinson et al., 1982; Robinson, 1984; Camp & Robinson, 1988b, a; van Haaren & Meyer, 1991b; Forgie & Stewart, 1994).

Following ovariectomy (OVX) of female rats the expression of sensitization to amphetamine is attenuated (Robinson et al., 1982; Robinson, 1984; Camp & Robinson, 1988b, a; Forgie and Stewart, 1994) or suppressed all together (van Haaren & Meyer, 1991b; Sircar & Kim, 1999).

Estradiol treatments in OVX rats enhance sensitization of locomotor activity induced by amphetamine or cocaine (Peris et al., 1991; Forgie & Stewart, 1994). These studies demonstrate that the neurobiological response to stimulant drugs is sexually dimorphic, but they do not address how this biological difference impacts sex differences in the motivation to take drugs.

Sex Differences in Stimulant Self-Administration in Animals

The animal model of human drug-taking behavior that has the most face validity is self-administration. In self-administration studies, animals are trained to bar press or nose poke in order to receive an i.v. infusion of a drug. The animal's pattern of drug taking can be studied during acquisition, maintenance, and relapse. It is also possible to manipulate the schedule of reinforcement in order to determine motivation to take a drug.

Sex differences have been reported during all phases of the addiction process as assessed using various self-administration paradigms (see Lynch et al., 2002a; Carroll et al., 2004b; Roth et al., 2004). When a low dose of drug is used, female rats acquire cocaine self-administration at a faster rate (Lynch & Carroll, 1999; Carroll et al., 2002; Hu et al., 2004). Further, when responding for low doses of cocaine is assessed under a schedule in which the number of responses required in order to obtain a cocaine infusion progressively increases, female rats reach much higher final ratios than do males suggesting that females are more motivated to obtain cocaine (Roberts et al., 1989a).

Similar sex differences have been observed under reinstatement testing conditions designed to parallel relapse in humans (Lynch & Carroll, 2000; Roth & Carroll, 2004b, a; Kippin et al., 2005; but see, Fuchs et al., 2005). It should be noted that sex differences are most robust at lower doses of cocaine; and at higher doses, differences are less evident. This literature has been reviewed extensively, so the review here will be brief. The reader is referred to recent reviews for additional information.

There has been a recent emphasis on developing animal cocaine self-administration procedures that model the transitional process from use/abuse to addiction (e.g., Ahmed & Koob, 1998; Tornatzky & Miczek, 2000; Roberts et al., 2002). Using a procedure similar to that developed by Roberts et al. (2002), female rats binge for a longer initial period of time, take more cocaine over a 7-day access period, and show a greater loss of diurnal control over cocaine intake than do males (Lynch & Taylor, 2004).

When the role of estradiol in binge-cocaine intake and subsequent motivational changes is examined, estradiol benzoate (EB) treatment increases the initial binge length and total levels of cocaine self-administration (Lynch & Taylor, 2005). In the experiment under discussion, OVX female rats with and without EB replacement were compared under a 24-hr discrete trial cocaine self-administration procedure (4 trials/hr, 1.5 mg/kg/infusion) over a 7-day period.

Results revealed that following a 1-day abstinence period, motivation to obtain cocaine was decreased in OVX rats treated with vehicle, but not in OVX rats treated with EB. These results show that estradiol influences both cocaine self-administration under high access conditions and that there are subsequent motivational changes resulting from such access. An important question remains as to how genetic sex and/or hormonal differences interact and whether differences in the biology of motivational function can explain sex differences that promote uncontrolled and dysregulated patterns of intake that are the hallmark of addiction.

Evidence from studies in both humans and animals indicate that ovarian hormones modulate self-administration of stimulants and thus may influence sex differences during different phases of cocaine addiction. In humans, the subjective effects of stimulants vary across the menstrual cycle (Justice & de Wit, 1999, 2000; Justice & De Wit, 2000). For example, several of the positive subjective effects of d-amphetamine such as euphoria, desire, increased energy and intellectual efficiency are potentiated during the follicular phase—when estradiol levels are low, at first, and rise slowly; progesterone levels are low—relative to the luteal phase when estradiol levels are moderate and progesterone levels are high. Additionally, administration of estradiol during the follicular phase further increases the subjective effects of d-amphetamine (Justice & de Wit, 2000). In contrast,

progesterone administered during the follicular phase has been reported to attenuate the subjective response to repeated self-administered cocaine (Sofuoglu et al., 2002).

Hormonal fluctuations in the rat estrous cycle likewise have been reported to influence behavioral responses to stimulants. Self-administration of cocaine varies as a function of estrous cycle phase (Roberts et al., 1989b). Female rats will also work harder for cocaine during the estrous phase of the cycle than during other phases of the cycle, and females work harder than male rats (Roberts et al., 1989b). The finding that the motivation to self-administer cocaine is greater during the estrous phase of the cycle may be related to the finding that stimulant-induced DA release is enhanced during estrus, relative to diestrus (Becker & Ramirez, 1980; Becker & Cha, 1989).

In contrast, sucrose self-administration does not vary across the estrous cycle (Hecht et al., 1999) suggesting that drug-taking behavior taps into a slightly different motivation circuit or that drugs of abuse are more effective at activating these neural circuits and so effects of the estrous cycle are observed.

Estradiol administration to OVX females affects many psychostimulant drug-induced behaviors, including self-administration (Verimer et al., 1981; Peris et al., 1991; Morissette & Di Paolo, 1993; Thompson & Moss, 1994; Grimm & See, 1997; Becker, 1999; Sircar & Kim, 1999; Quinones-Jenab et al., 2000; Freeman et al., 2001). For example, Hu et al. (2004) found that in OVX female rats, exogenous estradiol treatment alone was sufficient to facilitate acquisition of cocaine self-administration. Estradiol-facilitated cocaine self-administration has also been found in other studies (Roberts et al., 1989b; Freeman et al., 2001). Finally, acquisition of cocaine self-administration is markedly reduced by OVX and restored by estradiol replacement (Lynch et al., 2001).

In contrast to estradiol, the subjective effects of psychomotor stimulant drugs are negatively correlated with salivary progesterone levels in women (White, 2002). In rodents, progesterone inhibits cocaine-mediated behaviors, such as estradiol-enhanced locomotor activity and sensitization of cocaine-induced stereotyped behavior, compared to OVX females treated with estradiol. For example, Peris et al. (1991) reported that OVX female rats treated with estradiol had the greatest amount of striatal DA release following injections of amphetamine compared to OVX females treated with either progesterone alone or progesterone plus estradiol. Recently, it was reported that concurrent administration of progesterone with estradiol counteracts the effect of estradiol on acquisition of cocaine self-administration behavior (Jackson et al., 2005).

Taken together, a wealth of data now indicate that ovarian hormones contribute to sex differences in cocaine self-administration and that estradiol in particular is a key factor influencing the reinforcing effects of cocaine in female rats. Over the course of the estrous cycle and menstrual cycle, there are peaks and valleys during which females are more or less susceptible to the reinforcing properties of cocaine. The effect of progesterone may be similar to the hormonal influences on maternal behavior, where withdrawal from progesterone is necessary for the rapid onset of maternal behavior at parturition.

Castration (CAST) of males has been reported to enhance sensitization of amphetamine- or cocaine-induced psychomotor behavior (e.g., Robinson, 1984; Camp & Robinson, 1988a, b), although this result has not been found consistently (van Haaren & Meyer, 1991b; Forgie & Stewart, 1994).

It has been hypothesized that if CAST enhances the induction and/or expression of behavioral sensitization, that testosterone treatment should reverse this effect. This is not the case, however, as testosterone treatment has not been found to affect behavioral sensitization in CAST males (Forgie & Stewart, 1994). Furthermore, there is no effect of CAST on acquisition of cocaine self-administration behavior and a dose of estradiol that enhances self-administration in female rats has no effect on cocaine self-administration behavior in male rats (Jackson et al., 2005). Thus, the effects of estradiol on the acquisition of cocaine self-administration are sexually dimorphic.

Chromosomal Mechanisms Underlying Sex Differences in Motivation

Although gonadal hormones regularly account for sex differences in a variety of behaviors (Arnold & Gorski, 1984), it is also possible that some sex differences may be accounted for by the complement of sex chromosomes (XX vs. XY) alone or in combination with gonadal hormone influences. Such potential contributions become most evident in cases where sexual phenotype appears to be insensitive to the effects of sex hormones during development or in cases where sex differences develop before the onset of sex-specific patterns of gonadal secretions (Arnold et al., 2003). Until recently, parsing the influences of gonadal hormones and sex chromosome complement was extremely difficult. However, mouse models are now available in which gonadal hormone status (ovaries vs. testes) is independent of sex chromosome complement (XX vs. XY; see Chapter 3).

Mice with a deletion of the testis-determining *Sry* gene from the Y chromosome develop ovaries even when the Y chromosome is present. Absence of the *Sry* gene in these mice (XY⁻) as well as in normal females (XX) results in the development of ovaries and a gonadally female phenotype (Lovell-Badge & Robertson, 1990). These mice allow us to assess independently the influences of gonadal hormones and sex chromosome complement on the neurobiology of sex differences in both normal and pathological behavior (De Vries et al., 2002). There are no reports of sex differences in behaviors relevant to addiction where these two influences have been assessed independently. However, we have recently found that sex chromosome complement, independent of gonadal hormone status, influences the rate of habit formation (Quinn et al., 2006a).

Specifically, XX mice acquired a food-reinforced habit faster than XY mice, independent of gonadal hormone status. In addition, we have examined the well-documented sex difference in cocaine-induced locomotor sensitization, e.g., (van Haaren & Meyer, 1991a; Harrod et al., 2005) using a similar approach. We found that female mice show greater locomotor sensitization to cocaine compared to males, replicating the previous literature. Critically, this effect depended upon the gonadal hormone status rather than sex chromosome complement (Quinn et al., 2006b). Studies of other motivational processes, rather than food or drug motivated responding, using these mice would be of interest (Sanchez et al., 2006). Clearly sexual dimorphism in the development of habit formation could also have important implications for drug addiction (Everitt & Robbins, 2005).

Functional Roles of Cortico-Limbic-Striatal Circuits

Cortical and limbic glutamatergic inputs to the ventral striatum (from prefrontal, anterior cingulate, hippocampal and amygdalar cortices) modulate NAcc function and its subsequent outputs to motor circuits (O'Donnell & Grace, 1995; Moore et al., 1999; Haber et al., 2000). These limbic-striatal circuits are involved in emotional responsivity and motivational function that contribute to incentive learning. These effects are also critically dependent on DA and/or glutamatergic activity (Kelley, 2004). Specifically, the representation of the incentive value of stimuli and rewards, including drug-associated conditioned stimuli is mediated by the amygdala (Cador et al., 1989; Hiroi & White, 1991; Robbins & Everitt, 1996; Holland & Gallagher, 1999).

Lesions of the BLA impair the ability of conditioned stimuli to affect instrumental responding (Malkova et al., 1997; Balleine et al., 2003); and this area may thus be involved in establishing stimulus-reward associations that contribute to reward-motivated behavior, and for the transfer of information about the current incentive value of conditioned stimuli to instrumental responding (Everitt et al., 1999; Robbins & Everitt, 1999; Everitt et al., 2001). Moreover, the central nucleus of the amygdala is connected with hypothalamic and brainstem regions involved in autonomic and consummatory responses to incentive stimuli and in the acquisition of stimulus-reward associations (Parkinson et al., 2000; Cardinal et al., 2002).

By contrast, the NAcc DA innervation may mediate the behavioral impact of motivational state (Wyvell & Berridge, 2000, 2001) and conditioned reinforcers (Taylor & Robbins, 1984, 1986; Parkinson et al., 1999; Parkinson et al., 2000; Parkinson et al., 2001) on behavior. Indeed, the NAcc has been argued to mediate the influence of incentive information on reward-motivated behavior.

The prefrontal cortical (PFC) has been shown to play an important role in craving, reinstatement of drug-seeking and in higher-order processing of reward information/salience and drug cues in both humans and animals (London et al., 2000; Gottfried et al., 2003; Kalivas & McFarland, 2003; O'Doherty, 2004; Wilson et al., 2004). In combination with its well-described involvement in inhibitory control (Roberts & Wallis, 2000), the PFC is critical for decision-making and response-selection that is impaired in alcoholics and in drug addicts (Rogers et al., 1999; Bechara, 2003; Hildebrandt et al., 2006; Schoenbaum et al., 2006).

The nigrostriatal projection mediates a number of relevant functions such as processing of reward information, reward-related learning, goal-directed ac-

tions and the formation of habits (Gerdeman et al., 2003; Yin et al., 2004; Everitt & Robbins, 2005; Vanderschuren et al., 2005; Yin et al., 2005a; Yin et al., 2005b; Volkow et al., 2006; Yin et al., 2006).

Together, these regions appear to be part of a distributed network responsible for several levels of reward processing. Moreover, a number of studies have demonstrated adaptations in synaptic functions, intracellular signaling pathways and changes in dendritic morphology (Robinson & Kolb, 1999; Nestler, 2001) that may play a critical role in aberrant plasticity within these circuits (Berke & Hyman, 2000; Hyman & Malenka, 2001). Studies of sex differences and the regulation by estrogen within these circuits would provide critical information with regards aspects of motivational function associated with obesity and addiction that may differ between men and women.

SEX DIFFERENCES IN AMYGDALO-STRIATAL FUNCTION

Sex differences in motivation may be the result of sex-differences in reward-related learning mechanisms (and vice versa) that impact on various emotional and cognitive processes (Maren et al., 1994; Sandstrom et al., 1998; Wood & Shors, 1998; Frick & Gresack, 2003; Gresack & Frick, 2003, 2004; Jonasson, 2005; Gresack & Frick, 2006).

Of particular interest, studies in men and women have found that women exhibit greater recall of emotional memory and patterns of brain activation, most notably in the AMY; and that men and women are different, particularly, when processing both positive and negative emotional stimuli (Cahill et al., 2001; Canli et al., 2002; Klein et al., 2003; Wrase et al., 2003; Hamann & Canli, 2004; Hamann, 2005). This suggests that AMY-dependent emotional memory formation may occur via different (by degree) neural substrates in males and females, with the net result being enhanced memory strength in females at the time of retrieval.

Further evidence for enhanced responsiveness to positive emotional stimuli in females comes from research on reactivity to cues associated with drugs of abuse (see previous) where sexual dimorphism in reward-related learning may contribute to the sex differences. As noted, female cocaine users report higher levels of craving when exposed to drug-associated cues than males (Robbins et al., 1999a; Elman et al., 2001) and female smokers are more sensitive to the hedonic and reinforcing properties of cigarette-associated cues (Perkins et al., 2001). Similarly, in preclinical studies nicotine self-administration is potentiated by cues to a greater extent in female than male rats (Chaudhri et al., 2005). Neuroimaging studies are beginning to confirm gender-specific correlates of motivation and craving in cocaine dependent individuals (Kilts et al., 2004; Tucker et al., 2004; Li et al., 2005b; Li et al., 2005a).

Pavlovian learning processes are thought to participate in the process by which drug-associated cues come to control motivated behavior (see Everitt et al., 2001), and thus such sexual dimorphisms in cue reactivity may reflect sex differences in amydalo-striatal circuits that contribute to affective learning and subsequent motivational processing of emotional stimuli. Additionally, exposure to drugs of abuse, including amphetamine, cocaine, or nicotine, in male rats prior to the initiation of training enhances stimulus-reward learning (Hitchcott et al., 1997; Harmer & Phillips, 1998; Taylor & Jentsch, 2001; Olausson et al., 2003, 2004; Wiseman et al., 2005). Further studies using both male and female subjects are needed to characterize the potential interaction between sex and prior drug experience in this type of learning, as well as the involvement of gonadal hormones, and in anxiety-associated emotional learning (Toufexis et al., 2006).

Recently, the Taylor laboratory has directly examined whether females show enhanced appetitive emotional learning relative to males, measured by acquisition of food-reinforced stimulus-reward learning (Wiseman et al., unpublished observation). The investigators found that females exhibited facilitated learning on Pavlovian approach tasks relative to males. Ovariectomy, prior to training, resulted in impaired learning relative to sham-operated females, suggesting a role for circulating ovarian hormones in mediating the observed sex difference. These data suggest sexually dimorphic reward-related learning, which may contribute not only to sex differences in psychiatric disorders such as addiction, but also to eating disorders.

Interestingly, no published studies have investigated sex differences in cue-elicited eating and/or binge eating in animal models (Hagan et al., 2002; Petrovich et al., 2002; Holland & Petrovich, 2005; Lee et al., 2005; Petrovich et al., 2005; Ghitza et al., 2006; Petrovich et al., 2006) though such models often use female rats (Avena & Hoebel, 2003; Avena

et al., 2005). Sex differences in food motivational processes are known to exist and clinical evidence suggests that eating disorders are far more prevalent in women. Parallels between food and drug "addictive" disorders (see for review Trinko et al., 2007) and the biological parallels with respect to sex differences should be a focus of research.

We hypothesize that such sex differences in motivational function are also likely mediated by parallel limbic-striatal circuits (Jentsch & Taylor, 1999; Jentsch et al., 2000; Jentsch et al., 2002; Jentsch & Taylor, 2003). Moreover, sex differences in AMY structure and function have been demonstrated in both rodent and human studies (Nishizuka & Arai, 1981, 1983; Arai et al., 1985) (Cooke et al., 1999; Hamann, 2005). Further experiments using local manipulations of the AMY are required to directly test whether this structure mediates the sex difference observed in aspects of reward-related learning, as well as to identify which AMY subnuclei are involved. Given that females have greater oxytocin projections from the paraventricular nucleus to the NAcc shell and AMY than do males, it is possible that oxytocin and dopamine activation in the AMY and NAcc are involved in enhanced motivational function associated with stimulus-reward learning and/or emotional behavior, irrespective of whether the reward is food, drugs or formation of mother-infant bond.

SUMMARY

From this brief discussion it should be clear that there are sex differences in motivation. The pathways that we have proposed to mediate these sex differences in motivation have been inferred from studies that have approached the question of the neural basis of motivation from behavior-specific perspectives, rather from the perspective of investigating sex differences in motivation. This means that there are significant gaps in our knowledge, due to the lack of empirical data that would be generated from a systematic approach to the topic. Thus, some of the apparent sex differences may be due to a lack of data in one of the sexes. This indicates the need for additional experimental data generated from testing specific hypotheses about the neural bases for sex differences in motivation.

Studies of the response to cocaine in gonadectomized male and female rats provide the strongest data regarding the neural evidence for sex differences in

MOTIVATIONAL SYSTEMS

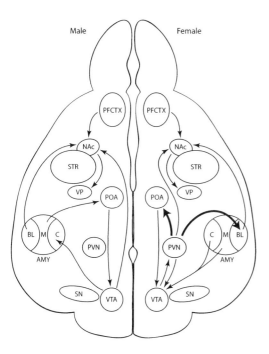

Figure 10.5. Sex differences in motivational systems. On the left are the neural systems critical for motivated behaviors in the male rat. On the right are the neural systems important for motivated behaviors in the female rat. The primary differences between males and females are in the vasopressin and oxytocin systems. In the male rat the vasopressin projections from medial amygdala to preoptic area modulates motivation, while in the female the oxytocin projection from the PVN to the POA and blAMY is modulating motivated behaviors.

motivation. These data indicate that there is an underlying sex difference due to sexually dimorphic development of the brain that, in part, mediates the sex difference in motivated behaviors.

Studies from mice in which the testes-determining *Sry* gene is deleted from the Y chromosome and inserted in an autosome indicate that these sex differences in motivation may, at least in part, be genetic in origin. The precise relationship between sex differences in learning and differences in motivation remains to be determined. It is possible that these learning differences may be due secondarily to primary differences in the motivational impact of the rewards that are being learned about, and consequently result from the motivational differences.

We hypothesize that the presence of the neural circuits that mediate maternal motivation, and in particular the greater oxytocin projection to the NAcc in females, may play an important role in this sex difference. In addition, there are effects of gonadal hormones that modulate the reward system. In particular, estradiol enhances the rewarding value of drugs, while progesterone counteracts the effect of estradiol. Ultimately research on the neurobiological mechanisms of sex differences in motivation will aid in the treatment and understanding of motivation-related pathologies for females and males.

Acknowledgments

The authors would like to thank Kent Berridge, Elaine Hull, Joseph Lonstein, and Robert Meisel for their helpful comments on an earlier version of this manuscript. We would also like to thank the USPHS for funding for research discussed in this chapter (NS48141 and DA12677 to JBB and DA15222, DA1171 and DA16556 to JRT) and the Society for Women's Health Research Isis Research Fund.

References

Acheson A, Farrar AM, Patak M, Hausknecht KA, Kieres AK, Choi S, et al. (2006). Nucleus accumbens lesions decrease sensitivity to rapid changes in the delay to reinforcement. *Behavioural Brain Research*, 173:217–228.

Adler NT. (1969). Effects of the male's copulatory behavior on successful pregnancy of the female rat. *J Comp Physiol Psychol*, 69:613–622.

Adler NT. (1974). The behavioral control of reproductive physiology. *Adv Behav Biol*, 11:259–286.

Adler NT. (1978). On the mechanisms of sexual behavior and their evolutionary constraints. In *Biological Determinants of Sexual Behavior* (Hutchison JB (Ed.), pp 657–694. New York: Wiley and Sons, Ltd.

Ahmed SH, Koob. GF (1998). Transition from moderate to excessive drug intake: change in hedonic set point. *Science*, 282:298–300.

Arai Y, Matsumoto A, Nishizuka M. (1985). Sexually dimorphic pattern in the hypothalamic and limbic brain. *Int J Neurol*, 19–20:133–143.

Arnold AP, Gorski RA. (1984). Gonadal steroid induction of structural sex differences in the central nervous system. *Annu Rev Neurosci*,7:413–442.

Arnold AP, Rissman EF, De Vries GJ. (2003). Two perspectives on the origin of sex differences in the brain. *Ann N Y Acad Sci*, 1007:176–188.

Avena NM, Hoebel BG. (2003). A diet promoting sugar dependency causes behavioral cross-sensitization to a low dose of amphetamine. *Neuroscience,* 122:17–20.

Avena NM, Long KA, Hoebel BG. (2005). Sugar-dependent rats show enhanced responding for sugar after abstinence: evidence of a sugar deprivation effect. *Physiol Behav,* 84:359–362.

Balleine BW, Killcross AS, Dickinson A. (2003). The effect of lesions of the basolateral amygdala on instrumental conditioning. *J Neurosci,* 23:666–675.

Baum MJ. (2002). Neuroendocrinology of sexual behavior in the male. In Becker JB, Breedlove SM, Crews D, McCarthy MM, (Eds.). *Behavioral Endocrinology,* 2nd Edition (pp 153–203). Cambridge: The MIT Press.

Bazzett TJ, Albin RL, Becker JB. (2000). Malonic acid and the chronic administration model of excitotoxicity. *Mitochondrial Inhibitors and Neurodegenerative Disorders,* 219–231.

Bechara A. (2003). Risky business: emotion, decision-making, and addiction. *J Gambl Stud,* 19:23–51.

Becker J, Ramirez VD. (1980). Dynamics of endogenous catecholamine release from brain fragments of male and female rats. *Neuroendocrinology,* 31:18–25.

Becker JB. (1999). Gender differences in dopaminergic function in striatum and nucleus accumbens. *Pharmacology Biochemistry and Behavior,* 64:803–812.

Becker JB, Ramirez VD. (1981). Sex differences in the amphetamine stimulated release of catecholamines from rat striatal tissue in vitro. *Brain Res,* 204:361–372.

Becker JB, Beer ME. (1986). The influence of estrogen on nigrostriatal dopamine activity: behavioral and neurochemical evidence for both pre- and postsynaptic components. *Behav Brain Res,* 19:27–33.

Becker JB, Cha JH. (1989). Estrous cycle-dependent variation in amphetamine-induced behaviors and striatal dopamine release assessed with microdialysis. *Behav Brain Res,* 35:117–125.

Becker JB, Rudick CN, Jenkins WJ. (2001). The role of dopamine in the nucleus accumbens and striatum during sexual behavior in the female rat. *J Neuroscience,* 21:3236–3241.

Berke JD, Hyman SE. (2000). Addiction, dopamine, and the molecular mechanisms of memory. *Neuron,* 25:515–532.

Bermant G. (1961). Response latencies of female rats during sexual intercourse. *Science,* 133:1771–1773.

Bermant G. (1967). Copulation in rats. *Psychology Today,* pp 52–60.

Bradley KC, Boulware MB, Jiang H, Doerge RW, Meisel RL, Mermelstein PM. (2005). Sexual experience generates distinct patterns of gene expression within the nucleus accumbens and dorsal striatum of female Syrian hamsters. *Genes, Brain and Behavior,* 4:31–44.

Brady KT, Randall CL. (1999). Gender differences in substance use disorders. *Psychiatr Clin North Am,* 22:241–252.

Bridges RS, Hay LE. (2005). Steroid-induced alterations in mRNA expression of the long form of the prolactin receptor in the medial preoptic area of female rats: effects of exposure to a pregnancy-like regimen of progesterone and estradiol. *Molecular Brain Research,* 140:10–16.

Brog JS, Salyapongse A, Deutch AY, Zahm DS. (1993). The patterns of afferent innervation of the core and shell in the "accumbens" part of the rat ventral striatum: immunohistochemical detection of retrogradely transported fluoro-gold. *J Comparative Neurology,* 338:255–278.

Brown AG, Leite RS, Strauss JF, III. (2004). Mechanisms underlying "functional" progesterone withdrawal at parturition. *Annals of the New York Academy of Sciences,* 1034:36–49.

Cador M, Robbins TW, Everitt BJ. (1989). Involvement of the amygdala in stimulus-reward associations: interaction with the ventral striatum. *Neurosciece,* 30:77–86.

Cahill., (2006). Why sex matters for neuroscience. *Nat Rev Neurosci,* 7:477–484.

Cahill L, Haier RJ, White NS, Fallon J, Kilpatrick L, Lawrence C, et al. (2001). Sex-related difference in amygdala activity during emotionally influenced memory storage. *Neurobiol Learn Mem,* 75:1–9.

Camp DM, Robinson TE. (1988a). Susceptibility to sensitization. I. Sex differences in the enduring effects of chronic D-amphetamine treatment on locomotion, stereotyped behavior and brain monoamines. *Behav Brain Res,* 30:55–68.

Camp DM, Robinson TE. (1988b). Susceptibility to sensitization. II. The influence of gonadal hormones on enduring changes in brain monoamines and behavior produced by the repeated administration of D-amphetamine or restraint stress. *Behav Brain Res,* 30:69–88.

Canli T, Desmond JE, Zhao Z, Gabrieli JD. (2002). Sex differences in the neural basis of emotional memories. *Proc Natl Acad Sci U S A,* 99:10789–10794.

Cardinal RN, Parkinson JA, Hall J, Everitt BJ. (2002). Emotion and motivation: the role of the amygdala, ventral striatum and prefrontal cortex. *Neurosci Biobehav Rev,* 26:321–352.

Carroll M, Lynch W, Roth M, Morgan A, Cosgrove K. (2004a). Sex and estrogen influence drug abuse. *Trends in Pharmacological Sciences,* 25:273–279.

Carroll ME, Morgan AD, Lynch WJ, Campbell UC, Dess NK. (2002). Intravenous cocaine and heroin self-administration in rats selectively bred for differential saccharin intake: phenotype and sex differences. *Psychopharmacology* (Berl), 161:304–313.

Carroll ME, Lynch WJ, Roth ME, Morgan AD, Cosgrove KP. (2004b). Sex and estrogen influence drug abuse. *Trends Pharmacol Sci,* 25:273–279.

Champagne F, Diorio J, Sharma S, Meaney M. (2001). Naturally occurring variations in maternal behavior in the rat are associated with differences in estrogen-inducible central oxytocin receptors. *Proc Natl Acad Sci USA,* 98:12736–12741.

Chaudhri N, Caggiula AR, Donny EC, Booth S, Gharib MA, Craven LA, et al. (2005). Sex differences in the contribution of nicotine and nonpharmacological stimuli to nicotine self-administration in rats. *Psychopharmacology* (Berl), 180:258–266.

Chudasama Y, Robbins TW. (2003). Dissociable contributions of the orbitofrontal and infralimbic cortex to pavlovian autoshaping and discrimination reversal learning: further evidence for the functional heterogeneity of the rodent frontal cortex. *J Neurosci*, 23:8771–8780.

Cooke BM, Tabibnia G, Breedlove SM. (1999). A brain sexual dimorphism controlled by adult circulating androgens. *Proc Natl Acad Sci USA*, 96:7538–7540.

Craig W. (1918). Appetites and aversions as constituents of instincts. *Biological Bulletin of Woods Hole*, 34:91–107.

Damsma G, Pfaus JG, Wenkstern D, Phillips AG, Fibiger HC. (1992). Sexual behavior increases dopamine transmission in the nucleus accumbens and striatum of male rats: comparison with novelty and locomotion. *Behavioral Neurosci*, 106:181–191.

De Vries GJ, Rissman EF, Simerly RB, Yang LY, Scordalakes EM, Auger CJ, et al. (2002). A model system for study of sex chromosome effects on sexually dimorphic neural and behavioral traits. *J Neurosci*, 22:9005–9014.

Di Paolo T, Poyet P, Labrie F. (1981). Effect of chronic estradiol and haloperidol treatment on striatal dopamine receptors. *Eur J Pharmacol*, 73:105–106.

Di Paolo T, Levesque D, Daigle M. (1986). A physiological dose of progesterone affects rat striatum biogenic amine metabolism. *Eur J Pharmacol*, 125:11–16.

Dluzen DE, Ramirez VD. (1984). Bimodal effect of progesterone on in vitro dopamine function of the rat corpus striatum. *Neuroendocrinol*, 39:149–155.

Dluzen DE, Ramirez VD. (1990). In vitro progesterone modulation of amphetamine-stimulated dopamine release from the corpus striatum of ovariectomized estrogen-treated female rats: response characteristics. *Brain Res*, 517:117–122.

Elman I, Karlsgodt KH, Gastfriend DR. (2001). Gender differences in cocaine craving among non-treatment-seeking individuals with cocaine dependence. *Am J Drug Alcohol Abuse*, 27:193–202.

Erskine MS. (1989). Solicitation behavior in the estrous female rat: a review. *Hormon Behav*,23:473–502.

Erskine MS. (1995). Prolactin release after mating and genitosensory stimulation in females. *Endocr Rev*, 16:508–528.

Erskine MS, Hanrahan SB. (1997). Effects of paced mating on c-fos gene expression in the female rat brain. *J Neuroendocrinology*, 9:903–912.

Erskine MS, Kornberg E, Cherry JA. (1989). Paced copulation in rats: effects of intromission frequency and duration on luteal activation and estrus length. *Physiol Behav*, 45:33–39.

Evans SM, Haney M, Fischman MW, Foltin RW. (1999). Limited sex differences in response to "binge" smoked cocaine use in humans. *Neuropsychopharmacology*, 21:445–454.

Everitt BJ. (1990). Sexual motivation: a neural and behavioural analysis of the mechanisms underlying appetitive and copulatory responses of male rats. *Neurosci Biobehav Rev*, 14:217–232.

Everitt BJ, Stacey P. (1987). Studies of instrumental behaviour with sexual reinforcement in male rats (*Rattus norvegicus*): II Effects of preoptic area lesions, castration and testosterone. *J Comparative Psychology*, 101:407–419.

Everitt BJ, Robbins TW. (2005). Neural systems of reinforcement for drug addiction: from actions to habits to compulsion. *Nat Neurosci*, 8:1481–1489.

Everitt BJ, Dickinson A, Robbins TW. (2001). The neuropsychological basis of addictive behaviour. *Brain Res Brain Res Rev*, 36:129–138.

Everitt BJ, Parkinson JA, Olmstead MC, Arroyo M, Robledo P, Robbins TW. (1999). Associative processes in addiction and reward. The role of amygdala-ventral striatal subsystems. *Ann N Y Acad Sci*, 877:412–438.

Ferguson J, Aldag J, Insel T, Young L. (2001). Oxytocin in the medial amygdala is essential for social recognition in the mouse. *J Neurosci*, 21:8278–8285.

Fernandes MS, Pierron V, Michalovich D, Astle S, Thornton S, Peltoketo H, et al. (2005). Regulated expression of putative membrane progestin receptor homologues in human endometrium and gestational tissues. *J Endocrinology*, 187:89–101.

Flanagan LM, Pfaus JG, Pfaff DW, McEwen BS. (1993). Induction of FOS immunoreactivity in oxytocin neurons after sexual activity in female rats. *Neuroendocrinology*, 58:352–358.

Forgie ML, Stewart J. (1994). Sex difference in amphetamine-induced locomotor activity in adult rats: role of testosterone exposure in the neonatal period. *Pharmacol, Biochem Behav*, 46.

Freeman WM, Brebner K, Lynch WJ, Robertson DJ, Roberts DC, Vrana KE. (2001). Cocaine-responsive gene expression changes in rat hippocampus. *J Neurosci*, 108:371–380.

Frick KM, Gresack JE. (2003). Sex differences in the behavioral response to spatial and object novelty in adult C57BL/6 mice. *Behav Neurosci*, 117:1283–1291.

Fuchs RA, Evans KA, Mehta RH, Case JM, See RE. (2005). Influence of sex and estrous cyclicity on conditioned cue-induced reinstatement of cocaine-seeking behavior in rats. *Psychopharmacology* (Berl), 179:662–672.

Garcia-Horsman P, Paredes RG. (2004). Dopamine antagonists do not block conditioned place preference induced by paced mating behavior in female rats. *Behavioral Neuroscience*, 118:356–364.

Gatewood JD, Wills A, Shetty S, Xu J, Arnold AP, Burgoyne PS, Rissman EF. (2006). Sex chromosome complement and gonadal sex influence aggressive and parental behaviors in mice. *J Neuroscience*, 26:2335–2342.

Gerdeman GL, Partridge JG, Lupica CR, Lovinger DM. (2003). It could be habit forming: drugs of abuse and striatal synaptic plasticity. *Trends Neurosci*, 26:184–192.

Ghitza UE, Gray SM, Epstein DH, Rice KC, Shaham Y. (2006). The anxiogenic drug yohimbine reinstates palatable food seeking in a rat relapse model: a role of CRF1 receptors. *Neuropsychopharmacology*, 31:2188–2196.

Gilman DP, Mercer LF, Hitt JC. (1979). Influence of female copulatory behavior on the induction of pseudopregnancy in the female rat. *Physiol Behav*, 22: 675–678.

Gordon JH. (1980). Modulation of apomorphine-induced stereotypy by estrogen: time course and dose response. *Brain Res Bull*, 5:679–682.

Gottfried JA, O'Doherty J, Dolan RJ. (2003). Encoding predictive reward value in human amygdala and orbitofrontal cortex. *Science*, 301:1104–1107.

Gresack JE, Frick KM. (2003). Male mice exhibit better spatial working and reference memory than females in a water-escape radial arm maze task. *Brain Res*, 982:98–107.

Gresack JE, Frick KM. (2004). Environmental enrichment reduces the mnemonic and neural benefits of estrogen. *Neuroscience*, 128:459–471.

Gresack JE, Frick KM. (2006). Post-training estrogen enhances spatial and object memory consolidation in female mice. *Pharmacol Biochem Behav*, 84:112–119.

Griffin ML, Weiss RD, Lange U. (1989). A comparison of male and female cocaine abuse. *Arch Gen Psychiatry*, 46:122–126.

Grimm JW, See RE. (1997). Cocaine self-administration in ovariectomized rats is predicted by response to novelty, attenuated by 17-beta estradiol, and associated with abnormal vaginal cytology. *Physiology & Behavior*, 61:755–761.

Gubernick DJ, Sengelaub DR, Kurz EM. (1993). A neuroanatomical correlate of paternal and maternal behavior in the biparental California mouse (Peromyscus californicus). *Behavioral Neuroscience*, 107: 194–201.

Haber SN, Fudge JL, McFarland NR. (2000). Striatonigrostriatal pathways in primates form an ascending spiral from the shell to the dorsolateral striatum. *J Neurosci*, 20:2369–2382.

Hagan MM, Wauford PK, Chandler PC, Jarrett LA, Rybak RJ, Blackburn K. (2002). A new animal model of binge eating: key synergistic role of past caloric restriction and stress. *Physiol Behav*, 77:45–54.

Hamann S. (2005). Sex differences in the responses of the human amygdala. *Neuroscientist*, 11:288–293.

Hamann S, Canli T. (2004). Individual differences in emotion processing. *Curr Opin Neurobiol*, 14:233–238.

Harmer CJ, Phillips GD. (1998). Enhanced appetitive conditioning following repeated pretreatment with d-amphetamine. *Behav Pharmacol*, 9:299–308.

Harrod SB, Booze RM, Welch M, Browning CE, Mactutus CF. (2005). Acute and repeated intravenous cocaine-induced locomotor activity is altered as a function of sex and gonadectomy. *Pharmacol Biochem Behav*, 82:170–181.

Hauser H, Gandelman R. (1985). Lever pressing for pups: evidence for hormonal influence upon maternal behavior of mice. *Horm Behav*, 19:454–468.

Hecht GS, Spear NE, Spear LP. (1999). Changes in progressive ratio responding for intravenous cocaine throughout the reproductive process in female rats. *Developmental Psychobiology*, 35:136–145.

Hildebrandt H, Brokate B, Hoffmann E, Kroger B, Eling P. (2006). Conditional responding is impaired in chronic alcoholics. *J Clin Exp Neuropsychol*, 28: 631–645.

Hiroi N, White NM. (1991). The lateral nucleus of the amygdala mediates expression of the amphetamine-produced conditioned place preference. *J Neurosci*, 11:2107–2116.

Hitchcott PK, Harmer CJ, Phillips GD. (1997). Enhanced acquisition of discriminative approach following intra-amygdala d-amphetamine. *Psychopharmacology* (Berl), 132:237–246.

Holland PC, Gallagher M. (1999). Amygdala circuitry in attentional and representational processes. *Trends Cognitive Science*, 3:65–73.

Holland PC, Petrovich GD. (2005). A neural systems analysis of the potentiation of feeding by conditioned stimuli. *Physiol Behav*, 86:747–761.

Hruska RE. (1988). 17ßEstradiol regulation of DA receptor interactions with G-proteins. *Soc Neurosci*, Abstr 14:454.

Hruska RE, Silbergeld EK. (1980). Increased dopamine receptor sensitivity after estrogen treatment using the rat rotation model. *Science*, 208:1466–1468.

Hu M, Crombag HS, Robinson TE, Becker JB. (2004). Biological basis of sex differences in the propensity to self-administer cocaine. *Neuropsychopharmacology*, 29:81–85.

Hyman SE, Malenka RC. (2001). Addiction and the brain: the neurobiology of compulsion and its persistence. *Nature Reviews Neuroscience*, 2:695–703.

Jackson LR, Robinson TE, Becker JB. (2005). Sex differences and hormonal influences on acquisition of cocaine self-administration in rats. *Neuropsychopharmacology*, 31(1):129–138.

Jenkins WJ, Becker JB. (2003a). Dynamic increases in dopamine during paced copulation in the female rat. *European Journal of Neuroscience*, 18:1997–2001.

Jenkins WJ, Becker JB. (2003b). Female rats develop conditioned place preferences for sex at their preferred interval. *Hormones and Behavior*, 43:503–507.

Jentsch JD, Taylor JR. (1999). Impulsivity resulting from frontostriatal dysfunction in drug abuse: implications for the control of behavior by reward-related stimuli. *Psychopharmacology*, (Berl) 146:373–390.

Jentsch JD, Taylor JR. (2003). Sex-related differences in spatial divided attention and motor impulsivity in rats. *Behav Neurosci*, 117:76–83.

Jentsch JD, Roth RH, Taylor JR. (2000). Role for dopamine in the behavioral functions of the prefrontal corticostriatal system: implications for mental disorders and psychotropic drug action. *Prog Brain Res*, 126:433–453.

Jentsch JD, Olausson P, De La Garza R, II, Taylor JR. (2002). Impairments of reversal learning and response perseveration after repeated, intermittent cocaine administrations to monkeys. *Neuropsychopharmacology*, 26:183–190.

Jonasson Z. (2005). Meta-analysis of sex differences in rodent models of learning and memory: a review of behavioral and biological data. *Neurosci Biobehav Rev*, 28:811–825.

Joyce JN, Smith RL, Van Hartesveldt C. (1982). Estradiol suppresses then enhances intracaudate dopamine-induced contralateral deviation. *Eur J Pharmacol*, 81:117–122.

Justice AJ, de Wit H. (1999). Acute effects of d-amphetamine during the follicular and luteal phases of the menstrual cycle in women. *Psychopharmacology* (Berl), 145:67–75.

Justice AJ, De Wit H. (2000). Acute effects of d-amphetamine during the early and late follicular phases of the menstrual cycle in women. *Pharmacol Biochem Behav*, 66:509–515.

Justice AJ, de Wit H. (2000). Acute effects of estradiol pretreatment on the response to d-amphetamine in women. *Neuroendocrinology*, 71:51–59.

Kalivas PW, McFarland K. (2003). Brain circuitry and the reinstatement of cocaine-seeking behavior. *Psychopharmacology* (Berl), 168:44–56.

Kandel DB, Warner MPP, Kessler RC. (1995). The epidemiology of substance abuse and dependence among women. In Wetherington CL, Roman AR, (Eds.), *Drug Addiction Research and the Health of Women* (pp. 105–130). Rockville, MD: US Department of Health and Human Services.

Karteris E, Zervou S, Pang Y, Dong J, Hillhouse EW, Randeva HS, Thomas P. (2006). Progesterone signaling in human myometrium through two novel membrane G protein-coupled receptors: potential role in functional progesterone withdrawal at term. *Molecular Endocrinology*, 20:1519–1534.

Kelley AE. (2004). Ventral striatal control of appetitive motivation: role in ingestive behavior and reward-related learning. *Neurosci Biobehav Rev*, 27:765–776.

Kilts CD, Gross RE, Ely TD, Drexler KP. (2004). The neural correlates of cue-induced craving in cocaine-dependent women. *Am J Psychiatry*, 161:233–241.

Kippin TE, Fuchs RA, Mehta RH, Case JM, Parker MP, Bimonte-Nelson HA, See RE. (2005). Potentiation of cocaine-primed reinstatement of drug seeking in female rats during estrus. *Psychopharmacology* (Berl), 182:245–252.

Klein S, Smolka MN, Wrase J, Grusser SM, Mann K, Braus DF, Heinz A/ (2003)/ The influence of gender and emotional valence of visual cues on fMRI activation in humans. *Pharmacopsychiatry*, 36(Suppl 3):S191–S194.

Kosten TA, Gawin FH, Kosten TR, Rounsaville BJ. (1993). Gender differeces in cocaine use and treatment response. *J Subst Abuse Treat*, 10:63–66.

Kosten TR, Rounsaville BJ, Kleber HD. (1985). Ethnic and gender differences among opiate addicts. *Int J Addict*, 20:1143–1162.

Lee A, Clancy S, Fleming AS. (2000). Mother rats bar-press for pups: effects of lesions of the mpoa and limbic sites on maternal behavior and operant responding for pup-reinforcement. [republished from Behav Brain Res. 1999;100(1–2):15–31; PMID: 102 12050]. *Behavioural Brain Research*, 108:215–231.

Lee AW, Brown RE. (2002). Medial preoptic lesions disrupt parental behavior in both male and female California mice (Peromyscus californicus). *Behavioral Neuroscience*, 116:968–975.

Lee HJ, Groshek F, Petrovich GD, Cantalini JP, Gallagher M, Holland PC. (2005). Role of amygdalo-nigral circuitry in conditioning of a visual stimulus paired with food. *J Neurosci*, 25:3881–3888.

Li CS, Kosten TR, Sinha R. (2005a). Sex differences in brain activation during stress imagery in abstinent cocaine users: a functional magnetic resonance imaging study. *Biol Psychiatry*, 57:487–494.

Li CS, Kemp K, Milivojevic V, Sinha R. (2005b). Neuroimaging study of sex differences in the neuropathology of cocaine abuse. *Gend Med*, 2:174–182.

Li M, Fleming AS. (2003). Differential involvement of nucleus accumbens shell and core subregions in maternal memory in postpartum female rats. *Behavioral Neuroscience*, 117:426–445.

London ED, Ernst M, Grant S, Bonson K, Weinstein A. (2000). Orbitofrontal cortex and human drug abuse: functional imaging. *Cereb Cortex*, 10:334–342.

Lonstein JS, Morrell JI. (2006). Neuroendocrinology and neurochemistry of maternal motivation and behavior. In Blaustein JD, (Ed.), *Behavioral Neurobiology (Stress, Memory, Agggression, Endocrine Influences)* 3rd Edition, in press. New York, NY.

Lonstein JS, Morrell JI. (2007). Neuroendocrinologya nd neurochemistry of maternal motivation and behavior. In Blaustein JA, (Ed.) *Behavioral Neurochemistry and Neuroendocrinology*, 3rd Edition, (p 954). Berlin: Springer-Verlag.

Lonstein JS, Simmons DA, Swann JM, Stern JM. (1998). Forebrain expression of c-fos due to active maternal behaviour in lactating rats. *Neuroscience*, 82:267–281.

Lonstein JS, Greco B, De Vries G, Stern JM, Blaustein JD. (2000). Maternal behavior stimulates c-fos activity within estrogen receptor alpha-containing neurons in lactating rats. *Neuroendocrinology*, 72:91–101.

Lonstein JS, Dominguez JM, Putnam SK, De Vries GJ, Hull EM. (2003). Intracellular preoptic and striatal monoamines in pregnant and lactating rats: possible role in maternal behavior. *Brain Research*, 970:149–158.

Lovell-Badge R, Robertson E. (1990). XY female mice resulting from a heritable mutation in the primary testis-determining gene, Tdy. *Development*, 109: 635–646.

Lynch WJ, Carroll ME. (1999). Sex differences in the acquisition of intravenously self-administered cocaine and heroin in rats. *Psychopharmacology* (Berl), 144:77–82.

Lynch WJ, Carroll ME. (2000). Reinstatement of cocaine self-administration in rats: sex differences. *Psychopharmacology*, (Berl) 148:196–200.

Lynch WJ, Taylor JR (2004) Sex differences in the behavioral effects of 24-h/day access to cocaine under a discrete trial procedure. *Neuropsychopharmacology* 29:943–951.

Lynch WJ, Taylor JR. (2005). Decreased motivation following cocaine self-administration under extended access conditions: effects of sex and ovarian hormones. *Neuropsychopharmacology*, 30:927–935.

Lynch WJ, Roth ME, Carroll ME. (2002a). Biological basis of sex differences in drug abuse: preclinical and clinical studies. *Psychopharmacology* (Berl), 164: 121–137.

Lynch WJ, Roth ME, Carroll ME. (2002b). Biological basis of sex differences in drug abuse: preclinical and clinical studies. *Psychopharmacology*, 164:121–137.

Lynch WJ, Roth ME, Mickelberg JL, Carroll ME. (2001). Role of estrogen in the acquisition of intravenously self-administered cocaine in female rats. *Pharmacol Biochem Behav*, 68:641–646.

Lynch WJ, Kiraly DD, Caldarone BJ, Picciotto MR, Taylor JR. (2006). Effect of cocaine self-administration on striatal PKA-regulated signaling in male and female rats. *Psychopharmacology* (Berl), 191(2): 263–271.

Malkova L, Gaffan D, Murray E. (1997). Excitotoxic lesions of the amygdala fail to produce impairment in visual learning for auditory secondary reinforcement but interfere with reinforcer devaluation effects in rhesus monkeys. *J Neuroscience*, 17:6011–6020.

Maren S, De Oca B, Fanselow MS. (1994). Sex differences in hippocampal long-term potentiation (LTP) and Pavlovian fear conditioning in rats: positive correlation between LTP and contextual learning. *Brain Res*, 661:25–34.

Martinez I, Paredes RG. (2001). Only self-paced mating is rewarding in rats of both sexes. *Hormones and Behavior*, 40:510–517.

Mattson BJ, Morrell JI. (2005). Preference for cocaine- versus pup-associated cues differentially activates neurons expressing either Fos or cocaine- and amphetamine-regulated transcript in lactating, maternal rodents. *Neuroscience*, 135:315–328.

Mattson BJ, Williams SE, Rosenblatt JS, Morrell JI. (2003). Preferences for cocaine- or pup-associated

chambers differentiates otherwise behaviorally identical postpartum maternal rats. *Psychopharmacology*, 167:1–8.

McCarthy MM, Becker JB. (2002). Neuroendocrinology of sexual behavior in the female. In Becker JB, Breedlove SM, Crews D, McCarthy MM, (Eds.) *Behavioral Endocrinology*, 2nd Edition, (pp 117–151). Cambridge, MA: MIT Press/Bradford Books.

McClintock MK. (1984). Group mating in the domestic rat as context for sexual selection: consequences for the analysis of sexual behavior and neuroendocrine responses. *Adv Study of Behav*, 14:1–50.

McClintock MK, Adler NT. (1977). The role of the female during copulation in wild and domestic Norway rats. *Behaviour*, LXVII:67–96.

Meisel RL, Mullins AJ. (2006). Sexual experience in female rodents: cellular mechanisms and functional consequences. *Brain Research*, 1126:56–65.

Meisel RL, Camp DM, Robinson TE. (1993). A microdialysis study of ventral striatal dopamine during sexual behaivor in female Syrian hamsters. *Behav Brain Res*, 55:151–157.

Meisel RL, Joppa MA, Rowe RK. (1996). Dopamine receptor antagonists attenuate conditioned place preference following sexual behavior in female Syrian hamsters. *Eur J Pharmacol*, 309:21–24.

Mendelson JH, Weiss R, Griffin M, Mirin SM, Teoh SK, Mello NK, Lex BW. (1991). Some special considerations for treatment of drug abuse and dependence in women. *NIDA Res Monogr*, 106:313–327.

Mermelstein PG, Becker JB. (1995). Increased extracellular dopamine in the nucleus accumbens and striatum of the female rat during paced copulatory behavior. *Behavioral Neuroscience*, 109:354–365.

Moore H, West AR, Grace AA. (1999). The regulation of forebrain dopamine transmission: relevance to the pathophysiology and psychopathology of schizophrenia. *Biol Psychiatry*, 46:40–55.

Morissette M, Di Paolo T. (1993). Effect of chronic estradiol and progesterone treatments of ovariectomized rats on brain dopamine uptake sites. *J Neurochem*, 60:1876–1883.

Nestler EJ. (2001). Molecular neurobiology of addiction. *Am J Addict*, 10:201–217.

Nishimori K, Young L, Guo Q, Wang Z, Insel T, Matzuk M. (1996). Oxytocin is required for nursing but is not essential for parturition or reproductive behavior. *Proc Natl Acad Sci U S A*, 93:11699–11704.

Nishizuka M, Arai Y. (1981). Sexual dimorphism in synaptic organization in the amygdala and its dependence on neonatal hormone environment. *Brain Res*, 212:31–38.

Nishizuka M, Arai Y. (1983). Male-female differences in the intra-amygdaloid input to the medial amygdala. *Exp Brain Res*, 52:328–332.

O'Doherty JP. (2004). Reward representations and reward-related learning in the human brain: insights from neuroimaging. *Curr Opin Neurobiol*, 14:769–776.

O'Donnell P, Grace AA. (1995). Synaptic interactions among excitatory affects to nucleus accumbens neurons: hippocampal gating of prefrontal cortical inputs. *J Neurosci*, 15:3622–3639.

Olausson P, Jentsch JD, Taylor JR. (2003). Repeated nicotine exposure enhances reward-related learning in the rat. *Neuropsychopharmacology*, 28:1264–1271.

Olausson P, Jentsch JD, Taylor JR. (2004). Nicotine enhances responding with conditioned reinforcement. *Psychopharmacology* (Berl), 171:173–178.

Oldenberger WP, Everitt BJ, De Jonge FH. (1992). Conditioned Place Preference Induced by Sexual Interaction in Female Rats. *Hormones and Behavior*, 26:214–228.

Paredes RG, Alonso A. (1997). Sexual behavior regulated (paced) by the female induces conditioned place preference. *Behavioral Neuroscience*, 111:123–128.

Paredes RG, Vazquez B. (1999). What do female rats like about sex? Paced mating. *Behavioural Brain Research*, 105:117–127.

Paredes RG, Martinez I. (2001). Naloxone blocks place preference conditioning after paced mating in female rats. *Behavioral Neuroscience*, 115:1363–1367.

Parkinson JA, Robbins TW, Everitt BJ. (2000). Dissociable roles of the central and basolateral amygdala in appetitive emotional learning. *Eur J Neurosci*, 12:405–413.

Parkinson JA, Olmstead MC, Burns LH, Robbins TW, Everitt BJ. (1999). Dissociation of effects of lesions of nucleus accumbens core and shell in appetitive Pavlovian approach behavior and the potentiation of conditioned reinforcement and locomotor activity by D-amphetamine. *J Neurosci*, 16:2401–2411.

Parkinson JA, Crofts HS, McGuigan M, Tomic DL, Everitt BJ, Roberts AC. (2001). The role of the primate amygdala in conditioned reinforcement. *J Neurosci*, 21:7770–7780.

Pecina S, Smith KS, Berridge KC. (2006). Hedonic hot spots in the brain. *Neuroscientist*, 12:500–511.

Pedersen C, Vadlamudi S, Boccia ML, Amico J. (2006). Maternal behavior deficits in nulliparous oxytocin knockout mice. *Genes Brain Behav*, 5:274–281.

Peris J, Decambre N, Coleman-Hardee M, Simpkins J. (1991). Estradiol enhances behavioral sensitization to cocaine and amphetamine-stimulated [3H]dopamine release. *Brain Res*, 566:255–264.

Perkins KA, Gerlach D, Vender J, Grobe J, Meeker J, Hutchison S. (2001). Sex differences in the subjective and reinforcing effects of visual and olfactory cigarette smoke stimuli. *Nicotine Tob Res*, 3:141–150.

Petrovich GD, Holland PC, Gallagher M. (2005). Amygdalar and prefrontal pathways to the lateral hypothalamus are activated by a learned cue that stimulates eating. *J Neurosci*, 25:8295–8302.

Petrovich GD, Setlow B, Holland PC, Gallagher M. (2002). Amygdalo-hypothalamic circuit allows learned cues to override satiety and promote eating. *J Neurosci*, 22:8748–8753.

Petrovich GD, Ross CA, Gallagher M, Holland PC. (2006). Learned contextual cue potentiates eating in rats. *Physiol Behav*, 28;90(2–3):362–367.

Pfaus JG, Phillips AG. (1991). Role of dopamine in anticipatory and consummatory aspects of sexual behavior in the male rat. *Behavioral Neurosci*, 105:727–743.

Pfaus JG, Damsma G, Wenkstern D, Fibiger HC. (1995). Sexual activity increases dopamine transmission in the nucleus accumbens and striatum of female rats. *Brain Res*, 693:21–30.

Pfaus JG, Damsma G, Nomikos GG, Wenkstern DG, Blaha CD, Phillips AG, et al. (1990). Sexual behavior enhances central dopamine transmission in the male rat. *Brain Res*, 530:345–348.

Pleim ET, Matochik JA, Barfield RJ, Auerbach SB. (1990). Correlation of dopamine release in the nucleus accumbens with masculine sexual behavior in rats. *Brain Res*, 524:160–163.

Polston EK, Heitz M, Barnes W, Cardamone K, Erskine MS. (2001). NMDA-mediated activation of the medial amygdala initiates a downstream neuroendocrine memory responsible for pseudopregnancy in the female rat. *J Neuroscience*, 21:4104–4110.

Quinn JJ, Hitchcott PK, Umeda EA, Arnold AP, Taylor JR. (in press). Sex chromosome complement regulates habit formation. *Nature Neuroscience*.

Quinn JJ, Hitchcott PK, Pesquera FR, Arnold AP, Taylor JR. (2006). Sex differences in habit formation and sensitization to cocaine: Independent contributions of chromosomal sex and gonadal sex. Third Annual Interdisciplinary Women's Health Research Symposium, National Institutes of Health.

Quinones-Jenab V, Perrotti LI, Mc Monagle J, Ho A, Kreek MJ. (2000). Ovarian hormone replacement affects cocaine-induced behaviors in ovariectomized female rats. *Pharmacology Biochemistry and Behavior*, 67:417–422.

Robbins SJ, Ehrman RN, Childress AR, O'Brien CP. (1999a). Comparing levels of cocaine cue reactivity in male and female outpatients. *Drug Alcohol Depend*, 53:223–230.

Robbins SJ, Ehrman RN, Childress AR, O'Brien CP. (1999b). Comparing levels of cocaine cue reactivity in male and female outpatients. *Drug Alcohol Depend*, 53:223–230.

Robbins TW, Everitt BJ. (1996). Neurobehavioural mechanisms of reward and motivation. *Curr Opin Neurobiol*, 6:228–236.

Robbins TW, Everitt BJ. (1999). Drug addiction: bad habits add up. *Nature*, 398:567–570.

Roberts AC, Wallis JD. (2000). Inhibitory control and affective processing in the prefrontal cortex: neuropsychological studies in the common marmoset. *Cereb Cortex*, 10:252–262.

Roberts DC, Bennett SA, Vickers GJ. (1989a). The estrous cycle affects cocaine self-administration on a progressive ratio schedule in rats. *Psychopharmacology* (Berl), 98:408–411.

Roberts DC, Brebner K, Vincler M, Lynch WJ. (2002). Patterns of cocaine self-administration in rats produced by various access conditions under a discrete trials procedure. *Drug Alcohol Depend*, 67:291–299.

Roberts DCS, Bennett SAL, Vickers GJ. (1989b). The estrous cycle affects cocaine self-administration on a progressive ratio schedule in rats. *Psychopharmacology*, 98:408–411.

Robinson TE. (1984). Behavioral sensitization: characterization of enduring changes in rotational behavior produced by intermittent injections of amphetamine in male and female rats. *Psychopharmacology (Berlin)*, 84:466–475.

Robinson TE, Kolb B. (1999). Alterations in the morphology of dendrites and dendritic spines in the nucleus accumbens and prefrontal cortex following repeated treatment with amphetamine or cocaine. *Eur J Neurosci*, 11:1598–1604.

Robinson TE, Becker JB, Presty SK. (1982). Long-term facilitation of amphetamine-induced rotational behavior and striatal dopamine release produced by a single exposure to amphetamine: sex differences. *Brain Res*, 253:231–241.

Rogers RD, Everitt BJ, Baldacchino A, Blackshaw AJ, Swainson R, Wynne K, et al. (1999). Dissociable deficits in the decision-making cognition of chronic amphetamine abusers, opiate abusers, patients with focal damage to prefrontal cortex, and tryptophan-depleted normal volunteers: evidence for monoaminergic mechanisms. *Neuropsychopharmacology*, 20:322–339.

Rosenblatt JS. (1992). Hormone-behavior relations in the regulation of maternal behavior. In Becker JB, Breedlove SM, Crews D, (Eds.), *Behavioral Endocrinology*, 1st Edition (pp 219–259). Cambridge, MA: MIT Press/Bradford Books.

Rosenblatt JS, Ceus K. (1998). Estrogen implants in the medial preoptic area stimulate maternal behavior in male rats. *Hormones and Behavior*, 33:23–30.

Rosenblatt JS, Hazelwood S, Poole J. (1996). Maternal behavior in male rats: effects of medial preoptic area lesions and presence of maternal aggression. *Hormones and Behavior*, 30:201–215.

Roth ME, Carroll ME. (2004a). Sex differences in the acquisition of IV methamphetamine self-administration and subsequent maintenance under a progressive ratio schedule in rats. *Psychopharmacology (Berl)*, 172:443–449.

Roth ME, Carroll ME. (2004b). Sex differences in the escalation of intravenous cocaine intake following long- or short-access to cocaine self-administration. *Pharmacol Biochem Behav*, 78:199–207.

Roth ME, Cosgrove KP, Carroll ME. (2004). Sex differences in the vulnerability to drug abuse: a review of preclinical studies. *Neurosci Biobehav Rev*, 28:533–546.

Saddoris MP, Gallagher M, Schoenbaum G. (2005). Rapid associative encoding in basolateral amygdala depends on connections with orbitofrontal cortex. *Neuron*, 46:321–331.

Sanchez H, Quinn JJ, Taylor JR. (2006). Sex differences in contextual fear conditioning: A role for dorsal hippocampus 17-estradiol. Society for Neuroscience, Online.

Sandstrom NJ, Kaufman J, Huettel SA (1998). Males and females use different distal cues in a virtual environment navigation task. *Brain Res Cogn Brain Res*, 6:351–360.

Schoenbaum G, Chiba AA, Gallagher M. (2000). Changes in functional connectivity in orbitofrontal cortex and basolateral amygdala during learning and reversal training. *J Neuroscience*, 20:5179–5189.

Schoenbaum G, Roesch MR, Stalnaker TA. (2006). Orbitofrontal cortex, decision-making and drug addiction. *Trends Neurosci*, 29:116–124.

Sell SL, Thomas ML, Cunningham KA. (2002). Influence of estrous cycle and estradiol on behavioral sensitization to cocaine in female rats. *Drug Alcohol Depend*, 67:281–290.

Sheehan PM. (2006). A possible role for progesterone metabolites in human parturition. *Australian and New Zealand Journal of Obstetrics and Gynaecology*, 46:159–163.

Sircar R, Kim D. (1999). Female gonadal hormones differentially modulate cocaine-induced behavioral sensitization in Fischer, Lewis and Sprague-Dawley rats. *J Pharmacol*, 289(1):54–65.

Sofuoglu M, Babb DA, Hatsukami DK. (2002). Effects of progesterone treatment on smoked cocaine response in women. *Pharmacol Biochem Behav*, 72:431–435.

Taylor JR, Robbins TW. (1984). Enhanced behavioural control by conditioned reinforcers following microinjections of d-amphetamine into the nucleus accumbens. *Psychopharmacology (Berl)*, 84:405–412.

Taylor JR, Robbins TW. (1986). 6-Hydroxydopamine lesions of the nucleus accumbens, but not of the caudate nucleus, attenuate enhanced responding with reward-related stimuli produced by intra-accumbens d-amphetamine. *Psychopharmacology (Berl)*, 90:390–397.

Taylor JR, Jentsch JD. (2001). Repeated intermittent administration of psychomotor stimulant drugs alters the acquisition of Pavlovian approach behavior in rats: differential effects of cocaine, d-amphetamine and 3,4- methylenedioxymethamphetamine ("Ecstasy"). *Biol Psychiatry*, 50:137–143.

Thompson TL, Moss RL. (1994). Estrogen regulation of dopamine release in the nucleus accumbens: genomic- and nongenomic-mediated effects. *J Neurochem*, 62:1750–1756.

Tornatzky W, Miczek KA. (2000). Cocaine self-administration "binges": transition from behavioral and autonomic regulation toward homeostatic dysregulation in rats. *Psychopharmacology (Berl)*, 148:289–298.

Toufexis DJ, Myers KM, Davis M. (2006). The effect of gonadal hormones and gender on anxiety and emotional learning. *Horm Behav*, 50:539–549.

Trinko R, Sears RM, Guarnieri DJ, DiLeone RJ. (2007). Neural mechanisms underlying obesity and addiction. *Physiol Behav*, In press Jan 16; [Epub ahead of print].

Tucker KA, Browndyke JN, Gottschalk PC, Cofrancesco AT, Kosten TR. (2004). Gender-specific vulnerability for rCBF abnormalities among cocaine abusers. *Neuroreport*, 15:797–801.

Van Etten ML, Anthony JC. (1999). Comparative epidemiology of initial drug opportunities and transitions to first use: marijuana, cocaine, hallucinogens and heroin. *Drug Alcohol Depend*, 54:117–125.

Van Etten ML, Neumark YD, Anthony JC. (1999). Male-female differences in the earliest stages of drug involvement. *Addiction*, 94:1413–1419.

van Haaren F, Meyer ME. (1991a). Sex differences in locomotor activity after acute and chronic cocaine administration. *Pharmacol Biochem Behav*, 39:923–927.

van Haaren F, Meyer M. (1991b). Sex differences in the locomotor activity after acute and chronic cocaine administration. *Pharmacol Biochem Behav*, 39:923–927.

Van Hartesveldt C, Cottrell GA, Meyer ME. (1989). Effects of intrastriatal hormones on the dorsal immobility response in male rats. *Pharmacol Biochem Behav*, 35:307–310.

Vanderschuren LJ, Di Ciano P, Everitt BJ. (2005). Involvement of the dorsal striatum in cue-controlled cocaine seeking. *J Neurosci*, 25:8665–8670.

Verimer T, Arneric SP, Long JP, Walsh BJ, Abou Zeit-Har MS. (1981). Effects of ovariectomy, castration, and chronic lithium chloride treatment on stereotyped behavior in rats. *Psychopharmacol*, 75:273–276.

Volkow ND, Wang GJ, Telang F, Fowler JS, Logan J, Childress AR, et al. (2006). Cocaine cues and dopamine in dorsal striatum: mechanism of craving in cocaine addiction. *J Neurosci*, 26:6583–6588.

Wang Z. (1994). Testosterone effects on development of vasopressin messenger RNA expression in the bed nucleus of the stria terminalis and medial amygdaloid nucleus in male rats. *Brain Res Dev Brain Res*, 79:147–150.

Wang Z, Ferris CF, De Vries GJ. (1994a). Role of septal vasopressin innervation in paternal behavior in prairie voles (*Microtus ochrogaster*). *Proc Natl Acad Sci USA*, 91:400–404.

Wang Z, Smith W, Major DE, De Vries GJ. (1994b). Sex and species differences in the effects of cohabitation on vasopressin messenger RNA expression in the bed nucleus of the stria terminalis in prairie voles (*Microtus ochrogaster*) and meadow voles (*Microtus pennsylvanicus*). *Brain Res*, 650:212–218.

Wetherington CL, Roman AR, (Eds.) (1995) Drug Addiction Research and the Health of Women. Rock-ville, MD: US Department of Health and Human Services.

White FJ. (2002). A behavioral/systems approach to the neuroscience of drug addiction. *J Neuroscience*, 22:3303–3305.

Wilson SJ, Sayette MA, Fiez JA. (2004). Prefrontal responses to drug cues: a neurocognitive analysis. *Nat Neurosci*, 7:211–214.

Wiseman SL, Lynch WJ, Olausson P, Taylor JR. (2005). Sex differences in reward-related learning after repeated nicotine exposure during adolescence. Society for Neuroscience, Online *Abstract Viewer/ Itinerary Planner*. *Washington, DC*.

Wood GE, Shors TJ. (1998). Stress facilitates classical conditioning in males, but impairs classical conditioning in females through activational effects of ovarian hormones. *Proc Natl Acad Sci U S A*, 95:4066–4071.

Wood W, Eagly AH. (2002). A cross-cultural analysis of the behavior of women and men: implications for the origins of sex differences. *Psychological Bulletin*, 128:699–727.

Wrase J, Klein S, Gruesser SM, Hermann D, Flor H, Mann K, Braus DF, Heinz A. (2003). Gender differences in the processing of standardized emotional visual stimuli in humans: a functional magnetic resonance imaging study. *Neurosci Lett*, 348:41–45.

Wright C, Beijer A, Groenewegen HJ. (1996). Basal amygdaloid complex afferent to the rat nucleus accumbens are compartmentally organized. *J Neurosci*, 16:1877–1893.

Wyvell CL, Berridge KC. (2000). Intra-accumbens amphetamine increases the conditioned incentive salience of sucrose reward: enhancement of reward "wanting" without enhanced "liking" or response reinforcement. *J Neurosci*, 20:8122–8130.

Wyvell CL, Berridge KC. (2001). Incentive sensitization by previous amphetamine exposure: increased cue-triggered "wanting" for sucrose reward. *J Neurosci*, 21:7831–7840.

Yin HH, Knowlton BJ, Balleine BW. (2004). Lesions of dorsolateral striatum preserve outcome expectancy but disrupt habit formation in instrumental learning. *Eur J Neurosci*, 19:181–189.

Yin HH, Knowlton BJ, Balleine BW. (2005a). Blockade of NMDA receptors in the dorsomedial striatum prevents action-outcome learning in instrumental conditioning. *Eur J Neurosci*, 22:505–512.

Yin HH, Knowlton BJ, Balleine BW. (2006). Inactivation of dorsolateral striatum enhances sensitivity to changes in the action-outcome contingency in instrumental conditioning. *Behav Brain Res*, 166:189–196.

Yin HH, Ostlund SB, Knowlton BJ, Balleine BW. (2005b). The role of the dorsomedial striatum in instrumental conditioning. *Eur J Neurosci*, 22:513–523.

Chapter 11

Sex Differences in Neuroplasticity

Csaba Leranth, Neil J. MacLusky, and Tibor Hajszan

The idea that the nervous system undergoes different plastic changes at all stages of development is not new. Almost 100 years ago, Ramon y Cajal suggested that neuronal connectivity in the adult brain could change as a consequence of mental activity (Ramon y Cajal, 1911). At that time, Cajal's idea was not accepted and until as late as the middle of the last century (Hebb, 1949), neuronal plasticity was only considered as a behavior- and adaptation-induced change in the transmission strength of existing synapses, without any concomitant morphological remodeling.

Since then, accumulating experimental evidence indicates that morphological neuroplasticity does indeed take place in the brain, which contributes to the functional adaptation to changing conditions in the external and internal environment. Although the magnitude and distribution of these neuroplastic alterations is more prominent in developing animals, the adult brain also retains a remarkable capacity for structural and functional modifications. It has become clear that several factors are able to influence neuroplasticity mechanisms. Among these, the gonadal steroids represent a group of circulating hormones that powerfully regulate cellular and morphological changes in the brain, resulting in sexually differentiated patterns of neuronal connectivity.

Throughout development, steroids exert a critical influence upon the architecture of numerous sex steroid-responsive areas in the brain, resulting in sexual dimorphisms at both morphological and physiological levels; as reviewed by MacLusky and Naftolin (1981). While these responses are most prominent in regions of the hypothalamus and preoptic area, that are involved in the control of neuroendocrine function and sex behavior (Raisman & Field, 1971, 1973; Gorski et al., 1978; Simerly et al., 1985), they are also observed in a number of other structures that subserve higher cognitive functions. For example, effects of gonadal steroids on the structure and function of the hippocampus are evident in rodents as early as the first postnatal week of life. Androgens produced by the testis mediate sexual differentiation of the hippocampus. In some strains of mice, males have more granule cells in the hippocampal dentate gyrus than females (Wimer & Wimer, 1989). Likewise, male rats have a larger and more asymmetric dentate gyrus than females (Roof & Havens, 1992; Roof, 1993), while sex differences have been demonstrated in the apical dendritic structure and the dendritic branching patterns of CA3 pyramidal neurons. Because the apical dendrites of CA3 pyramidal cells are the targets of afferent mossy fibers from the granule cells, these observations are consistent with the hypothesis that there is increased input from the dentate gyrus in males, as compared to females (Parducz & Garcia-Segura, 1993).

Initially, gonadal hormone-induced neuroplastic responses were viewed as being confined to early development, during developmental "critical periods" for sexual differentiation. During the past decade, this view has had to be revised as several studies have shown that gonadal hormones are still capable of activating structural and functional alterations in the adult central nervous system. The first direct evidence regarding the spine growth promoting effect of estrogen was presented more than a decade ago (Gould et al., 1990). Using the Golgi impregnation technique, these authors showed that estrogen administration to adult, ovariectomized rats results in a dramatic increase in the number of CA1 area pyramidal cell apical dendritic spines per unit dendritic length.

In a concomitant study, using electron microscopic stereological calculation, Woolley and McEwen (Woolley & McEwen, 1992) have demonstrated that, even during the ovarian cycle there is a fluctuation in the density of spine synapses in the stratum radiatum of the CA1 hippocampal subfield. Recent studies have also demonstrated that administration of male hormones to both gonadectomized male and female animals has the same synaptoplastic effects in the hippocampus as estrogen in females (Leranth et al., 2003; Hajszan et al., 2004; Leranth et al., 2004a; MacLusky et al., 2006). However, there are major sex differences in the effectiveness and mechanisms of actions of the gonadal hormones, between males and females.

The purpose of this chapter is to review these differences, to indicate where areas of uncertainty still remain, and suggest possible future avenues of research to explore the underlying mechanisms and potential neurological significance of these morphological responses to gonadal steroid exposure. Because the majority of the work in this field to date has focused on the CA1 area of the hippocampus, this review will also focus on sex differences in CA1 responses to androgen and estrogen. It is becoming clear, however, that many of the changes that have been reported for CA1 probably also apply to other areas of the hippocampus, as well as regions of the neocortex. Some examples of these responses will also be cited, as directions for future investigation.

METHODOLOGICAL CONSIDERATIONS

Theoretically, many potential approaches are available to examine the regulation of dendritic synaptic plasticity, including calculating the number of spines on unit lengths of dendrites of Golgi-impregnated, biocytin- or Lucifer yellow-filled neurons (Gould et al., 1990; Kretz et al., 2004; Hao et al., 2006), or measurement of the total number of profiles immunolabeled for biochemical markers of spines and synapses (Rune et al., 2002; Tang et al., 2004). These methods provide data of interest in terms of biochemical and structural effects of gonadal hormones, e.g., morphological changes in the dendritic arbor and shape of spines. However, they only indirectly reflect spine synapse numbers and may under some circumstances give a misleading impression of changes in the number of spine synapses. Procedures carried out at the light microscopic level do not allow determination of the proportion of the measured markers or spines that is really associated with synapses and, more specifically, with spine synapses. There are several reports showing that expression of synaptic marker molecules can change without alterations in synapse density (Harrison, 2004).

As described below, in some regions of the hippocampus, Golgi-based estimation of pyramidal dendritic spine density appears to give data at odds with direct measures of spine synapse density. For this reason, we feel that nothing gives a better insight into the relationship between hippocampal function and spine synapse remodeling than direct measurement of the number of spine synapses in a precisely defined sampling area. The most reliable approach to achieve this is the electron microscopic stereological calculation of the total number of spine synapses, which we have used extensively over the last few years. For the details of this EM stereology technique, see MacLusky et al. (2006).

SYNAPTOPLASTIC EFFECTS OF FEMALE AND MALE GONADAL STEROIDS IN THE HIPPOCAMPUS AND CEREBRAL CORTEX OF GONADECTOMIZED MALE AND FEMALE RATS

Synaptoplastic Effect of Estrogen in the Hippocampal CA1 and CA3 Subfields and Dentate Gyrus of Ovariectomized Female Rats

The first hard evidence for morphological changes in the adult brain was provided in an elegant work performed by Woolley and Gould in Bruce McEwen's laboratory (Gould et al., 1990) that demonstrated an increase in the number of CA1 area pyramidal cell apical dendritic spines in ovariectomized rats, following estrogen administration. Subsequent studies confirmed that the observed dendritic changes re-

flected effects on the density of spine synaptic contacts (Woolley & McEwen, 1992).

Intriguingly, these initial experiments suggested that the effects of estrogen might be region specific, confined to the CA1 area of the hippocampus. Thus, while changes in dendritic structure were observed after estrogen in CA1, they were not detected in CA3. Because of the inherent limitations of the Golgi impregnation used in this study, however, it could not be determined with confidence whether or not density in CA3 synapses was affected by estrogen treatment. In fact, follow up experiments applying the unbiased electron microscopic stereological calculation have demonstrated that estrogen administration to ovariectomized rats also results in a significant increase of apical dendritic spine synapses in the stratum radiatum of the CA3 hippocampal subfield (Fig. 11.1), as well as in the stratum moleculare of the dentate gyrus. Therefore, the effects of estrogen on dendritic spine synapse density in the hippocampus may involve all the principal cell fields, not just the CA1 subfield in which dendritic morphological responses are particularly prominent.

Sex Differences in the Synaptoplastic Effects of Estrogen and Androgen in the Hippocampus of Gonadectomized Male Rats

While numerous studies have demonstrated that, during the female reproductive cycle, physiological levels of the ovarian steroids greatly influence the density of pyramidal cell dendritic spines and spine synapses in the CA1 subfield of the hippocampus (Gould et al., 1990; Woolley et al., 1990; Woolley & McEwen, 1992; Leranth et al., 2000a; Leranth et al., 2002), until quite recently almost nothing was known about the responses of the male. The hippocampus is rich in androgen receptor-expressing cells (Simerly et al., 1990) indicating that it is a target for testosterone action. In the CA1 area, the androgen receptors appear to be primarily located in pyramidal neurons (Kerr et al., 1995). The rat hippocampus also contains low levels of aromatase (MacLusky et al., 1994), the enzyme converting testosterone to estrogen. Thus, effects of circulating testosterone could be mediated either via actions of the steroid on androgen receptors, or via conversion to estrogen. Morphological studies suggest that androgens and estrogens both modulate hippocampal structure in the male. In the CA1 area,

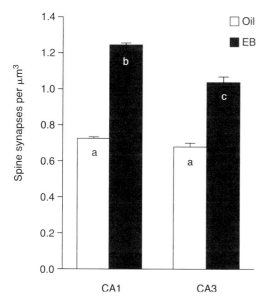

Figure 11.1. Effects of 2-day estrogen (EB) treatment on CA1 and CA3 spine synapse density of ovariectomized rats. The result of unbiased electron microscopic stereological calculation demonstrate that a 2-day EB administration to ovariectomized rats results in a significant (P<.05) increase in the spine synapse density in the stratum radiatum of both the CA1 and CA3 hippocampal subfields. Columns labeled with the same letters are not statistically different.

spine density peaks at puberty in male mice and this increase can be prevented by prepubertal castration (Meyer et al., 1978).

Orchidectomy reduces the density of CA1 area pyramidal cell spines in male rats, an effect that is partially reversed by estrogen administration (Lewis et al., 1995). These previous studies, however, used techniques (light microscopic examination of Golgi impregnated material) that do not provide information about synaptic connectivity. Therefore, we set out to determine the effects of testosterone and estrogen on the density of spine synapses on CA1 area pyramidal cells in gonadectomized male rats.

One week following gonadectomy, different groups of adult rats received the aromatizable androgen testosterone propionate (TP), the nonaromatizable androgen 5α-dihydrotestosterone (DHT), or estradiol benzoate (EB) treatment. Control animals were sham operated and received only sesame oil injections. The results of the statistical analyses provided evidence of different effects of the various hormone treatments on the density of spine synapses in the CA1 region (Fig. 11.2). The highest density of CA1 area pyramidal cell spine synapses was calculated in TP- or DHT-treated rats. A slightly, but not significantly lower synaptic density was observed in the sham-gonadectomized control group. Significantly lower (~50%) spine synapse densities were observed in the gonadectomized oil-treated and EB-treated rats.

These observations demonstrate that in adult male rats, the integrity of CA1 area pyramidal cell spine synapses depends on the presence of circulating testosterone. Gonadectomy dramatically reduces the number of spine synapses, a response that is reversed by treatment with either testosterone or the nonaromatizable androgen DHT. By contrast, estrogen

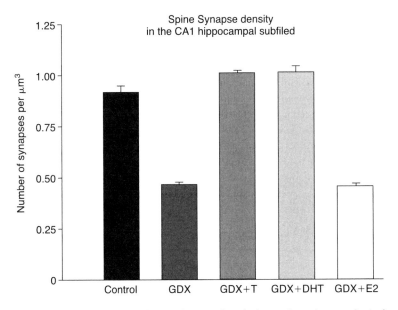

Figure 11.2. Bar graph shows the result of the unbiased stereological calculation of spine synapse density in the stratum radiatum of the CA1 subfield of control, gonadectomized (GDX), gonadectomized plus testosterone-treated (GDX+T), gonadectomized plus dihydrotestosterone-treated (GDX+DHT), and gonadectomized plus estrogen-treated (GDX+E2) male rats. There is no significant difference between the density values of spine synapses between the Control, GDX+T, and GDX+DHT animals. However, the spine synapse density of the GDX and GDX+E2 rats is significantly ($P<.001$) lower (48%) than that of control animals. Reprinted with permission from from Leranth C, Petnehazi O, MacLusky, NJ. (2003). Gonadal hormones affect spine synaptic density in the CA1 hippocampal subfield of male rats. *J Neuroscience*, 23:1588–1592.

administration has no significant effect on CA1 spine synapse density in gonadectomized animals.

These data also indicate a striking sexual dimorphism in the response mechanisms that maintain normal hippocampal CA1 structure. In the female, estrogen is a potent modulator of CA1 spine synapse density (Gould et al., 1990; Woolley et al., 1990; Woolley & McEwen, 1992; Leranth et al., 2000a; Leranth et al., 2002). In the male, however, the dramatic loss of hippocampal CA1 spine synapse density after gonadectomy is not significantly affected by short-term estrogen treatment. By contrast, treatment with testosterone or DHT completely reverses the post-orchidectomy decline in hippocampal spine synapse numbers. The lack of effect of estrogen administration and the comparable responses observed with testosterone and DHT strongly suggest that the effect of testosterone is mediated via androgen per se, rather than by conversion of the androgen to estrogen. The apparent lack of response to systemic estrogen administration in these experiments was somewhat unexpected, in view of previous data indicating effects of estrogen treatment on dendritic structure in males (Lewis et al., 1995), particularly since the doses of estrogen used in this previous study were identical to those used here.

In this previous study, however, the effects of estrogen treatment on dendritic spine density, while statistically significant, were quantitatively much smaller than the effect of gonadectomy. Thus, spine density on the primary apical dendrites of CA1 pyramidal neurons was reduced by almost 50% following gonadectomy (Lewis et al., 1995), a response consistent with the almost 50% decrease in the number of spine synapses observed in the present study. By contrast, estrogen treatment induced only an approximately 10% increase in dendritic spine density (Lewis et al., 1995) and no significant change in the number of spine synapses per μm^3.

Synaptoplastic Effect of Aromatizable and Non-aromatizable Androgen Hormones in the Hippocampal CA1 Area of Ovariectomized Female Rats

During the female reproductive cycle, the preovulatory surge of ovarian steroid hormone release induces an increase in the density of pyramidal cell dendritic spines and spine synapses in the CA1 subfield of the hippocampus (Gould et al., 1990; Woolley et al., 1990; Woolley & McEwen, 1992). This response is mediated at least in part by estrogen secretion: In ovariectomized females, estrogen treatment restores CA1 synapse density to levels close to those normally observed at proestrus (McEwen & Woolley, 1994; Leranth et al., 2000a; Leranth & Shanabrough, 2001). Estradiol is not the only ovarian hormone released during the preovulatory period, however. Testosterone circulates during the estrous cycle at levels substantially higher than those of estradiol and also peaks at proestrus (Rush & Blake, 1982).

As discussed above, CA1 spine synapse density in male rats is dependent on the continued presence of testosterone. Thus, castration reduced CA1 synapse density by almost 50%, an effect that was completely reversed by only two days of treatment with either testosterone or the nonaromatizable androgen, DHT (Leranth et al., 2003). While these data clearly indicate the potential for testosterone to contribute to the regulation of synapse number in cycling females, whether such responses actually occur in females remained uncertain because the responses of the male and female hippocampus to gonadal steroids were known to be sexually differentiated. The distributions of both estrogen (Rainbow et al., 1982; Brown et al., 1988) and androgen (Roselli, 1991) receptors in the brain are sexually dimorphic. Sex differences in the structure and function of the rodent hippocampus have been reported by a number of laboratories (Lewis et al., 1995; Patchev & Almeida, 1996; Tabibnia et al., 1999; Shors & Miesegaes, 2002). Administration of estrogen to ovariectomized female rats dramatically increases CA1 spine synapse density (see above), while the same treatment in castrated males is without effect (Leranth et al., 2003). The possibility therefore had to be considered that the effects of testosterone on hippocampal structure might not be the same in females as it is in males.

In fact, the female does indeed respond to testosterone with an increase in CA1 spine synapse numbers; but the underlying mechanisms are probably different than those in the male. Figure 11.3 illustrates the results of experiments in which ovariectomized rats were treated for two days with TP or DHT, with or without previous administration of the aromatase inhibitor, letrozole. Although short-term treatment with TP reversed the loss of CA1 area pyramidal spine synapses observed in ovariectomized rats, this response appeared to be almost entirely mediated via intermediate formation of estrogen. Thus, administration of letrozole almost completely

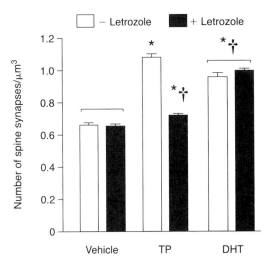

Figure 11.3. Pyramidal cell spine synapse densities in the CA1 stratum radiatum of ovariectomized (OVX) rats. Open bars: an increase in spine synapse density was observed after testosterone-propionate (TP) treatment. A slightly smaller increase in synaptic density was observed in dihydrotestosterone (DHT)-injected animals. Significant differences were observed between the OVX+DHT group and both the OVX + vehicle controls and OVX+TP animals. Solid bars: pretreatment with letrozole (1 mg, s.c.) 1 hr before the steroid or vehicle injections had no effect on synapse density in the OVX + vehicle animals, almost completely blocked the response to TP, but had no effect on the response to DHT. Reprinted with permission from Leranth C, Hajszan T, MacLusky, NJ. (2004). Androgens increase synaptic density in the CA1 hippocampal subfield of ovariectomized female rat. *J Neuroscience*, 24:495–499. *Significantly different from OVX vehicle-injected rats;†significantly (P<.05) different from the OVX+TP group without letrozole pretreatment. Histogram bars linked by square brackets are not significantly different from each other. Reproduced with permission from Leranth C, Hajszan T, MacLusky NJ. (2004a). Androgens increase spine synapse density in the CA1 hippocampal subfield of ovariectomized female rats. *J Neurosci*, 24:495–499.

blocked the synaptic response to TP. While the effects of testosterone appear to be almost entirely mediated via intermediate estrogen biosynthesis, the female retains the capacity to also respond to androgen without aromatization. Thus, despite the fact that the dose of letrozole used was very high, sufficient to completely shut off estrogen formation, a statistically significant effect of TP was still observed in the pres-

ence of letrozole. Moreover, treatment with the nonaromatizable androgen DHT also increased CA1 spine synapse density, in a letrozole-independent fashion, although it did not completely reproduce the effect of TP (Leranth et al., 2004a).

The functional consequences of androgen-induced increases in CA1 synaptic density remain to be determined. Effects of estrogen on hippocampal synaptogenesis have been correlated with the positive effects of this hormone on cognitive behavior (Cordoba Montoya & Carrer, 1997; Luine, 1997). Synaptic responses to androgen could play a similar role. Enhancement of cognitive performance by androgen has been demonstrated in laboratory animals (Flood et al., 1995; Hart, 2001) (also see Chapter 12).

While androgen replacement in postmenopausal women has not generally been reported to have significant effects on measures of cognition (Huppert & Van Niekerk, 2001), higher endogenous free testosterone levels have been positively associated with cognitive performance, in both men and women (Barrett-Connor et al., 1999; Neave et al., 1999; Yaffe et al., 2002). Positive effects on memory of androgen supplementation have been reported in young women (Postma et al., 2000; Ross et al., 2003), as well as in postmenopausal women receiving simultaneous high-dose estrogen treatment (Wisniewski et al., 2002).

Androgen may also ameliorate the effects of neurodegenerative disease states. Cognitive deficits in female mice expressing the human apolipoprotein E4 gene, a known risk factor for Alzheimer's disease, are reversed by androgen treatment (Raber et al., 2002); while in men, circulating testosterone concentrations have been reported to be lower in patients with Alzheimer's disease (Hogervorst et al., 2001).

UNDERLYING MECHANISMS: LOCAL VERSUS DISTANT EFFECTS, STEROID RECEPTORS AND OTHER POTENTIAL CONTRIBUTORS TO SYNAPTOPLASTIC RESPONSES

The mechanisms responsible for the synaptoplastic effects of gonadal steroids, and by extension the cellular basis for the existence of sex differences in these responses remain largely unknown. A large number of studies have been performed over the last few years in an attempt to elucidate these mechanisms; the resultant data have raised as many questions as they have answered. In many cases, we remain almost completely in the dark regarding the receptors mediating the effects of the steroids, let alone how the signals resulting from activation of these receptors lead to such dramatic changes in spine synapse density. In considering these issues, we will first focus on anatomical studies that have attempted to define the brain area(s) at which the steroids act. Next, we will turn to the receptor systems that may be involved. Finally, we will present very new experimental evidence, which suggests potential cellular mechanisms that may be essential for new synapse formation.

Local versus Distant Effects: Where Does Estrogen Act?

The cellular targets of the gonadal hormones that are directly involved in the synaptoplastic effects remain ill defined. In vivo experiments have shown that the action of estrogen on hippocampal remodeling is glutamate dependent and that estrogen increases the sensitivity of CA1 pyramidal cells to N-methyl-D-aspartate (NMDA) receptor mediated synaptic inputs (Gazzaley et al., 1996; Woolley et al., 1997). However, it is not known whether this estrogen action is associated exclusively with the hippocampus or is, at least partly, a transneuronal, indirect effect mediated via estrogen activation of subcortical structures. In support of a direct estrogenic action on the hippocampus are the observations of some levels of estrogen receptor-β in a small population of principal cells (Shughrue et al., 1997; Shughrue & Merchenthaler, 2000), nuclear estrogen receptor-α in a limited number of interneurons located in the dentate hilar area and stratum radiatum of the CA1 in adults (Weiland et al., 1997), estrogen receptor mRNA-containing cells in the hippocampus (Simerly et al., 1990) and the observation of a non-genomic estrogen action in the hippocampus (Moss & Gu, 1999), perhaps via estrogen-binding sites that have been detected in hippocampal plasma membrane preparations (Toran-Allerand et al., 2002).

Furthermore, in vitro studies using cultured hippocampal slices and dissociated hippocampal cells have shown that estradiol increases CA1 pyramidal cell spine density (Murphy & Segal, 1997), which involves increased NMDA-dependent Ca^{++} transients in these spines (Pozzo-Miller et al., 1999). There is also in vitro evidence that links phosphorylation of the cyclic AMP response element-binding protein to estrogen induced spine formation (Murphy & Segal, 1997; Segal & Murphy, 1998). Finally, the idea of direct hippocampal action by estrogen is further reinforced by the important in vitro morphological and electrophysiological findings that prolonged (one day) estradiol administration to cultured hippocampal cells results in a decrease in the density of GABA cells and GABAergic inhibition, as well as massive increases in spine density (Murphy et al., 1998b); these changes are associated with an estrogen-induced decrease of brain-derived neurotrophic factor (Murphy et al., 1998a).

At the same time, it must be recognized that subcortical structures are known to play major roles in the regulation of hippocampal function. Neurons in subcortical areas, including cholinergic cells in the medial septum/diagonal band of Broca (MSDB), supramammillary area (SUM), and the median raphe (MR) serotonin cells contain nuclear estrogen receptor (Leranth et al., 1999; Shughrue et al., 2000). These subcortical structures are associated with the generation/regulation of hippocampal theta activity and long-term potentiation, and hippocampal theta activity in conjunction with long-term potentiation is believed to be involved in memory processes (Vertes & Kocsis, 1997).

In an attempt to determine the extent to which extrinsic as well as intrinsic factors may contribute to the neuroplastic effects of estrogens on the hippocampus, adult female rats were ovariectomized and the fimbria/fornix was transected (FFX), unilaterally. One group of animals was only sham operated (control). One week later, the animals were treated systemically daily, for two days with estrogen and were sacrificed 48 h after the second injection. Figure 11.4 shows that unilateral fimbria/fornix transection itself, which disconnects the ipsilateral hippocampus from the majority of its subcortical inputs and, by necessity, eliminates the commissural connections between the left and right hippocampi, does not extensively influence the density of spine synapses. Confirming previous observations (see above), estrogen replacement to ovariectomized rats resulted in a dramatic increase (~50%) in the density of spine synapses in the stratum radiatum of the CA1 subfield of the Ammon's horn. However, this increased density of spine synapses could only be observed in the hippocampi in which the subcortical connections remained intact (those contralateral to the fimbria/fornix transection).

These observations suggest that while there may be local effects of estrogen within the hippocampus itself, the ability to respond to estrogen administration

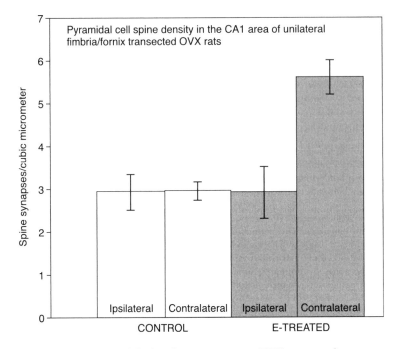

Figure 11.4. Unilateral fimbria fornix transection (FFX) prevents the synapto-plastic effects of estrogen administration in the hippocampus ipsilateral to FFX, but has no negative effect on the contralateral hippocampus. Open bars show CA1 area spine synapse densities in the ipsi- and contralateral hippocampi of ovariectomized (OVX) + oil-treated animals (control). Solid bars represent spine synapse density values in the ipsi- and contralateral hippocampi of FFX and OVX + estrogen-treated rats. The spine density is the same low in the ipsi- and contralateral hippocampi of the controls as in the hippocampus ipsilateral to the FFX of estrogen-treated animals. In contrast, systemic estrogen administration results in a significant (P<.001) ~50% increase in the density of spine synapses in the CA1 area contralateral to the FFX.

with an increase in CA1 spine synapse density is absolutely dependent on the integrity of afferent subcortical connections, suggesting that at least a major component of the effect may be mediated indirectly, via effects of the estrogen on neurons that project to the hippocampus via the fimbria/fornix (Leranth et al., 2000a).

A large number of subcortical structures that contain estrogen sensitive neurons are known to project to the hippocampus. We have suggested that these neurons might be the MSDB cholinergic cells, the calretinin/glutamate containing SUM neurons and/or the MR serotonin cells, because they express nuclear estrogen receptors (Leranth et al., 1999; Shughrue et al., 2000). The available experimental evidence supports this hypothesis. Implanting estrogen-releasing cannulas into these three subcortical areas resulted in a significant increase (~30%–50%) in CA1 area spine

synapse density (Leranth & Shanabrough, 2001; Lam & Leranth, 2003; Prange-Kiel et al., 2004).

Furthermore, following elimination of the MSDB cholinergic system by 192-IgG saporin injection, local estrogen administration into the MSDB was ineffective in restoring spine synapse density (Lam & Leranth, 2003). The positive synaptoplastic effects of local estrogen administration into the SUM and MSDB were expected. Both the MSDB cholinergic and a large population of SUM neurons that project to the hippocampus contain estrogen receptors and stimulation of these brain regions has major facilitatory effect on the electric activity of the hippocampus, via direct (SUM) and indirect (MSDB) stimulation of principal neurons (Freund & Antal, 1988; Vertes & Kocsis, 1997).

By contrast, the observation that local estrogen implantation into the MR has a major synaptoplastic

Spine synapse density in stratum radiatum of CA1
following E implant into the MR of OVX rats

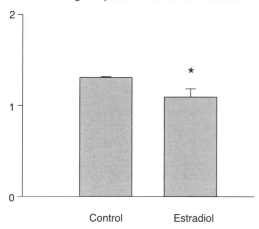

Figure 11.5. Bar graph demonstrates the spine synapse density in the CA1 area stratum radiatum of ovariectomized (OVX) rats. The spine synapse density is increased after local administration of estrogen into the median raphe (MR). The increase of 47.1% is significant (*$P<.02$). Reprinted with permission from Prange-Kiel J, Rune GM, Leranth C. (2004). Median raphe mediates estrogenic effects to the hippocampus in female rats. *Eur J Neuroscience*, 19:309–317.

effect in the hippocampus (Fig. 11.5) was unexpected. Previous studies have shown that serotonin depletion results in a decrease of spine density in the hippocampus (Alves et al., 2002), electrical stimulation of the MR results in the desynchronization of the hippocampal EEG, and the inhibition of the serotonergic neurons in the MR evokes a constant theta rhythm (Vertes & Kocsis, 1997). Based on the morphology, two mechanisms are suggested by which MR neurons influence the hippocampus. A population of MR serotonergic neurons project directly to the hippocampus and terminate mainly on a distinct population of GABAergic interneurons located in the strata radiatum and oriens (Freund et al., 1990). These GABAergic cells, in turn, exert inhibitory action on the input sector (apical and basal dendrites) of pyramidal cells (Gulyas & Freund, 1996).

On the other hand, MR neurons heavily innervate the MSDB (Leranth & Vertes, 1999) and exert a robust stimulatory effect on parvalbumin containing septo-hippocampal GABAergic neurons (Alreja, 1996). These GABAergic neurons, in turn, selectively innervate hippocampal basket and chandelier cells

(Freund & Antal, 1988). Basket and chandelier cells are known to have inhibitory effects on the output sector (soma and axon hillock) of pyramidal neurons (Freund & Buzsaki, 1996). Thus, estrogen-induced serotonergic stimulation of parvalbumin containing GABAergic neurons in the MSDB results in a disinhibition of the pyramidal cells (Freund & Antal, 1988). Thus, the synaptoplastic effect in the CA1 region is not only or even not at all mediated by serotonin fibers projecting directly to the hippocampus, but the indirect innervation via the MSDB may be the critical factor.

Local versus Distant Effects: Where Does Androgen Act?

In the case of androgen, similar uncertainties exist about the site of androgen action. While there is no question that indirect effects are possible, via androgen sensitive projections to the hippocampus, the potential for direct effects cannot be ruled out. Nuclear androgen receptors are widely distributed throughout the brain, including the pyramidal cell layer of the Ammon's horn, particularly CA1 (Sar et al., 1990; Simerly et al., 1990), as well as in extranuclear sites, in pyramidal cell dendritic spines (Tabori et al., 2005). However, when compared to the above-detailed observations in females, considerably less information is available about the potential role of afferent subcortical input in the male.

As shown in Figure 11.6, FFX does not produce the same effect on hippocampal responses to testosterone as it does in females with respect to estrogen. In hippocampi ipsilateral to FFX, testosterone replacement is still capable of inducing a significant rise on CA1 spine synapse density, but this increase is significantly less than that observed on the contralateral side of the brain (Kovacs et al., 2003). These data suggest that the effects of testosterone on CA1 synaptogenesis in the male may include components of both local androgen action, and distal effects on neurons projecting to the hippocampus via the fimbria/fornix.

Unfortunately, there is as yet no information on the potential subcortical targets for androgen action. In terms of local effects, a number of mechanisms exist within the hippocampus that could potentially mediate such responses. The hippocampus is rich in androgen receptors, while metabolites of testosterone and DHT, such as 5α-androstan-3α,17β-diol, may directly modulate hippocampal GABA$_A$ receptor function (Edinger & Frye, 2004). It is also possible

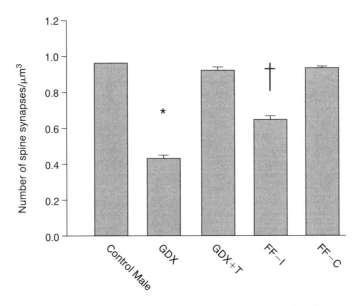

Figure 11.6. Bar graph shows the density of pyramidal cell spine synapses in the CA1 stratum radiatum of the hippocampi of control male, gonadectomized (GDX) and GDX + testosterone-replaced (GDX+T) rats. Approximately equal, high spine synapse densities are present in the hippocampi of control males, GDX+T males, and fimbria/fornix (FF)-transected testosterone-replaced males contralateral to the FF transection (FF-C). The spine synapse density is significantly lower in the hippocampi of GDX+T rats ipsilateral to FF transection (FF-I) than in the aforementioned groups, but not as low as in the GDX rats. *Significantly (P<.05) different from control intact males; †significantly (P<.05) different from both control intact and GDX males. Reprinted with permission from Kovacs EG, MacLusky NJ, Leranth C. (2003). Effects of testosterone on hippocampal CA1 spine synaptic density in the male rat are inhibited by fimbria-fornix transection. *Neuroscience*, 122:807–810.

that there might be indirect effects of testosterone on CA1 via afferents that remain intact after FFX, e.g., from the entorhinal cortex or other regions of the hippocampus.

The sites of testosterone action in females have not so far been explored. However, it seems likely that the sites are different from those in males, because the sites involve different cellular mechanisms. As mentioned previously, testosterone action in the female is highly dependent on local estrogen biosynthesis in the brain, since administration of an aromatase inhibitor almost completely blocks the response to testosterone (Fig 11.3). This contrasts with the situation in the male, in which estrogen has no significant effect on hippocampal spine synapse density (Fig. 11.2). Because the actions of estrogen in females are dependent

on sub-cortical afferent input, a reasonable hypothesis is that the effects of testosterone in females will also prove to be dependent on sub-cortical afferent connections. This remains to be established experimentally.

Role of the Androgen Receptor in Mediating Hippocampal Synaptoplastic Effects

Estrogen and androgen receptor systems: Despite extensive research, the cellular and molecular mechanisms underlying gonadal steroid-induced remodeling of hippocampal spine synapses remain obscure. Estrogen receptors (ERs) are relatively well-defined, as estrogen acts primarily via the nuclear receptors

ERα and ERβ, as well as via ERs in association with extranuclear components of the neuron (Blaustein, 1992; Shughrue & Merchenthaler, 2000; Vasudevan et al., 2001; Toran-Allerand et al., 2002). Androgens, by contrast, may interact with a number of receptor systems in the brain, including androgen receptors, the GABA$_A$ receptor, and even ERα and ERβ. The basis for this diversity is the fact that circulating androgens are subject to extensive local metabolism in target tissues, which results in the formation of a wide range of bioactive metabolites.

Local androgen metabolism: The actions of gonadal steroids in the brain reflect a complex interplay of circulating endocrine, as well as local paracrine mechanisms. The key enzymes involved in androgen metabolism, including the aromatase enzyme necessary for the conversion of testosterone to estrogen, are all expressed in the brain, to varying extents (Zwain et al., 1997; Zwain & Yen, 1999; Baulieu et al., 2001). Androgens extensively use these local metabolic pathways to exert their broad spectrum of action because they are natural substrates for the synthesis of several biologically active metabolites. For example, while the weak aromatizable androgen, dehydroepiandrosterone (DHEA) and its principal circulating metabolite, DHEA-sulfate are known to exert a wide range of direct effects on neuronal function (Ueda et al., 2001; Kaasik et al., 2003; Sullivan & Moenter, 2003), DHEA is also extensively converted by 17β-hydroxysteroid-dehydrogenase to androst-5-ene-3β,17β-diol (androstenediol), and by the CYP7B enzyme to 7α-hydroxy-DHEA, which both have significant estrogenic bioactivity (Littlefield et al., 1990; Martin et al., 2004). DHEA may also act, at least in part, via conversion to testosterone and its derivatives in androgen target tissues (Labrie et al., 2003).

The principal aromatizable testicular androgen, testosterone is irreversibly converted in target tissues, including the brain, to estradiol by the aromatase enzyme (testosterone metabolism is reviewed by, e.g., (Reddy, 2004b). As mentioned, this conversion seems to play a significant role in the CA1 synaptogenic effect of testosterone in female rats. Testosterone can also be metabolized via 5α-reduction and the product of this conversion is the nonaromatizable androgen, DHT. DHT is more potent than testosterone in most bioassays of androgenic activity. Production of DHT from testosterone is irreversible and the necessary enzyme, 5α-reductase is widely expressed in the brain (Pelletier et al., 1994).

In both male and female rats, DHT can induce CA1 spine synapse formation with a magnitude equal to or greater than that observed following physiological estrogen exposure. Further metabolism of DHT results in the formation of 5α-androstane-3α,17β-diol (3αA-diol), as well as its 3β-isomer (3βA-diol), both of which express biological activities that are distinct from those of their parent steroids. The enzymes necessary for these conversions of DHT are expressed mainly in the glial cells of the brain (Pelletier et al., 1995; Zwain & Yen, 1999; Ibanez et al., 2003), and DHT metabolites synthesized in the periphery can also easily cross the blood-brain barrier, as well. Synthesis of the A-diols is reversible, but the conversion of 3βA-diol back to DHT occurs less readily than that of 3αA-diol (Reddy, 2004b). While the A-diols show limited affinity toward the androgen receptor (Roselli et al., 1987; Reddy, 2004b), 3αA-diol can modulate GABA action at the GABA$_A$ receptor (Reddy, 2004a) and 3βA-diol is a potent activator of ERβ (Pak et al., 2005).

The obvious hypothesis to explain the action of androgens on CA1 spine synapse density was that these effects are mediated via activation of nuclear androgen receptors, as this receptor type is widely expressed in pyramidal neurons throughout the hippocampus (Sar et al., 1990; Simerly et al., 1990). Two basic approaches have been used to test this hypothesis: studying of the effects of androgen receptor antagonists, such as the non-steroid androgen receptor antagonist flutamide; and examining the effects of sex steroids in animals lacking functional androgen receptors, such as the naturally occurring testicular feminization mutant (tfm) rat. These experiments have yielded the most surprising results so far.

The Effect of Flutamide

In gonadectomized males, DHEA and DHT both increased CA1 spine synapse density by around 100% when compared to oil-injected gonadectomized rats. Letrozole pretreatment had no significant effect on the response to DHEA. Surprisingly, flutamide did not block the actions of DHEA and DHT; instead, it increased spine synapse density when it was administered either alone or in combination with the hormones (Figs. 11.7, 11.8 upper panel). Similar responses to flutamide were observed in ovariectomized females (Fig. 11.9) (MacLusky et al., 2004).

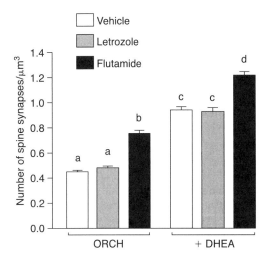

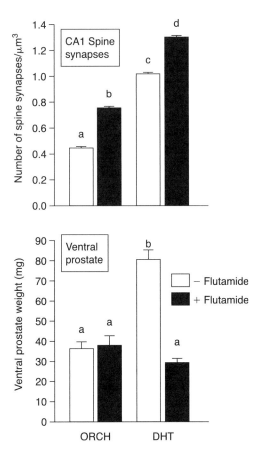

Figure 11.7. Effect of dehydroepiandrosterone (DHEA) treatment ± flutamide or letrozole on the density of pyramidal cell spine synapses in the CA1 stratum radiatum of orchidectomized (ORCH) male rats. DHEA increased spine synapse density, a response that was augmented by pretreatment with flutamide but unaffected by pretreatment with letrozole. Results of individual group comparisons are presented as letters above the histogram bars, in which bars with the same letter represent results that are not significantly different from one another. Different letters denote statistically significant (P<0.05) differences in mean synapse density. Reprinted with permission from MacLusky NJ, Hajszan T, Leranth C. (2004). Effects of DHEA and flutamide on hippocampal CA1 spine synapse density in male and female rats: implication for the role of androgens in maintenance of hippocampal structure. *Endocrinology*, 145:4154–4161.

In contrast to its apparent androgen agonist activity in the hippocampus, flutamide had no effect on ventral prostate weight when injected alone; and completely eliminated the prostate weight gain induced by DHT in this bioassay (Fig. 11.8, lower panel) (MacLusky et al., 2004). These results confirmed previous observation of DHT effects in male rats and also demonstrated that the potential of DHEA to induce hippocampal synaptic remodeling in males is similar to that in females (Hajszan et al., 2004).

The lack of letrozole effect on this DHEA response in the male reconfirmed the observation that the actions of aromatizable androgens in hippocampal synaptogenesis are sexually differentiated, being heavily

Figure 11.8. Effects of 5α-dihydrotestosterone (DHT) alone or in combination with flutamide on hippocampal synapse density and ventral prostate weight in castrate (ORCH) male rats. Rats were gonadectomized and 1 week later, steroid and flutamide treatments were initiated. Top panel: Density of pyramidal cell spine synapses in the CA1 stratum radiatum. Administration of flutamide (5 mg) s.c. 1 h before the steroid or vehicle injections significantly (P<.001) increased synapse density. Lower panel: Ventral prostate weight. In the prostate, flutamide alone had no significant effect but completely blocked the response to DHT. Results of individual group comparisons are presented as letters above the histogram bars. Different letters denote statistically significant (P<.05) differences in mean synapse density and prostate weight. Reprinted with permission from MacLusky NJ, Hajszan T, Leranth C. (2004). Effects of DHEA and flutamide on hippocampal CA1 spine synapse density in male and female rats: implication for the role of androgens in maintenance of hippocampal structure. *Endocrinology*, 145:4154–4161.

dependent on local conversion to estrogen in females, but completely independent of aromatization in the male. However, the effects of flutamide suggest that androgen regulation of CA1 spine synapse density may occur via a mechanism different from that responsible for the anabolic effect of androgen in tissues of the reproductive tract, in which flutamide acts as a nuclear androgen receptor antagonist (Richie, 1999). These observations, however, could not be construed as evidence for androgen receptor-independent action of androgens on hippocampal spine synapse density, because of evidence that flutamide can exert androgen agonist effects via membrane-associated androgen receptors (Lee et al., 2002) or even via nuclear androgen receptors, depending on the availability of receptor coactivator proteins (Miyamoto et al., 1998).

Studies with Tfm Males

To further test the role of androgen receptors in the actions of androgen on hippocampal spine synapse formation, we used the Tfm rat model. The Tfm rat expresses a defective androgen receptor gene on the X chromosome (Yarbrough et al., 1990), leading to an essentially complete loss of developmental responses to androgen in the reproductive tract. Groups of Tfm and littermate wild-type male rats were gonadectomized and treated with estrogen, the nonaromatizable androgen DHT and flutamide; and the total number of CA1 area spine synapses was calculated. As expected, DHT induced a more than two-fold increase in the number of CA1 spine synapses in wild-type animals. Estrogen treatment, however, had no significant effect on the number of spine synapses in the CA1, in either wild-type or Tfm males (Fig. 11.10).

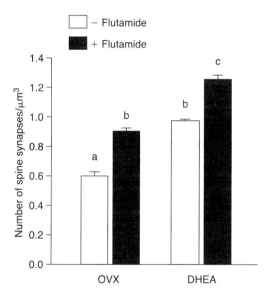

Figure 11.9. Effect of dehydroepiandrosterone (DHEA) treatment ± flutamide on the density of pyramidal cell spine synapses in the CA1 stratum radiatum of ovariectomized (OVX) female rats. DHEA increased spine synapse density, a response that was augmented by pretreatment with flutamide. Results of individual group comparisons are presented as letters above the histogram bars. Different letters denote statistically significant ($P<.05$) differences in mean synapse density. Reprinted with permission from MacLusky NJ, Hajszan T, Leranth C. (2004). Effects of DHEA and flutamide on hippocampal CA1 spine synapse density in male and female rats: implication for the role of androgens in maintenance of hippocampal structure. *Endocrinology*, 145:4154–4161.

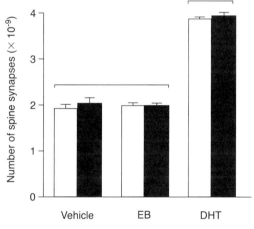

Figure 11.10. Effects of treatment of castrated male rats with estradiol benzoate (EB), 5α-dihydrotestosterone (DHT) or the sesame oil injection vehicle on the total number of dendritic spine synapses in the CA1 stratum radiatum. Columns represent means +/–SEM of results from three animals in each treatment group. Data for wild-type males (open bars) and testicular feminization mutant (Tfm) males (solid bars) are indistinguishable. Histogram bars linked by horizontal brackets are not significantly different from one another. Histogram bars that are not linked by brackets are significantly ($P<.05$) different from each other. Reprinted with permission from MacLusky NJ, Hajszan T, Johansen J-A, Jordan CL, Leranth C. (2006). Androgen effects on hippocampal CA1 spine synapse numbers are retained in tfm male rats with defective androgen receptors. *Endocrinology*, 147:2392–2398.

Flutamide induced a partial response (Fig. 11.11) almost identical to that we previously described with flutamide in gonadectomized Sprague-Dawley rats (see previous).

Surprisingly, despite the almost complete loss of functional androgen receptors in Tfm males, there was no impairment whatsoever of the CA1 spine synapse response to flutamide or DHT in these animals (Figs. 11.10, 11.11). Thus, the profound deficiency in nuclear androgen receptor-mediated responses in the Tfm males, which blocks masculine differentiation of normal secondary sexual characteristics (Yarbrough et al., 1990), appears to have no significant effect on DHT or flutamide-induced increases in the number of CA1 spine synapses. These data further support the hypothesis that androgen regulation of CA1 spine synapse formation may involve distinct response mechanisms, independent of the classical nuclear androgen receptor system. The persistent androgen response in Tfm males cannot be ascribed to androgen action via estrogen receptors, as has recently been demonstrated (Pak et al., 2005), because the Tfm male, like the wild-type male, does not respond to estrogen with an increase in the number of CA1 spine synapses.

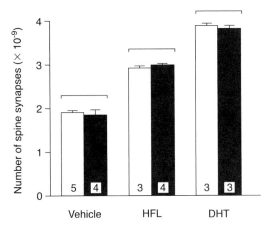

Figure 11.11. Effects of treatment of castrate male rats with hydroxyflutamide (HFL), 5α-dihydrotestosterone (DHT) or the sesame oil injection vehicle on the total number of dendritic spine synapses in the CA1 stratum radiatum. Columns represent means +/–SEM of results from the numbers of animals indicated in the inset boxes at the base of each histogram bar. Data for wild-type males (open bars) and testicular feminization mutant (Tfm) males (solid bars) are indistinguishable. Histogram bars linked by horizontal brackets are not significantly different from one another. Histogram bars that are not linked by brackets are significantly (P<.05) different from each other. Reprinted with permission from MacLusky NJ, Hajszan T, Johansen J-A, Jordan CL, Leranth C. (2006). Androgen effects on hippocampal CA1 spine synapse numbers are retained in tfm male rats with defective androgen receptors. *Endocrinology*, 147:2392–2398.

REMODELING OF SPINE SYNAPSES
IN THE PREFRONTAL CORTEX

Are the Synaptoplastic Effects
of Gonadal Hormones Confined
to the Hippocampus?

While much of the work on the synaptoplastic effects of gonadal steroids so far has focused on the CA1 region of the hippocampus, it is important to recognize that these effects are clearly not confined to that area and may indeed involve many other regions of the brain. Extensive studies over the last 20 years have demonstrated considerable hormone-induced synaptic plasticity in the hypothalamus, which may contribute to changes in the neuroendocrine regulation of sexually-differentiated patterns of gonadotropin release (Fernandez-Galaz et al., 1997; Kalra et al., 1997; Parducz et al., 2006).

Other regions of the brain involved in mnemonic functions may also be affected. For example, there is growing evidence that the prefrontal cortex (PFC) retains considerable sensitivity to hormone-induced

plasticity in adulthood. Recent human clinical and animal behavioral studies suggest that estrogen replacement enhances performance not only on hippocampus-associated memory tests, but also on working memory tasks that are reliant on the PFC (Duff & Hampson, 2000; Keenan et al., 2001; Rapp et al., 2003).

It is well established that phencyclidine administration to monkeys and rats (an animal model of schizophrenia) impairs attention and performance of PFC-dependent object retrieval/detour tasks (Jentsch et al., 1997); and has been shown that the number of spine synapses in the PFC of phencyclidine-treated male rats is significantly lower when compared to controls (Hajszan et al., 2006). Taken together, it appears that, similar to the events in the hippocampus, spine synapse remodeling in the PFC is also associated with alterations of PFC-related memory test performance.

It has been demonstrated that experimental manipulations of the levels of gonadal hormones results in morphological alterations in the PFC of rodents (Kritzer & Kohama, 1998, 1999). Changing levels of estrogen have a great influence on the total number of spines in the PFC of non-human primates (Tang et al., 2004), similar to androgen in the PFC of rodents (see next section).

Effects of Androgen and Estrogen on Spine Synapse Formation in the PFC of Wild-type and Tfm Male rats

Intriguingly, the relative contributions from androgen and estrogen receptors to the synaptoplastic effects of androgens may be different not only between males and females, but also between different regions of the brain. Very recent studies on the effects of androgens on spine synapse remodeling in the male PFC have surprisingly demonstrated somewhat different patterns of response from those observed in CA1. The effects of androgen and estrogen administration on spine synapse numbers in the PFC of wild-type and Tfm male rats were investigated. All rats were gonadectomized and one week later, the following treatment groups were tested: DHT/wild-type, EB/wild-type, oil/wild-type, DHT/tfm, EB/tfm, and oil/tfm. Hormone or vehicle injection (s.c.) was administered daily for two days. Two days after the second injection, animals were sacrificed and the total number of spine synapses was calculated in PFC layer 3. The results are summarized in Figure 11.12.

When compared to oil-treated wild-type controls, administration of the nonaromatizable androgen hormone, DHT to wild-type animals resulted in a surprisingly high (136%) increase in the number of spine synapses, while administration of EB to wild-type animals elicited a 56.4% increase. Although this effect of EB was considerably ($P<.01$) reduced compared to that of DHT in wild-type animals, it still represented a statistically significant ($P<.03$) increase as compared to wild-type oil controls. In Tfm male rats, administration of DHT resulted in a markedly smaller, but still significant 62.6% increase in the number of spine synapses, while administration of EB led to a 123.1% increase. This effect of EB in Tfm males was significantly larger than those of both oil and DHT in Tfm rats. The number of spine synapses

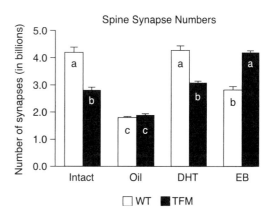

Figure 11.12. Effects of administration of sesame oil (Oil), 5α-dihydrotestosterone (DHT) and estradiol-benzoate (EB) to castrated wild-type (WT, open bars) and testicular feminization mutant (Tfm, solid bars) male rats on the number of spine synapses in the medial prefrontal cortex. Intact male rats were untreated and gonadally intact. Columns labeled with the same letter are statistically indistinguishable (Newman-Keuls multiple comparison test).

was significantly less in DHT-treated Tfm males than in DHT-treated wild-type rats, while EB administration elicited the formation of significantly more spine synapses in Tfm males than in wild-type animals. The number of spine synapses in EB-treated Tfm males was statistically indistinguishable from that of DHT-treated wild-type rats.

These observations demonstrate that remodeling of spine synapses in the PFC of male rats, in contrast to the male hippocampus (Leranth et al., 2003) is under the control of *both* androgen and estrogen, which may potentially explain why these gonadal hormones have both been reported to enhance cognitive function, in males as well as females (Kampen & Sherwin, 1996; Friedman, 2000; Janowsky et al., 2000; Postma et al., 2000; Cordova et al., 2004). Whether or not similar patterns of response are observed in females remains to be determined; but it seems possible that there may be differences in the synaptoplastic effects of the hormones on the PFC in the two sexes. One possible explanation for the reduced efficacy of estradiol in the PFC of the wild-type as opposed to the Tfm male is that the response of the normal male may have been partially impaired as a result of androgen-induced sexual differentiation. However, further studies will be needed to test this hypothesis.

SYNAPTOPLASTIC EFFECTS
OF FEMALE AND MALE HORMONES
IN THE HIPPOCAMPUS
OF NON-HUMAN PRIMATES

Synaptoplastic Effect of Estrogen in the Hippocampal CA1 Area of Ovariectomized Non-human Primates

As discussed, data accumulated in the past decade have demonstrated that experimental manipulations, as well as physiological changes in the levels of circulating gonadal hormones during the ovarian cycle, greatly influence the density of pyramidal cell spine synapses in the CA1 hippocampal subfield of rats (Gould et al., 1990; Woolley et al., 1990; Woolley & McEwen, 1992, 1994; Gazzaley et al., 1996; Woolley et al., 1997; Woolley, 1998).

Elevated levels of estrogen and androgen are associated with an increased density of spine synapses. A vitally important question, in terms of the relevance of these findings to human beings, is whether similar changes also occur in the primate brain. Major differences have been shown in the morphology and functional connections of the hippocampus between primates and rats. Furthermore, rats have a 4-day ovarian cycle, while humans have a 28-day menstrual cycle. However, the monkey and human hippocampus are structurally similar, (Rosene & Van Hoesen, 1987), while monkeys and humans both have a menstrual cycle with a true luteal phase, as opposed to the much shorter estrous cycle observed in rats. Therefore, determining whether hormonal manipulations influence synaptic plasticity in the brain of non-human primates should provide a good indication of whether similar changes are likely in the human.

Indirect evidence suggests that estrogen effects on dendritic spine synapse density may well be similar in rats and in a representative primate, the rhesus monkey. Using light and electron microscopic immunostaining for the spine-associated protein, spinophilin, the total number of spines was calculated in layers I-IV of the PFC and in layer I of the visual cortex of ovariectomized and estrogen-replaced monkeys. It has been shown that in layer I of the PFC of estrogen-replaced ovariectomized animals, the number of spines is 55% higher than in the same layer of ovariectomized monkeys. Other layers of the PFC are not affected by estrogen. Furthermore, no differences were observed in the number of spines of layer I in the visual cortex (Tang et al., 2004).

In another elegant study performed in the same laboratory (Hao et al., 2006), the authors analyzed the possible beneficial effects of estrogen (administered every 3 weeks for 2–3 years) in the PFC of aged (~22 years old), ovariectomized non-human primates. Cyclic administration of estrogen to these aged animals did not affect several parameters, such as total dendritic length and branching. However, most importantly, estrogen treatment increased apical and basal dendritic spine density and induced a shift toward smaller spines, a response linked to spine motility, NMDA-mediated activity, and learning. These observations clearly demonstrate that the aged PFC remains responsive to long-term cyclic estrogen treatment and may contribute to the cognitive benefits that were observed in the same animals in a previous study (Rapp et al., 2003).

Direct evidence for estrogen regulation of hippocampal spine synapse density in a primate was obtained in our own laboratory. Female African green monkeys (*Cercopithecus aethiops sabaeus*) of reproductive age without stigmata of advanced age were used. All of the animals were ovariectomized, and one group of monkeys received two 4-cm estrogen-filled (100% estradiol-benzoate) silastic capsules that were implanted below the skin of the back, at the time of ovariectomy. The other animals were implanted with empty silastic capsules. One month later, all of the animals were sacrificed and the density of pyramidal cell apical dendritic spine synapses was calculated in the CA1 stratum radiatum (Fig. 11.13). There was a striking difference in the density of spine synapses between the two groups of monkeys (Leranth et al., 2002). The average synapse density in estrogen-replaced animals was 1.13 ± 0.16 spine synapse / μm^3. The same value for the non-estrogen-replaced animals was more than 40% less (0.66 ± 0.11 spine synapse / μm^3).

This finding indicates that estrogen is essential in maintaining the morphological integrity of the primate hippocampus. These data, together with additional observations on the beneficial effects of estrogen on other brain structures of the monkey, including the nigrostriatal dopamine cells (Leranth et al., 2000b) and dopamine innervation of the prefrontal cortex (Kritzer & Kohama, 1998), further support the view that despite the endocrinological differences that exist between primates and rodents,

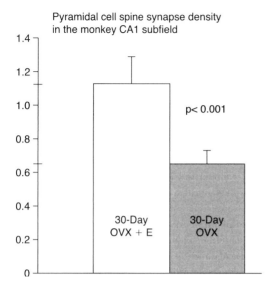

Figure 11.13. Bar graph shows the result of unbiased stereological calculation of the density of CA1 area spine synapses in the monkey. The 30-day ovariectomized animals (30-Day OVX) have a significantly ($P<.001$) lower (40%) density of CA1 area pyramidal cell pine synapses than the 30-day ovariectomized plus estrogen-replaced monkeys (30-Day OVX + E). Reprinted with permission from Leranth C, Shanabrough M, Redmond DE Jr. (2002). Gonadal hormones are responsible for maintaining the integrity of spine synapses in the CA1 hippocampal subfield of female non-human primates. *J Comp Neurol*, 447:34–42.

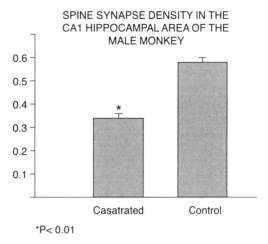

Figure 11.14. Bar graphs show a significant ($P<$ .001) difference between the apical dendritic spine synapses of CA1 area pyramidal cells in the hippocampus of castrated and gonadally-intact (control) monkeys. The spine synapse density in control animals is 40% higher than in the castrated monkeys. Reprinted with permission from Leranth C, Prange-Kiel J, Frick KM, Horvath TL. (2004). Low CA1 spine synapse density is further reduced by castration in male non-human primates. *Cereb Cortex*, 14:503–510.

the effects of estrogen on cortical anatomy may well have been evolutionarily conserved.

Gonadectomy Reduces the Density of Spine Synapses in the Hippocampal CA1 Subfield of Male Non-human Primates

Androgens also appear to have significant stimulatory effects on spine synapse density in the primate CA1. Figure 11.14 shows the results of a study in which male St. Kitts vervet monkeys were examined either gonadally intact, or 1 month after castration. In the castrate animals, there was a significant 40% decrease in spine synapse density compared to intact animals. This observation indicates that similar to male rodents, normal levels of circulating androgen hormones are required for the maintenance of hip-

pocampal spine synapse density (Leranth et al., 2004b).

SPECIES AND SEX DIFFERENCES IN SPINE SYNAPSE DENSITY OF RODENTS AND NON-HUMAN PRIMATES

Intriguingly, comparison of CA1 spine synapse densities in rats and monkeys reveals a great deal of similarity, not only in basal synapse densities and the effects of hormone treatment, but also in the expression of sex differences. In rats, similar to monkeys, experimental manipulations of circulating gonadal hormone levels have no effect on pyramidal cell density in either female or male animals. In contrast, gonadectomy has a significant effect on the density of the dendritic spine synapses of pyramidal cells in both female and male rats, as well as female and male monkeys (Table 11.1).

In percentage terms, the magnitude of the synaptoplastic effect of female and male gonadal hormones is

Table 11.1. CA1 Area Spine Synapse Densities in Male and Female Rodents
and Non-human Primates

Animals	Gonadectomized	Control	Difference	Source
Female rat	$0.71/\mu m^3$	$1.08/\mu m^3$	34%	(Leranth et al., 2000a)
Male rat	$0.45/\mu m^3$	$0.9/\mu m^3$	50%	(Leranth et al., 2003)
Female monkeys	$0.65/\mu m^3$	$1.15/\mu m^3$	40%	(Leranth et al., 2002)
Male monkeys	$0.34/\mu m^3$	$0.58/\mu m^3$	40%	(Leranth et al., 2004b)

similar in rats (50%) and monkeys (40%) of both genders. The absolute spine synapse density values of estrogen-replaced female rats ($1.08 / \mu m^3$) and monkeys ($1.15 / \mu m^3$) are also very similar.

On the other hand, there are marked differences between the absolute values of spine synapse densities of gonadally-intact male rats ($0.9 / \mu m^3$) and monkeys ($0.58 / \mu m^3$). More importantly, there are major differences in both species between the spine synapse density values of females and males, regardless of the levels of circulating gonadal hormones. Both gonadally intact ($0.58 / \mu m^3$) and castrated males ($0.34 / \mu m^3$) have about 48% fewer spine synapses than estrogen-replaced ($1.15 / \mu m^3$) and ovariectomized ($0.65 / \mu m^3$) female monkeys, respectively. Furthermore, the spine synapse density in the gonadally intact, control male monkey hippocampus ($0.58 / \mu m^3$) is more than 10% lower than in the ovariectomized female monkey ($0.65 / \mu m^3$).

DO EFFECTS OF GONADAL STEROIDS ON SYNAPTIC PLASTICITY UNDERLIE CHANGES IN COGNITIVE PERFORMANCE?

The above mentioned sex differences raise important questions regarding the potential links between spine synapse density and cognitive performance. There is extensive evidence that gonadal steroids influence cognitive function. For example in humans, a positive relationship has been reported between testosterone levels and several types of memory, particularly in older men (Gouchie & Kimura, 1991; Barrett-Connor et al., 1999; Silverman et al., 1999; Moffat et al., 2002; Cherrier et al., 2003; Janowsky, 2006). Men with lower testosterone levels tend to have impaired memory relative to those with higher levels (Barrett-Connor et al., 1999; Moffat et al., 2002). We have suggested as well as others that the basis for these

differences may well be found in the synaptoplastic effects of gonadal steroids on the brain, but is this really the case? Is there really a simple and direct relationship between synapse density and cognitive performance? Table 11.1 suggests that this is unlikely. In gonadally-intact male monkeys, the density of CA1 synapses remains at or below the level observed in ovariectomized females, and greatly below the levels observed in estrogen-replaced females. There is no evidence that overall cognitive performance in the two sexes parallels these substantial differences in overall synapse density.

Other examples of apparent dissociation between the synaptoplastic effects of the hormones and functional differences can also be cited. It is generally accepted that hippocampal long-term potentiation (LTP) is associated with synaptic plasticity and memory, and electrophysiological experiments have demonstrated that estrogen-induced elevated spine synapse density in ovariectomized rats is associated with augmented CA1 LTP (Cordoba Montoya & Carrer, 1997; Foy et al., 1999; Good et al., 1999; Ito et al., 1999). In contrast, testosterone administration to castrated male rats has been reported to have an opposite, negative effect on CA1 LTP (Harley et al., 2000), in spite of the fact that testosterone dramatically increases hippocampal spine synapse density in both male rats (Leranth et al., 2003) and monkeys (Leranth et al., 2004b).

Sex differences favoring males have been observed in some hippocampus-dependent memory tasks (Williams et al., 1990; Williams & Meck, 1991; Roof & Havens, 1992; Roof, 1993). Because males excel at some hippocampus-dependent memory tasks, despite having fewer CA1 spine synapses than females, it is tempting to speculate that either spine density has little to do with hippocampal-dependent memory processing, or that both LTP and gonadal hormones induce synaptic sprouting without causal relationships. On the other hand, the organizational effects of steroid hormones on the brain may necessitate that females have a greater density of CA1 spine synapses to compensate for spine reductions or other alterations elsewhere in the brain. High spine synapse density could actually be detrimental (e.g. by producing excessive disorganized input to the dendrite). Alternatively, absolute numbers of dendritic synapses may not be the most important factor in the relationship between synapse density and cognitive performance, but rather the nature of the synapses and both the nature and magnitude of the changes induced by gonadal hormone exposure.

These uncertainties highlight what is probably the most important remaining question in this field: namely, whether changes in synapse number are really important for maintenance of cognitive function, or merely reflect trophic effects of the hormones in the brain that contribute to other aspects of hippocampal function. While it seems reasonable to suppose that changes in synapse number are involved in the cognitive effects of the steroids, it also remains possible that other changes induced by the hormones (including regulation of protein synthesis and the synthesis and degradation of key neurotransmitters) could be quantitatively more important.

At the present time, there remain no definitive data to distinguish between these possibilities. However, very recent data from studies of the cellular mechanisms mediating synaptic plasticity provide circumstantial evidence to suggest that the ability to regulate synapse density may indeed play a critical role in cognitive function. Several authors have suggested that remodeling and subsequent stabilization of dendritic spines and their synapses represent a mechanism of how memories are made and stored (Kandel, 2001; Kasai et al., 2003). Although in recent years, some studies have demonstrated very tight correlation between gonadal steroid-induced cognitive and CA1 spine synapse changes, even under conditions of rapid hormonal response (Luine et al., 2003; MacLusky et al., 2005), doubts still remain as to whether these responses are functionally related, or whether they represent distinct and separable aspects of overall, hormone-elicited events in the brain. The key question is whether gonadal steroid-induced cognitive and memory improvement is a function of proliferation of CA1 spines and their synapses. Testing this hypothesis presents severe theoretical and practical problems, however, since the mechanisms that underlie spine synapse formation are so fundamental that arresting them may lead to the loss of vital cellular functions and consequently to problems in interpreting the observations.

One approach to this problem is based on the rationale that signaling mechanisms triggered by gonadal steroids should ultimately converge upon the molecular machinery that underlies spine motility. Spine motility means not only spine growth and retraction, but also it may be involved in spine synapse formation, as already existing spines may establish new synapses by moving to contact the presynaptic structure (Yankova et al., 2001). Conversely, spines can eliminate their synapses without being retracted, simply by moving away from the presynaptic bouton (these events also illustrate, parenthetically, why the number of dendritic spines is an insufficient measure of spine synapses). Thus, if remodeling of spine synapses contributes to the cognitive effects of gonadal steroids, interfering with spine motility may impair both CA1 spine synapse formation and hormone-induced enhancement of hippocampus-dependent memory. Recent studies indicate that spine motility is driven by actin-based mechanisms (for review see Matus et al., 2000), raising the possibility that by preventing actin rearrangement, one can halt spine motility and hence, impair cognitive function. Earlier studies have shown that blocking actin polymerization decreases spine plasticity (Fischer et al., 1998), blocks long-term depression (Chen et al., 2004), and does indeed impair cognitive function (Fischer et al., 2004).

A recent study from the Picciotto laboratory has shown similar impairments in β-adducin knock-out male and female mice (Rabenstein et al., 2005). Adducins are capable of translating inputs from different signaling pathways into cytoskeletal changes. Adducins cap, bundle, and promote spectrin binding to actin filaments (Gardner & Bennett, 1987; Mische et al., 1987; Kuhlman et al., 1996). Several intracellular signaling mechanisms are known to remove adducin complexes from the barbed ends of actin filaments, allowing them to polymerize or depolymerize (Matsuoka et al., 1996; Kimura et al., 1998; Matsuoka et al., 1998). This supports the idea that adducin mediates cytoskeletal changes associated with synaptic activity. β-Adducin knock-out animals have been found to be impaired in several electrophysiological measures, such as LTP, paired-pulse facilitation, and posttetanic potentiation (Rabenstein et al., 2005).

In addition, lack of β-adducin resulted in generalized learning deficiencies in the fear conditioning and Morris water maze paradigms. Based on these data, the β-adducin knock-out mouse seems to be a particularly useful model for future studies to test hypotheses regarding the functional connection between CA1 spine synapse formation and enhancement of hippocampus-dependent memory by gonadal steroids.

Lack of β-adducin Prevents the CA1 Synaptogenic Effect of Estrogen in Ovariectomized Female Mice

To determine whether β-adducin knock-out female mice respond to estrogen treatment with increased CA1 spine synapse formation, adult β-adducin knock-out and littermate wild-type female mice were ovariectomized and one week later, they were treated with 1 µg/mouse/day EB, or the 100 µl /mouse/day sesame oil vehicle in the form of daily s.c. injections for two days. Two days later, the animals were sacrificed and their CA1 spine synapse density was calculated using the electron microscopic stereology method. As Figure 11.15 shows, EB administration increased CA1 spine synapse density in wild-type mice compared to oil-treated animals, while this effect was abolished in the knock-out animals.

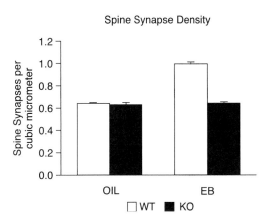

Figure 11.15. Effect of estrogen treatment (EB) on CA1 spine synapse density in wild-type and β-adducin knock-out ovariectomized female mice. Open bars represent spine synapse density in wild-type animals, while solid bars show the spine synapse density in β-adducin knock-out mice. The results indicate that disrupted actin regulation prevents CA1 spine synapse changes in response to estrogen.

These results indicate that disrupted actin regulation prevents CA1 spine synapse changes in response to estrogen. Although it might be argued that lack of CA1 synaptogenic response to estrogen could be due to disrupted estrogen signaling, the normal reproductive capacity and sexual function of β-adducin knock-out mice suggests an unimpaired endocrine status. Together with the data of Rabenstein et al. (Rabenstein et al., 2005), these observations suggest that the β-adducin knock-out mouse may provide a good model for future studies, to test the hypothesis that CA1 spine synapse formation may contribute to hormone-induced enhancement of spatial memory.

CONCLUSIONS

The data presented in this short review illustrate more than anything else how much still remains to be learned about the effects of gonadal steroids on synaptic plasticity in the male and female brain. While the list of structures affected by these steroids in terms of changes in dendritic spine synapse numbers continues to grow, and it becomes increasingly clear that the regulatory mechanisms in different regions of the brain and in the two sexes are probably different, we remain almost completely in the dark regarding the cellular mechanisms involved. The available evidence suggests that there may be common final signaling mechanisms, involving changes in activation of NMDA receptor-dependent pathways, mediating the effects of both estrogens and androgens (Woolley & McEwen, 1994; Romeo et al., 2005). The nature of the ER involved (membrane as opposed to nuclear), as well as the nature of the receptor systems that mediate the actions of androgens, however, remains largely a matter of conjecture. While we can be fairly confident that the actions of circulating testosterone in females are largely mediated via intermediate estrogen formation, the effects of this steroid in males, and indeed the effects of nonaromatizable androgens in both sexes, are mediated via mechanisms that remain obscure. Understanding these mechanisms could conceivably be useful for treatment of human neurodegenerative disorders, since the fact that the mechanisms mediating the neurotrophic effects of gonadal steroids seem to have different ligand specificity than their non-neural counterparts opens the door to potentially creating drugs with gonadal hormonal activity that can target neurotrophic pathways in the brain. It will also be very important, in future studies, to clearly establish whether the sex differences in response to androgen and estrogen that are observed in rodents are also seen in primates, because this could have a major impact on the design of potential future hormone replacement therapies.

References

Alreja M. (1996). Excitatory actions of serotonin on GABAergic neurons of the medial septum and diagonal band of Broca. *Synapse*, 22:15–27.

Alves SE, Hoskin E, Lee SJ, Brake WG, Ferguson D, Luine V, et al. (2002). Serotonin mediates CA1 spine density but is not crucial for ovarian steroid regulation of synaptic plasticity in the adult rat dorsal hippocampus. *Synapse*, 45:143–151.

Barrett-Connor E, Goodman-Gruen D, Patay B. (1999). Endogenous sex hormones and cognitive function in older men. *J Clin Endocrinol Metab*, 84:3681–3685.

Baulieu EE, Robel P, Schumacher M. (2001). Neurosteroids: beginning of the story. *Int Rev Neurobiol*, 46:1–32.

Blaustein JD, (1992). Cytoplasmic estrogen receptors in rat brain: immunocytochemical evidence using three antibodies with distinct epitopes. *Endocrinology*, 131:1336–1342.

Brown TJ, Hochberg RB, Zielinski JE, MacLusky NJ. (1988). Regional sex differences in cell nuclear estrogen-binding capacity in the rat hypothalamus and preoptic area. *Endocrinology*, 123:1761–1770.

Chen Y, Bourne J, Pieribone VA, Fitzsimonds RM. (2004). The role of actin in the regulation of dendritic spine morphology and bidirectional synaptic plasticity. *Neuroreport*, 15:829–832.

Cherrier MM, Rose AL, Higano C. (2003). The effects of combined androgen blockade on cognitive function during the first cycle of intermittent androgen suppression in patients with prostate cancer. *J Urol*, 170:1808–1811.

Cordoba Montoya DA, Carrer HF. (1997). Estrogen facilitates induction of long term potentiation in the hippocampus of awake rats. *Brain Res*, 778:430–438.

Cordova M, Jacome L, Lachman V, Luine VN. (2004). Castration impairs and gonadal hormones restore recognition memory in rats. ENDO Meeting: P2–214.

Duff SJ, Hampson E. (2000). A beneficial effect of estrogen on working memory in postmenopausal women taking hormone replacement therapy. *Horm Behav*, 38:262–276.

Edinger KL, Frye CA. (2004). Testosterone's analgesic, anxiolytic, and cognitive-enhancing effects may be due in part to actions of its 5alpha-reduced metabolites in the hippocampus. *Behav Neurosci*, 118: 1352–1364.

Fernandez-Galaz MC, Morschl E, Chowen JA, Torres-Aleman I, Naftolin F, Garcia-Segura LM. (1997). Role of astroglia and insulin-like growth factor-I in gonadal hormone-dependent synaptic plasticity. *Brain Res Bull*, 44:525–531.

Fischer A, Sananbenesi F, Schrick C, Spiess J, Radulovic J. (2004). Distinct roles of hippocampal de novo protein synthesis and actin rearrangement in extinction of contextual fear. *J Neurosci*, 24:1962–1966.

Fischer M, Kaech S, Knutti D, Matus A. (1998). Rapid actin-based plasticity in dendritic spines. *Neuron*, 20:847–854.

Flood JF, Farr SA, Kaiser FE, La Regina M, Morley JE. (1995). Age-related decrease of plasma testosterone in SAMP8 mice: replacement improves age-related impairment of learning and memory. *Physiol Behav*, 57:669–673.

Foy MR, Xu J, Xie X, Brinton RD, Thompson RF, Berger TW. (1999). 17beta-estradiol enhances NMDA receptor-mediated EPSPs and long-term potentiation. *J Neurophysiol*, 81:925–929.

Freund TF, Antal M. (1988). GABA-containing neurons in the septum control inhibitory interneurons in the hippocampus. *Nature*, 336:170–173.

Freund TF, Buzsaki G. (1996). Interneurons of the hippocampus. *Hippocampus*, 6:347–470.

Freund TF, Gulyas AI, Acsady L, Gorcs T, Toth K. (1990). Serotonergic control of the hippocampus via local inhibitory interneurons. *Proc Natl Acad Sci USA*, 87:8501–8505.

Friedman G. (2000). The effects of estrogen on short-term memory in genetic men. *J Am Med Dir Assoc*, 1:4–7.

Gardner K, Bennett V. (1987). Modulation of spectrin-actin assembly by erythrocyte adducin. *Nature*, 328:359–362.

Gazzaley AH, Weiland NG, McEwen BS, Morrison JH. (1996). Differential regulation of NMDAR1 mRNA and protein by estradiol in the rat hippocampus. *J Neurosci*, 16:6830–6838.

Good M, Day M, Muir JL. (1999). Cyclical changes in endogenous levels of estrogen modulate the induction of LTD and LTP in the hippocampal CA1 region. *Eur J Neurosci*, 11:4476–4480.

Gorski RA, Gordon JH, Shryne JE, Southam AM. (1978). Evidence for a morphological sex difference within the medial preoptic area of the rat brain. *Brain Res*, 148:333–346.

Gouchie C, Kimura D. (1991). The relationship between testosterone levels and cognitive ability patterns. *Psychoneuroendocrinology*, 16:323–334.

Gould E, Woolley CS, Frankfurt M, McEwen BS. (1990). Gonadal steroids regulate dendritic spine density in hippocampal pyramidal cells in adulthood. *J Neurosci*, 10:1286–1291.

Gulyas AI, Freund TF. (1996). Pyramidal cell dendrites are the primary targets of calbindin D28k-immunoreactive interneurons in the hippocampus. *Hippocampus*, 6:525–534.

Hajszan T, MacLusky NJ, Leranth C. (2004). Dehydroepiandrosterone increases hippocampal spine synapse density in ovariectomized female rats. *Endocrinology*, 145:1042–1045.

Hajszan T, Leranth C, Roth RH. (2006). Subchronic phencyclidine treatment decreases the number of dendritic spine synapses in the rat prefrontal cortex. *Biol Psychiatry*, 15;60(6):639–644.

Hao J, Rapp PR, Leffler AE, Leffler SR, Janssen WG, Lou W, et al. (2006). Estrogen alters spine number and morphology in prefrontal cortex of aged female rhesus monkeys. *J Neurosci*, 26:2571–2578.

Harley CW, Malsbury CW, Squires A, Brown RA. (2000). Testosterone decreases CA1 plasticity in vivo in gonadectomized male rats. *Hippocampus*, 10:693–697.

Harrison PJ. (2004). The hippocampus in schizophrenia: a review of the neuropathological evidence and its pathophysiological implications. *Psychopharmacology* (Berl), 174:151–162.

Hart BL. (2001). Effect of gonadectomy on subsequent development of age-related cognitive impairment in dogs. *J Am Vet Med Assoc*, 219:51–56.

Hebb DO. (1949). *The Organization of Behavior*. New York: Wiley.

Hogervorst E, Williams J, Budge M, Barnetson L, Combrinck M, Smith AD. (2001). Serum total testosterone is lower in men with Alzheimer's disease. *Neuro Endocrinol Lett*, 22:163–168.

Huppert FA, Van Niekerk JK. (2001). Dehydroepiandrosterone (DHEA) supplementation for cognitive function. Cochrane Database Syst Rev: CD000304.

Ibanez C, Guennoun R, Liere P, Eychenne B, Pianos A, El-Etr M, Baulieu EE, Schumacher M. (2003). Developmental expression of genes involved in neurosteroidogenesis: 3beta-hydroxysteroid dehydrogenase/delta5-delta4 isomerase in the rat brain. *Endocrinology*, 144:2902–2911.

Ito K, Skinkle KL, Hicks TP. (1999). Age-dependent, steroid-specific effects of oestrogen on long-term potentiation in rat hippocampal slices. *J Physiol*, 515 (Pt 1):209–220.

Janowsky JS. (2006). The role of androgens in cognition and brain aging in men. *Neuroscience*, 138:1015–1020.

Janowsky JS, Chavez B, Orwoll E. (2000). Sex steroids modify working memory. *J Cogn Neurosci*, 12:407–414.

Jentsch JD, Redmond Jr DE, Elsworth JD, Taylor JR, Youngren KD, Roth RH. (1997). Enduring cognitive deficits and cortical dopamine dysfunction in monkeys after long-term administration of phencyclidine. *Science*, 277:953–955.

Kaasik A, Safiulina D, Kalda A, Zharkovsky A. (2003). Dehydroepiandrosterone with other neurosteroids preserve neuronal mitochondria from calcium overload. *J Steroid Biochem Mol Biol*, 87:97–103.

Kalra SP, Horvath T, Naftolin F, Xu B, Pu S, Kalra PS. (1997). The interactive language of the hypothalamus for the gonadotropin releasing hormone (GNRH) system. *J Neuroendocrinol*, 9:569–576.

Kampen DL, Sherwin BB. (1996). Estradiol is related to visual memory in healthy young men. *Behav Neurosci*, 110:613–617.

Kandel ER. (2001). The molecular biology of memory storage: a dialogue between genes and synapses. *Science*, 294:1030–1038.

Kasai H, Matsuzaki M, Noguchi J, Yasumatsu N, Nakahara H. (2003). Structure-stability-function relationships of dendritic spines. *Trends Neurosci*, 26: 360–368.

Keenan PA, Ezzat WH, Ginsburg K, Moore GJ. (2001). Prefrontal cortex as the site of estrogen's effect on cognition. *Psychoneuroendocrinology*, 26:577–590.

Kerr JE, Allore RJ, Beck SG, Handa RJ. (1995). Distribution and hormonal regulation of androgen receptor (AR) and AR messenger ribonucleic acid in the rat hippocampus. *Endocrinology*, 136:3213–3221.

Kimura K, Fukata Y, Matsuoka Y, Bennett V, Matsuura Y, Okawa K, et al. (1998). Regulation of the association of adducin with actin filaments by Rho-associated kinase (Rho-kinase) and myosin phosphatase. *J Biol Chem*, 273:5542–5548.

Kovacs EG, MacLusky NJ, Leranth C. (2003). Effects of testosterone on hippocampal CA1 spine synaptic density in the male rat are inhibited by fimbria/fornix transection. *Neuroscience*, 122:807–810.

Kretz O, Fester L, Wehrenberg U, Zhou L, Brauckmann S, Zhao S, et al. (2004) Hippocampal synapses depend on hippocampal estrogen synthesis. *J Neurosci*, 24:5913–5921.

Kritzer MF, Kohama SG. (1998). Ovarian hormones influence the morphology, distribution, and density of tyrosine hydroxylase immunoreactive axons in the dorsolateral prefrontal cortex of adult rhesus monkeys. *J Comp Neurol*, 395:1–17.

Kritzer MF, Kohama SG. (1999). Ovarian hormones differentially influence immunoreactivity for dopamine beta- hydroxylase, choline acetyltransferase, and serotonin in the dorsolateral prefrontal cortex of adult rhesus monkeys. *J Comp Neurol*, 409:438–451.

Kuhlman PA, Hughes CA, Bennett V, Fowler VM. (1996). A new function for adducin. Calcium/calmodulin-regulated capping of the barbed ends of actin filaments. *J Biol Chem*, 271:7986–7991.

Labrie F, Luu-The V, Labrie C, Belanger A, Simard J, Lin SX, Pelletier G. (2003). Endocrine and intracrine sources of androgens in women: inhibition of breast cancer and other roles of androgens and their precursor dehydroepiandrosterone. *Endocr Rev*, 24: 152–182.

Lam TT, Leranth C. (2003). Role of the medial septum diagonal band of Broca cholinergic neurons in oestrogen-induced spine synapse formation on hippocampal CA1 pyramidal cells of female rats. *Eur J Neurosci*, 17:1997–2005.

Lee YF, Lin WJ, Huang J, Messing EM, Chan FL, Wilding G, Chang C. (2002). Activation of mitogen-activated protein kinase pathway by the antiandrogen hydroxyflutamide in androgen receptor-negative prostate cancer cells. *Cancer Res*, 62:6039–6044.

Leranth C, Vertes RP. (1999). Median raphe serotonergic innervation of medial septum/diagonal band of Broca (MSDB) parvalbumin-containing neurons: possible involvement of the MSDB in the desynchronization of the hippocampal EEG. *J Comp Neurol*, 410:586–598.

Leranth C, Shanabrough M. (2001). Supramammillary area mediates subcortical estrogenic action on hippocampal synaptic plasticity. *Exp Neurol*, 167:445–450.

Leranth C, Shanabrough M, Horvath TL. (1999). Estrogen receptor-alpha in the raphe serotonergic and supramammillary area calretinin-containing neurons of the female rat. *Exp Brain Res*, 128:417–420.

Leranth C, Shanabrough M, Horvath TL. (2000a). Hormonal regulation of hippocampal spine synapse density involves subcortical mediation. *Neuroscience*, 101:349–356.

Leranth C, Shanabrough M, Redmond DEJ. (2002). Gonadal hormones are responsible for maintaining the integrity of spine synapses in the CA1 hippocampal subfield of female nonhuman primates. *J Comp Neurol*, 447:34–42.

Leranth C, Petnehazy O, MacLusky NJ. (2003). Gonadal hormones affect spine synaptic density in the CA1 hippocampal subfield of male rats. *J Neurosci*, 23: 1588–1592.

Leranth C, Hajszan T, MacLusky NJ. (2004a). Androgens increase spine synapse density in the CA1 hippocampal subfield of ovariectomized female rats. *J Neurosci*, 24:495–499.

Leranth C, Prange-Kiel J, Frick KM, Horvath TL. (2004b). Low CA1 spine synapse density is further reduced by castration in male non-human primates. *Cereb Cortex*, 14:503–510.

Leranth C, Roth RH, Elsworth JD, Naftolin F, Horvath TL, Redmond Jr DE. (2000b). Estrogen is essential for maintaining nigrostriatal dopamine neurons in primates: implications for Parkinson's disease and memory. *J Neurosci*, 20:8604–8609.

Lewis C, McEwen BS, Frankfurt M. (1995). Estrogen-induction of dendritic spines in ventromedial hypothalamus and hippocampus: effects of neonatal aromatase blockade and adult GDX. *Brain Res Dev Brain Res*, 87:91–95.

Littlefield BA, Gurpide E, Markiewicz L, McKinley B, Hochberg RB. (1990). A simple and sensitive microtiter plate estrogen bioassay based on stimulation of alkaline phosphatase in Ishikawa cells: estrogenic action of delta 5 adrenal steroids. *Endocrinology*, 127:2757–2762.

Luine VN. (1997). Steroid hormone modulation of hippocampal dependent spatial memory. *Stress*, 2:21–36.

Luine VN, Jacome LF, Maclusky NJ. (2003). Rapid enhancement of visual and place memory by estrogens in rats. *Endocrinology*, 144:2836–2844.

MacLusky NJ, Naftolin F. (1981). Sexual differentiation of the central nervous system. *Science*, 211:1294–1302.

MacLusky NJ, Hajszan T, Leranth C. (2004). Effects of dehydroepiandrosterone and flutamide on hippocampal CA1 spine synapse density in male and female rats: implications for the role of androgens in maintenance of hippocampal structure. *Endocrinology*, 145:4154–4161.

MacLusky NJ, Walters MJ, Clark AS, Toran-Allerand CD. (1994). Aromatase in the cerebral cortex, hippocampus, and mid-brain: ontogeny and developmental implications. *Mol Cell Neurosci*, 5:691–698.

MacLusky NJ, Luine VN, Hajszan T, Leranth C. (2005). The 17alpha and 17beta isomers of estradiol both induce rapid spine synapse formation in the CA1 hippocampal subfield of ovariectomized female rats. *Endocrinology*, 146:287–293.

MacLusky NJ, Hajszan T, Johansen JA, Jordan CL, Leranth C. (2006). Androgen effects on hippocampal CA1 spine synapse numbers are retained in Tfm male rats with defective androgen receptors. *Endocrinology*, 147:2392–2398.

Martin C, Ross M, Chapman KE, Andrew R, Bollina P, Seckl JR, Habib FK. (2004). CYP7B generates a selective estrogen receptor beta agonist in human prostate. *J Clin Endocrinol Metab*, 89:2928–2935.

Matsuoka Y, Hughes CA, Bennett V. (1996). Adducin regulation. Definition of the calmodulin-binding domain and sites of phosphorylation by protein kinases A and C. *J Biol Chem*, 271:25157–25166.

Matsuoka Y, Li X, Bennett V. (1998). Adducin is an in vivo substrate for protein kinase C: phosphorylation in the MARCKS-related domain inhibits activity in promoting spectrin-actin complexes and occurs in many cells, including dendritic spines of neurons. *J Cell Biol*, 142:485–497.

Matus A, Brinkhaus H, Wagner U. (2000). Actin dynamics in dendritic spines: a form of regulated plasticity at excitatory synapses. *Hippocampus*, 10:555–560.

McEwen BS, Woolley CS. (1994). Estradiol and progesterone regulate neuronal structure and synaptic connectivity in adult as well as developing brain. *Exp Gerontol*, 29:431–436.

Meyer G, Ferres-Torres R, Mas M. (1978). The effects of puberty and castration on hippocampal dendritic spines of mice. A Golgi study. *Brain Res*, 155:108–112.

Mische SM, Mooseker MS, Morrow JS. (1987). Erythrocyte adducin: a calmodulin-regulated actin-bundling protein that stimulates spectrin-actin binding. *J Cell Biol*, 105:2837–2845.

Miyamoto H, Yeh S, Wilding G, Chang C. (1998). Promotion of agonist activity of antiandrogens by the androgen receptor coactivator, ARA70, in human prostate cancer DU145 cells. *Proc Natl Acad Sci USA*, 95:7379–7384.

Moffat SD, Zonderman AB, Metter EJ, Blackman MR, Harman SM, Resnick SM. (2002). Longitudinal assessment of serum free testosterone concentration predicts memory performance and cognitive status in elderly men. *J Clin Endocrinol Metab*, 87:5001–5007.

Moss RL, Gu Q. (1999). Estrogen: mechanisms for a rapid action in CA1 hippocampal neurons. *Steroids*, 64:14–21.

Murphy DD, Segal M. (1997). Morphological plasticity of dendritic spines in central neurons is mediated by activation of cAMP response element binding protein. *Proc Natl Acad Sci USA*, 94:1482–1487.

Murphy DD, Cole NB, Segal M. (1998a.) Brain-derived neurotrophic factor mediates estradiol-induced dendritic spine formation in hippocampal neurons. *Proc Natl Acad Sci USA*, 95:11412–11417.

Murphy DD, Cole NB, Greenberger V, Segal M. (1998b). Estradiol increases dendritic spine density by reducing GABA neurotransmission in hippocampal neurons. *J Neurosci*, 18:2550–2559.

Neave N, Menaged M, Weightman DR. (1999). Sex differences in cognition: the role of testosterone and sexual orientation. *Brain Cogn*, 41:245–262.

Pak TR, Chung WC, Lund TD, Hinds LR, Clay CM, Handa RJ. (2005). The androgen metabolite, 5alpha-androstane-3beta, 17beta-diol, is a potent modulator of estrogen receptor-beta1-mediated gene transcription in neuronal cells. *Endocrinology*, 146:147–155.

Parducz A, Garcia-Segura LM. (1993). Sexual differences in the synaptic connectivity in the rat dentate gyrus. *Neurosci Lett*, 161:53–56.

Parducz A, Hajszan T, Maclusky NJ, Hoyk Z, Csakvari E, Kurunczi A, et al. (2006). Synaptic remodeling induced by gonadal hormones: neuronal plasticity as a mediator of neuroendocrine and behavioral responses to steroids. *Neuroscience*, 138:977–985.

Patchev VK, Almeida OF. (1996). Gonadal steroids exert facilitating and "buffering" effects on glucocorticoid-mediated transcriptional regulation of corticotropin-releasing hormone and corticosteroid receptor genes in rat brain. *J Neurosci*, 16:7077–7084.

Pelletier G, Luu-The V, Labrie F. (1994). Immunocytochemical localization of 5 alpha-reductase in rat brain. *Mol Cell Neurosci*, 5:394–399.

Pelletier G, Luu-The V, Labrie F. (1995). Immunocytochemical localization of type I 17 beta-hydroxysteroid dehydrogenase in the rat brain. *Brain Res*, 704:233–239.

Postma A, Meyer G, Tuiten A, van Honk J, Kessels RP, Thijssen J. (2000). Effects of testosterone administration on selective aspects of object-location memory in healthy young women. *Psychoneuroendocrinology*, 25:563–575.

Pozzo-Miller LD, Inoue T, Murphy DD. (1999). Estradiol increases spine density and NMDA-dependent Ca2+ transients in spines of CA1 pyramidal neurons from hippocampal slices. *J Neurophysiol*, 81:1404–1411.

Prange-Kiel J, Rune GM, Leranth C. (2004). Median raphe mediates estrogenic effects to the hippocampus in female rats. *Eur J Neurosci*, 19:309–317.

Rabenstein RL, Addy NA, Caldarone BJ, Asaka Y, Gruenbaum LM, Peters LL, et al. (2005). Impaired synaptic plasticity and learning in mice lacking beta-adducin, an actin-regulating protein. *J Neurosci*, 25:2138–2145.

Raber J, Bongers G, LeFevour A, Buttini M, Mucke L. (2002). Androgens protect against apolipoprotein E4-induced cognitive deficits. *J Neurosci*, 22:5204–5209.

Rainbow TC, Parsons B, McEwen BS. (1982). Sex differences in rat brain oestrogen and progestin receptors. *Nature*, 300:648–649.

Raisman G, Field PM. (1971). Sexual dimorphism in the preoptic area of the rat. *Science*, 173:731–733.

Raisman G, Field PM. (1973). Sexual dimorphism in the neuropil of the preoptic area of the rat and its dependence on neonatal androgen. *Brain Res*, 54:1–29.

Ramon y Cajal S. (1911). *Histologie du Système Nerveux de l'Homme et des Vertèbrès*. Paris: Maloine.

Rapp PR, Morrison JH, Roberts JA. (2003). Cyclic estrogen replacement improves cognitive function in aged ovariectomized rhesus monkeys. *J Neurosci*, 23:5708–5714.

Reddy DS. (2004a). Anticonvulsant activity of the testosterone-derived neurosteroid 3alpha-androstanediol. *Neuroreport*, 15:515–518.

Reddy DS. (2004b). Testosterone modulation of seizure susceptibility is mediated by neurosteroids 3alpha-androstanediol and 17beta-estradiol. *Neuroscience*, 129:195–207.

Richie JP. (1999). Anti-androgens and other hormonal therapies for prostate cancer. *Urology*, 54:15–18.

Romeo RD, Staub D, Jasnow AM, Karatsoreos IN, Thornton JE, McEwen BS. (2005). Dihydrotestosterone increases hippocampal N-methyl-D-aspartate binding but does not affect choline acetyltransferase cell number in the forebrain or choline transporter levels in the CA1 region of adult male rats. *Endocrinology*, 146:2091–2097.

Roof RL. (1993). The dentate gyrus is sexually dimorphic in prepubescent rats: testosterone plays a significant role. *Brain Res*, 610:148–151.

Roof RL, Havens MD. (1992). Testosterone improves maze performance and induces development of a male hippocampus in females. *Brain Res*, 572:310–313.

Roselli CE. (1991). Sex differences in androgen receptors and aromatase activity in microdissected regions of the rat brain. *Endocrinology*, 128:1310–1316.

Roselli CE, Horton LE, Resko JA. (1987). Time-course and steroid specificity of aromatase induction in rat hypothalamus-preoptic area. *Biol Reprod*, 37:628–633.

Rosene DL, Van Hoesen GW. (1987). The hippocampal formation of the primate brain. A review of some comparative aspects of cytoarchitecture and connections. *Cereb Cortex*, 6:345–456.

Ross JL, Roeltgen D, Stefanatos GA, Feuillan P, Kushner H, Bondy C, Cutler Jr GB. (2003). Androgen-responsive aspects of cognition in girls with Turner syndrome. *J Clin Endocrinol Metab*, 88:292–296.

Rune GM, Wehrenberg U, Prange-Kiel J, Zhou L, Adelmann G, Frotscher M. (2002). Estrogen up-regulates estrogen receptor alpha and synaptophysin in slice cultures of rat hippocampus. *Neuroscience*, 113:167–175.

Rush ME, Blake CA. (1982). Serum testosterone concentrations during the 4-day estrous cycle in normal and adrenalectomized rats. *Proc Soc Exp Biol Med*, 169:216–221.

Sar M, Lubahn DB, French FS, Wilson EM. (1990). Immunohistochemical localization of the androgen receptor in rat and human tissues. *Endocrinology*, 127:3180–3186.

Segal M, Murphy DD. (1998). CREB activation mediates plasticity in cultured hippocampal neurons. *Neural Plast*, 6:1–7.

Shors TJ, Miesegaes G. (2002). Testosterone in utero and at birth dictates how stressful experience will affect learning in adulthood. *Proc Natl Acad Sci USA*, 99:13955–13960.

Shughrue PJ, Merchenthaler I. (2000). Estrogen is more than just a "sex hormone": novel sites for estrogen action in the hippocampus and cerebral cortex. *Front Neuroendocrinol*, 21:95–101.

Shughrue PJ, Lane MV, Merchenthaler I. (1997). Comparative distribution of estrogen receptor-alpha and -beta mRNA in the rat central nervous system. *J Comp Neurol*, 388:507–525.

Shughrue PJ, Scrimo PJ, Merchenthaler I. (2000). Estrogen binding and estrogen receptor characterization (ERalpha and ERbeta) in the cholinergic neurons of the rat basal forebrain. *Neuroscience*, 96:41–49.

Silverman I, Kastuk D, Choi J, Phillips K. (1999). Testosterone levels and spatial ability in men. *Psychoneuroendocrinology*, 24:813–822.

Simerly RB, Swanson LW, Gorski RA. (1985). The distribution of monoaminergic cells and fibers in a periventricular preoptic nucleus involved in the control of gonadotropin release: immunohistochemical evidence for a dopaminergic sexual dimorphism. *Brain Res*, 330:55–64.

Simerly RB, Chang C, Muramatsu M, Swanson LW. (1990). Distribution of androgen and estrogen receptor mRNA-containing cells in the rat brain: an in situ hybridization study. *J Comp Neurol*, 294:76–95.

Sullivan SD, Moenter SM. (2003). Neurosteroids alter gamma-aminobutyric acid postsynaptic currents in gonadotropin-releasing hormone neurons: a possible mechanism for direct steroidal control. *Endocrinology*, 144:4366–4375.

Tabibnia G, Cooke BM, Breedlove SM. (1999). Sex difference and laterality in the volume of mouse dentate gyrus granule cell layer. *Brain Res*, 827: 41–45.

Tabori NE, Stewart LS, Znamensky V, Romeo RD, Alves SE, McEwen BS, Milner TA. (2005). Ultrastructural evidence that androgen receptors are located at extranuclear sites in the rat hippocampal formation. *Neuroscience*, 130:151–163.

Tang Y, Janssen WG, Hao J, Roberts JA, McKay H, Lasley B, et al. (2004). Estrogen replacement increases spinophilin-immunoreactive spine number in the prefrontal cortex of female rhesus monkeys. *Cereb Cortex*, 14:215–223.

Toran-Allerand CD, Guan X, MacLusky NJ, Horvath TL, Diano S, Singh M, et al. (2002). ER-X: a novel, plasma membrane-associated, putative estrogen receptor that is regulated during development and after ischemic brain injury. *J Neurosci*, 22:8391–8401.

Ueda H, Yoshida A, Tokuyama S, Mizuno K, Maruo J, Matsuno K, Mita S. (2001). Neurosteroids stimulate G protein-coupled sigma receptors in mouse brain synaptic membrane. *Neurosci Res*, 41:33–40.

Vasudevan N, Kow LM, Pfaff DW. (2001). Early membrane estrogenic effects required for full expression of slower genomic actions in a nerve cell line. *Proc Natl Acad Sci USA*, 98:12267–12271.

Vertes RP, Kocsis B. (1997). Brainstem-diencephalo-septohippocampal systems controlling the theta rhythm of the hippocampus. *Neuroscience*, 81:893–926.

Weiland NG, Orikasa C, Hayashi S, McEwen BS. (1997). Distribution and hormone regulation of estrogen receptor immunoreactive cells in the hippocampus of male and female rats. *J Comp Neurol*, 388:603–612.

Williams CL, Meck WH. (1991). The organizational effects of gonadal steroids on sexually dimorphic spatial ability. *Psychoneuroendocrinology*, 16:155–176.

Williams CL, Barnett AM, Meck WH. (1990). Organizational effects of early gonadal secretions on sexual differentiation in spatial memory. *Behav Neurosci*, 104:84–97.

Wimer CC, Wimer RE. (1989). On the sources of strain and sex differences in granule cell number in the dentate area of house mice. *Brain Res Dev Brain Res*, 48:167–176.

Wisniewski AB, Nguyen TT, Dobs AS. (2002). Evaluation of high-dose estrogen and high-dose estrogen plus methyltestosterone treatment on cognitive task performance in postmenopausal women. *Horm Res*, 58:150–155.

Woolley CS. (1998). Estrogen-mediated structural and functional synaptic plasticity in the female rat hippocampus. *Horm Behav*, 34:140–148.

Woolley CS, McEwen BS. (1992). Estradiol mediates fluctuation in hippocampal synapse density during the estrous cycle in the adult rat. *J Neurosci*, 12: 2549–2554.

Woolley CS, McEwen BS. (1994). Estradiol regulates hippocampal dendritic spine density via an

N-methyl-D-aspartate receptor-dependent mechanism. *J Neurosci*, 14:7680–7687.

Woolley CS, Gould E, Frankfurt M, McEwen BS. (1990). Naturally occurring fluctuation in dendritic spine density on adult hippocampal pyramidal neurons. *J Neurosci*, 10:4035–4039.

Woolley CS, Weiland NG, McEwen BS, Schwartzkroin PA. (1997). Estradiol increases the sensitivity of hippocampal CA1 pyramidal cells to NMDA receptor-mediated synaptic input: correlation with dendritic spine density. *J Neurosci*, 17:1848–1859.

Yaffe K, Lui LY, Zmuda J, Cauley J. (2002). Sex hormones and cognitive function in older men. *J Am Geriatr Soc*, 50:707–712.

Yankova M, Hart SA, Woolley CS. (2001). Estrogen increases synaptic connectivity between single pre-synaptic inputs and multiple postsynaptic CA1 pyramidal cells: a serial electron-microscopic study. *Proc Natl Acad Sci U S A*, 98:3525–3530.

Yarbrough WG, Quarmby VE, Simental JA, Joseph DR, Sar M, Lubahn DB, et al. (1990). A single base mutation in the androgen receptor gene causes androgen insensitivity in the testicular feminized rat. *J Biol Chem*, 265:8893–8900.

Zwain IH, Yen SS. (1999). Neurosteroidogenesis in astrocytes, oligodendrocytes, and neurons of cerebral cortex of rat brain. *Endocrinology*, 140:3843–3852.

Zwain IH, Yen SS, Cheng CY. (1997). Astrocytes cultured in vitro produce estradiol-17beta and express aromatase cytochrome P-450 (P-450 AROM) mRNA. *Biochim Biophys Acta*, 1334:338–348.

Chapter 12

Sex Differences in Cognitive Function in Rodents

Victoria Luine and Gary Dohanich

Characteristics that exist in "two kinds or forms" between genders are known as *sexual dimorphisms* and can be either *qualitative* or *quantitative* in nature. Qualitative differences are based on characteristics unique to each gender such as the display of mounting behavior during mating by male rodents versus the display of the sexual posture known as lordosis by female rodents. On the other hand, quantitative sexual dimorphisms are based on the degree to which a characteristic is expressed by each gender such as the higher percentage of body fat in females than males, or the greater amount of body hair on men than women.

In regard to learning and memory, both qualitative and quantitative dimorphisms are present. Quantitative differences are evident in the rate and accuracy for solving specific tasks (see Quantitative Differences in Spatial Memory). Qualitative dimorphisms include sex differences in the strategies by which cognitive tasks are performed/solved and sex differences in cognitive responses to stress (see Qualitative Differences in Spatial Memory).

Quantitative sex differences are sometimes small in magnitude, with the largest differences usually constituting no more than one standard deviation unit. Thus, quantitative cognitive differences between the sexes appear to be within the normal range of performance. For example, in a task where females perform better than males (quantitative dimorphism), the average score of females is higher than males, but the normal distribution of the sexes overlap. Thus, the performance of many females is lower than the performance of many males. Although these small quantitative differences may be inconsequential it can be argued that qualitative sexual dimorphisms have important repercussions for a species and may have contributed to its evolutionary success. Specifically, qualitative sex differences such as opposite cognitive responses to stress (chronic stress impairs male, but enhances female performance in many cognitive tasks) as well as different strategies for forming cognitive maps of space (females and males may use differing strategies when learning the same task) constitute major differences in patterns of behavior. Thus, qualitative sexual dimorphisms in cognition and behavior may afford each sex with the requisite tools that provide an edge for their mutual survival and for the survival of their progeny.

This chapter reviews cognitive function in rodents within this context of qualitative and quantitative sex differences in performance. Whether these sex differences impact day-to-day functioning, contribute to the successful evolution of a species, and can be accounted for by mechanisms underlying cognitive function are explored.

OVERVIEW OF LEARNING AND MEMORY

Learning—defined historically by psychologists—is a relatively permanent change in behavior as a result of experience. This definition suggests that learning and associated memory can be quantified by recording changes in behavior. Researchers have faithfully applied this technique to measure learning and memory in various species, including humans. Behavioral measurement of learning and memory is complex, however, and the study of sex differences in species other than humans presents special problems. First, although learning and memory are inextricably linked, these are distinct processes that are not defined sharply in the scientific literature. Second, learning or memory can only be inferred from behavioral performance on cognitive tasks. Third, emerging evidence indicates that male and female mammals learn and remember information differently. Therefore, direct comparisons of performance on specific cognitive tasks can be misleading or at least confounded. Finally, hormone levels in adults, often cyclic in nature, add another layer of complexity to the study of gender differences in cognition.

Learning and memory are highly interdependent processes that include the *acquisition, consolidation, retention,* and *retrieval* of information. Each of these elements can be studied and manipulated using contemporary behavioral techniques. Learning to solve a particular cognitive task depends on diverse factors. During the *acquisition phase* of learning, subjects must adopt a strategy or solution appropriate to the task that allows information to be acquired for storage and later retrieval. Some investigators propose distinct, though interconnected, learning and mem-

ory systems that subserve specific cognitive strategies (Poldrack & Packard, 2003; Gold, 2004; Kesner & Rogers, 2004; Squire, 2004).

A successful strategy can be as simple as learning to turn right on every trial to obtain a reward—known as an *egocentric strategy*—or as complex as developing a cognitive map of the surrounding environment to locate the reward—known as an *allocentric strategy*. Selection of a successful strategy depends not only the demands of the cognitive task, but on the experience, gender, and hormonal profile of the learner (Packard, 1999; Chang & Gold, 2003a; Korol, 2004). Acquisition is further complicated by the novelty of the training environment, which can cause subjects to be distracted, anxious, or confused (Saucier et al., 1996; Cain et al., 1996; Cain, 1997, 1998).

Acclimating or pretraining subjects by exposing them to the learning environment and the demands of the task prior to acquisition can reduce the impact of non-mnemonic factors during acquisition of a cognitive task (Beiko et al., 1997; Cain, 1997; Hoh & Cain, 1997). Additionally, the rate at which learning proceeds can be affected by such factors as massed versus distributed training trials, the saliency of cues that aid learning, and the nature of reinforcements that motivate learning (Hodges, 1996). An important implication for the current discussion of sex differences is the potential for a wide range of variables to have dissimilar consequences for the acquisition of information by male and female mammals.

As training proceeds, information becomes encoded and retained as memory during the consolidation phase. *Consolidation*, first inferred from the retrograde amnesia experienced by patients following brain trauma or surgery (Milner, 1959), can be facilitated or inhibited in rats by manipulations applied within one or two hours after training (McGaugh & Izquierdo, 2000). However, consolidation continues to be a poorly understood process that may require as little as several hours for some memories in rats to several years for certain types of memories in humans (McGaugh, 2000; Rosenbaum et al., 2001; Frankland & Bontempi, 2005).

Inspired by selective cognitive deficits typical of human amnesia, researchers have divided memory into a series of overlapping, but non-synonymous categories such as *declarative and procedural, associate and non-associative, working and reference, short-term and long-term* (Squire, 1987). In the study of non-human cognition, *working memory* is defined traditionally as a flexible form of short-term memory for information that is useful within a single trial set for durations of minutes to hours (Baddeley & Hitch, 1974). *Reference memory*, in contrast, is an inflexible form of long-term memory for information that is useful across trial sets often persisting over many days (Olton & Papas, 1979).

Although the use of the working and reference paradigm has been abandoned by some investigators, this model has significant historical value and continues to be applied by some researchers who study the impacts of gender and hormones on cognition. Working memory and reference memory can be demonstrated empirically in a variety of cognitive tasks. In *spatial* tasks that depend on three-dimensional relationships between environmental stimuli, reference memory allows subjects to develop associations between static elements of the task; for example, swimming to the same location of a pool on each trial to escape the aversive environment of a water maze or visiting only the arms of a radial maze that are always baited.

Working memory, in contrast, allows subjects to solve a task with varying parameters; for example, learning the new location for escape on the first swim of each day to allow escape on subsequent trials or remembering which arms of a radial maze were visited previously during the course of a daily trial set. In *non-spatial* tasks that do not depend on three-dimensional cues in the surrounding environment, reference memory allows subject to learn inflexible elements of the task; for example, learning to always choose the novel object to obtain food reward in an object recognition task. Working memory in an object recognition task informs the subject which of two objects was presented on the previous trial allowing the correct choice of the novel object.

The spatial and non-spatial tasks described above have been employed in various versions in the study of cognition in male and female rodents. Currently, there are more questions than answers endemic to the issue of gender differences in learning and memory. For example, are sex differences in cognitive performance reliable? Do sex differences in performance of cognitive tasks reflect actual sex differences in learning and memory? Do sex differences reflect differences in cognitive ability between the sexes or differences in cognitive style? Are sex differences in learning and memory important? In the sections that follow, these intriguing questions are considered within the context of a rich, but complex, scientific literature.

PHYSIOLOGICAL AND NEURAL BASES FOR SEXUAL DIMORPHISMS

Differences in the cognitive function of males and females have been reported by many investigators. Potential sex differences in cognitive performance can be caused by a variety of factors; the three most commonly studied are genetic constitution, hormonal regulation of development, and hormonal influences in adulthood. These factors have profound effects on the development and expression of reproductive functions, and as a logical extension could play a role in establishing differences in performance of males and females on tasks of learning and memory.

The *Sry* gene on the Y chromosome (sex-determining region) directs the expression of a high-mobility-group protein that drives the medulla of the fetal genital ridge toward testicular development (Berta et al., 1990; Harley & Goodfellow, 1994). In the absence of the *Sry* gene and its expressed protein, the cortex of the genital ridge becomes an ovary. Steroid and peptide hormones secreted by the fetal and neonatal testes further sculpt masculine characteristics both peripherally and centrally, a process that continues during adolescence (Sisk & Zehr, 2005).

As a consequence of this early organization, tissues are not only shaped but also primed to respond to various hormones that predominate in adult males and females. These *organizational* events leave lasting imprints during development that are later manifest as sex differences, which in some (but not all) cases can be modulated by circulating hormones in adulthood, through *activational* effects (McCarthy & Konkle, 2005).

Since the seminal report by Phoenix et al. (1959), the impact of testicular secretions on development of the reproductive brain and subsequent sexual behaviors has been recognized. Structural dimorphisms in male and female phenotypes of most mammals are evident, ranging from differences in external genitalia to tissue composition. Correspondingly, sex differences in total volume, neuronal number and density, glial number, axonal length, and dendritic length, spine density and neural connectivity are well-documented (De Vries, 2002; De Vries & Simerly, 2002; Simerly, 2002; Cooke & Woolley, 2005a). The influences of genetic and hormonal factors on the development of structures not typically implicated in reproduction have been confirmed, most notably in the rodent hippocampus.

Historically, the hippocampus has been the primary focus of investigators who study the neurobiology of learning and memory. Although much remains to be learned about the role of hippocampus in cognition, the profound impact of this structure on various forms of learning and memory is well established (Squire, 1992; Zola-Morgan & Squire, 1993; Eichenbaum, 1999; Hasselmo, 1999; O'Keefe, 1999; Taube, 1999). However, sex differences in the morphometry of hippocampal subregions in rats, mice, and voles are much smaller in magnitude than sex differences in the structures implicated in reproduction (Madeira et al., 1991; Roof & Havens, 1992; Galea et al., 1999; Tabibnia et al., 1999; Andrade et al., 2000). For example, the volume of the hippocampus typically is less than 20% larger in male rats and voles compared to female conspecifics while the volumes of some nuclei vary by as much as 500% between males and females (McCarthy & Konkle, 2005; see also Chapter 2, McCarthy and Arnold in this book).

Importantly, the effects of gender on hippocampal structure interact with hormonal status in adult rodents. Dendritic spine density and synapse number in CA1 pyramidal neurons of the female dorsal hippocampus fluctuate by approximately 30% across the 4-day estrous cycle in rats (Woolley at al., 1990; Woolley & McEwen, 1992), fluctuations that are dependent on cyclic release of the ovarian steroids, estrogen and progesterone (Gould et al., 1990; Woolley & McEwen, 1992, 1993; Leranth et al., 2000; Adams et al., 2001; MacLusky et al., 2005). In addition, ovariectomy is associated with a 48% decrease in spine density in CA1 basal dendrites (Wallace et al., 2006).

These activational effects of ovarian steroids on hippocampal connectivity involve the formation of new synaptic connections (Yankova et al., 2001) and are dependent on GABAergic, cholinergic, glutamatergic, and neurotrophic factors (Weiland, 1992a,b; Murphy & Segal, 1996; Woolley et al., 1997; Murphy et al., 1998a,b; Leranth et al., 2000; Daniel & Dohanich, 2001; Rudick & Woolley, 2001, 2003; Lam & Leranth, 2003; Rudick et al., 2003).

Gonadectomy of male rats reduced spine synapse density by 50%, and normal density can be restored by replacement with testosterone or dihydrotestosterone, the latter being an androgen that (unlike testosterone) cannot be metabolized to estrogen (Leranth et al., 2003; MacLusky et al., 2006). Both androgens restore spine density in the hippocampus of ovariectomized females although testosterone is somewhat more effective than dihydrotestosterone (Leranth et al., 2004). However, unlike females, estradiol treatment in males does not affect spine synapse density in the hippocampus (Leranth et al., 2003). Moreover, males do not undergo cyclic gonadal hormone changes like females. Thus, organizational and activational modifications of hippocampal connectivity by steroids in males and females follow different patterns that may lay the foundation for the expression of sex differences in cognition. See Chapter 11 by Leranth et al. in this book for further information on this topic. Alterations in dendritic morphology also are influenced by variables such as subject age, rearing conditions, and environmental stressors (see Psychological Performance Parameters).

Sex differences in other structures associated with cognitive function (including cortical regions) have been reported, but provide little evidence of the robust volumetric and structural differences between the sexes typical of reproductive brain areas (Juraska, 1984, 1991, 1992; Seymoure & Juraska, 1992). Sex differences in the amygdala seem to be region-specific and dependent on circulating levels of adult hormones, rather than sexual genotype or early hormonal influences (Cooke et al., 1999, 2003; Cooke & Woolley, 2005b). The volume of the medial nucleus of the amygdala is reliably larger in male rats than females (Mizukami et al., 1983; Hines et al., 1992). The medial nucleus is implicated strongly in sexual and social behaviors (Baum & Everitt, 1992), and medial amygdaloid circuits may be important contributors to sex differences in freezing behavior and contextual fear conditioning.

The profound differences between genders demonstrated in peripheral and central tissues regulating reproduction are associated with striking differences in the sexual behaviors displayed during mating by rodents. Therefore, it might be predicted that the circumscribed impact of gender and hormones on structures involved in cognitive function would be paralleled by relatively subtle sex differences in the performance of learning and memory tasks, particularly for quantitative measures of cognitive performance. This prediction has some empirical support as discussed in the next section.

SEXUAL DIMORPHISMS IN SPATIAL MEMORY TASKS

Commonly Used Spatial Memory Tasks

As indicated above, the hippocampus has been the most studied neural structure involved in learning and memory. Spatial memory, dependent on an intact hippocampus, is the most widely assessed form of cognition in rodents. Numerous tasks have been developed for measurement of hippocampal-dependent, spatial memory, and all tasks are based on the innate ability of rodents to use key landmarks and the hippocampus to construct "mental maps" of their environment (Mumby et al., 2002).

In the widely applied radial arm maze task developed by Olton and colleagues, subjects receive a food reward at the end of arms of the maze (mazes include from 8–17 arms). This task also relies on the natural foraging strategy of rats, and the ability to complete a trial without re-entering arms depends on building a cognitive map of the cues around the maze and remembering the arms entered using the cues (Olton & Samuelson, 1976). The Morris water maze uses a similar spatial context, requiring subjects to learn the location of an invisible escape platform in a large pool (typically 2 meters in diameter) (Morris, 1981, 1984).

Recognition memory tasks, which rely on the natural predisposition of rodents to seek novelty, can also be configured to assess spatial memory. For object placement tests, subjects are exposed to two identical objects in a sample trial before a variable inter-trial delay is given. In the recognition/retention trial following the delay, one object is moved to a new location. Memory is assessed by determining whether the subject spends more time exploring the object at the new as compared to the old location (Ennaceur & Aggleton, 1994; Ennaceur et al., 1997). Object placement assesses only short-term or working memory, but not acquisition (there are no contingency rules to learn). Thus, this place recognition task can be contrasted to other spatial tasks which are commonly configured to measure acquisition and reference memory, but not (usually) working memory.

Another widely employed maze for assessing spatial learning, memory, and strategy is the T-maze. In this task, the subject is rewarded with food by visiting one baited arm of a T-shaped maze. The sequence may involve visiting the alternate arm from the previous trial or visiting the same arm as in the previous trial. Criterion to successful performance (e.g., 9 correct visits to the baited arm in 10 trials) measures acquisition of the task. In addition, a probe trial can be incorporated to determine the type of strategy used to solve the task (Restle, 1957).

Quantitative Sex Differences in Spatial Memory—How Large and How Reliable?

In general, sex differences reported in acquisition or retention of spatial information in radial arm mazes and water mazes—males outperform females—are typically small in magnitude and are somewhat inconsistent across the literature (Dohanich, 2002; see Fig. 12.1). Furthermore, sex differences in performance on spatial tasks can be reduced or eliminated by pretraining, additional training, or cue manipulations. A meta-analysis by Jonasson (2005) indicated that male superiority in spatial performance on radial arm maze and water maze tasks is affected by the species, as indeed the strain of rodent under study.

On the radial arm maze task, when a subject revisits a baited arm during a trial, an error of working memory occurs. If a subject visits an arm that is never baited with a reward, an error of reference memory occurs. When sex differences have been reported in radial arm maze experiments, males often make fewer errors of working and reference memory (see Fig. 12.1; Einon, 1980; Tees et al., 1981; Mishima et al., 1986; Williams et al., 1990; Roof, 1993; Endo et al., 1994; Luine & Rodriguez, 1994; Lund & Lephart, 2001; Lund et al., 2001; LaBuda et al., 2002). However, numerous experiments have failed to find significant sex differences in these measures of performance (Einon, 1980; Juraska et al., 1984; Maier & Pohorecky, 1986; Kobayashi et al., 1988; Endo et al., 1994; Kolb & Cioe, 1996).

Performance on radial mazes, especially working memory, is also affected by other factors, and these factors may differentially affect the response of the genders. Ovariectomized rats and mice made more working memory errors than gonadally-intact rats and mice or ovariectomized rats treated with estradiol (Luine & Rodriguez, 1994; Daniel et al., 1997, 2006; Luine et al, 1998; Wilson et al., 1999). Yet, male rats castrated as adults still made fewer errors and had better choice accuracy than females castrated as adults (Luine & Rodriguez, 1994, see also Fig. 12.1), sug-

A Radial Arm Maze   **B** Object Placement

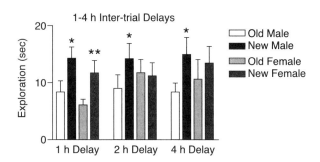

C Morris Water Maze

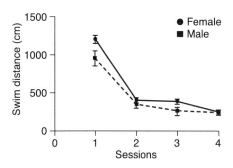

Figure 12.1. Quantitative sex differences in spatial memory tasks. (A). Radial-arm maze: Choice accuracy parameters (number correct choices in first 8 choices and choice with the first mistake) are shown for gonadectomized male (open bars, n = 5) and female (closed bars, n = 5) rats. Bars represent average ± SEM for 20 trials. Data analyzed by 2-way repeated measures ANOVA (Sex × Trial) and a significant sex effect, $*P<.05$; $**P<.01$ showed that males had higher scores than females. Data from Luine and Rodriquez, 1994. (B). Object placement. Bar graphs show performance of males (n = 8) and females (n = 8) as time (sec) spent with objects at old and new locations (see figure for bar designations). Rats viewed two identical objects and then an inter-trial delay of 1, 2, or 4 hours was given. Following the inter-trial delay, one object was moved to a new location. Data analyzed by 2-way ANOVA (Sex × Object), and differences between time at old and new objects within sexes was tested by paired t-test where $*P<.05$; $**P<.01$. Male performance was better than female performance since significantly more time was spent exploring at the new location for all inter-trial delays while females spent more time at new location only at the shortest inter-trial delay. Data from Bisagno et al., 2003. (C). Water maze. Place discrimination is shown as swim distance to reach the submerged platform across sessions for males (squares, n = 10) and females (circles, n = 12). Entries represent average ± SEM for 5 trials in each session. Data analyzed by 2-way ANOVA (Sex × session), and significant sex (P<.001) and sex × session (p0.01) effects were found. Data is for 6-months old rats. From Markowska, 1999.

gesting that these quantitative sex differences may reflect both organizing and activating effects of hormones. Additionally, both male and female rats housed in enriched, social environments made fewer working memory errors compared to rats housed alone in non-enriched environments (Juraska et al., 1984).

Estrogen improved working memory performance on a radial water maze when administered to ovari-

ectomized mice housed under non-enriched conditions, but not ovariectomized mice housed in an enriched environment (Gresack & Frick, 2004). Thus, a complex array of variables can influence performance on the radial arm maze task and possibly affect males and females differentially.

On the water maze task, rodents learn to find a small platform submerged beneath the surface of an opaque solution in a circular pool. On each trial, subjects are introduced to the pool from different compass points and use extramaze or intramaze cues to locate the hidden escape platform. In the reference memory version of the water maze, the platform location is fixed across all trials and all days. Probe trials are often given after training, during which the platform is removed and the time spent in proximity to the former location of the platform is used as a measure of retention.

Sex differences in this task are similar to those of the radial arm maze. Male rats and mice reached asymptotic performance in fewer trials and spent more time in the platform quadrant than females in some studies (see Fig. 12.1; Kelly et al., 1988; Berger-Sweeney et al., 1995; Perrot-Sinal et al., 1996; Markowska, 1999), and male mice outperformed females on a radial arm version of the water maze task (Gresack & Frick, 2003). However, a number of reports failed to find sex differences in water maze performance in rats and mice (Bucci et al., 1995; Kolb & Cioe, 1996; Perrot-Sinal et al., 1996; Healey et al., 1999; Lukoyanov et al., 1999; Markowska, 1999) and a female advantage was reported in mice (Lamberty & Gower, 1988; Frick et al., 2000).

Sex differences in water maze performance appear to be affected by various factors including age (Markowksa, 1999; Frick et al., 2000; Warren & Juraska, 2000). Interestingly, ovariectomized rats often performed better than intact females or ovariectomized rats treated with estrogen and progesterone during acquisition of the water maze task (Frye, 1995; Galea et al., 1995, 2000; Warren & Juraska, 1997, 2000; Daniel et al., 1999; Chesler & Juraska, 2000). In comparison, female mice were impaired, enhanced, or not affected by the presence of estrogen (Fugger et al., 1998; Wilson et al., 1999; Rissanen et al., 1999).

In the working memory version of the water maze, the platform is moved to a new location for each daily trial set (Steele & Morris, 1999). Although there have been no direct comparisons of males and females on working memory in the water maze task, estrogen treatment strongly enhanced retention in ovariectomized rats when females were required to remember the daily location of the submerged platform for one or two hours (Sandstrom & Williams, 2001, 2004; Daniel et al., 2005). Additionally, estradiol treatment enhanced working memory performance of ovariectomized rats during acquisition on the radial arm version of the water maze task (Bimonte et al., 1999).

Quantitative differences in performance between the sexes have been found in the object placement task (see Fig. 12.1). Males can successfully discriminate between objects at old and new locations with inter-trial delays (time between the sample and recognition trials) of up to 4 hours, while females can only discriminate at shorter inter-trial delays (approximately 1–2 hours) (Beck & Luine, 2002; Bisagno et al., 2003; Bowman et al., 2003). Like other spatial memory tasks, estradiol enhanced performance of the object placement task in ovariectomized female rats and in mice at doses that also increased dendritic spine density in CA1 of the hippocampus (Luine et al, 2003; Li et al., 2004; Jacome et al., submitted).

To summarize, quantitative sex differences in performance on classic rodent spatial tasks are reported, but these differences are often small in magnitude and not always consistent among studies. Generally, male rodents, gonadally intact or not, display better working and reference memory than female counterparts; however, a number of reports have not confirmed these sex differences. Additionally, female performance is affected by circulating levels of estrogen, and in some cases progesterone. Estradiol typically improves working memory performance in female rodents, but impairs or fails to affect reference memory performance especially in combination with progesterone.

QUALITATIVE SEX DIFFERENCES IN SPATIAL MEMORY

In solving radial arm maze and water maze tasks, male and female rats often apply different strategies which can be reflected quantitatively as sex differences in the rate and accuracy of learning a task. Williams and colleagues (Williams et al., 1990; Williams & Meck, 1991) were among the first to investigate sex differences in spatial memory performance using a radial arm maze. They demonstrated a quantitative difference in performance on a 12-arm maze, with females requiring more choices to achieve a criterion than males and making more working and reference memory errors than males during acquisition. Nevertheless, both sexes reached the same level of steady state performance by twelve trials.

These quantitative sex differences in maze performance were shown to be due to the organizing influence of estradiol on male brains during the perinatal period since neonatally castrated males and estradiol-treated females performed like control females and males, respectively (Williams et al., 1990). Later studies in gonadally-intact and gonadectomized rats confirmed both the sex differences in radial arm maze performance and prenatal hormone effects on performance (Luine & Rodriguez, 1994; Bowman et al., 2004).

The nature of the sex differences in performance was investigated by removing cues surrounding the maze and by altering the geometry of the room using drapes that followed the rectangular contours of the room or enclosed the maze in a circle (Williams et al., 1990). Performance of males and neonatally estradiol-treated females was disrupted by alteration of the geometry of the room but not movable landmarks. In contrast, the performance of control females and neonatally castrated males was not disrupted by either alteration of geometry or landmarks.

Williams et al. (1990) concluded that females construct a detailed cognitive map of all cues in the room, presumably in the hippocampus, which makes acquisition of the task slower but allows sustained, accurate performance even when cues are removed (see Fig. 12.2). On the other hand, males appear to map only a few cues and utilize a "vectoring approach," that is, use the geometric properties of the shape of the environment in relation to only a few cues. Hence males rapidly map and acquire the task, but male performance plummets when the environment is even minimally altered.

The superior performance of males compared to females during acquisition in the water maze task is indicated by the longer latencies required by females to find a submerged platform over early training trials. However, this performance difference also appears to reflect a difference in learning strategy between the sexes (see Fig. 12.2). Females show more thigmotaxis, a tendency to swim close to the walls and not venture into the open, center area of the pool (Korol, 2004). Even when the platform is visible, females will often not take a direct course to the platform, a pattern typically displayed by males (Beiko et al., 2004; see Fig. 12.2). Hence, longer latencies to locate the hidden platform by females may reflect a strategy difference in solving the task, rather than delayed acquisition of the task.

The T-maze or plus maze task allows for more direct assessment of strategy use by rodents (Restle, 1957; Tolman et al., 1947). After a subject reaches a criterion of successful performance (e.g., 9 correct visits to the baited arm of the T-maze in 10 trials), the strategy used can be probed by rotating the start arm 180° (see Fig. 12.2). Subjects that continue to visit the same location on the probe trial are using a place or allocentric strategy; subjects that continue to turn left (or right) on the probe trial are using a response or egocentric strategy. Permanent lesions or transient inactivation of the male hippocampus during training inhibited use of a place strategy while lesions or inactivation of the striatum during training inhibited use of a response strategy (Packard & McGaugh, 1996; Chang & Gold, 2003b).

Almost 90% of male rats initially adopted a place strategy in some studies depending on the arrangement of cues, but many of these place learners changed to response learners using an egocentric strategy after continued training (Packard & McGaugh, 1996; Chang & Gold, 2003a). No direct comparisons of male and female rats have been made of strategy use on T-mazes, but Korol et al. (2004) found that female rats often utilize both strategies depending on the stage of their reproductive cycle. During the proestrus phase of the estrous cycle, female rats utilized predominantly a place strategy, while during the estrous phase females predominantly used a response strategy (see Fig. 12.2). Thus, T-maze performance appears to show a sex difference in strategy use and may provide a useful model for probing the nature and basis for the qualitative sex differences displayed in spatial memory tasks.

HORMONAL EFFECTS ON QUALITATIVE SEX DIFFERENCES IN SPATIAL MEMORY

Exposure of animals to stressors and the resultant release of corticosterone are associated with numerous physiological changes, as well as effects on neural function and behavior (McEwen, 2001, 2002). Stress also evokes striking, qualitative differences in cognitive function in males and females. When exposed to 21 days of daily restraint (6 hours per day), males show impaired performance on spatial memory tasks, including object placement (Beck & Luine, 1999, 2002), radial arm maze (Luine et al., 1994), Y-maze (Conrad et al., 1996), and water maze (Kitraki et al., 2004).

Females, on the other hand, show enhanced performance on all these tasks following the same 21 days

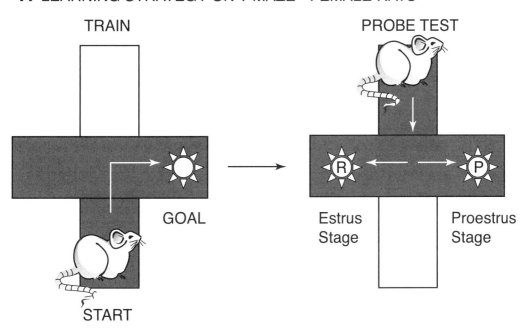

A LEARNING STRATEGY ON T-MAZE - FEMALE RATS

TRAIN

PROBE TEST

GOAL

START

Estrus
Stage

Proestrus
Stage

Figure 12.2. Qualitative sex differences in spatial memory tasks. (A). Learning strategy on T-Maze: female rats. Female rats were trained to find food reward (goal) on a T-maze. During training, the start and goal arms remained constant so that subjects could use either a place strategy (P, go to a specific place-arm) or a response strategy (R, turn right). During the probe trial, the maze was turned 180 degrees, and the strategy used during training assessed. As indicated in probe figure, Korol et al., (2004) reported that rats at proestrus were significantly more likely to use a place strategy (71%) while rats in estrus were significantly more likely to use a response strategy (71%). (B). Learning strategy on T-maze: male rats. Male rats were trained to find food reward (goal) on a T-maze. During training, the start and goal arms remain constant so that subjects could use either a place strategy (P, go to a specific place-arm) or a response strategy (R, turn right). During the probe trial, the maze was rotated 180 degrees, and the strategy used during training assessed. As indicated in probe figure, Packard and McGaugh, (1996) reported that 90% of male rats used a place strategy. (C). Learning strategy on radial-arm maze: female rats. A female rat is depicted as being in the center of a radial-arm maze and looking at cues in the room. Cues, both landmarks such as a plant, telephone or microscope, and geometry of the room such as cupboards which make angles, are used to make a cognitive map for exploration and remembrance of arms explored. Females make a detailed map of all landmarks and geometry which is depicted by the arrows emanating from the eyes and going to all cues (See Williams et al., [1990] for further information and discussion). (D). Learning strategy on radial-arm maze: male rats. A male rat is depicted in the same environment as the female in (C). Males do not make a detailed map of all landmarks and geometry, but use mainly geometry of the room with a few landmarks to make a cognitive map (See Williams et al., [1990] for further discussion). The detailed map made by females (C) contributes to their slower acquisition of the task as compared to males; see Figure 12.1. (E). Learning strategy on Morris water maze: male and female rats. Female rats often employ a thigmostaxic strategy on early trials when learning the water maze task. The strategy to swim near the edge of the pool increases the time and distance required to find the hidden platform. In contrast, male rats often search near the center of the pool and locate the platform in less time and distance than females.

Figure 12.2. (*continued*)

B LEARNING STRATEGY ON T-MAZE - MALE RATS

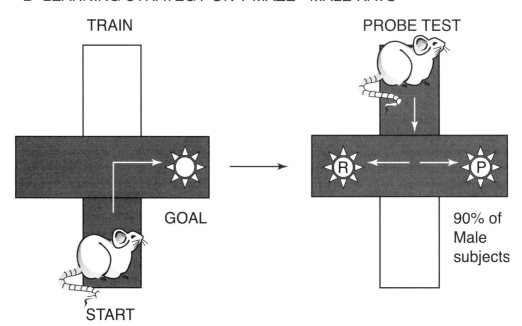

TRAIN

PROBE TEST

GOAL

START

90% of
Male
subjects

C SPATIAL MAPPING BY FEMALE RATS ON RAM

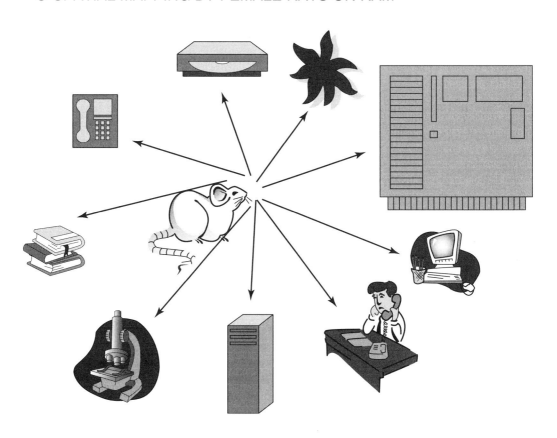

D SPATIAL MAPPING BY MALE RATS ON RAM

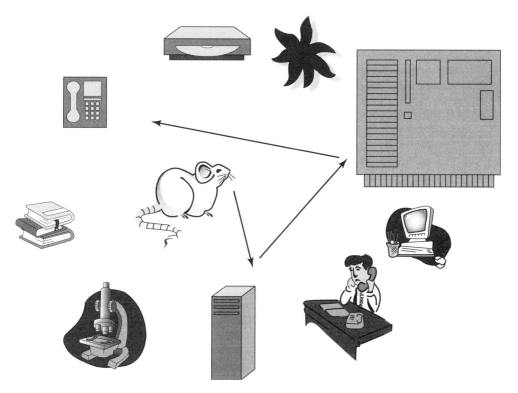

E SPATIAL MAPPING BY MALE AND FEMALE RATS IN WATER MAZE

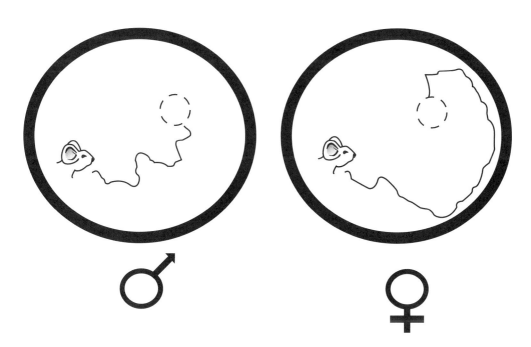

Figure 12.2. (*continued*)

of restraint stress (see Fig. 12.3; Bowman et al., 2001; Beck & Luine, 2002; Luine 2002; Bowman et al., 2003; Conrad et al., 2003; Kitraki et al., 2004). Sex differences in response to stress also are maintained at shorter stress intervals (Luine et al., 1996; Conrad et al., 2004; Bowman, 2005). In addition, estradiol appears to influence the stress response, since ovariectomized rats failed to show enhanced radial arm maze performance following 21 days of daily restraint stress (Bowman et al., 2002).

However, ovariectomy does not completely reverse the sex difference in response to stress, as ovariectomized rats were not impaired by restraint stress as is the case with males. Thus, chronic stress causes opposite effects on performance of spatial memory tasks in males and females. In these studies, the rats displaying sex differences in the behavioral effects of stress also showed related sex differences in stress effects on activity of monoaminergic systems in the hippocampus, frontal cortex, and amygdala (Luine et al., 2001; Bowman et al., 2003), and other studies have found sex differences in stress effects on morphology of hippocampal neurons (Galea et al., 1997; McLaughlin et al., 2006).

Another series of intriguing studies indicates that learning strategies used by female rats are also affected profoundly by gonadal hormones. Korol and associates have highlighted the qualitative versus quantitative dichotomy for sexual differences in cognition by focusing on " . . . *what* and *how* information is learned, and thus not only *how much* is learned . . ." (Korol, 2004). Ovariectomized rats treated with estrogen for 2 days prior to training reached a performance criterion in fewer training trials on a T-maze task that required the use of an allocentric or place strategy compared to ovariectomized rats treated with a vehicle (Korol & Kolo, 2002). Equally interesting, females without estrogen reached the criterion in fewer trials when learning depended on an egocentric or response strategy compared to females receiving estrogen. Similarly, gonadally-intact female rats were more likely to select a place strategy to solve the T-maze task (Restle, 1957) when estrogen levels were elevated naturally at proestrus, and more likely to select a response strategy when estrogen levels were low at estrus (Korol et al., 2004; see Fig. 12.3).

Taken together, these studies suggest that the learning strategy employed by female rats depends on circulating levels of estrogen. Estrogen biases females to use allocentric strategies that create three-dimensional relationships between stimuli in the surrounding environment ("go to this place") and depend primarily on hippocampal processing. Females with insufficient estrogen, following ovariectomy or during estrus, are biased to use egocentric strategies that guide learning by internal or proprioceptive cues ("turn right") and depend primarily on striatal processing.

Furthermore, the use of an allocentric strategy was associated with an increase in acetylcholine release in the hippocampus during training (Marriott & Korol, 2003), while inhibition of the hippocampus by enhanced GABAergic activity induced a shift from an allocentric strategy to an egocentric strategy (Korol, 2004). These neuropharmacological findings are supported by earlier evidence that estradiol promotes cholinergic and inhibits GABAergic neurotransmission in the female hippocampus (Luine, 1985; Luine et al., 1997; Murphy et al., 1998; Gibbs & Aggarwal, 1998; Gibbs, 2000; Gibbs et al., 2004).

Several other reports confirm the effects of estrogen on the use of learning strategies by female rats. Ovariectomized rats treated with estradiol required fewer days to master a place version of a radial arm maze task than a response version (Davis et al., 2005). Additionally, ovariectomized rats treated with vehicle outperformed females treated with estradiol on a response version of the task.

Daniel and Lee (2004) reported that chronic estradiol implants impaired learning in ovariectomized rats when the only cue available to guide escape to a submerged platform was a landmark within the pool. Alternatively, ovariectomized rats without estradiol replacement were impaired when this intrapool landmark was unavailable.

These studies support the hypothesis proposed by Daniel (2006) that estrogen facilitates the use of hippocampal strategies that allow female rats to establish flexible relationships between the stimuli in a learning environment, such as the relationships between extramaze cues and the location of a goal. Alternatively, the lack of estrogen promotes the use of striatal strategies that establish inflexible relationships between a single stimulus, such an intramaze landmark, and a response (Daniel, 2006). The effects of gonadal hormones on learning strategy selection and use by males have not yet been reported. Future experiments will be necessary; not only to compare male and female learning strategies directly, but to deter-

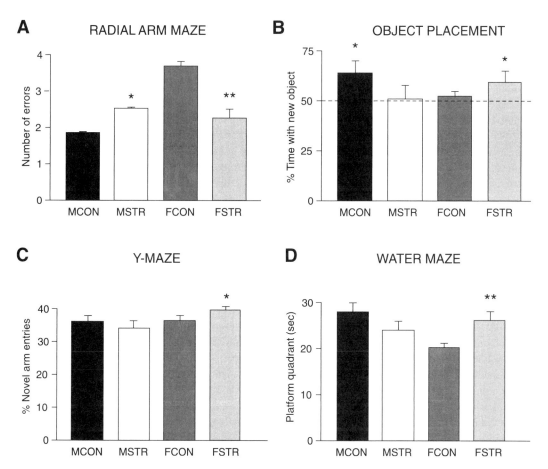

Figure 12.3. Sex differences in chronic-stress effects on spatial memory tasks. (A). Radial-arm maze. Male and female rats were stressed (STR) or not (CON) by 6 h/day of restraint for 21 days. The total number of errors made in completing the radial-arm maze task (average ± SEM) is shown. Separate experiments in the sexes were performed and analyzed by 2-way repeated measures ANOVA (group × trials), and significant group effects were found: *P<.05, MSTR different from MCON; **P<.001, FSTR different from FCON. Stressed male performance is decreased as compared to non-stress while performance in stressed females is enhanced. Male data from Luine et al., (1994), and female data from Bowman et al., (2001). (B). Object Placement. Males and females were stressed (STR) or not (CON) by 6 h/day of restraint for 21 days. The percentage of time spent exploring the object in the new location in trials with a 4 h inter-trial delay between the sample trial and the recognition trial is shown. Dashed line at 50% indicates chance discrimination (same amount of time spent exploring object at the old and new location). Ability to discriminate between old and new locations in each group was tested by paired t-test where *P<.05, **P<.01. Control males were able to discriminate between locations, but stress impaired male performance. Control females did not significantly discriminate; however, stress enhanced their performance and stressed females were able to successfully discriminate between locations. Data from Beck and Luine, (2002). (C). Y-Maze. Male and female rats were stressed (STR) or not (CON) by 6 h/day of restraint for 21 days. Data represent the percentage of entries made into the novel arms during a 2–5 min. trial. Stressed females entered the novel arm more than the start and other arms indicating enhanced memory (Wilcoxon, where *P<.05) whereas control and stressed males did not. Data from Conrad et al., (2003). (D). Morris water maze. Male and female rats were stressed (STR) or not (CON) by 6 h/day of restraint for 21 days. Data are the mean ± SEM of time spent in target quadrant (quadrant where platform was located) during the 60 s probe trial (platform is removed). Stress enhanced female performance since more time was spent by stressed subjects in the target quadrant than control females (** P<.005). Stressed males did not spend more time in the target quadrant, and not shown on the graph is the result that stressed males spent significantly more time in the opposite quadrant than control males. Thus, stress impaired male performance. Data from Kitraki et al., (2004).

mine if similar mechanisms underlie the implementation of these strategies by each gender.

Although the idea that there are different types of learning dates back to at least the nineteenth century (Squire, 1987), only a few investigators have explored the proposal that learning strategies might differ between males and females, an important hypothesis that is supported by growing empirical evidence.

SEX DIFFERENCES IN NON-SPATIAL MEMORY TASKS

Fewer studies have examined possible sex difference in memory tasks that are not dependent on the hippocampus, and most were conducted many years ago. However, Shors and colleagues have extensively investigated the classical conditioning paradigms of eyeblink responses in relation to sex differences.

In eyeblink response conditioning, subjects learn to associate a conditioned stimulus (CS) such as a white noise burst with the unconditioned stimulus (US), a periorbital shock. Eyeblinks occurring after CS onset, but prior to the US onset are considered conditioned responses (CR). Unlike spatial learning and memory tasks, females acquire this task in fewer trials than males (Fig. 12.4). Female rats registered approximately 80% CRs in the first 200 trials while males showed only approximately 50% CRs (Wood & Shors, 1998). As is the pattern with other cognitive tasks, further training equalizes performance between the sexes.

In addition to this quantitative difference in performance, qualitative sex differences were reported in acquisition following stress. Twenty-four hours following a 30-minute session of 30 tail shocks, acquisition of the CR was facilitated in males but impaired in females (Fig. 12.4). In the first 200 trials, stressed males showed 80% CRs while stressed females showed only 20% CRs, a large difference in the percentages of CRs and a dramatic reversal from the superior performance of females in the non-stressed state (Shors et al., 2000; Shors, 2004). The opposite effects of stress on male and female performance in the eyeblink conditioning task are paralleled by the opposite effects of this stress on dendritic spine density in the CA hippocampal region of male and female rats (Shors et al., 2001).

Shors and colleagues have also investigated trace eyeblink conditioning. In this paradigm, the CS and US are separated by a longer interval, and thus a memory "trace" of the CS must be maintained by the subjects (Beylin & Shors, 1998). Hippocampal lesions prevented acquisition and short-term retention of the conditioned response indicating that trace eyeblink conditioning is a hippocampal dependent, nonspatial memory task (Beylin & Shors, 1998). Like regular eyeblink conditioning, females acquired the task faster and showed approximately 50% CRs as compared to approximately 20% CRs in males. Trace eyeblink conditioning is likewise affected by acute stress and is associated with female impairments and male enhancements in acquisition. Like the sex differences in the response to stress for spatial memory tasks, circulating estradiol appears to contribute to the sex differences in eyeblink conditioning paradigms (Leuner et al., 2004; Wood & Shors, 1998); however, it is unknown whether a qualitative/strategy difference exists between the sexes in acquisition of this task.

Avoidance conditioning has traditionally involved placing a subject in a two-compartment box where a shock is received in one compartment (distinguished by light intensity or other cues) but not in the adjacent compartment. Typically, shocks are administered, and subjects are tested for their latency to enter the shock compartment 24 h later. Avoidance paradigms can be active such that the subject must leave or escape the shock compartment (*active avoidance conditioning*) or passive such that the subject must remain in the non-shock compartment to avoid shock (*passive avoidance conditioning*).

Quantitative sex differences have been reported using both paradigms. For active avoidance, intact or gonadectomized females acquired the behavior in fewer trials than gonadectomized males, and neonatal treatment of females with androgens resulted in behavior like that of males (van Haaren et al., 1990). Thus, this sex difference in avoidance responding appears to be organized but not activated by gonadal hormones. In passive avoidance paradigms, males generally condition in fewer trials, but some exceptions have been found (van Haaren et al., 1990). Testosterone appears to enhance or activate avoidance responding since gonadectomy impaired male but not female performance. Unlike active avoidance, organizational effects of testosterone on performance of passive avoidance have not been reported.

Object recognition is a task that does not rely on conditioning or either positive or negative

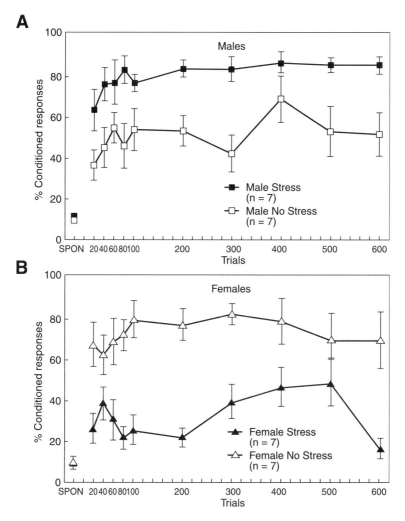

Figure 12.4. Eyeblink conditioning: sex differences and stress effects. (A). Males—The Percent Conditioned Responses (CRs) is plotted for control males and males who received 30 min of tail shock stress (see legend). Control males show approximately 40% conditioned responses which is lower than control females, approximately 70%, see (B). Exposure to the stressor facilitated acquisition of the CR 24 h after stressor cessation. (B). Females—The Percent Conditioned Responses is plotted for control females and females who received 30 min of tail shock stress (see legend). Control females show approximately 70% conditioned responses which is higher than control males (see A). Exposure to the same stressor impaired female acquisition of the CR 24 h after stressor cessation. Unstressed females elicited more CRs than unstressed males during the first day of training (1–300 trials), but were not significantly different from each other by the second day of training (301–600 trials). Reprinted with permission from Wood GE, Shors TJ. (1998). Stress facilitates classical conditioning in males, but impairs classical conditioning in females though activational effects of ovarian hormones. *Proc Natl Acad Sci USA*, 7:4066–4071.

reinforcement, but this task relies on the exploratory nature of rats and interest in novelty. Subjects are presented objects in the sample trial, and following delays of minutes to hours, they are presented the old object and a new object in a recognition/retention trial. If subjects explore the new object more then the old object, then they are considered to have remembered the old object (see section on object placement for a more detailed description). No quantitative sex differences have been identified in this task; males and females discriminate objects after inter-trial delays of 4 h equally well (Beck & Luine, 2002; Bisagno et al., 2003a,b).

Performance is thus unlike object placement (spatial memory task) in which males successfully discriminate with longer inter-trial delays than females. Interestingly, like the object placement and eye blink conditioning tasks, a sex difference in performance following chronic stress is present: male object recognition performance was impaired but female performance was not when 21 days of daily restraint stress was given (Beck & Luine, 2002; Luine 2002; Bowman et al., 2003). Thus, object recognition does not show quantitative sex differences, but qualitative sex differences are evident following stress.

Thus, a number of memory tasks, which are not dependent on major input from the hippocampus, show substantial quantitative performance differences between the sexes. Some of these differences are dependent on alterations in brain by gonadal hormones during the perinatal, critical period for brain sexual differentiation. Whether these quantitative differences emanate from qualitative differences in strategies used by the sexes remains to be investigated. Other parameters may also contribute to these sex differences and are discussed in the following section.

PSYCHOLOGICAL PERFORMANCE PARAMETERS VERSUS COGNITIVE DIFFERENCES

Do sex differences in cognitive performance actually reflect sex differences in the processes and underlying mechanisms of learning and memory? Non-mnemonic variables can affect performance on cognitive tasks, but these variables are considered to be outside the primary domain of learning and memory systems. Gender and hormones can affect a wide range of non-mnemonic variables including sensory and percep-

tion processes, motor activities, affective states, and regulatory functions (see Fig. 12.5; Dohanich, 2002). In particular, the effects of gender and hormones on the hypothalamic-pituitary-adrenal axis can influence cognition profoundly by modulating stress responses and anxiety levels. Furthermore, housing conditions, single or group (Beck & Luine, 2002) and enriched or non-enriched (Daniel et al., 1999), also have sexually dimorphic impacts on performance of cognitive tasks.

Non-mnemonic factors can be most intrusive to learning during acquisition of cognitive tasks, particularly during early trials when subjects become anxious in the testing environment and experiment with different strategies to solve the problem at hand. Consequently, performance during training may reflect these processes rather than learning itself. Acclimation or pretraining allows subjects to become familiar with the demands of the task and various aspects of learning the task, as well as handling by experimenters, transport to the testing room, and the novelty of the learning environment (Saucier et al., 1996; Cain et al., 1996; Cain, 1997, 1998).

Pretraining can reduce the influence of these variables on performance (Beiko et al., 1997; Cain, 1997; Hoh & Cain, 1997); and not surprisingly, when rats were pretrained adequately before actual training, males and females learned some maze tasks at similar rates (Bucci et al., 1995). That males and females typically achieve the same level of performance after sufficient training/acclimation in radial arm mazes and water mazes, and continue to perform similarly after tasks have been learned also supports the hypothesis that quantitative sex differences may result from non-mnemonic factors or strategy selection than actual differences in cognitive ability.

Variations in performance across the estrous cycle of female rats (Warren & Juraska, 1997) also were eliminated by handling and pre-exposure to a water maze (Berry et al., 1997). Further, female rats with higher levels of estrogen and progesterone performed poorly on the initial trials of a water maze task because they swam near the pool wall more than females with low levels of these hormones although both groups reached the same level of performance on later trials (Korol, 2004). The initial thigmotaxic strategy, less effective in this task, may have been caused by hormone dependent effects on anxiety in early trials or attending to less relevant cues such as the pool wall (Korol, 2004).

However, pretraining does not eliminate sex differences in all cognitive tasks, and sex differences are

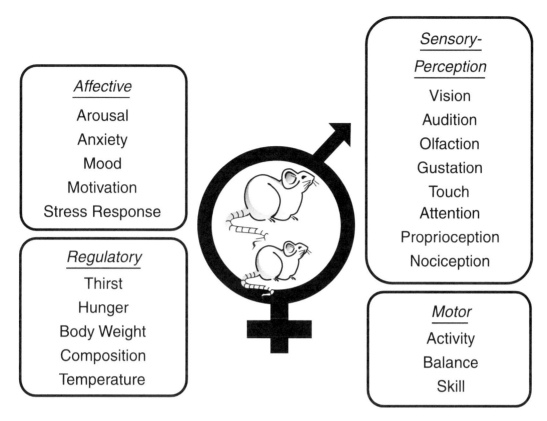

Figure 12.5. Non-nmemonic effects on memory performance. Male and female rodents display sex differences over a wide range of affective, regulatory, sensory-perception, and motor functions which could influence performance of tasks.

present in not only acquisition but in short-term memory for the tasks. As discussed earlier, male rodents discriminate location in the object placement task better than females (males can discriminate at longer inter-trial delays, and thus exhibit better working memory of places in the task). Better male performance is present despite extensive pretraining/acclimation/habituation trials on the open field and on the task itself (Beck & Luine, 2002; Bisagno et al., 2003a,b). Likewise, acquisition of radial arm maze performance can remain superior in male as compared to female rats despite extensive behavioral evaluations being conducted before radial arm maze trials (Bowman et al., 2004).

The demands and contingencies of specific tasks may constitute another important variable which obscures or confounds measurement of sex differences. For example, object placement does not depend on reinforcement of any variety (aversive or positive), while the water maze task presents an aversive component (possibility of drowning) if the invisible, sanctuary platform is not found. Compounding the possibility of drowning, the generally tepid or sometimes cold water may provide additional stress to the subject. Thus, performance of this task may be susceptible to several potent, non-mnemonic variables. A recent study showed release of stress levels of corticosterone across trials which did not habituate (Engelhardt, et al, 2006), and other recent studies illuminate a number of confounds that this aversive task engenders in subjects (Frick et al., 2004; Rubinow et al., 2004). The radial arm maze requires food deprivation, and hormones, notably estradiol, influence food intake (see Dohanich, 2002), which could impact performance on this task.

Lastly, it is also relevant to consider the origin of behavioral tasks when assessing possible sex differences in performance. When behavioral psychologists develop tasks to measure specific behaviors, extensive control experiments are completed to investigate possible contingencies that directly influence task performance and to identify other extraneous parameters that may indirectly affect performance (Olton et al., 1978, 1979). Unfortunately, male rats and mice were the targeted subjects for all tasks currently utilized in almost all learning and memory assessments. Thus, most of the tasks currently in use to mitigate (or enhance) the effects of mnemonic and non-mnemonic variables are biased toward males.

ARE SEX DIFFERENCES IN LEARNING AND MEMORY IMPORTANT?

There can be few objections to the conclusion that gender and hormones play definitive roles in processes critical to successful reproduction, but current scientific literature provides less compelling examples of differences in cognitive ability between the sexes. Alternatively, the effects of gender and hormones on non-mnemonic variables that can affect cognitive function and on the choice of strategies used to learn a task are both intriguing and germane. These variables, however, require further and systematic investigation for validation.

A discussion of the importance of sex differences in the performance of cognitive tasks can be approached from two perspectives. An *evolutionary* model explains the emergence of sex differences in cognition as adaptive to the reproductive success of the male and female members of a species. A *utilitarian* model acknowledges gender differences in learning styles rather than in cognitive ability, and promotes policies and practices that recognize these differences in educational settings.

The evolution of distinct cognitive systems seems to be a reasonable prediction because the male and female members of many species often face different challenges in the quest to reproduce and nurture offspring. Several evolutionary models have been proposed to explain why sex differences in cognitive systems might have emerged. In some species in which the reproductive success of males is related to range size, males might be expected to have better cognitive ability than females. According to the male-range hypothesis, males with large ranges will find more females with which to mate and/or be selected by females based on the area of their territories. Superior male spatial ability might also be predicated on the

navigational and agonistic demands faced by male members of some species (Ecuyer-Dab & Robert, 2004). In support of this theory, polygamous male voles have larger hippocampal volumes than females (Jacobs et al., 1990). However, whether similar structural differences translate into superior spatial ability in other mammals has not been confirmed definitively.

Other hypotheses to explain putative sex differences in cognitive function focus on the roles of adaptive pressures unique to females. The *female foraging* hypothesis proposes that female members of some species must search their environments to nourish themselves and their offspring more commonly than their male counterparts and therefore should display better spatial ability (Eals & Silverman, 1997; He et al., 1997). The *fertility and parental care* hypothesis proposes that less mobile females, especially during periods of fertility and maternity, are at less risk, and therefore should display less developed spatial ability (Sherry & Hampson, 1997).

As extension of this hypothesis, Ecuyer-Dab and Robert (2004) proposed that maternity favors limited navigation and familiarity with local cues in the immediate environment reducing risks to mothers and their offspring. The *female communication* hypothesis proposes that females of some species benefit by diverting more cognitive capacity to non-spatial processes, such as communication, especially during periods of mating (Desmond & Levy, 1997).

Finally, the *female range* hypothesis emerged from the early field research of Calhoun (1962) who observed that wild female rats explore and mark an area beyond their normal territory the night before reaching sexual receptivity in order to attract mates (Cooke & Woolley, 2005a). Therefore, enhanced spatial cognition during this precopulatory phase of the estrous cycle might provide a reproductive advantage to females by attracting more potential mates. Although each of these evolutionary explanations is intriguing, convincing support has not been forthcoming. Nevertheless, the differences in environmental pressures faced by mammalian species leads to the proposition that sex differences in cognitive function also vary across species, shaped by the unique natural history of each species. Therefore, attempts to draw broad conclusions about the evolution of sex differences in cognition across species may be unwarranted. However, the advantages provided by enhanced cognition to successful reproduction, gestation, and maternity must be considered by investigators in their attempts to understand the putative sex differences in cognitive functioning.

CONCLUSIONS

Much has been written and debated regarding the existence and significance of sex differences in cognitive function (Kimura, 1999). Generalizations about superior spatial ability in males versus superior verbal ability in females abound and are often accepted by the public as scientific fact. The unfortunate consequence of these widely-held beliefs is that stereotypes have emerged that create barriers to both males and females in their social and professional lives. If contemporary research on species other than humans reveals any constructive findings about sex differences in cognition it is that males and females learn and remember information using distinct strategies.

Furthermore, many of the sex differences in cognition in rodents discussed in this chapter are small in magnitude and appear to be within the normal range of performance for males, and some of these sex differences disappear with pre-exposure to the learning environment, with additional training, or with altering the features of the task being learned. Thus, male and female rodents typically reach identical levels of performance on most cognitive tasks although their rates and strategies of learning may differ.

Another important, emerging concept is that hormones exert sexually dimorphic effects on cognitive function. Males and females show distinctly different responses to chronic stress on a variety of tasks, and females show different cognitive strategies depending on the level of circulating gonadal hormones. Thus, possible sex differences in cognition must be approached with a wider view than just simple quantification of performance, and definitive conclusions regarding the nature and scope of cognitive sex differences await results of such detailed and more sophisticated studies.

References

Adams MM, Shah RA, Janssen WG, Morrison JH. (2001). Different modes of hippocampal plasticity in response to estrogen in young and aged female rats. *Proc Natl Acad Sci USA*, 98:8071–8076.

Andrade JP, Madeira MD, Paula-Barbosa MM. (2000). Sexual dimorphism in the subiculum of the rat hippocampal formation. *Brain Res*, 875:125–137.

Baddeley AD, Hitch GJ. (1974). Working memory. In Bower GA (Ed.), *The psychology of learning and motivation: advances in research and theory* Vol. 8, (pp. 47–90). New York: Academic Press.

Baum MJ, Everitt BJ. (1992). Increased expression of c-fos in the medial preoptic area after mating in male rats: role of afferent inputs from the medial amygdala and midbrain central tegmental field. *Neuroscience*, 50:627–646.

Beck KD, Luine VN. (1999). Food deprivation modulates chronic stress effects on object recognition in male rats: role of monoamines and amino acids. *Brain Res*, 830:56–71.

Beck KD, Luine VN. (2002). Sex differences in behavioral and neurochemical profiles after chronic stress: role of housing conditions. *Physiol Behav*, 75:661–673.

Beiko J, Candusso L, Cain DP. (1997). The effects of nonspatial water maze pretraining in rats subjected to serotonin depletion and muscarinic receptor antagonism: a detailed behavioural assessment of spatial performances. *Behav Brain Res*, 88:201–211.

Beiko J, Lander R, Hampson E, Boon F, Cain DP. (2004). Contribution of sex differences in the acute stress response to sex differences in water maze performance in the rat. *Behav Brain Res*, 151:239–253.

Berger-Sweeney J, Arnold A, Gabeau D, Mills J. (1995). Sex differences in learning and memory in mice: effects of sequence of testing and cholinergic blockade. *Behav Neurosci*, 109:859–873.

Berry B, McMahan R, Gallagher M. (1997). Spatial learning and memory at defined points of the estrous cycle: effects on performance of a hippocampal-dependent task. *Behav Neurosci*, 111:267–274.

Berta P, Hawkins JR, Sinclair AH, Taylor A, Griffiths BL, Goodfellow PN, et al. (1990). Genetic evidence equating SRY and the testis-determining factor. *Nature*, 348:448–450.

Beylin AV, Shors TJ. (1998). Stress enhances excitatory trace eyeblink conditioning and opposes acquisition of inhibitory conditioning. *Behav Neurosci*, 112:1327–1338.

Bimonte HA, Denenberg VH (1999) Estradiol facilitates performance as working memory load increases. *Psychoneuroendocrinology*, 24:161–173.

Bisagno V, Bowman R, Luine V. (2003a). Functional aspects of estrogen neuroprotection. *Endocrine*, 21:33–41.

Bisagno V, Ferguson D, Luine VN. (2003b). Chronic D-amphetamine induces sexually dimorphic effects on locomotion, recognition memory, and brain monoamines. *Pharmacol Biochem Behav*, 74:859–867.

Bowman RE. (2005). Stress-induced changes in spatial memory are sexually differentiated and vary across the lifespan. *J Neuroendocrinol*, 17:526–535.

Bowman RE, Zrull MC, Luine VN. (2001). Chronic restraint stress enhances radial arm maze performance in female rats. *Brain Res*, 904:279–289.

Bowman RE, Ferguson D, Luine VN. (2002). Effects of chronic restraint stress and estradiol on open field activity, spatial memory, and monoaminergic neurotransmitters in ovariectomized rats. *Neuroscience*, 113:401–410.

Bowman RE, Beck KD, Luine VN. (2003). Chronic stress effects on memory: sex differences in performance and monoaminergic activity. *Horm Behav*, 43:48–59.

Bowman RE, MacLusky NJ, Sarmiento Y, Frankfurt M, Gordon M, Luine VN. (2004). Sexually dimorphic effects of prenatal stress on cognition, hormonal responses, and central neurotransmitters. *Endocrinology*, 145:3778–3787.

Bucci, DJ, Chiba AA, Gallagher M. (1995). Spatial learning in male and female Long-Evans rats. *Behav Neurosci*, 109:180–183.

Cain DP. (1997). Prior non-spatial pretraining eliminates sensorimotor disturbances and impairments in water maze learning caused by diazepam. *Psychopharmacology* (Berl), 130:313–319.

Cain DP. (1998). Testing the NMDA, long-term potentiation, and cholinergic hypotheses of spatial learning. *Neurosci Behav Revs*, 22:181–193.

Cain DP, Saucier D, Hall J, Hargreaves, EL, Boon, EF. (1996). Detailed behavioral analysis of water maze acquisition under APV or CNQX: contribution of sensorimotor disturbances to drug-induced acquisition deficits. *Behav Neurosci*, 110:86–102.

Calhoun JB. (1962). Population density and social pathology. *Sci Am*, 206:139–148.

Chang Q, Gold PE. (2003a). Switching memory systems during learning: changes in patterns of brain acetylcholine release in the hippocampus and striatum in rats. *J Neurosci*, 23:3001–3005.

Chang Q, Gold PE. (2003b). Intra-hippocampal lidocaine injections impair acquisition of a place task and facilitate acquisition of a response task in rats. *Behav Brain Res*, 144:19–24.

Chesler EJ, Juraska JM. (2000). Acute administration of estrogen and progesterone impairs the acquisition of the spatial Morris water maze in ovariectomized rats. *Horm Behav*, 38:234–242.

Conrad CD, Galea LA, Kuroda Y, McEwen BS. (1996). Chronic stress impairs rat spatial memory on the Y maze, and this effect is blocked by tianeptine pretreatment. *Behav Neurosci*, 110:1321–1334.

Conrad CD, Grote KA, Hobbs RJ, Ferayorni A. (2003). Sex differences in spatial and non-spatial Y-maze performance after chronic stress. *Neurobio Learn Mem*, 79:32–40.

Conrad CD, Jackson JL, Wieczorek L, Baran SE, Harman JS, Wright RL, Korol DL. (2004). Acute stress impairs spatial memory in male but not female rats: influence of estrous cycle. *Pharmacol Biochem Behav*, 78:569–579.

Cooke BM, Woolley CS. (2005a). Gonadal hormone modulation of dendrites in the mammalian CNS. *J Neurobiol*, 64:34–46.

Cooke BM, Woolley CS (2005b) Sexually dimorphic synaptic organization of the medial amygdala. *J Neurosci* 25:10759–10767.

Cooke BM, Tabibnia G, Breedlove SM. (1999). A brain sexual dimorphism controlled by adult circulating androgens. *Proc Natl Acad Sci USA*, 96:7538–7540.

Cooke BM, Breedlove SM, Jordan CL. (2003). Both estrogen receptors and androgen receptors contribute to testosterone-induced changes in the morphology of the medial amygdala and sexual arousal in male rats. *Horm Behav*, 43:336–346.

Daniel JM. (2006). Effects of estrogen on cognition: what have we learned from basic research? *J Neuroendocrinol*, 18:787–795.

Daniel JM, Dohanich GP. (2001). Acetylcholine mediates the estrogen-induced increase in NMDA receptor binding in CA1 of the hippocampus and the associated improvement in working memory. *J Neurosci*, 21:6949–6956.

Daniel JM, Lee CD. (2004). Estrogen replacement in ovariectomized rats affects strategy selection in the Morris water maze. *Neurobiol Learn Mem*, 82:142–149.

Daniel JM, Fader AJ, Spencer AL, Dohanich GP. (1997). Estrogen enhances performance of female rats during acquisition of a radial arm maze. *Horm Behav*, 32:217–225.

Daniel JM, Roberts SL, Dohanich GP. (1999). Effects of ovarian hormones and environment on radial maze and water maze performance of female rats. *Physiol Behav*, 66:11–20.

Daniel JM, Hulst JL, Lee CD. (2005). Role of hippocampal M2 muscarinic receptors in the estrogen-induced enhancement of working memory. *Neuroscience*, 132:57–64.

Daniel JM, Hulst JL, Berbling JL. (2006). Estradiol replacement enhances working memory in middle-aged rats when initiated immediately after ovariectomy but not after a long-term period of ovarian hormone deprivation. *Endocrinology*, 147:607–614.

Davis DM, Jacobson TK, Aliakbari S, Mizumori SJ. (2005). Differential effects of estrogen on hippocampal- and striatal-dependent learning. *Neurobiol Learn Mem*, 84:132–137.

Desmond NL, Levy WB. (1997). Ovarian steroidal control of connectivity in the female hippocampus: an overview of recent experimental findings and speculations on its functional consequences. *Hippocampus*, 7:239–245.

De Vries GJ. (2004). Minireview: Sex differences in adult and developing brains: compensation, compensation, compensation. *Endocrinology*, 145:1063–1068.

De Vries GJ, Simerly RB. (2002). Anatomy, development, and function of sexually dimorphic neural circuits in the mammalian brain. In Pfaff DW, Arnold AP, Etgen AM, Farbach SE, Rubin RT, (Eds.), *Hormones, brain and behavior*, (pp.137–191). San Diego: Academic Press.

Dohanich GP. (2002). Gonadal steriods, learning and memory. In Pfaff DW, Arnold AP, Etgen AM, Farbach SE, Rubin RT, (Eds.) *Hormones, brain and behavior* (pp. 265–327). San Diego: Academic Press.

Eals M, Silverman I. (1997). The hunter-gatherer theory of spatial sex differences: proximate factors mediating the female advantage in recall of object arrays. *Ethol Sociobiol*, 15:95–105.

Ecuyer-Dab I, Robert M. (2004). Have sex differences in spatial ability evolved from male competition for mating and female concern for survival? *Cognition*, 91:221–257.

Eichenbaum H. (1999). Neurobiology. The topography of memory. *Nature*, 402:597–599.

Einon D. (1980). Spatial memory and response strategies in rats: age, sex and rearing differences in performance. *Quarterly J of Exp Psychology*, 32:473–489.

Endo Y, Mizuno T, Fujita K, Funabashi T, Kimura F. (1994). Soft-diet feeding during development enhances later learning abilities in female rats. *Physiol Behav*, 56:629–633.

Ennaceur A, Aggleton JP. (1994). Spontaneous recognition of object configurations in rats: effects of fornix lesions. *Exp Brain Res*, 100:85–92.

Ennaceur A, Neave N, Aggleton JP. (1997). Spontaneous object recognition and object location memory in rats: the effects of lesions in the cingulate cortices, the medial prefrontal cortex, the cingulum bundle and the fornix. *Exp Brain Res*, 113:509–519.

Englemann M, Ebner K, Landgraf R, Wotjak CT. (2006). Effects of Morris water maze testing on the neuroendocrine stress response and intrahypothalamic release of vasopressin and oxytocin in the rat. *Horm Behav*, 50: 496–501.

Frankland PW, Bontempi B. (2005). The organization of recent and remote memories. *Nat Rev Neurosci*, 6:119–130.

Frick KM, Burlingame LA, Arters JA, Berger-Sweeney J. (2000). Reference memory, anxiety and estrous cyclicity in C57BL/6NIA mice are affected by age and sex. *Neuroscience*, 95:293–307.

Frick KM, Fernandez SM, Bennett JC, Prange-Kiel J, Maclusky NJ, Leranth CS. (2004). Behavioral training interferes with the ability of gonadal hormones to increase CA1 spine synapse density in ovariectomized female rats. *Eur J Neurosci*, 19:1–7.

Frye CA. (1995). Estrus-associated decrements in a water maze task are limited to acquisition. *Physiol Behav*, 57:5–14.

Fugger HN, Cunningham SG, Rissman EF, Foster TC. (1998). Sex differences in the activational effect of ER-alpha on spatial learning. *Horm Behav*, 34:163–170.

Galea LAM, Kavaliers M, Ossenkopp KP, Hampson E. (1995). Gonadal hormones and spatial learning in the Morris water-maze in the male and female meadow vole, Microtus pennsylanicus. *Horm Behav*, 29:106–125.

Galea LA, McEwen BS, Tanapat P, Deak T, Spencer RL, Dhabhar FS. (1997). Sex differences in dendritic atrophy of CA3 pyramidal neurons in response to chronic restraint stress. *Neuroscience*, 81:689–697.

Galea LAM, Perrot-Sinal TS, Kavaliers M, Ossenkopp KP. (1999). Relations of hippocampal volume and detate gyrus width to gonadal hormone levels in male and female meadow voles. *Brain Res*, 821:383–391.

Galea LAM, Ormerod BK, Sampath S, Kostaras X, Wilkie DM, Phelps MT. (2000). Spatial working memory and hippocampal size across pregnancy in rats. *Horm Behav*, 37:86–95.

Gibbs RB. (2000). Basal forebrain cholinergic neurons are necessary for estrogen to enhance acquisition of a delayed matching-to-position T-maze task. *Horm Behav*, 42:245–257.

Gibbs RB, Aggarwal P. (1998). Estrogen and basal forebrain cholinergic neurons: implications for brain aging and Alzheimer's disease-related cognitive decline. *Horm Behav*, 334:98–111.

Gibbs RB, Gabor R, Cox T, Johnson DA. (2004). Effects of raloxifene and estradiol on hippocampal acetylcholine release and spatial learning in the rat. *Psychoneuroendocrinology*, 29:741–748.

Gold, PE. (2004). Coordination of multiple memory systems. *Neurobiol Learn Mem*, 82:230–242.

Gould E, Woolley CS, Frankfurt M, McEwen BS. (1990). Gonadal steroids regulate dendritic spine density in hippocampal pyramidal cells in adulthood. *J Neurosci*, 10:1286–1291.

Gresack JE, Frick KM. (2003). Male mice exhibit better spatial working and reference memory than females in a water-escape radial arm maze task. *Brain Res*, 982:98–107.

Gresack JE, Frick KM. (2004). Environmental enrichment reduces the mnemonic and neural benefits of estrogen. *Neuroscience*, 128:459–471.

Harley VR, Goodfellow PN. (1994). The biochemical role of SRY in sex determination. *Mol Reprod Dev*, 39:184–193.

Hasselmo ME. (1999). Neuromodulation and the hippocampus: memory function and dysfunction in a network simulation. *Prog Brain Res*, 121:3–18.

He D, Reneker DH, Mattice WL, James TW, Kimura D. (1997). Sex differences in remembering the locations of objects in an array: location-shifts versus location-exchanges. *Evol Hum Behav*, 18:155–163.

Healy SD, Braham SR, Braithwaite VA. (1999). Spatial working memory in rats: no differences between the sexes. *Proc R Soc Lond*, 266:2303–2308.

Hines M, Allen LS, Gorski RA. (1992). Sex differences in subregions of the medial nucleus of the amygdala and the bed nucleus of the stria terminalis of the rat. *Brain Res*, 579:321–326.

Hodges, H. (1996). Maze procedures: the radial-arm and water maze compared. *Brain Res Cogn Brain Res*, 3:167–181.

Hoh TE, Cain DP. (1997). Fractionating the nonspatial pretraining effect in the water maze task. *Behav Neurosci*, 111:1285–1291.

Jacobs LF, Gaulin SJ, Sherry DF, Hoffman GE. (1990). Evolution of spatial cognition: sex-specific patterns of spatial behavior predict hippocampal size. *Proc Natl Acad Sci USA*, 87:6349–6352.

Jacome, LF, Inagaki T, Mohan G, Arellanos A, MacLusky N, Luine VN. (submitted). Estrogenic enhancements of memory are mediated by ERO in ovariectomized rats.

Jonasson Z. (2005). Meta-analysis of sex differences in rodent models of learning and memory: a review of behavioral and biological data. *Neurosci Biobehav Rev*, 28:811–825.

Juraska JM. (1984). Sex differences in developmental plasticity in the visual cortex and hippocampal dentate gyrus. *Prog Brain Res*, 61:205–214.

Juraska JM. (1991). Sex differences in "cognitive" regions of the rat brain. *Psychoneuroendocrinology*, 16:105–109.

Juraska JM. (1992). Sex differences in dendritic response to differential experience in the rat visual cortex. *Brain Res*, 295:27–34.

Juraska JM, Henderson C, Muller J. (1984). Differential rearing experience, gender, and radial maze performance. *Dev Psychobiol*, 17:209–215.

Kelly SJ, Goodlett CR, Hulsether SA, West JR. (1988). Impaired spatial navigation in adult female but not adult male rats exposed to alcohol during the brain growth spurt. *Behav Brain Res*, 27:247–257.

Kesner RP, Rogers J. (2004). An analysis of independence and interactions of brain substrates that subserve multiple attributes, memory systems, and underlying processes. *Neurobiol Learn Mem*, 82:199–215.

Kimura D. (1999). *Sex and Cognition*. Cambridge, MA: MIT Press.

Kitraki E, Kremmyda O, Youlatos D, Alexis MN, Kittas C. (2004). Gender-dependent alterations in corticosteroid receptor status and spatial performance following 21 days of restrain stress. *Neuroscience*, 125:47–55.

Kobayashi S, Kametani H, Ugawa Y, Osanai M. (1988). Age difference of response strategy in radial maze performance of Fischer-344 rats. *Physiol Behav*, 42:277–280.

Kolb B, Cioe J. (1996). Sex-related differences in cortical function after medial frontal lesions in rats. *Behav Neurosci*, 110:1271–1281.

Korol DL (2004) Role of estrogen in balancing contributions from multiple memory systems. *Neurobiol Learn Mem*, 82:309–323.

Korol DL, Kolo LL. (2002). Estrogen-induced changes in place and response learning in young adult female rats. *Behav Neurosci*, 116:411–420.

Korol DL, Malin EL, Borden KA, Busby RA, Couper-Leo J. (2004). Shifts in preferred learning strategy across the estrous cycle in female rats. *Horm Behav*, 45:330–338.

LaBuda CJ, Mellgren RL, Hale RL. (2002). Sex differences in the acquisition of a radial maze task in the CD-1 mouse. *Physiol Behav*, 76:213–217.

Lam LL, Leranth C. (2003). Role of the medial septum diagonal band of Broca cholinergic neurons in oestrogen-induced spine synapse formation on hippocampal CA1 pyramidal cells of female rats. *Eur J Neurosci*, 17:1997–2005.

Lamberty Y, Gower AJ. (1988). Investigation into sex-related differences in locomotor activity, place learning and passive avoidance responding in NMRI mice. *Physiol Behav*, 44:787–790.

Leranth C, Shanabrough M, Horvath TL. (2000). Hormonal regulation of hippocampal spine synapse density involves subcortical mediation. *Neuroscience*, 101:349–356.

Leranth C, Petnehazy O, MacLusky NJ. (2003). Gonadal hormones affect spine synaptic density in the CA1 hippocampal subfield of male rats. *J Neurosci*, 23:1588–1592.

Leranth C, Hajszan T, MacLusky NJ. (2004). Androgens increase spine synapse density in the CA1 hippocampal subfield of ovariectomized female rats. *J Neurosci*, 24:495–499.

Leuner B, Mendolia-Loffredo S, Shors TJ. (2004). High levels of estrogen enhance associative memory formation in ovariectomized females. *Psychoneuroendocrinology*, 29:883–890.

Li C, Brake WG, Romeo RD, Dunlop JC, Gordon M, Buzescu R, et al. (2004). Estrogen alters hippocampal dendritic spine shape and enhances synaptic protein immunoreactivity and spatial memory in female mice. *Proc Natl Acad Sci USA*, 101:2185–2190.

Luine VN. (1985). Estradiol increases choline acetyltransferase activity in specific basal forebrain nuclei and projection areas of female rats. *Exp Neurol*, 89:484–490.

Luine VN. (1994). Steroid hormone influences on spatial memory. *Ann NY Acad Sci*, 743:201–211.

Luine VN, Villegas M, Martinez C, McEwen BS. (1994). Repeated stress causes reversible impairments of spatial memory performance. *Brain Res*, 639:167–170.

Luine VN. (1997). Steroid hormone modulation of hippocampal dependent spatial memory. *Stress*, 2:21–36.

Luine VN, Richards ST, Wu VY, Beck KD. (1998). Estradiol enhances learning and memory in a spatial memory task and effects levels of monoaminergic neurotransmitters. *Horm Behav*, 34:149–162.

Luine VN. (2002). Sex differences in chronic stress effects on memory in rats. *Stress*, 5:205–216.

Luine VN, Rodriguez M. (1994). Effects of estradiol on radial arm maze performance of young and aged rats. *Behav Neural Biol*, 62:230–236.

Luine V, Martinez C, Villegas M, Magarinos AM, McEwen B. (1996). Restraint stress reversibly enhances spatial memory performance. *Physiology and Behavior*, 59:27–32.

Luine V, Beck K, Bowman R, Kneavel M (2001) Sex differences in chronic stress effects on cognitive function and brain neurochemistry. In Handa RJ, Hayaski S, Terasawas E, Kawata M, (Eds.), *Neuroplasticity, development and steroid hormone action*. Boca Raton, FL: CRC Press.

Luine VN, Jacome LF, MacLusky NJ. (2003). Rapid enhancement of visual and place memory by estrogens in rats. *Endocrinology*, 144:2836–2844.

Lukoyanov NV, Andrade JP, Dulce Madeira M, Paula-Barbosa MM. (1999). Effects of age and sex on the water maze performance and hippocampal cholinergic fibers in rats. *Neurosci Lett*, 269:141–144.

Lund TD, Lephart ED. (2001). Manipulation of prenatal hormones and dietary phytoestrogens during adulthood alter the sexually dimorphic expression of visual spatial memory. *BMC Neurosci*, 2:21.

Lund TD, West TW, Tian LY, Bu LH, Simmons DL, Setchell KD, et al. (2001). Visual spatial memory is enhanced in female rats (but inhibited in males) by dietary soy phytoestrogens. *BMC Neurosci*, 2:20.

MacLusky NJ, Luine VN, Hajszan T, Prange-Kiel J, Leranth C. (2005). The 17α and β isomers of estradiol both induce rapid spine synapse formation in the CA1 hippocampal subfield of ovariectomized female rats. *Endocrinology*, 146:287–293.

MacLusky NJ, Hajszan T, Prange-Kiel J, Leranth C. (2006). Androgen modulation of hippocampal synaptic plasticity. *Neuroscience*, 138:957–965.

Madeira MD, Sousa N, Paula-Barbosa MM. (1991). Sexual dimorphism in the mossy fiber synapses of the rat hippocampus. *Exp Brain Res*, 87:537–545.

Maier DM, Pohorecky LA. (1986). The effect of ethanol and sex on radial arm maze performance in rats. *Pharmacol Biochem Behav*, 25:703–709.

Markowska AL. (1999). Sex dimorphisms in the rate of age-related decline in spatial memory: relevance to alterations in the estrous cycle. *J Neurosci*, 19:8122–8133.

Marriott LK, Korol DL. (2003). Short-term estrogen treatment in ovariectomized rats augments hippocampal acetylcholine release during place learning. *Neurobiol Learn Mem*, 80:315–322.

McCarthy MM, Konkle AT. (2005). When is a sex difference not a sex difference? *Front Neuroendocrinol*, 26:85–102.

McEwen BS. (2001). Plasticity of the hippocampus: adaptation to chronic stress and allostatic load. *Ann NY Acad Sci*, 933:265–277.

McEwen BS. (2002). Sex, stress and the hippocampus: allostasis, allostatic load and the aging process. *Neurobiol Aging*, 23:921–939.

McGaugh JL. (2000). Memory—a century of consolidation. *Science*, 14:248–251.

McGaugh JL, Izquierdo I. (2000). The contribution of pharmacology to research on the mechanisms of memory formation. *Trends Pharmacol Sci*, 21:208–210.

McLaughlin KJ, Baran SE, Wright RL, Conrad CD. (2005). Chronic stress enhances spatial memory in ovariectomized female rats despite CA3 dendritic retraction: possible involvement of CA1 neurons. *Neuroscience*, 135:1045–1054.

Milner B. (1959). The memory defect in bilateral hippocampal lesions. *Psychia Res Rep*, 11:43–52.

Mishima N, Higashitani F, Teraoka K, Yoshioka R. (1986). Sex differences in appetitive learning of mice. *Physiol Behav*, 37:263–268.

Mizukami S, Nishizuka M, Arai Y. (1983). Sexual difference in nuclear volume and its ontogeny in the rat amygdala. *Exp Neurol*, 79:569–275.

Morris RGM. (1981). Spatial localisation does not depend on the presence of local cues. *Learning Motivation*, 12:239–260.

Morris RGM. (1984). Developments of a water-maze procedure for studying spatial learning in the rat. *J Neurosci Methods*, 11:47–60.

Mumby DG, Gaskin S, Glenn MJ, Schramek TE, Lehmann H. (2002). Hippocampal damage and exploratory preferences in rats: memory for objects, places, and contexts. *Learn Mem*, 2002 9:49–57.

Murphy DD, Segal M. (1996). Regulation of dendritic spine density in cultured rat hippocampal neurons by steroid hormones. *J Neurosci*, 16:4059–4068.

Murphy DD, Cole NB, Greenberger V, Segal M. (1998a). Estradiol increases dendritic spine density by reducing GABA neurotransmission in hippocampal neurons. *J Neurosci*, 18:2550–2559.

Murphy DD, Cole NB, Segal M. (1998b). Brain-derived neurotrophic factor mediates estradiol-induced dendritic spine formation in hippocampal neurons. *Proc Natl Acad Sci USA*, 95:11412–11417.

O'Keefe J. (1999). Do hippocampal pyramidal cells signal non-spatial as well as spatial information? *Hippocampus*, 9:352–364.

Olton DS, Papas BC. (1979). Spatial memory and hippocampal system function. *Neuropsychologia*, 17:669–681.

Olton DS, Samuelson RJ. (1976). Remberance of places passed: spatial memory in rats. *J Exper Psychol: Anim Behav Procs* 2:97–116.

Olton DS, Walker JA, Gage FH. (1978). Hippocampal connections and spatial discrimination. *Brain Res*, 130:295–308.

Olton DS, Becker JT, Handlemann GE. (1979). Hippocampus, space and memory. *Brain Behav Sci*, 2:313–365.

Packard MG. (1999). Glutamate infused posttraining into the hippocampus or caudate-putamen differentially strengthens place and response learning. *Proc Natl Acad Sci USA*, 96:12881–12886.

Packard MG, McGaugh JL. (1996). Inactivation of hippocampus or caudate nucleus with lidocaine differentially affects expression of place and response learning. *Neurobiol Learn Mem*, 65:65–72.

Perrot-Sinal TS, Kostenuik MA, Ossenkopp KP, Kavaliers M. (1996). Sex differences in performance in the Morris water maze and the effects of initial nonstationary hidden platform training. *Behav Neurosci*, 110:1309–1320.

Phoenix CH, Goy RW, Gerall AA, Young WC. (1959). Organizing action of prenatally administered testosterone propionate on the tissues mediating mating behavior in the female guinea pig. *Endocrinology*, 65:369–382.

Poldrack RA, Packard MG. (2003). Competition among multiple memory systems: converging evidence from animal and human brain studies. *Neuropsychologia*, 41:245–251.

Restle F. (1957). Discrimination of cues in mazes: a resolution of the place-vs.-response question. *Psychol Rev*, 64:217–228.

Rissanen A, Puolivali J, van Groen T, Riekkinen P Jr. (1999). In mice tonic estrogen replacement therapy improves non-spatial and spatial memory in a water maze task. *Neuroreport*, 10:1369–1372.

Roof RL, Havens MD. (1992). Testosterone improves maze performance and induces development of a male hippocampus in females. *Brain Res*, 572:310–313.

Roof RL. (1993). Neonatal exogenous testosterone modifies sex difference in radial arm and Morris water maze performance in prepubescent and adult rats. *Behav Brain Res*, 53:1–10.

Rosenbaum RS, Winocur G, Moscovitch M. (2001). New views on old memories: re-evaluating the role of the hippocampal complex. *Behav Brain Res*, 127:183–197.

Rubinow MJ, Arseneau LM, Beverly JL, Juraska JM. (2004). Effect of the estrous cycle on water maze acquisition depends on the temperature of the water. *Behav Neurosci*, 118:863–868.

Rudick CN, Woolley CS. (2001). Estrogen regulates functional inhibition of hippocampal CA1 pyramidal cells in the adult female rat. *J Neurosci*, 21:6532–6543.

Rudick CN, Woolley CS. (2003). Selective estrogen receptor modulators regulate phasic activation of hippocampal CA1 pyramidal cells by estrogen. *Endocrinology*, 144:179–187.

Rudick CN, Gibbs RB, Woolley CS. (2003). A role for the basal forebrain cholinergic system in estrogen-induced disinhibition of hippocampal pyramidal cells. *J Neurosci*, 23: 4479–4490.

Sandstrom NJ, Williams CL. (2001). Memory retention is modulated by acute estradiol and progesterone replacement. *Behav Neurosci*, 115:384–393.

Sandstrom NJ, Williams CL. (2004). Spatial memory retention is enhanced by acute and continuous estradiol replacement. *Horm Behav*, 45:128–135.

Saucier D, Hargreaves EL, Boon F, Vanderwolf CH, Cain DP. (1996). Detailed behavioral analysis of

water maze acquisition under systemic NMDA or muscarinic antagonism: nonspatial pretraining eliminates spatial learning deficts. *Behav Neurosci*, 110:103–116.

Seymoure P, Juraska JM. (1992). Sex differences in cortical thickness and the dendritic tree in the monocular and binocular subfields of the rat visual cortex at weaning age. *Brain Res Dev Brain Res*, 69:185–189.

Sherry DGH, Hampson E. (1997). Evolution and the hormonal control of sexually-dimorphic spatial abilities in humans. *Trends Cogn Sci*, 1:50–56.

Shors TJ. (2004). Learning during stressful times. *Learn Mem*, 11:137–144.

Shors TJ, Beylin AV, Wood GE, Gould E. (2000). The modulation of Pavlovian memory. *Behav Brain Res*, 110:39–52.

Shors TJ, Chua C, Falduto J. (2001). Sex differences and opposite effects of stress on dendritic spine density in the male versus female hippocampus. *J Neurosci*, 21:6292–6297.

Simerly R. (2002). Wired for reproduction: organization and development of sexually dimorphic circuits in the mammalian forebrain. *Annu Rev Neurosci*, 25: 507–536.

Sisk CL, Zehr JL. (2005). Pubertal hormones organize the adolescent brain and behavior. *Front Neuroendocrinol*, 26:163–174.

Steele RJ, Morris RG. (1999). Delay-dependent impairment of a matching-to-place task with chronic and intrahippocampal infusion of the NMDA-antagonist D-AP5. *Hippocampus*, 9:118–136.

Squire LR. (1987). *Memory and Brain*. New York: Oxford University Press.

Squire LR. (1992). Memory and the hippocampus: a synthesis from findings with rats, monkeys, and humans. *Psychol Rev*, 99:195–231.

Squire LR. (2004). Memory systems of the brain: a brief history and current perspective. *Neurobiol Learn Mem*, 82:171–177.

Tabibnia G, Cooke BM, Breedlove SM. (1999). Sex difference and laterality in the volume of mouse dentate gyrus granule cell layer. *Brain Res*, 827: 41–45.

Taube JS. (1999). Some thoughts on place cells and the hippocampus. *Hippocampus*, 9:452–457.

Tees RC, Midgley G, Nesbit JC. (1981). The effect of early visual experience on spatial maze learning in rats. *Dev Psychobiol*, 14:425–438.

Tolman EC. (1949). There is more than one kind of learning. *Psych Rev*, 56:144–155.

van Haaren F, van Hest A, Heinsbroek RP. (1990). Behavioral differences between male and female rats: effects of gonadal hormones on learning and memory. *Neurosci Biobehav Rev*, 14:23–33.

Wallace M, Luine V, Arellanos A, Frankfurt M. (2006). Ovariectomized rats show decreased recognition memory and spine density in hippocampus and prefrontal cortex. *Brain Research*, 1126:176–182.

Warren SG, Juraska JM. (1997). Spatial and nonspatial learning across the rat estrous cycle. *Behav Neurosci*, 111:259–266.

Warren SG, Juraska JM. (2000). Sex differences and estropausal phase effects on water maze performance in aged rats. *Neurobio Learn Mem*, 74:229–240.

Weiland NG (1992a). Estradiol selectively regulates agonist binding sites on the N-methyl-D-aspartate receptor complex in the CA1 region of the hippocampus. *Endocrinology*, 131:662–668.

Weiland NG. (1992b). Glutamic acid decarboxylase messenger ribonucleic acid is regulated by estradiol and progesterone in the hippocampus. *Endocrinology*, 131:2697–2702.

Williams CL, Barnett AM, Meck WH. (1990). Organizational effects of early gonadal secretions on sexual differentiation in spatial memory. *Behav Neurosci*, 104:84–97.

Williams CL, Meck WH. (1991). The organizational effects of gonadal steroids on sexually dimorphic spatial ability. *Psychoneuroendocrinology*, 16:155–176.

Wilson IA, Puolivali J, Heikkinen T, Riekkinen P. (1999). Estrogen and NMDA receptor antagonism: effects upon reference and working memory. *Eur J Pharmacol*, 381:93–99.

Wood GE, Shors TJ. (1998). Stress facilitates classical conditioning in males, but impairs classical conditioning in females through activational effects of ovarian hormones. *Proc Natl Acad Sci U S A*, 7:4066–4071.

Woolley CS, Gould E, Frankfurt M, McEwen BS. (1990). Naturally occurring fluctuation in dendritic spine density on adult hippocampal pyramidal neurons. *J Neurosci*, 10:4035–4039.

Woolley CS, McEwen BS. (1992). Estradiol mediates fluctuations in hippocampal synapse density during the estrous cycle in the adult rat. *J Neurosci*, 12:2549–2554.

Woolley CS, McEwen BS. (1993). Roles of estradiol and progesterone in regulation of hippocampal dendritic spine density during the estrous cycle in the rat. *J Comp Neurol*, 336:293–306.

Woolley CS, Weiland NG, McEwen BS, Schwartzkroin PA. (1997). Estradiol increases the sensitivity of hippocampal CA1 pyramidal cells to NMDA receptor-mediated synaptic input: correlation with dendritic spine density. *J Neurosci*, 17:1848–1859.

Yankova M, Hart SA, Woolley CS. (2001). Estrogen increases synaptic connectivity between single presynaptic inputs and multiple postsynaptic CA1 pyramidal cells: a serial electron-microscopic study. *Proc Natl Acad Sci USA*, 98:3525–3530.

Xiao L, Jordan CL. (2002). Sex differences, laterality, and hormonal regulation of androgen receptor immunoreactivity in rat hippocampus. *Horm Behav*, 42:327–336.

Zola-Morgan S, Squire LR. (1993). Neuroanatomy of memory. *Ann Rev Neurosci*, 16:547–563.

Chapter 13

Sex Differences in Energy Metabolism, Obesity, and Eating Behavior

Nori Geary and Jennifer Lovejoy

This chapter introduces the most important aspects of sex differences in energy metabolism, obesity, and eating behavior. The ordering of these topics has a certain logical appeal as, first, energy metabolism ultimately determines body weight and, second, both metabolism and obesity, or, more properly, adiposity, are considered to be important controls of eating. A wide range of evidence indicates that there are physiologically important sex differences in energy metabolism, obesity, and eating behavior both in animals and humans. Relevant data come from basic animal research, basic and clinical human research, and epidemiology. Because a comprehensive review of each of these areas is far beyond the scope of this chapter, we cover the field selectively and with a somewhat uneven emphasis. In each area, however, we include illustrative highlights of important discoveries, growth points, and open issues.

SEX DIFFERENCES IN ENERGY METABOLISM

Several lines of evidence suggest that females have lower energy expenditure than males (adjusted for body composition differences) and that fat storage tends to be increased in females under a variety of conditions. While there is a plausible evolutionary argument for why females may benefit from a greater capacity to store body fat in order to maintain reproductive competence during times of famine (Hoyenga & Hoyenga, 1982), there is no question that in modern times of abundant, highly energy-dense food sources and minimal physical activity, such a trait would have more negative health consequences than evolutionary benefit.

Whole Body Energy Expenditure

A number of studies suggest that whole body energy expenditure (EE) is lower in women than in men. For example, in a population of age-matched men and women in their 60s, sleeping metabolic rate was 11.2% lower in women, and total daily EE was 8.7% lower in women than in men after adjusting for lean body mass and physical activity covariates (Morio et al., 1997). Similarly, total daily EE was 14% lower in Caucasian women than in Caucasian men and 18% lower in African-American women than in African-American men after adjusting for lean body mass (Carpenter et al., 1998). These differences were due to sex differences in both resting EE and physical activity EE.

Dionne et al. (1999) observed that for any given fat mass, women had a lower EE than men independent of fat-free mass; as described below, this may be due to sex differences in abdominal fat deposition. Finally, in a cross-sectional study of men and women aged 18 to 87 years, the decline in resting EE with age was greater in women (–80.3 kJ/day/year) than in men (–46.9 kJ/day/ year) (Roubenoff et al., 2000), thus suggesting that women would be more likely to gain body weight with aging if they do not reduce energy intake.

Gonadal steroid hormone levels are an important factor in resting EE, although it is not clear whether they fully account for the sex differences in resting EE. This is because in adults of both sexes, deficiencies in gonadal steroids reduce resting EE. This has been shown elegantly in studies in which GnRH antagonists have been used to suppress gonadal steroid secretion. Acute hypogonadalism produced in this way reduced resting EE by 5% in premenopausal women (Day et al., 2005) and by 9% in young men (Mauras et al., 1998). The physiological role of gonadal steroids in maintaining resting EE in women was significantly higher in premenopausal women than in postmenopausal women who were not taking hormone replacement therapy (HRT), whereas there was no difference in resting EE between premenopausal women and postmenopausal HRT users (Reimer et al., 2005).

Furthermore, Meijer et al. (1992) measured an 8% increase in sleeping EE, the major component of resting EE, in women who were in the luteal phase of the menstrual cycle in comparison to women in the follicular phase. In contrast, another component of EE, the postprandial thermic effect of food, which is quantitatively much smaller than resting EE, was reported to decrease ~15% during the luteal phase of the menstrual cycle as compared to the follicular phase (Tai, Castillo & Pi-Sunyer, 1997).

Sex differences in energy metabolism appear even in young children. Kirkby et al. (2004), reporting on a study of 307 healthy 5-year olds, found that resting EE was 6% lower in girls than in boys after adjusting for fat-free mass and other anthropometric variables. Similarly, in the Baton Rouge Children's Study, which examined 114 African-American and Caucasian boys and girls aged ~12 years, total daily EE and resting EE were significantly lower in girls than in boys after adjusting for anthropometric variables and Tanner stage (DeLany et al., 2004). There was also a tendency for a lower activity EE in girls compared to boys after adjusting for body composition differences. Whether such prepubertal sex differences are due to early developmental, organizational effects of gonadal hormones, in utero metabolic imprinting, or other causes remains to be established.

It is also important to note, for reasons that remain unclear, not all studies have detected sex differences in energy expenditure after adjusting for absolute differences in fat free mass, either in adults (Bucholz et al., 2001; Klausen et al. 1997; Tarnopolsky, 1999) or children (Grund et al., 2000).

In many species of rodents, physical activity EE is controlled by estradiol secretion and normally varies markedly across the estrous cycle. In most rodents and many other species in which female sexual receptivity is periodic, the period of increased sexual receptivity is defined as estrus and the ovarian cycle is called the estrous cycle. Estrus also refers to the day(s) of the cycle when this occurs, which in rats and mice, is the final day of the 4- or 5-d cycle. Unfortunately, the usual convention for labeling cycle days has the confusing consequence that behavioral estrus does not occur during the nominal estrus day, but rather during proestrus (Asarian & Geary, 2002; Becker et al., 2005; Eckel et al, this volume). For that reason, we refer here to the period of increased sexual receptivity as "behavioral estrus."

One of the oldest findings in behavioral neuroendocrinology is that female rats typically run three to five times as much during the night of behavioral estrus (when ovulation occurs and they are fertile) than during any other phase of the ovarian cycle (Geary, 2006; Wang, 1923). Ovariectomy eliminates this pattern and cyclic estradiol treatment reinstates it, indicating an activational hormonal control of locomotor activity (Wade, 1972; Asarian & Geary, 2006).

Early, organizational effects of gonadal hormones on brain development, however, are also important. The specific neural mechanisms mediating these effects have been investigated by several groups (i.e., Fahrbach et al., 1985; Gentry and Wade, 1976; Roy et al., 1990; Stewart & Rodaros, 1999).

One important issue is that different forms of spontaneous physical activity seem to have different neuroendocrine controls. For example, in comparing estrogenic regulation of physical activity in male and female knock-out mice lacking either the estrogen-receptor (ER)α or ERβ gene, Ogawa et al. (2003) found that running wheel activity was mediated by ERα in both males and females, whereas the mediation of open-field activity differed by both genetic background and sex. As physical activity EE is emerging as a crucial factor in human obesity (Levine et al., 2005), determining whether these findings in rodents have any human counterpart is an urgent research question.

Intermediary Metabolism

In addition to sex differences in overall EE and physical activity EE, there are sex differences in the intermediary metabolism of energy substrates both in exercising and non-exercising individuals (reviewed in Horton & Braun, 2004; Mittendorfer, 2005; Tarnopolsky, 1999). Following meals, plasma triglyceride (TG) levels are higher in men than women, even when subjects are matched for fasting plasma TG (Jensen, 1995). This may be due in large part to an increased uptake of plasma TG into skeletal muscle in women (Jensen, 1995), which in turn could also account for the greater intramyocellular fat content in women (Steffensen et al., 2002). A preliminary study suggested that estrogen may regulate intromyocellular fat content in postmenopausal women, as estrogen-deficient women had higher intromyocellular fat content than women taking exogenous estrogen replacement therapy (Lovejoy et al., 2003).

There are also sex differences in postprandial TG uptake into adipose tissue, with more TG taken into the visceral organs in men and into the subcutaneous adipose tissue in women (Romanskie et al., 2000). This latter difference in TG metabolism would of course contribute to sex differences in regional body fat distribution. Another sex difference emerges during fasting, when plasma glucose levels fall more in women than men, apparently because of a reduced CNS response to reduced blood glucose and a consequently reduced autonomic response, especially reduced secretion of the so-called counter-regulatory hormones glucagon and epinephrine (Davis et al., 2000b).

Several other sex differences in regional fatty acid storage, mobilization, and oxidation have been reported that may contribute to the observed sex differences in normal and disordered whole-body metabolism. For example, whereas abdominal adipose tissue of men and women were equally responsive to β-adenergic stimulation of lipolysis, men appeared to have more abdominal α-2 receptor-mediated antilipolytic function (Hellstrom et al., 1996; Leibel & Hirsch, 1987). Basal fat oxidation, adjusted for fat-free mass, was also lower in women than in men whereas postprandial fat storage in subcutaneous adipose tissue was higher in women (Blaak, 2001). In children aged 6–16 y, the effects of adaptation to a high-fat/low-carbohydrate diet on substrate oxidation were less pronounced in girls than in boys (Trueth et al., 2003). These findings all support the idea that fat storage generally tends to be increased in females compared to males.

The situation changes during exercise, when females oxidize proportionally more fat and less carbohydrate and amino acids than do males. This has been documented across a wide range of exercise intensities in several methodologically rigorous studies that carefully matched level of fitness training, percent body fat, dietary history, phase of menstrual cycle, etc. (Horton & Braun, 2004). Interestingly, one study in which microdialysis was used to measure lipolysis in abdominal and femoral subcutaneous adipose tissue and in the quadriceps femoris muscle, most of the sex difference in fueling energy metabolism during exercise occurred because women utilized much more intramyocellular lipid than did men (Boschman et al., 2002). Nevertheless, despite the increased utilization of intramyocellular lipid during exercise, both trained and untrained women had higher basal levels of intramycellular lipid than men (Steffensen et al., 2002). As intramyocellular lipid increases with body adiposity and is associated with a high risk for decreased insulin sensitivity, this may be a reason that increased adiposity disproportionally increases women's risk for type 2 diabetes mellitus (T2DM) (Bray, 2004).

The sex difference in metabolic fuel utilization during exercise appears to be largely due to differences in circulating 17β-estradiol (D'Eon & Braun, 2002; Tarnopolsky & Ruby, 2001). Consistent with this, the effect is larger during the luteal phase of the menstrual cycle (~d 20), when estradiol levels are high, than during the mid-follicular stage (~d 9), when estradiol levels are lower (DeVries et al., 2006).

Neuroendocrine and Metabolic Responses to Hypoglycemia

An interesting and clinically relevant sex difference occurs in the neuroendocrine response to hypoglycemia. Hypoglycemia is a serious complication of insulin therapy in type 1 diabetes mellitus (T1DM). As described above, normal women tend to have blunted secretion of glucagon and epinephrine during fasts, which suggests that women with T1DM would suffer from acute hypoglycemic episodes more often than men with T1DM. This, however, was not the case in a study by Davis and colleagues (2000a).

Although endogenous glucose production did indeed increase less as women with T1DM became hypoglycemic, they had a greater lipolytic response, which spares glucose, and apparently were more consciously sensitive to the development of autonomic symptoms than were men, which would presumably facilitate the initiation of behavioral countermeasures, i.e., carbohydrate ingestion. Tests of estradiol treatment in postmenopausal women suggest that estradiol is the culprit in the decreased neuroendocrine and metabolic responses to hypoglycemia in women (Sanoval et al., 2003). The variable that the brain actually responds to during hypoglycemia, however, may be lactate produced by glycolysis in glial cells (Patil & Briski, 2005). Whether there are sex differences in the response to or production of brain lactate, however, has not yet been tested.

Estrogen Receptor Mechanisms

Two nuclear estrogen receptors (ER) exist, ERα and ERß; the two isoforms are products of separate genes (located on chromosomes 6 and 14, respectively, in humans). Complexes of estradiol with either ERα or ERß act as transcriptional modulators by binding directly or indirectly to estradiol response elements in the promoter regions of many genes. The relative contributions of these various mechanism to the myriad biological functions of estrogens is a matter of intense research (for reviews, see [Couse & Korach, 1999; Koehler et al., 2005]).

Both male and female transgenic mice with null deletions of the ERα gene have insulin insensitivity

and impaired glucose tolerance (Heine et al., 2000; Ohlsson et al., 2000). A probable mechanism has recently been discovered. One of insulin's most important effects is to regulate glucose transport in skeletal muscle by translocating the glucose transporter-4 (GLUT4) to the cell membrane. Barros et al. (2006) reported that, in both sexes, skeletal muscle GLUT4 expression is positively regulated by ERα and negatively regulated by ERß, suggesting functional imbalances in these ERs could alter glucose homeostasis, affect insulin sensitivity, and increase the vulnerability to increased T2DM; indeed, these disorders were discovered in a man lacking ERα (Smith et al., 1994).

SEX DIFFERENCES IN OBESITY

Epidemiology of Obesity in Men and Women

Obesity is currently a global epidemic. According to the World Health Organization, non-communicable diseases related to overweight and obesity account for 60% of global deaths and 47% of the global burden of disease (WHO, 2002). In the United States, 65% of American adults are classified as overweight (Body Mass Index >25 kg/m^2) or obese (BMI >30 kg/m^2) (Hedley et al., 2004). This is a very significant public health concern as obesity is associated with life-threatening chronic and expensive comorbidities, including T2DM, cardiovascular disease, osteoarthritis, asthma, and some cancers.

Important sex differences in the prevalence of obesity exist that may be relevant to both obesity prevention and treatment efforts. The prevalence of overweight and obesity are consistently higher in females than in males in many countries around the world (Table 13.1).

The most recent national survey indicates that in the U.S.A. 33% of adult women vs. 28% of adult men are obese (Hedley et al., 2004). This sex difference is even more marked when one considers morbid or type III obesity (BMI >40 kg/m^2), which in the United States affects twice as many women as men (Flegal et al., 2002; Hedley et al., 2004) (Table 13.2g).

Both rates of obesity in women and sex differences in prevalence are strikingly high in minority groups in the United States, including Mexican Americans, African Americans, and Native Americans. For ex-

Table 13.1. Sex Differences in Global Obesity Prevalence

Country	Year Data Collected	Males	Females
Albania	2001	22.8	35.6
Australia	2000	19.3	22.2
Brazil	1997	6.9	12.5
Czech Republic	1997/8	24.7	26.2
England	2004	22.7	23.8
Germany	2002	22.5	23.3
Guyana	2000	14.3	26.9
Indonesia	2001	1.1	3.6
Israel	1999–2001	19.9	25.7
Jordan	1994–6	32.7	59.8
Mexico	2000	19.4	29
Oman	2000	16.7	23.1
Peru	1998–2000	16	23
South Africa	1998	10.1	27.9
Spain	1990–2000	13.4	15.8
Thailand	1997	3.5	8.8
Turkey	2001–2	16.5	29.4

Data are % BMI >30 kg/m^2

Source: International Obesity Task Force (www.iotf.org)

ample, over 50% of African-American women aged 40 y and older have BMI >30 kg/m^2 while ~15% have BMI >40 kg/m^2 versus ~30% and ~3 % in African-American men, respectively (Hedley et al., 2004). Finally, it should also be noted that at every level of BMI, women have a greater percentage of body fat than do men, thus a woman's risk of being "overfat" is higher even at BMIs within the nominally normal range.

Regional Fat Distribution

Sex differences in regional fat distribution in humans have been recognized since the early 1900s. Men tend to deposit more fat in the abdominal area (including

Table 13.2. Prevalence of Extreme Obesity (BMI >40 kg/m^2) in the U.S.A., 1999–2002.

Sex	White Non-Hispanic	Black Non-Hispanic	Mexican American
Men	3.3 ± 0.5	3.4 ± 0.6	2.9 ± 0.7
Women	5.5 ± 0.5	13.5 ± 1.2	5.7 ± 0.9

Data are for adults, 20 y of age or older. Data modified from Hedley et al., 2004.

both subcutaneous and intra-abdominal or visceral fat) and premenopausal women typically deposit more fat in the gluteo-femoral area. Reproductive steroids clearly influence body fat distribution in women (Bjorntop, 1993; Lovejoy et al., 1996; Wajchenberg, 2000). Specifically, estrogens appear to promote gluteo-femoral fat accumulation, whereas androgens appear to promote abdominal fat accumulation in both premenopausal (Pasquali et al., 1993) and post-menopausal Caucasian women (Lovejoy et al., 1996). At menopause, there is a shift in the ratio of androgens to estrogens—ovarian estrogen production ceases while adrenal androgen production continues. Consequently, abdominal fat mass tends to increase during the time of perimenopause and persists into the postmenopausal years unless exogenous estrogen replacement therapy is used.

The mechanisms mediating the effects of sex hormones on regional fat distribution are unknown. Candidates include changes in lipoprotein lipase activity in different fat depots in premenopausal compared to postmenopausal women (Rebuffe-Scrive et al., 1986) and changes in leptin or insulin signaling (Clegg et al., 2006). Clegg and colleagues (2006) have recently reported that sex differences in body fat distribution analogous to those in humans occur in rats (Clegg et al., 2006). That is, as in postmenopausal human females, ovariectomy increased the amount of visceral fat, but decreased the amount of subcutaneous fat in rats. Interestingly, these changes were reversed by either peripheral or central estradiol treatment, suggesting a potential brain mediated control of regional fat distribution. In male rats, orchiectomy decreased the amount of visceral fat and increased the amount of subcutaneous fat.

Effects of Oophorectomy and Menopause

The marked hyperphagia and increased adiposity produced in rats and other animals by ovariectomy and their reversal by estradiol are well documented. Comparable data in women are much more limited and are confounded by a number of factors. For example, some studies suggest that women who undergo hysterectomy/oophorectomy have a higher rate of obesity pre-surgery, thus confounding potential analyses of obesity and/or weight gain related to surgical removal of the ovaries (Howard et al., 2005). Nonetheless, the Study of Women's Health Across the Nation (SWAN), a US survey of ~13,000 women of varying ethnicity, found that body weight was significantly higher in women who had surgical menopause (BMI 28.5 ± 0.1 kg/m^2) than in premenopausal women (26.2 ± 0.1 kg/m^2); peri- and postmenopausal women had intermediate values (Matthews et al. 2001).

The majority of data in humans on sex hormone deficiency and obesity relates to natural menopause and indicate that menopause is associated with a modest increase in body weight independent of aging. In the Pasquali et al. (1993) population study in Italy, the BMI of perimenopausal and postmenopausal women was significantly higher than that of premenopausal women, even after adjusting for age, diet, activity, and smoking habits. Aloia et al. (1995) applied a 4-compartment model of body composition analysis to 155 Caucasian women aged 51 ± 14 y and found that menopause was associated with a gain in body fat and an increased rate of change in body fat. Toth et al. (2000) reported that body weight was 6% higher and percent of body fat 17% higher in postmenopausal women compared to similarly aged (47 vs 51 y, n = 53) premenopausal women. In addition, the body fat difference remained significant after adjusting for age and body weight.

In contrast, the 3-y longitudinal study of middle-aged women by Wing et al. (1991) found no difference in mean weight gain of women who remained premenopausal compared to those who underwent menopause. However, the average weight gain in perimenopausal women was 2.25 kg, and 20% of the population gained 4.5 kg or more, suggesting that, even apart from menopause, weight gain is a significant issue for middle-aged women.

Decreased estrogen after surgical or natural menopause appears to have a stronger effect on regional body fat distribution than on total body adiposity. For example, using dual-energy X-ray absorptiometry (DEXA), Svendsen et al. (1995) found increased upper body or trunk fat in postmenopausal women independent of the effects of aging. Similarly, several studies using CT scans indicate that visceral fat increases after menopause (Kotani et al., 1994; Hunter et al., 1996; Toth et al., 2000). Lovejoy and Smith (unpublished results) observed that the increase in visceral fat mass actually occurs 1–2 years prior to the cessation of menses, suggesting that reduced secretion or altered patterns of reproductive hormone secretion during the perimenopause are sufficient to trigger changes in regional fat distribution.

Effects of Exogenous Sex Steroids

The effects of exogenous sex steroids on obesity and eating behavior have been examined in relation to postmenopausal HRT and premenopausal oral contraceptive use. HRT tends to slightly reduce the increases in BMI seen with aging in women. One of the largest prospective studies to examine the effects of HRT on body weight is the Postmenopausal Estrogen/Progestin Intervention (PEPI) trial. This randomized, placebo-controlled clinical trial of 875 women found that women assigned to estrogen replacement (with or without progestin) gained on average 1.0 kg less at the end of 3 years than women in the placebo group and also had a 1.2 cm smaller gain in waist girth (Espeland et al., 1997).

In the SWAN study (Matthews et al., 2001), HRT use was associated with lower BMI independent of ethnicity (26.5 vs. 27.3 kg/m^2) and HRT users were less likely to be obese than were non-HRT users (22.6% vs. 27.2%). In contrast, however, the Rancho Bernardo population study, in which women were studied over 15 y, found no significant difference between estrogen-users and non-users in BMI after adjusting for other confounding factors (Kritz-Silverstein & Barrett-Connor, 1996).

In addition to its association with reduced body weight, HRT use is also associated with reduced accumulation of intra-abdominal fat. Using DEXA, Haarbo et al. (1991) reported that HRT prevented the increase in intra-abdominal fat seen in placebo-treated postmenopausal women over a 2-year period. Similarly, Sites et al. (2001) found that HRT users had significantly lower body fat mass (by DEXA) and visceral abdominal adipose tissue (by CT scan) compared to non-users. After adjusting for total body fatness, there was still a trend for lower visceral fat in the HRT users. Munoz et al. (2002) also observed that postmenopausal women receiving HRT had lower visceral adipose tissue mass by CT scan than did those not receiving HRT. All in all, these studies suggest that both body weight and intra-abdominal fat distribution are strongly influenced by ovarian steroids.

The data on the effects of hormonal contraceptives on body weight are mixed. A systematic review of 42 randomized, controlled trials of combination estrogen-progestin contraceptives concluded that the majority of evidence does not indicate a major effect of oral contraceptives on body weight in reproductive-age women (Gallo et al., 2004). Of concern, however, are several studies showing that both adolescent girls (age 12–18 yr) and young women (age 18–35 yr) are at significant risk of weight gain from the use of depot medroxyprogesterone for contraception (Bonny et al., 2006; Mangan et al., 2002; Clark et al., 2005). A very closely related progestin, megestrol is used as an appetite stimulant in anorectic cancer patients, and seems similarly effective in both men and women (Berenstein & Ortiz, 2005; Pasqual López et al., 2004). The mechanisms of action of these progestins are not fully explained; it may be that their effects differ from those of natural progesterone (Schindler et al., 2003).

Unfortunately, there are only limited data on the effects of exogenous testosterone on body composition in healthy men with reduced endogenous testosterone due to aging and/or obesity. One seminal study was conducted by Marin et al. (1992), who administered oral testosterone or placebo for 8 months to healthy, abdominally obese middle-aged men. Testosterone treatment significantly reduced visceral abdominal fat without changing total body fat or lean mass. Lovejoy et al. (1995) conducted a 9-month clinical trial comparing testosterone injections with an oral androgen (oxandrolone) or placebo in obese, middle-aged men undergoing weight loss. The oral androgen decreased visceral fat significantly more than the injected testosterone or placebo.

More recently, Simon et al. (2001) conducted a 3-month, randomized, controlled trial in healthy, overweight men comparing testosterone, dihydrotestosterone, and placebo. These investigators observed that androgen treatment caused a slight increase in body weight relative to placebo, with no effect on waist to hip ratio. Unfortunately, this study did not use imaging methodology to examine intra-abdominal fat, so it is unknown whether the relative amount of visceral versus subcutaneous abdominal fat changes with androgen treatment. Further research is needed to understand the effects of exogenous androgens on body composition in men.

Lastly, some interesting data have been obtained on the effects of exogenous steroids on adiposity in transsexual individuals. Elbers et al. (1997, 1999) performed imaging studies of both male-to-female (M-F) and female-to-male (F-M) transsexual patients treated with exogenous steroids. In healthy, young F-M transsexuals, long-term (3-year) testosterone administration was associated with a relative increase in visceral fat by 47% as measured by MRI (Elbers et al. 1997). Exogenous testosterone also decreased subcu-

taneous adiposity in F-M transsexuals in the short-term, although this effect did not persist after long-term treatment. In contrast, treatment of M-F transsexuals with exogenous estradiol for 1 year increased all subcutaneous fat depots and decreased visceral fat (Elbers et al., 1999).

Thus, overall, while the results vary depending on the type of exogenous steroid administered and on the patient population, the data suggest, in general, that estrogens decrease visceral fat and androgens increase visceral fat in women, while both estrogens and androgens may decrease visceral fat in men.

Estrogen Receptor Mechanisms

Adiposity has been reported in humans and in mice with disordered ER function. Both male and female transgenic mice with null deletions of the ERα gene become obese by 3 months of age (Heine et al., 2000; Ohlsson et al., 2000). The cause of the increased adiposity has not been identified. Whether metabolic effects, as described previously, changes in food intake, or both are involved is unclear (no significant increase in food intake was detected in the reports cited, but food intake was measured after the animals were already obese, not while they were becoming obese).

In humans, abnormal adiposity has been associated with a polymorphism of the human ERα gene in which guanidine is substituted for adenine in exon one (Okura et al., 2003; Yamada et al., 2002). In a cross-sectional study of over 2000 Japanese women, premenopausal women with the GG genotype had increased fat mass and increased waist-to-hip ratio compared to AA genotype; AG genotype women were intermediate. The polymorphism did not affect adiposity in postmenopausal women or in men. Thus, polymorphisms of the ERα gene may disrupt an activational effect of estradiol that affects body adiposity in women.

SEX DIFFERENCES IN HUMAN EATING

A considerable body of research reveals systematic relationships between gonadal steroid hormones and the control of food intake and body weight in females of many mammalian species, including rats, hamsters, guinea pigs, baboons, monkeys, and humans (reviewed by Asarian & Geary, 2006; Geary, 2004a;

Wade, 1972). In most species, food intake in females is decreased by elevations in estrogens. Progesterone has limited effect on eating behavior except in pharmacological doses in rats (Wade, 1975), and even a pharmacological dose had no effect on food intake in women (Pelkman et al., 2001). In males of many species, testosterone stimulates food intake and weight gain (Asarian & Geary, 2006).

Food Intake During the Menstrual Cycle

In women, appetite ratings and daily food intake are lowest during the peri-ovulatory period, defined as 2 days before to 2 days after the LH surge, when plasma estrogens peak (Gong et al., 1989; Lyons et al., 1989; Buffenstein et al., 1995) (Fig. 13.1). Some studies also demonstrate that average daily food intake is lower during the follicular phase, especially the later follicular phase, during which estrogen secretion increases, than during the luteal phase (Buffenstein et al., 1995; Pelkman et al., 2001). Both estrogens and progesterone are elevated through much of the luteal phase. Overall, the data suggest that women may eat about 10% less during one-third to one-half of the cycle, an amount more than sufficient to affect energy balance (Fig. 13.1).

The cyclic change in eating apparently does not occur during anovulatory cycles (Barr et al., 1995; Rock et al., 1996) and can be suppressed in women whose eating behavior is under strong cognitive restraint (Dye & Blundell, 1997).

Effects of Gonadal Hormones on Food Selection

Available data on the effects of gonadal hormones on food selection in humans are limited. Tarasuk and Beaton (1991) reported that energy intake is greater during the ten premenstrual days than during the 10 postmenstrual days mainly because of increased in intake of fat, without a significant increase in carbohydrate intake. Similarly, Geiselman and Lovejoy (unpublished results) recently compared macronutrient preferences in middle-aged premenopausal women across the menstrual cycle and observed that fat intake was significantly higher in the luteal phase than the follicular phase. Consistent with these data from normally cycling women, Eck et al. (1997) found that women using high estrogen/high progesterone oral

contraceptives ingested more fat and less carbohydrate than non-users. On the other hand, Bowen and Grunberg (1990) report increased intake of sweets or sweet/fat combination foods during the luteal phase.

Several factors complicate identifying sex differences in food selection (Bowen et al., 2003; Buffenstein et al., 1995; Dye & Blundell, 1997; Geary, 2004a). One is that nutritional physiology and hedonics may at least sometimes exert distinct, and potentially antagonistic, effects on food selection, and relatively few studies have measured both preference and actual intakes. An exception is Bowen and Grunberg's (1990) report that both preference for and (acute) intake of sweet fat foods (e.g., coffee cake, chocolate) were significantly higher during the luteal phase than the follicular phase, whereas there were no differences in either measure for salty (e.g., ham, salted peanuts) or bland (e.g., cheese, unsalted peanuts) foods.

Another factor is that learning and cognition, which clearly exert major influences on human food selection, may be the source of sex differences. For example, American and European women display greater interest in healthy eating and in weight control than do men (Bowen et al., 2003; Westenhoefer, 2005). Not surprisingly, learned influences are often culturally bound. For example, American women who identified themselves as chocolate cravers reported more cravings perimenstrually, but Spanish women who craved chocolate similarly did not, suggesting a cultural component to this phenomenon (Zellner et al., 2004).

We know of no studies of the effects of testosterone on nutrient selection in men. In women, a population-based longitudinal study of 611 women found no association between circulating testosterone concentrations and dietary macronutrient intake (Sowers et al., 2001).

Finally, it is worth noting that increasingly sophisticated functional brain imaging methods are opening up new possibilities for the study of sex differences in the brain mechanisms of eating in humans. In particular, there seem to be sex-specific brain responses to food stimuli (Del Parigi et al., 2002; Uher et al., 2006). Particularly exciting are differences in areas of the ventral forebrain that have recently been implicated in the mediation of the subjective experience of pleasure and pain (Craig, 2002; Kringelbach, 2005).

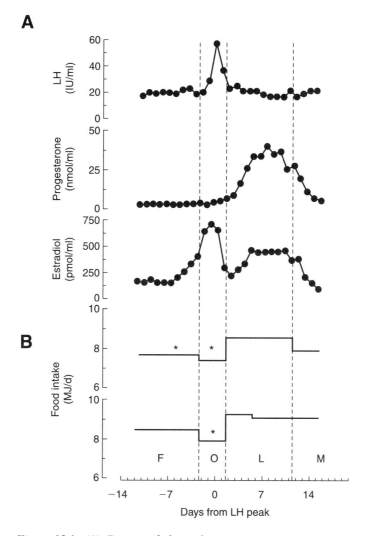

Figure 13.1. (A). Patterns of plasma hormone concentrations across the menstrual cycle in women. Phases of the cycle: F = follicular; O = peri-ovulatory; L = luteal; M = menstrual (data adapted, with permission, from Ross et al., 1970; Thorneycroft et al., 1971). (B). Food intakes, measured by weighing, across the menstrual cycle, shown as averages over the periods indicated (data adapted with permission from (upper) Gong et al., 1989, and (lower) Lyons et al., 1989. *Significantly different from food intake during the luteal phase. Reprinted with permission from Geary N. (2004). The estrogenic inhibition of eating. In Stricker EM, Woods S. (Eds.), *Neurobiology of food and fluid Intake*, 2nd edition. New York: Springer.

Sex Differences in Anorexia Nervosa and Bulimia Nervosa

Although a complete review of the literature on human eating disorders and their treatment is beyond the scope of this chapter, it is worth briefly noting the prominent sex differences in anorexia and bulimia nervosa. Shortly after the first formal recognition of these eating disorders, it was recognized that their prevalence was substantially greater in women than

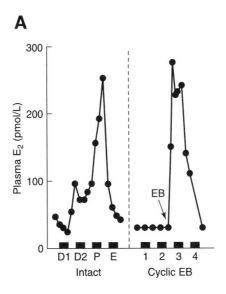

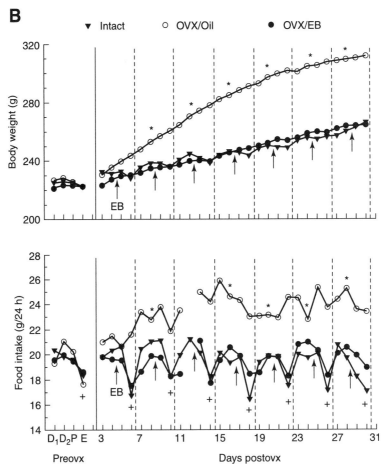

Figure 13.2. (A). Patterns of plasma estradiol concentration in: **left**, intact cycling rats (from Smith et al., 1975) and, **right**, in ovariectomized rats during the ninth cycle of a cyclic estradiol treatment regimen, in

men. While the importance of physiological factors in the etiology of eating disorders remains controversial, there is no question that sex hormones play some role in the onset (typically at puberty) and may have other influences in mediating the progression of eating disorders.

A number of abnormalities in the circulating levels of estradiol, testosterone, and adrenal androgens in females with anorexia nervosa and bulimia nervosa have been reported (e.g. Monteleone et al., 2001). These changes appear to be secondary to the dramatic changes in nutritional status and body composition, especially loss of body fat, associated with this disorder, however, because weight gain to within 5% of normal body weight in women with anorexia nervosa is usually associated with normalization circulating levels of LH, FSH, and estradiol, and normal ovarian morphology (Treasure et al., 1988).

On the other hand, Brambilla et al. (2003) reported that a subset of weight-stabilized women with previous anorexia nervosa remain amenorrheic with low circulating levels of estradiol and leptin compared to age and weight matched controls, consistent with the idea that there may be a primary defect in sex steroid function in some women with anorexia. Tomova and Kumanov (1999) reported that males with anorexia nervosa had lowered testosterone levels, but did not assess whether this effect was secondary to altered body composition.

A recent study by Klump et al. (2006) suggests that the sex difference in eating disorder prevalence may be due to both prenatal, organizational effects of sex hormones on the brain and postnatal, activational effects. These investigators found a significant positive relationship between finger-length ratios, a somatic marker of prenatal testosterone exposure, and disordered eating in 113 adult female twins. In an unrelated community sample of women, the investigators also observed that higher levels of circulating estradiol were associated with disordered eating symptoms.

Thus, while eating disorders clearly have complex and multifactorial causes, the effects of sex hormones on eating behavior, as well as their organizational effects on the brain in utero, may have significant relevance for the sex differences in their prevalence and possibly their treatment.

SEX DIFFERENCES IN EATING IN RATS AND MICE

Food Intake During the Estrous Cycle

As described earlier, rats and mice have 4–5 d ovarian cycles. Food intake decreases ~25% during the night following the LH surge, when ovulation and behavioral estrus occur, in comparison to the other nights of the cycle (about 80%–90% of food intake occurs nocturnally in rats and mice) (for reviews see [Asarian & Geary, 2006; Geary, 2004a]) (Fig. 13.2).

Plasma concentration of estradiol peaks just before the LH surge and is very low during estrus, i.e., plasma estradiol is actually low in the phase of the cycle when rats and mice eat least. Exogenous estradiol also inhibits feeding in ovariectomized rats only after a delay of 12–36 h (Geary and Asarian, 2002). The reason for this is unknown. Estradiol's effect on sexual responsivity in female rats is similarly delayed (Lee et al., 2006; Parsons et al., 1982). The cyclic decrease in food intake is due to a decrease in the size of spontaneous meals; meal number actually increases (Asarian & Geary, 2002; Blaustein & Wade, 1976; Drewett, 1974).

which 2 μg estradiol benzoate was subcutaneously injected on d 3 of each 4-d cycle (at arrow; modified with permission from Asarian and Geary, 2002). Thicker parts of abscissa indicate 12-h dark periods. Abbreviations: D1 = diestrus 1; D2 = diestrus 2; P = preoestrus; E = estrus. (B). Body weights (**upper**) and food intakes (**lower**) in intact rats, in ovariectomized rats receiving cyclic estradiol treatment (OVX/EB), at arrows, and in untreated ovariectomized rats (OVX/Oil). Abbreviations are as (A). Data to the left of the solid vertical lines are prior to ovariectomy; dashed vertical lines divide the 4-d estrus cycles and treatment cycles. +Food intake during E or d 4 significantly less than during D2 or d 2, respectively. *Food intake or body weight significantly less in intact and estradiol-treated ovariectomized rats than in untreated ovariectomized rats during the same cycle. Reprinted with permission from Asarian L, Geary N. (2002). Cyclic estradiol treatment normalizes body weight and restores physiological patterns of spontaneous feeding and sexual receptivity in ovariectomized rats. *Hormones & Behavior*, 42:461–471.

Effects of Gonadectomy and Gonadal Steroid Hormones on Food Intake and Obesity

Gonadectomy unveils another sex difference in the control of food intake and body weight in rats and mice. As discovered almost a century ago (Stotsenburg, 1913), ovariectomy leads to excess weight gain and adiposity. Although metabolic effects contribute under some conditions, the cause is usually increased food intake (Tattelin & Gorski, 1971; Geary, 2004a). Orchiectomy has the opposite effect on reductions in eating and body weight, at least in young animals (Asarian & Geary, 2006; Wallen et al., 2001).

The effects of gonadectomy on eating in males and females are also expressed differently in spontaneous meal patterns. Ovariectomy increases meal size (Asarian & Geary, 2002; Blaustein & Wade, 1976; Chai et al., 1999), whereas orchiectomy decreases meal frequency. During the initial 3–5 weeks postovariectomy, increased food intake leads to a 20%–30% increase in fat mass in young adults. After this dynamic period, food intake returns to near the control level and there is no further excess weight gain. This reduction in total food intake is due solely to a decrease in meal frequency; meal size in ovariectomized rats remains elevated permanently.

The effects of gonadectomy on eating and body weight in rats and mice are apparently due to testosterone in males (Chai et al., 1999; Wallen et al., 2001) and estradiol in females (Asarian & Geary, 2006; Geary, 2004a; Wade, 1972). Asarian and Geary (2002) demonstrated that a nearly physiological 4-day cyclic regimen of estradiol was sufficient to produce apparently normal cyclic patterns of spontaneous meal size and number and daily food intake in rats (Fig. 13.2). Levels of GnRH, LH, FSH, and prolactin do not correlate with eating in female rats; rather, they increase both when eating decreases in the peri-ovulatory period and when eating increases after ovariectomy. Furthermore, elimination of LH, FSH, and prolactin by hypophysectomy did not increase eating in female rats (and did not eliminate the inhibitory effect of estradiol on eating) (Wade & Zucker, 1970). Cyclic changes in food intake in rats do not appear attributable to differing food selection (Bartness & Waldbillig, 1984; Geiselman et al., 1981; Heisler et al., 1999).

Estrogen Receptor Mechanisms

Both molecular genetic and pharmacological tools have been used to investigate the ER subtype mediating the effects of estradiol on feeding. Estradiol treatment had no effect on food intake or body weight gain in ovariectomized mice with null mutations of the ERα gene, indicating that ERα is necessary for the estrogenic inhibition of eating and that ERβ alone is not sufficient for it (Geary, 2004a; Geary et al., 2001). Consistent with this, an ERα-selective agonist inhibited eating in ovariectomized rats, whereas an ERβ-selective agonist did not (Roesch, 2005). In another study, however, inhibition of ERβ synthesis in the brain by intracerebroventricular injection of ERβ antisense oligodeoxynucleotides decreased the inhibitory effect of estradiol on eating in ovariectomized rats (Liang et al., 2002). This apparent contradiction awaits resolution.

SEX DIFFERENCES IN THE PHYSIOLOGICAL CONTROLS OF EATING

The Three "Rs" of the Physiological Control of Eating

Current understanding indicates that eating is controlled by a neural network that is widely distributed throughout the brainstem, diencephalon, and telencephalon; and that the traditional practice of assigning hunger and satiety to "centers" in the hypothalamus or elsewhere is inappropriate and misleading (Berthoud, 2002; Smith, 2000). Nevertheless, some degree of functional localization has emerged in this neural network. Thus, three at least partially independent types of controls of eating seem to be processed in part in anatomically distinct, albeit richly interconnected, functional nodes in the brainstem, hypothalamus, and ventral telencephalon (Berthoud, 2002).

As a heuristic and rough first approximation, the functional controls of eating exerted by these areas may be considered the three "Rs" of eating—reflex, regulation, and reward—respectively. In addition, and especially in humans, the pervasive influences of learning and cognition fundamentally modify the basic biological controls of eating, so even the most potent "R" controls are best considered as simply the foundation of a fantastically elaborated structure, mirrored perhaps in the relative increase in cerebral cortex at the expense of the brainstem, hypothalamus, and ventral telencephalon during human phylogeny.

An important point for the physiological analysis of the three Rs is that each of them includes sensory mechanisms reaching outside the brain—for example, the olfactory, gustatory, and oropharyngeal sensory nerves carrying information used to evaluate the hedonic reward or palatability of food, the neural and hormonal feedbacks from GI and metabolic reflex controls of eating, and the hormonal signals thought to provide regulatory feedbacks from adipose tissue function. These sensory mechanisms are the input or feedback signals for the central neural networks that control eating. Research programs beginning with analyses of such signals represent a sort of bottom-up (or outside-in) approach, in contrast to more top-down (or inside-out) approaches, based for example, on brain lesion neuropharmacological studies. Examples of both are included in the next sections.

How are sex differences in these systems mediated? Because the three R mechanisms originate in the periphery, sex differences could arise from differences in the peripheral (neural and non-neural) mechanisms generating the signals, in the brain mechanisms processing and responding to the signals, or in both. The mechanisms so far described involve the second possibility, i.e., gonadal hormones appear to act in the brain to alter the central processing of neural signals controlling eating.

Cholecystokinin (CCK)

The prototypical molecule associated with reflexive control of eating is CCK, a peptide secreted from the small intestine during meals. Of the many signals hypothesized to be involved in the gastrointestinal and metabolic control of eating, CCK is the one that has been shown most convincingly to operate under normal physiological circumstances in both rats and humans (for references to the data reviewed in this section, see Asarian & Geary, 2006; Beglinger & Degan, 2004; Geary, 2004ab; Moran & Kinzig, 2004). Furthermore, at least in rats, there is a prominent sex difference in CCK's satiating action.

In both experimental animals and humans, administration of CCK at meal onset decreases meal size with little effect on the following intermeal interval.

In humans, acute injection of CCK increases the perception of fullness (the closest commonly used name for satiation), decreases the perception of hunger, and produces neither physical nor subjective side effects. Studies with selective CCK receptor antagonist indicate that the satiating effect of CCK is mediated by low-affinity CCK_A receptors (alternatively known as CCK-1 receptors); use of CCK_A receptor antagonists show clearly that in both rats and humans acute interference with CCK signaling increases meal size, blocks the satiating effect induced by intraduodenal infusions fat (which is the most important CCK secretogogue), and increases the perception of hunger in humans.

A reflex, as conceived originally by DesCartes, is a specific unlearned response to a specific stimulus. The satiating action of CCK can be considered reflexive because (a) very specific food stimuli elicit CCK secretion, (b) CCK secretion leads to a neural sensory signal, and (c) the processing of this signal in the CNS results in a fixed response, satiation. CCK satiation depends on an innately organized, relatively local neural network in the brainstem because it persists in rats in which the entire forebrain has been disconnected, i.e., in animals no longer capable of forebrain-mediated spontaneous or goal-directed behaviors, which begin eating only when brought in contact with food—(Grill & Kaplan, 1992; Grill & Smith, 1988). This localization fits with the facts that the CCK satiation signal originates in the abdomen and projects via vagal afferents to the brainstem (specifically, to the nucleus tractus solitarius [NTS]) and that the brainstem contains both the motor pattern generators and motor neurons that organize and effect the coordinated movements of biting, licking, chewing and swallowing once food contacts the mouth (Blessing, 1997).

CCK satiation also exhibits sex differences. In females, the modulation of CCK satiation by estradiol plays a major role in the peri-ovulatory decrease in eating. For example, in intact rats the de-satiating effect of CCK_A receptor antagonism was much larger during behavioral estrus than during diestrus, and in estradiol-treated ovariectomized rats the de-satiating effect was larger on the day that modeled estrus than on the day that modeled diestrus (Asarian & Geary, 1999; Eckel & Geary, 1999). These effects appear to result from altered neural processing rather than increased CCK secretion because exogenous estradiol also increased the satiating potency of exogenous CCK in ovariectomized rats (Geary et al., 1994). As a result of this cyclic effect, CCK appears to elicit more satiation in male rats than female rats, except at estrus, when the effect is comparable.

Four further results indicate that the neural processing mediating the estradiol-CCK interaction occurs in the brainstem: (a) Experiments mapping brain activity with c-Fos immmunocytochemistry indicate that estradiol increases c-Fos expression in the NTS after either food ingestion, intraduodenal fat infusion, or CCK injection (Eckel & Geary, 2001; Eckel et al., 2002); (b) the effect of CCK on NTS c-Fos depends on ERα in mice Geary et al., 2001); (c) many NTS cells that express c-Fos in response to intraduodenal fat infusions also express ERα (Asarian & Geary, 2007); and (d), as most recently discovered (Thammacharoen et al., 2007), local administration of estradiol to the surface of the brainstem just over the NTS was sufficient both to decrease eating and to increase CCK-induced c-Fos in the caudal NTS of ovariectomized rats. These data indicate that one mechanism through which estradiol decreases eating in rats is by increasing the satiating action of CCK.

In addition to the estradiol-mediated sex differences in *sensitivity* to CCK, it is possible that a sex difference in CCK *secretion* also contributes to sex differences. This is because it has recently been reported that food ingestion results in markedly higher plasma levels of CCK in women than in men (Nolan et al., 2003).

Finally, it should be reiterated that discussion of CCK satiation in terms of *reflex action* is heuristic. The reflex is an abstraction; reflexes do not exist in pure form in nature. More specifically, when CCK satiation is studied in the neurologically intact animal, things change importantly. One change that might be related to another sex difference in CCK satiation involves the role of hypothalamic 5-HT$_{2C}$ serotonin receptors (Poeschla et al., 1993).

Ghrelin

Ghrelin is another gut peptide with a reflex-like effect on eating. Ghrelin is unique among gut hormones in that it is secreted (from the stomach) in response to emptying, rather than filling, of the gut, and it stimulates eating, rather than inhibiting it (Geary, 2004b; Ueno et al., 2005; van der Lely et al., 2004).

We (Clegg et al., 2007) reported that ghrelin stimulates less during behavioral estrus than during other phases of the ovarian cycle in females, less in intact

females than in ovariectomized females, and less in estradiol-treated ovariectomized females than untreated females. These data suggest that changes in the eating-stimulatory potency of endogenous ghrelin may contribute to both the tonic and the cyclic inhibitory effects of estradiol on eating. The mediating mechanisms, however, remain unclear.

Insulin and Leptin

It has long been clear that animals change how they eat in response to increases or decreases in energy balance, sometimes in a manner that maintains normal weight. This phenomenon led to the theory of "behavioral regulation of energy homeostasis" or, because adipose tissue is the only quantitatively important energy store, "behavioral regulation of body weight." Although it can be debated whether body adiposity is truly regulated within a narrow physiological envelope by the control of eating, it is certainly clear that changes in adiposity change the activity of signaling systems that influence eating and that the concept of regulation provides a useful organizing principle.

The two best understood adiposity signals controlling eating are the hormones insulin and leptin, and the action of each displays sex differences in rats. Interestingly, the direction of the differences is opposite: exogenous leptin inhibits eating more potently in intact females than in males; whereas exogenous insulin inhibits eating more potently in males. Estradiol treatment increases this effect of leptin in females and decreases the effect of insulin (Ainslie et al., 2001; Clegg et al., 2003, 2006).

Furthermore, the secretion of both hormones is also affected by sex. For example, basal plasma leptin concentration increased more with increasing adiposity in women than in men and more in premenopausal than postmenopausal women (Rosenbaum et al., 1996). Whether there are sex differences in the influence of adiposity signals on eating, however, remains uncertain. Nevertheless, some questions remain. Endogenous leptin is secreted by the adipocytes into the peripheral circulation, and effects similar to those reported by Ainslie et al. (2001) and Clegg et al. (2003) have not been reported after peripherally administered leptin (see Chen & Heiman, 2001; Pelleymounter et al., 1999). Additionally, sex differences have not been found in the eating-inhibitory action of hypothalamic α-melanocyte-stimulating hormone (α-MSH), which is puzzling because α-MSH is a key neuronal mediator of leptin's eating-inhibitory action (reviewed in Asarian & Geary, 2006; Geary, 2004a).

Further work with these adiposity signals is urgently warranted. First, because very little research so far has involved leptin or insulin antagonism, which is a gold-standard of physiological function in endocrinology (Geary, 2004b), and future studies may well suggest different conclusions. Second, several lines of evidence suggest that adiposity signals normally function to detect and correct *deficits* in body adiposity rather than *surfeits* of adiposity (Schwartz et al., 2003), a direction so far neglected.

Insulin and leptin may also be involved in determining the different pattern of regional deposition of adiposity in males and females, at least in rats. Initial evidence for this is the Clegg et al. (2006) report that leptin administration led to relatively greater increase in subcutaneous than visceral fat, insulin administration led to relatively greater increases in visceral than subcutaneous fat, and these actions were increased by estradiol in females and testosterone in males.

Finally, it should be noted that at present the very best evidence for the a physiological role of leptin concerns the link between energy balance and fertility, where leptin plays crucial physiological roles in the control in pubertal development in both sexes (Chehab et al., 2002) and in the control of GnRH secretion and ovulation in women (Welt et al., 2004).

Forebrain Reward Mechanisms

Food reward, the third R, is defined in different contexts as the capacity of food to stimulate continued eating during the meal, to elicit positive hedonic experiences, or to reinforce learning. This section reviews the first of these functions, i.e., effects of flavor on eating. Sweet taste and other flavors provide potent positive feedback signals during meals that stimulate further eating and increase meal size. Although it is clear that caudal brainstem mechanisms are sufficient to mediate the potentiation of intake of sweet solutions in rats (i.e., Grill & Kaplan, 1992), in the neurologically-intact animal this effect of food is thought to be mediated by more rostral, especially ventral telencephalic, structures. Indeed, food reward is a very active area of research, and we seem to be at least on the verge of new insights about forebrain reward network functions in animals and humans alike. What remains very much unclear is the extent and importance of sex differences in food reward.

Sweet taste is the prototypical food reward. Although some investigators have reported sex differences in the effects of sucrose and other sugars on eating in rats, others have not (reviewed in Asarian & Geary, 2006; Geary, 2004a). One complication is that few studies have controlled for possible sex differences in gastrointestinal or postabsorptive handling of the ingesta that might obscure the effects of reward on eating. When gastrointestinal and postabsorptive effects were minimized by testing the effects of estradiol on sham feeding of sucrose in ovariectomized rats with gastric cannulas, estradiol did not decrease sham intake of any sucrose solution tested, although it did decrease real intake of some solutions. These data indicate that estradiol does not inhibit eating in rats by decreasing the rewarding effect of sweet taste.

Rats avidly ingest solutions of 3% glucose and 0.25%–0.75% saccharine; and beginning around puberty, female rats consume more of such solutions than males (Valenstein et al., 1967; Zucker, 1969). This difference is reduced by ovariectomy and reinstated by treatment with both estradiol and progesterone, but not by either hormone alone. This dependence on both estradiol and progesterone suggests that this phenomenon may be a useful model of changes in eating during the luteal phase in women.

Fat is another flavor preferred by rats and, as in the case of sweet, there are conflicting reports as to the existence in sex differences (Asarian & Geary, 2006; Geary, 2004a). Also as with sucrose, however, estradiol treatment did not decrease sham intake of corn oil emulsifications in ovariectomized rats, but did decrease real intake of some of the same solutions.

Serotonin

Of the many CNS neurochemical signaling molecules involved in the control of eating, serotonin (5-hydroxytryptamine [5-HT]) appears at present to have the most interesting links to sex: (a) the 5-HT agonist fenfluramine inhibited eating more in female rats than in male rats (Eckel et al., 2005); (b) fenfluramine inhibited eating more during behavioral estrus than during behavioral diestrus (Eckel et al., 2005); and (c) the eating-inhibitory effect of fenfluramine was increased by estradiol treatment in ovariectomized rats (Rivera & Eckel, 2005; but see also Souquet & Rowland, 1990).

$5-HT_{1A}$ receptors, which are autoreceptors on 5-HT neurons whose activation decreases 5-HT function, have been directly implicated implicated in this sex difference: (a) stimulation of 5-HT_{1A} receptors with 8-OH-DPAT stimulated eating less during behavioral proestrus and behavioral estrus than during behavioral diestrus in cycling rats (Uphouse et al., 1991); and (b) the eating-stimulatory effect of 8-OH-DPAT was decreased by estradiol treatment, and unaffected by progesterone treatment, in ovariectomized rats (Salamanca & Uphouse, 1992).

5-HT_{2C} receptors also may be involved in this sex difference because the non-selective 5-HT agonist mCPP did not inhibit eating in transgenic mice with null mutations of the 5-HT_{2C} receptor gene (these mice also become obese) (Tecott et al., 1995); and because the satiating effect of CCK, which displays sex differences depends on hypothalamic 5-HT_{2C} receptor function (Poeschla et al., 1993) and is absent in 5-HT_{2C} receptor knockout mice (Geary, unpublished data).

The amygdala is another site mediating sex differences in the eating action of 5-HT, although the data are not entirely consistent. On the one hand, (a) estradiol increased eating- and CCK-induced expression of c-Fos in the central nucleus of the amygdala (Eckel & Geary, 2001, Eckel et al., 2002); (b) infusions of the 5-HT receptor antagonist metergoline directly into the posterior basolateral amygdala increased diurnal eating less during behavioral diestrus than during the day after behavioral estrus (Parker et al., 2002); and (c) female rats were more hyperphagic following amygdala lesions than were male rats (although the effects of amygdala lesions and of ovariectomy appeared additive and, therefore, independent) (King et al., 2003).

It is also interesting to note that when rats were fed more palatable foods or were fed different macronutrients separately, there were no cyclic variations in the effect of 5-HT on eating (Heisler et al., 1999; Parker et al., 2002). These data may be relevant to the hypothesis that 5-HT controls food selection during luteal or the menstrual phases of the human cycle (Dye and Blundell, 1997; Heisler et al., 1999).

In summary, numerous data relate 5-HT to sex differences in eating, at least in rats. There are no comparably strong data for any other central signaling molecule (Asarian & Geary, 2006; Geary, 2004a).

CONCLUSION

The studies reviews in this chapter illustrate the existence of a range of physiologically important sex dif-

ferences in energy metabolism, obesity, and eating behavior. Sex differences in both the epidemiology and the biology of adiposity indicate, especially in the current environment of increasing overweight and obesity, that one major focus for basic and clinical research in energy metabolism and eating behavior should be analysis of sex differences and the role of sex hormones as direct or indirect modulators of eating and of adiposity. While acknowledging the challenges of studying sex differences, we believe the studies reviewed in this chapter illustrate ways that these challenges can be overcome, so as to lead to the discovery of important phenomena and open fruitful avenues for crucial future research.

Acknowledgment

The authors thank the Society for Women's Health Research, in particular its formation of the Isis Fund Metabolism Network," which provided the venue for the conversations that initiated this chapter.

References

Ainslie DA, Morris MJ, Wittert G, Turnbull H, Proietto J, Thorburn AW. (2001). Estrogen deficiency causes central leptin insensitivity and increased hypothalamic neuropeptides Y. *Int J Obes*, 25:1680–1688.

Aloia JF, Vaswani A, Russo L, Sheehan M, Flaster E. (1995). The influence of menopause and hormonal replacement therapy on body cell mass and body fat mass. *Am J Obstet Gynecol*, 172:896.

Asarian L, Geary N. (2002). Cyclic estradiol treatment normalizes body weight and restores physiological patterns of spontaneous feeding and sexual receptivity in ovariectomized rats. *Horm Behav*, 42:461–471.

Asarian L, Geary N. (2007). Estradiol enhances CCK-dependent lipid-induced satiation and activates ERα-expressing cells in the NTS of ovariectomized rats. *Endocrinology* (in press).

Asarian L, Geary N. (2006). Modulation of appetite by gonadal steroid hormones. *Proc Roy Soc B 361: 1251–1563.*

Barr SI, Janelle KC, Prior JC. (1995). Energy intakes are higher during the luteal phase of ovulatory menstrual cycles. *Am J Clin Nutr*, 61:39–43.

Barros RP, Machado UF, Warner M, Gustafsson J-Å. (2006). Muscle GLUT4 regulation by estrogen receptors ERbeta and ERalpha. *Proc Natl Acad Sci USA*, 103:1605–1608.

Bartness TJ, Waldbillig RJ. (1984). Dietary self-selection in intact, ovariectomized, and estradiol-treated female rats. *Behav Neurosci*, 98:125–137.

Becker JB, Arnold AA, Berkley KJ, Blaustein JB, Eckel LA, Hampson E, et al. (2005) Strategies and methods for research on sex differences in brain and behavior. *Endocrinol*, 146:1650–1673.

Beglinger C, Degen L. (2004). Fat in the intestine as a regulator of appetite—role of CCK. *Physiol Behav*, 83:617–621.

Berenstein EG, Ortiz Z. (2005). Megestrol acetate for the treatment of anorexia-cachexia syndrome. *Cochrane Database Syst Rev*, 2005:CD004310.

Berthoud HR. (2002). Multiple neural systems controlling food intake and body weight. *Neurosci Biobehav Rev*, 26:393–428.

Bjorntorp P. (1993). Visceral obesity: a 'civilization syndrome.' *Obesity Res*, 1:206–222.

Blaak E. (2001). Gender differences in fat metabolism. *Curr Opin Clin Nutr Metab Care*, 4:499–502.

Blaustein J D, Wade GN. (1976). Ovarian influences on the meal patterns of female rats. *Physiol Behav*, 17:201–208.

Blessing WW. (1997). The lower brainstem and bodily homeostasis. New York: Oxford University Press.

Bonny AE, Ziegler J, Harvey R, Debanne SM, et al. (2006). Weight gain in obese and nonobese adolescent girls initiating depot medroxyprogesterone, oral contraceptive pills, or no hormonal contraceptive method. *Arch Pediatr Adolesc Med*, 160:40–45.

Boschmann M, Rosenbaum M, Leibel R, Segal KR. (2002). Metabolic and hemodynamic responses to exercise in subcutaneous adipose tissue and skeletal muscle. *Int J Sports Med*, 23: 537–543.

Bowen D, Green P, Vizenor N, Vu C, Kreuter P, Rolls B. (2003). Effects of fat content on fat hedonics: cognition or taste? *Physiol Behav*, 78: 247–253.

Bowen DJ, Grunberg NE. (1990). Variations in food preference and consumption across the menstrual cycle. *Physiol Behav*, 47:287–291.

Brambilla F, Monteleone L, Bortolotti F, Dalle-Grave R, et al. (2003). Persistent amenorrhea in weight-recovered anorexics: psychological and biological aspects. *Psychiatry Res*, 118:249–257.

Braun B, Horton TJ. (2001). Endocrine regulation of exercise substrate utilization in women compared to men. *Ex Sport Sci Rev*, 29:149–154.

Bray GA. (2004). Medical consequences of obesity. *J Clin Endo Metab*, 89:2583–2589.

Bucholz AC, Rafii M, Pencharz PB. (2001). Is resting metabolic rate different between men and women? *Br J Nutr*, 86:641–646.

Buffenstein R, Poppitt SD, McDevitt RM, Prentice AM. (1995). Food intake and the menstrual cycle: a retrospective analysis, with implications for appetite research. *Physiol Behav*, 58:1057–1077.

Carpenter WH, Fonong T, Toth MJ, Ades PA, et al. (1998). Total daily energy expenditure in free-living older African-Americans and Caucasians. *Am J Physiol*, 274:E96–E101.

Chehab FF, Qiu J, Mounzih K, Ewart-Toland A, Ogus S. (2002). Leptin and reproduction. *Nutr Rev*, 60:S39–S46.

Chai JK, Blaha V, Meguid MM, Laviano A, Yang ZJ, Varma M. (1999). Use of orchiectomy and testosterone replacement to explore meal number-to-meal size relationship in male rats. *Am J Physiol*, 276:R1366–R1373.

Chen Y, Heiman ML. (2001). Increased weight gain after ovariectomy is not a consequence of leptin resistance. *Am J Physiol*, 280:E315–E322.

Clark MK, Dillon JS, Sowers M, Nichols S. (2005). Weight, fat mass, and central distribution of fat increase when women use depot medroxyprogesterone acetate for contraception. *Int J Obesity*, 29: 1252–1259.

Clegg DJ, Brown LM, Zigman JM, Kemp CJ, Strader AD, Benoit SC, Woods SC, Geary N. (2007). Estradiol-dependent decrease I the orexigenic potency of ghrelin in female rats. *Diabetes* 56:1051–1058.

Clegg DJ, Brown LM, Woods SC, Benoit SC. (2006). Gonadal hormones determine sensitivity to central leptin and insulin. *Diabetes*, 55:978–987.

Clegg DJ, Riedy CA, Blake Smith KA, Benoit SC, Woods SC. (2003). Differential sensitivity to central leptin and insulin in male and female rats. *Diabetes*, 52: 682–687.

Couse JF, Korach KS. (1999). Estrogen receptor null mice: what have we learned and where will they lead us? *Endocrine Review*, 20:358–417.

Craig AD. (2002). How do you feel? Interoception: the sense of the physiological condition of the body. *Nat Rev Neurosci*, 3:655–666.

Davis SN, Fowler S, Costa F. (2000a). Hypoglycemic counterregulatory responses differ between men and women with type 1 diabetes. *Diabetes*, 49:65–72.

Davis SN, Shavers C, Costa F. (2000b). Differential gender responses to hypoglycemia are due to alterations in CNS drive and not glycemic thresholds. *Am J Physiol*, 279:E1054–E1063.

Day DS, Gozansky WS, van Pelt RE, Schwartz RS, Kohrt WM. (2005). Sex hormone suppression reduces resting energy expenditure and beta-adrenergic support of resting energy expenditure. *J Clin Endocrinol Metab*, 90:3312–3317.

DeLany JP, Bray GA, Harsha DW, Volaufova J. (2004). Energy expenditure in African-American and white boys and girls in a 2-y follow-up of the Baton Rouge Children's Study. *Am J Clin Nutr*, 79:268–273.

Del Parigi A, Chen K, Gautier JF, Salbe AD, Pratley RE, Ravussin E, et al. (2002). Sex differences in the human brain's response to hunger and satiation. *Am J Clin Nutr*, 75:1017–1022.

D'Eon T, Braun B. (2002). The roles of estrogen and progesterone in regulating carbohydrate and fat utilization at rest and during exercise. *J Women's Health & Gender Based Med*, 11:225–237.

Devries MC, Hamedeh MJ, Phillips SM, Tarnopolsky MA. (2006). Menstrual cycle phase and sex influence muscle glycogen utilization and glucose turnover during moderate-intensity endurance exercise. *Am J Physiol*, 291:R1220–R1228.

Dionne I, Despres JP, Bouchard C, Tremblay A. (1999). Gender differences in the effect of body composition on energy metabolism. *Int J Obesity*, 23:312–319.

Drewett RF. (1974). The meal patterns of the oestrous cycle and their motivational significance. *Quart J Exp Psych*, 26:489–494

Dye L, Blundell JE. (1997). Menstrual cycle and appetite control: implications for weight regulation. *Hum Reprod*, 12:1142–1151.

Eck LH, Bennett AG, Egan BM, Ray JW, et al. (1997). Differences in macronutrient selections in user and non-users of an oral contraceptive. *Am J Clin Nutr*, 65:419–424.

Eckel LA, Geary N. (2001). Estradiol treatment increases feeding-induced c-Fos expression in the brains of ovariectomized rats. *Am J Physiol*, 281:R738–R746.

Eckel LA, Houpt TA, Geary N. (2002). Estradiol replacement increases CCK-induced c-Fos expression in the brains of ovariectomized rats. *Am J Physiol*, 283: R1378–R1385.

Eckel LA, Rivera HM, Atchley DP. (2005). The anorectic effect of fenfluramine is influenced by sex and stage of the estrous cycle in rats. *Am J Physiol*, 288:R1486–R1491.

Elbers JM, Asscheman H, Seidell JC, Megens JA, Gooren LJ. (1997). Long-term testosterone administration increases visceral fat in female to male transsexuals. *J Clin Endocrinol Metab*, 82:2044–2047.

Elbers JM, Asscheman H, Seidell JC, Gooren LJ. (1999). Effects of sex steroid hormones on regional fat depots as assessed by magnetic resonance imaging in transsexuals. *Am J Physiol*, 276:E317–E325.

Espeland MA, Stefanick ML, Kritz-Silverstein D, Fineberg SE, et al. (1997). Effect of postmenopausal hormone therapy on body weight and waist and hip girths. Postmenopausal Estrogen-Progestin Interventions Study Investigators. *J Clin Endocrinol Metab*, 82(5):1549–1556.

Fahrbach SE, Meisel RL, Pfaff DW. (1985). Preoptic implants of estradiol increase wheel running but not the open field activity of female rats. *Physiol Behav*, 35: 985–992.

Flegal KM, Carroll MD, Ogden CL, Johnson CL. (2002). Prevalence and trends in obesity among US adults, 1999–2000. *JAMA*, 288:1723–1727.

Gallo MF, Grimes DA, Schulz KF, Helmerhorst FM. (2004). Combination estrogen-progestin contraceptives and body weight: systematic review of randomized controlled trials. *Obstet Gynecol*, 103:359–373.

Geary N. (2004a). The estrogenic inhibition of eating. In Sticker EM, Woods SC (Eds.), *Handbook of behavioral neurobiology*, Vol 14, Neurobiology of Food and Fluid Intake, 2nd Ed. (pp. 307–345), New York NY: Kluver Academic/Plenum.

Geary N. (2004b). Endocrine controls of eating: CCK, leptin, and ghrelin. *Physiol Behav*, 81:719–733.

Geary N. (2004c). On Gerard P. Smith's scientific character and thought. *Physiol Behav*, 82:159–166.

Geary N. (2006). Curt Richter and the female rat. *Appetite* (in press).

Geary N, Asarian L, Korach KS, Pfaff DW, Ogawa S. (2001). Deficits in E2-dependent control of feeding, weight gain, and cholecystokinin satiation in ER-α null mice. *Endocrinology*, 142:4751–457.

Geiselman PJ, Martin JR, VanderWeele DA, Novin D. (1981). Dietary self-selection in cycling and neonatally ovariectomized rats. *Appetite*, 2:87–101.

Gentry RT, Wade GN. (1976). Sex differences in sensitivity of food intake, body weight, and running-wheel activity to ovarian steroids in rats. *J Comp Physiol Psychol*, 90:747–754.

Gong EJ, Garrel D, Calloway DH. (1989). Menstrual cycle and voluntary food intake. *Am J Clin Nutr*, 49:252–258.

Grill HJ, Kaplan JM. (1992). Sham feeding in intact and chronic decerebrate rats. *Am J Physiol*, 262:R1070–R1074.

Grill HJ, Smith GP. (1988). Cholecystokinin decreases sucrose intake in chronic decerebrate rats. *Am J Physiol*, 254:R853–R856.

Grund A, Vollbrecht H, Frandsen W, Krause H, et al. (2000). No effect of gender on different components of daily energy expenditure in free living prepubertal children. *Int J Obesity*, 24: 299–305.

Haarbo J, Marslew U, Gotfredsen A, Christiansen C. (1991). Postmenopausal hormone replacement therapy prevents central distribution of body fat after menopause. *Metabolism*, 40(12):1323–1326.

Hedley AA, Ogden CL, Johnson CL, Carroll MD, Curtin LR, Flegal KM. (2004). Prevalence of overweight and obesity among US children, adolescents, and adults, 1999–2002. *JAMA*, 291:2847–2850.

Heine PA, Taylor JA, Iwamoto GA., Lubahn DB, Cooke PS. (2000). Increased adipose tissue in male and female estrogen receptor-alpha knockout mice. *Proc Natl Acad Sci (USA)*, 97:12729–12734.

Heisler LK, Kanarek RB, Homoleski B. (1999). Reduction of fat and protein intakes but not carbohydrate intake following acute and chronic fluoxetine in female rats. *Pharmacol BiochemBehav*, 63: 377–385.

Hellstrom L, Blaak E, Hagstrom-Toft E. (1996) Gender differences in adrenergic regulation of lipid mobilization during exercise. *Int J Sports Med*, 17:439–447.

Horton T, Braun B. (2004) Sex based differences in substrate metabolism. In Miller V, Hay M (Eds.), *Principles of sex-based differences in physiology* (pp 208–227). Amsterdam:Elsevier.

Howard BV, Kuller L, Langer R, Manson JE, et al. (2005). Risk of cardiovascular disease by hysterectomy status, with and without oophorectomy. *Circulation*, 111:1462–1470.

Hoyenga KB, Hoyenga KT. (1982). Gender and energy balance: sex differences in adaptation to feast and famine. *Physiol Behav*, 28:545–563.

Hunter GR, Kekes-Szabo T, Trueth MJ, et al. (1996). Intra-abdominal adipose tissue, physical activity, and cardiovascular risk in pre- and postmenopausal women. *Int J Obes*, 20:860–865.

Jensen MD. (1995). Gender differences in regional fatty acid metabolism before and after meal ingestion. *J Clin Invest*, 96:2297–3303.

Jones ME, Thorburn AW, Britt KL, Hewitt N, Wreford G, Proietto J, et al. (2000). Aromatase-deficient (ArKO) mice have a phenotype of increased adiposity. *Proc Natl Acad Sci (USA)*, 97:12735–12740.

King BM, Rollins BL, Grundmann SJ, Olivier LG. (2003). Excessive weight gains in female rats with transactions of the stria terminalis. *Physiol Behav*, 78:563–568.

Kirkby J, Metcalf BS, Jeffery AN, O'Riordan CF, et al. (2004). Sex differences in resting energy expenditure and their relation to insulin resistance in children (Early Bird 13). *Am J Clin Nutr*, 80:430–435.

Klausen B, Toubro S, Astrup A. (1997). Age and sex effects on energy expenditure. *Am J Clin Nutr*, 65:895–907.

Klump KL, Gobregge KL, Perkins PS, Thorne D, et al. (2006). Preliminary evidence that gonadal hormones organize and activate disordered eating. *Psychol Med*, 36(4):539–546.

Koehler KF, Helguero LA, Haldosén L-A, Warner M, Gustafsson J-Å. (2005). Reflections on the discovery and significance of estrogen receptor β. *Endo Rev*, 26:465–478.

Kotani K, Tokunaga K, Fujioka S, Kobatake T, Keno Y, et al. (1994). Sexual dimorphism of age-related changes in whole-body fat distribution in the obese. *Int J Obesity*, 18:207–212.

Kringelbach ML. (2005). The human orbitofrontal cortex: linking reward to hedonic experience. *Nat Rev Neurosci*, 6:691–702.

Kritz-Silverstein D, Barrett-Connor E. (1996). Long-term postmenopausal hormone use, obesity, and fat distribution in older women. *JAMA*, 275(1):46–49.

Lee AW, Devidze N, Pfaff DW, Zhou J. (2006). Functional genomics of sex hormone-dependent neuroendocrine systems: specific and generalized actions in the CNS. *Prog Brain Res*, 158:243–2271.

Leibel RL, Hirsch J. (1987). Site- and sex-related differences in adrenoreceptor status of human adipose tissue. *J Endocrinol Metab*, 64:1205–1210.

Levine JA, Lanningham-Foster LM, McCrady SK, Krizan AC, Olson LR, Kane PH, et al. (2005). Intra-individual variation in posture allocation: possible role in human obesity. *Science*, 307:584–586.

Liang Y-Q, Akishita M, Kim S, Ako J, Hashimoto M, Ijima K, et al. (2002) Estrogen receptor β is involved in the anorectic action of estrogen. *Int J Obes*, 26:1103–1109.

Lissner L, Stevens J, Levitsky DA, Rasmussen KM, Strupp BJ. (1988). Variation in energy intake during the menstrual cycle: implications for food-intake research. *Am J Clin Nutr*, 48:956–962.

Lyons PM, Truswell AS, Mira M, Vizzard J, Abraham SF. (1989). Reduction of food intake in the ovulatory phase of the menstrual cycle. *Am J Clin Nutr*, 49:1164–1168.

Lovejoy JC, Bray GA, Greeson CS, Klemperer M, et al. (1995). Oral anabolic steroid treatment, but not parenteral androgen treatment, decreases abdominal fat in obese, older men. *Int J Obesity*, 19:614–624.

Lovejoy JC, Bray GA, Bourgeois MO, Macchiavelli R, et al. (1996). Exogenous androgens influence body composition and regional body fat distribution in obese postmenopausal women. *J Clin Endocrinol Metab*, 81:2198–2203.

Lovejoy JC, Smith SR, Larson-Meyer DE, Xie H. (2003). Intramuscular lipid stores in perimenopausal African-American and Caucasian women and relation to estrogen levels. *Obesity Research*, 11(Supplement 1):A4.

Mangan SA, Larsen PG, Hudson S. (2002). Overweight teens at increased risk for weight gain while using depot medroxyprogesterone acetate. *J Pediatr Adolesc Gynecol*, 15:79–82.

Marin P, Holmang S, Jonsson L, Sjostrom L, et al. (1992). The effects of testosterone treatment on body composition and metabolism in middle-aged obese men. *Int J Obesity*, 16:991–997.

Matthews KA, Abrams B, Crawford S, et al. (2001). Body mass index in mid-life women: relative influence of menopause, hormone use, and ethnicity. *Int J Obesity*, 25: 863–873.

Mauras N, Hayes V, Welch S, Rini A, Helgeson K, Dokler M, Veldhuis JD, Urban RJ. (1998). Testosterone deficiency in young men: marked alterations in whole body protein kinetics, strength, and adiposity. *J Clin Nutr Metab*, 83:1886–1892.

Meijer GA, Janssen GM, Westerterp KR, Verhoeven F, Saris WH, ten Hoor F. (1991). The effect of a 5-month endurance-training programme on physical activity: evidence for a sex difference in the metabolic response to exercise. *Eur J Appl Physiol Occup Physiol*, 62:11–17.

Meijer GA, Westerterp KR, Saris WH, ten Hoor F. (1992). Sleeping metabolic rate in relation to body composition and the menstrual cycle. *Am J Clin Nutr*, 55:637–640.

Mittendorfer B. (2005). Sexual dimorphism in human lipid metabolism. *J Nutr*, 135:681–686.

Monteleone P, Luisi M, Colurcio B, Casarosa E, et al. (2001). Plasma levels of neuroactive steroids are increased in untreated women with anorexia nervosa or bulimia nervosa. *Psychosom Med*, 63:62–68.

Moran TH, Kinzig KP. (2004). Gastrointestinal satiety signals II. Cholecystokinin. *Am J Physiol*, 286:G183–G188.

Morio B, Beaufrere B, Montaurier C, Verdier E, et al. (1997). Gender differences in energy expended during activities and in daily energy expenditure of elderly people. *Am J Physiol*, 273:E321–E327.

Munoz J, Derstine A, Gower BA. (2002). Fat distribution and insulin sensitivity in postmenopausal women: influence of hormone replacement. *Obes Res,* 10(6):424–431.

Nolan LJ, Guss JL, Liddle RA, Pi-Sunyer FX, Kissileff HR. (2003). Elevated plasma cholecystokinin and appetitive ratings after consumption of a liquid meal in humans. *Nutr,* 19:553–557.

Ogawa S, Chan J, Gustafsson J-A, Korach KS, Pfaff DW. (2003). Estrogen increases locomotor activity in mice through estrogen receptor α: specificity for the type of activity. *Endocrinol,* 144:230–239.

Ohlsson C, Hellberg N, Parini P, Vidal O, Bohlooly M, Rudling M, et al. (2000). Obesity and disturbed lipoprotein profile in estrogen receptor-alpha-deficient male mice. *Biochem Biophys Res Comm,* 278:640–645.

Okura T, Koda M, Ando F, Niino N, Ohta S, Shimokata H. (2003). Association of poymorphisms in the estrogen receptor α gene with body fat distribution. *Int J Obes,* 27:1020–1027.

Pagotto U, Gambineri A, Pelusi C, Genghini S, et al. (2003). Testosterone replacement therapy restores normal ghrelin in hypogonadal men. *J Clin Endocrinol Metab,* 88:4139–4143.

Parker GC, Bishop C, Coscina DV. (2002). Estrous cycle and food availability affect feeding induced by amygdala 5-HT receptor blockade. *Pharmacol Biochem Behav,* 71:701–707.

Parsons B, McEwen BS, Pfaff DW. (1982). A discontinuous schedule of estradiol treatment is sufficient to activate progesterone-facilitated feminine sexual behavior and to increase cytosol receptors for progestins in the hypothalamus of the rat. *Endocrinol,* 110:613–619.

Pascual Lopez A, Roque i Figuls M, Urrutia Cuchi G, Berenstein EG, Almenar Pasies B, Balcells Alegre M, Herdman M. (2004). Systematic review of megestrol acetate in the treatment of anorexia-cachexia syndrome. *J Pain Symptom Manage,* 27:360–369.

Pasquali R, Casimirri F, Cantobelli S, Labate AMM, et al. (1993). Insulin and androgen relationships with abdominal body fat distribution in women with and without hyperandrogenism. *Horm Res,* 39:179–187.

Patil GD, Briski KP. (2005). Lactate is a critical "sensed" variable in caudal hindbrain monitoring of CNS metabolic status. *Am J Physiol,* 289:R1777–R1786.

Pelkman CL, Chow M, Heinbach RA, Rolls BJ. (2001). Short-term effects of a progestational contraceptive drug on food intake, resting energy expenditure, and body weight in young women. *Am J Clin Nutr,* 73: 19–26.

Pelleymounter MA, Baker MB, McCaleb M. (1999). Does estradiol mediate leptin's effects on adiposity and body weight? *Am J Physiol,* 276:E955–E963.

Poeschla B, Gibbs J, Simansky KJ, Greenberg D, Smith GP. (1993). Cholecystokinin-induced satiety depends on activation of 5-HT1C receptors. *Am J Physiol,* 264: R62–R64.

Rebuffe-Scrive M, Eldh J, Hafstrom L-O, Bjorntorp P. (1986). Metabolism of mammary, abdominal, and femoral adipocytes in women before and after menopause. *Metabolism,* 35:792.

Reimer RA, Debert CT, House JL, Poulin MJ. (2005). Dietary and metabolic differences in pre- versus post-menopausal women taking or not taking hormone replacement therapy. *Physiol Behav,* 84:303–312.

Rivera HM, Boersma G, Eckel LA. (2005). Estradiol's inhibitory effect on food intake is attenuated by antagonism of central, but not peripheral, estrogen receptors. *Appetite,* 44:374.

Rivera HM, Eckel LA. (2005). The anorectic effect of fenfluramine is increased by estradiol in ovariectomized rats. *Physiol Behav,* 86:331–337.

Rock CL, Gorenflow DW, Drewnowski A, Demitrack MA. (1996). Nutritional characteristics, eating pathology, and hormonal status in young women. *Am J Clin Nutr,* 64:566–571.

Roesch DM. (2005). Effects of selective estrogen receptor agonists on food intake and body weight in rats. *Physiol Behav,* 87:39–44.

Romanskie S, Nelson R, Jensen MD. (2000). Meal fatty acid uptake in adipose tissue: gender effects in nonobese humans. *Am J Physiol,* 279:E445–E462.

Rosenbaum M, Nicholson M, Hirsch J, Heymsfeld SB, Gallagher D, Chu F, Leibel R. (1996). Effects of gender, body composition, and menopause on plasma concentration of leptin. *J Clin Endocrinol Metab,* 81:3424–3427.

Ross GT, Cargille CM, Lipsett MB, Rayford PL, Marshall JR, Strott CA, Rodbard D. (1970). Pituitary and gonadal hormones in woman during spontaneous and induced ovulatory cycles. *Rec Prog Horm Res,* 26:1–62.

Roubinoff R. Hughes VA, Dallal GE, Nelson ME, et al. (2000). The effect of gender and body composition method on the apparent decline in lean mass-adjusted resting metabolic rate with age. *J Gerontol A Biol Sci Med Sci,* 55:M757–M760.

Roy EJ, Buyer DR, Licari VA. (1990). Estradiol in the striatum: effects on behavior and dopamine receptors but no evidence for membrane steroid receptors. *Brain Res Bull,* 25:221–227.

Salamanca S, Uphouse L. (1992). Estradiol modulation of the hyperphagia induced by the 5-HT1A agonist, 8-OH-DPAT. *Pharmacol Biochem Behav,* 43:953–935.

Sandoval DA, Ertl AC, Richardson A, Tate DB, Davis SN. (2003). Estrogen blunts neuroendocrine and metabolic responses to hypoglycemia. *Diabetes,* 52:1749–1755.

Schwartz MW, Woods SC, Seeley RJ, Barsh GS, Baskin DG, Leibel RL. (2003). Is the energy homeostasis system inherently biased toward weight gain? *Diabetes,* 52:232–238.

Schindler AE, Campagnoli C, Druckmann R, Huber J, Pasqualini JR, Schweppe KW, et al. (2003). Classification and pharmacology of progestins. *Maturitas*, 46(Suppl 1):S7–S16.

Simon D, Charles M-A, Lahlou N, Nahoul K, et al. (2001). Androgen therapy improves insulin sensitivity and decreases leptin level in healthy adult men with low plasma total testosterone. *Diabetes Care*, 24:2149–2151.

Sites CK, Brochu M, Tchernof A, Poehlman ET. (2001). Relationship between hormone replacement therapy use with body fat distribution and insulin sensitivity in obese postmenopausal women. *Metabolism*, 50:835–840.

Smith EP, Boyd J, Frank GR, Takahashi H, Cohen RM, Specker B, et al. (1994) Estrogen resisitance caused by a mutation in the estrogen receptor gene in a man. *N Engl J Med*, 331:1056–1061.

Smith GP. (2000). The controls of eating: a shift from nutritional homeostasis to behavioral neuroscience. *Nutr*, 16:814–820.

Smith MS, Freeman ME, Neill JD. (1975). The control of progesterone secretion during the estrous cycle and early pseudopregnancy of the rat: prolactin, gonadotropin and steroid levels associated with rescue of the corpus luteum of pseudopregnancy. *Endocrinol*, 96:219–226.

Souquet A-M, Rowland NE. (1990). Dexfenfluramine: action with estradiol on food intake and body weight in ovariectomized rats. *Am J Physiol*, 258:R211–R215.

Sowers MF, Beebe JL, McConnell D, Randolph J, Jannausch M. (2001). Testosterone concentrations in women aged 25–50 years: associations with lifestyle, body composition, and ovarian status. *Am J Epidemiol*, 153:256–264.

Steffensen CH, Roepstorff C, Madsen M, Kiens B. (2002). Myocellular triacylglycerol breakdown in females but not males during exercise. *Am J Physiol*, 282: E364–E642.

Stewart J, Rodaros D. (1999). The effects of gonadal hormones on the development and expression of the stimulant effects of morphine in male and female rats. *Behav Brain Res*, 102:89–98.

Stotsenburg JM. (1913). The effect of spaying and semi-spaying young albino rats (*mus norvergicus albinus*) on the growth in body weight and body length. *Anat Rec*, 7:183–194.

Svendsen OL, Hassager C, Christiansen C. (1995). Age- and menopause-associated variations in body composition and fat distribution in healthy women as measured by dual-energy X-ray absorptiometry. *Metabolism*, 44:369–373.

Tai MM, Castillo TP, Pi-Sunyer FX. (1997). Thermic effect of food during each phase of the menstrual cycle. *Am J Clin Nutr*, 66(5):1110–1115.

Tarasuk V, Beaton GH. (1991). Menstrual-cycle patterns in energy and macronutrient intake. *Am J Clin Nutr*, 53(2):442–447.

Tarnopolsky M (Ed.). (1999). *Gender differences in metabolism*. Boca Raton FL:CRC Press.

Tarnopolsky MA, Ruby BC. (2001). Sex differences in carbohydrate metabolism. *Curr Opin Clin Nutr Metab Care*, 4:521–526.

Tarttelin MF, Gorski RA. (1973). The effects of ovarian steroids on food and water intake and body weight in the female rat. *Acta Endocrinol*, 72:551–568.

Tecott, LH, Sun LM, Akana AF, Strack AM, Lowenstein DH, Dallman MF, Julius D. (1995). Eating disorder and epilepsy in mice lacking 5-HT$_{2C}$ serotonin receptors. *Nature*, 374:542–546.

Thammacharoen S, Lutz T, Geary N, Asarian L. (2007). Hindbrain administration of estradiol inhibits feeding and activates ERα-expressing cells in the NTS of ovariectomized rats. *Appetite*, 46:387.

Thorneycroft IH, Mishell DR Jr, Stone SC, Kharma KM, Nakamura RM. (1971). The relation of serum 17-hydroxyprogesterone and estradiol-17-beta levels during the human menstrual cycle. *Am J Obst Gynecol*, 111:947–951.

Tomova A, Kumanov P. (1999). Sex differences and similarities of hormonal alterations in patients with anorexia nervosa. *Andrologia*, 31:143–147.

Toth MJ, Tchernof A, Sites CK, Poehlman ET. (2000). Effect of menopausal status on body composition and abdominal fat distribution. *Int J Obesity*, 24: 226–231.

Treasure JL, Wheeler M, King EA, Gordon PA, Russell GF. (1988). Weight gain and reproductive function: ultrosonographic and endocrine features of anorexia nervosa. *Clin Endocrinol* (Oxf) 29:607–616.

Trueth MS, Sunehag AL, Trautwien LM, Bier DM, Haymond MW, Butte NF. (2003). Metabolic adaptation to high-fat and high-carbohydrate diets in children and adolescents. *Am J Clin Nutr*, 77:479–489.

Ueno H, Yamaguchi H, Kangawa K, Nakazato M. (2005). Ghrelin: a gastric peptide that regulates food itake and energy homeostasis. *Reg Pep*, 126:11–19.

Uher R, Treasure J, Heining M, Brammer MJ, Campbell IC. (2006). Cerebral processing of food-related stimuli: effects of fasting and gender. *Behav Brain Res*, 169:111–119.

Uphouse L, Salamanca S, Caldarola-Pastuszka M. (1991). Gender and estrous cycle differences in the response to the 5-HT1A agonist 8-OH-DPAT. *Pharmacol Biochem Behav*, 40:901–906.

Van der Lely AJ, Tschöp M, Heiman ML, Ghigo E. (2004). Biological, physiological, pathophysiological and pharmacological aspects of ghrelin. *Endocr Rev*, 25:426–457.

Valenstein ES, Kakolewski JW, Cox VC. (1967). Sex differences in taste preference for glucose and saccharin solutions. *Science*, 156:942–943.

Wade GN. (1972). Gonadal hormones and behavioral regulation of body weight. *Physiol Behav*, 8:523–534.

Wade GN. (1975). Some effects of ovarian hormones on food intake and body weight in female rats. *J Comp Physiol Psychol*, 88:183–193.

Wade GN, Zucker I. (1970). Development of hormonal control over food intake and body weight in female rats. *J Comp Physiol Psychol*, 70:213–220.

Wajchenberg BL. (2000). Subcutaneous and visceral adipose tissue: their relation to the metabolic syndrome. *Endocr Rev*, 21(6):697–738.

Wallen WJ, Belanger MP, Wittnich C. (2001). Sex hormones and the selective estrogen receptor modulator tamoxifen modulate weekly body weights and food intakes in adolescent and adult rats. *J Nutr*, 131:2351–2357.

Wang G. (1923) The relation between "spontaneous" activity and the oestrous cycle in the white rat. *Comp Psychol Monogr* 2: 1–40.

Welt CK, Chan JL, Bullen J, Murphy R, Smith P, DePaoli AM, Karalis A, Mantzoros CS. (2004). Recombinant human leptin in women with hypothalamic amenorrhea. *N Eng J Med*, 351: 987–97.

Westenhoefer J. (2005). Age and gender dependent profile of food choice. *Forum Nutr*, 57:44–51.

Wing RR, Matthews KA, Kuller LH, Meilahn EN, Plantinga PL. (1991). Weight gain at the time of menopause. *Arch Intern Med*, 151:97–102.

World Health Organization. (2002). The world health report 2002: Reducing risks, promoting healthy life. Geneva, World Health Organization.

Yamada Y, Ando F, Niino N, Shimokata H. (2002). Association of polymorphisms of the estrogen receptor alpha gene with bone mineral density in community-swelling Japanese. *Int J Mol Med* 80:452–460.

Zellner DA, Garriga-Trillo A, Centeno S, Wadsworth E. (2004). Chocolate craving and the menstrual cycle. *Appetite*, 42:119–121.

Zucker I. (1969). Hormonal determinants of sex differences in saccharin preference, food intake and body weight. *Physiol Behav*, 4:595–602.

Chapter 14

Sex Differences in Children's Play

Sheri A. Berenbaum, Carol Lynn Martin,
Laura D. Hanish, Phillip T. Briggs,
and Richard A. Fabes

Step on to any playground anywhere on the planet and you will see boys and girls playing in different worlds. They differ in what they are doing, with whom they are doing it, and how they are doing it. These differences emerge early in life, and are among the largest of non-reproductive physical or psychological sex differences. Sex differences in play have led many scholars to suggest that boys and girls grow up and live in separate cultures (Maccoby, 1998). The differences have considerable significance for mental health, social relationships, and cognition across the life span.

What are these differences? How do they come about? What do they mean for the world outside of play? What can they tell us about sex differences in other characteristics? These questions are the focus of this chapter.

THE NATURE AND MAGNITUDE OF SEX DIFFERENCES IN CHILDREN'S PLAY

Boys and girls differ in several aspects of play including, interest and play with specific toys and activities, the sex of their play partners, and the styles they use when playing with toys and with friends. Males and females of other species differ in aspects of their play as well.

Toys and Activities: What Do Boys and Girls Do?

Studies across cultures document that girls more than boys are interested in and engage with dolls and doll accessories, arts and crafts, kitchen toys, fashion, and make-up, whereas boys more than girls are interested in and engage with transportation toys, electronics, blocks (especially complex building sets), and sports (Ruble et al., 2006). These differences earn toys the sex-typed labels of "boys' toys" and "girls' toys."

Sex differences in toy play are well-documented by 2 years of age for some toys, such as girls' preferences for dolls and boys' preferences for toy trucks and tools (Fagot et al., 1986; Campbell & Shirley, 2002). Nevertheless, questions remain about the exact age at which the differences emerge and for which toys (Ruble et al., 2006). The range and scope of sex-differentiated toy and activity play increases in early childhood (Maccoby, 1998). In preschool, girls prefer to play with dolls and kitchen sets, and to have fantasy play that involves relationships, household roles, and romance, whereas boys prefer to play with cars, trucks, and blocks, and to have fantasy play that involves superheroes, danger, and aggression. Boys also play video games increasingly more than girls from 2 to 7 years, and girls begin to spend more time in chores than do boys at age 3 to 4 (Huston et al., 1999).

The magnitude of sex differences in toy and activity preferences among preschool children is illustrated in a study in which children were observed daily for 3 months, and their activities, affective displays, and play partners were recorded (Martin, Fabes, & Hanish, 2006, unpublished data). Table 14.1 shows the significant and sizable differences in

Table 14.1. Sex Differences in Preschoolers' Time Spent Playing with Toys and Activities: Mean Proportion of Total Interactions[a]

	Boys (N = 32)	Girls (N = 23)	Size of Sex Difference, d
Boy-Preferred Toys/Activities			
Balls	.018 (.015)	.009 (.010)	.66**
Bikes	.021 (.017)	.010 (.011)	.74**
Blocks	.078 (.045)	.032 (.023)	1.05***
Play figure male	.009 (.009)	.001 (.002)	1.01***
Pretend play male	.022 (.020)	.004 (.005)	1.01***
Trucks	.018 (.017)	.005 (.004)	.92***
Total Boy-Preferred Toys/Activities	.166 (.055)	.059 (.031)	1.51***
Girl-Preferred Toys/Activities			
Board Games	.020 (.013)	.029 (.023)	−.54*
Crayons	.049 (.047)	.083 (.048)	−.68*
Play figure female	.001 (.002)	.013 (.012)	−1.24***
Kitchen play	.009 (.011)	.016 (.013)	−.53*
Pretend play female	.002 (.004)	.020 (.005)	−1.31***
Puzzles	.009 (.007)	.016 (.013)	−.62*
Total Girl-Preferred Toys/Activities	.090 (.048)	.176 (.055)	−1.30***
Neutral Toys/Activities			
Books	.068 (.024)	.070 (.033)	−.09
Clay	.018 (.013)	.022 (.014)	−.34
Computers	.014 (.022)	.012 (.019)	.11
Digging	.021 (.015)	.021 (.016)	.01
Fantasy play neutral	.010 (.007)	.014 (.010)	−.42
Music	.034 (.020)	.039 (.019)	−.30
Pretend neutral play	.028 (.016)	.029 (.013)	−.10
Phone	.002 (.003)	.002 (.003)	−.10
Toy animals	.012 (.014)	.011 (.011)	.30
TV	.001 (.001)	.001 (.002)	−.14
Total Neutral Toys/Activities	.209 (.049)	.221 (.050)	−.24

[a]Number of sampled intervals including each activity divided by the total number of observations per child
Sex differences significant by t-tests, *P < .05, **P < .01, ***P < .001.

the proportion of interactions in which boys and girls played with specific toys and activities. Sex differences are described in standard deviation units, *d* (mean of boys minus mean of girls divided by average standard deviation, Cohen, 1988). For total play with girls' and boys' toys and activities, the sex differences were very large, −1.3 and 1.5. Expressed in another way, child sex accounted for about one-third of the variation in toy and activity play.

Large and varied sex differences continue into middle and late childhood and adolescence, encompassing interests and hobbies, household chores, and sports involvement, as measured by self-reported preferences and time use (Etaugh & Liss, 1992; McHale et al., 2004a). The sex differences in activities continue and expand in scope as children move through adolescence: compared to boys, girls spend more time in relationship-oriented activities, personal care, and household chores, and less time in sports and male-typical activities (e.g., building things) (McHale et al., 2004b; Ruble et al., 2006).

There is considerable interest in children whose play and activity interests are not typical for their sex because of associations with sexual orientation, cognitive abilities, and emotional adjustment (as discussed later in the chapter). Cross-sex play decreases in middle childhood and is more common in girls than in boys. About one-quarter of boys and one-third of girls engage in multiple cross-sex behaviors at least occasionally (Sandberg et al., 1993). Studies of tomboys suggest within-group variability: some exhibit extreme cross-sex play, whereas other play with both girls' and boys' toys (Zucker & Bradley, 1995; Bailey et al., 2002).

A key question concerns the dimensions underlying sex differences in children's toy and activity preferences, which probably reflect the actions and qualities afforded by toys. Boys' and girls' toys differ on several dimensions, with boys' toys higher in symbolic play, sociability, competition, aggressiveness, dangerousness, and constructiveness, and girls' toys higher in domestic skills, nurturance, and attractiveness (Blakemore & Centers, 2005). We know little about the ways in which these or other dimensions contribute to sex differences in toy play.

Juvenile monkeys also show sex-differentiated preferences for human sex-typed toys (Alexander & Hines, 2002; Hassett et al., 2004). In fact, the sex-based preferences of rhesus monkeys for wheeled vs. plush toys are similar to the sex-based preferences of human children for boys' versus girls' toys (Hassett et al., 2004). This suggests that children's toy choices partly reflect inherent sex-differentiated preferences for characteristics that underlie the toys.

Play Partners: With Whom Do Boys and Girls Play?

The term *sex segregation* is used to characterize children's tendencies to interact preferentially with peers of the same sex. It begins at a young age (Serbin et al., 1994), with girls segregating earlier than boys. For example, in one observational study, girls preferred same-sex peers by 27 months, but boys did not show preferences for another year (LaFreniere et al., 1984). By 3 to 4 years of age, both boys and girls spend the majority of their social interactions with members of the same sex (Maccoby & Jacklin, 1987; Fabes et al., 1997). This preference is seen across method (e.g., observation, self-report) (Bukowski et al., 1993; Fabes, 1994), countries (Omark et al., 1975) and species (Barbu, 2006), including primates (Bernstein et al., 1993), rats (Meaney & Stewart, 1981), cats (Caro, 1981) and ungulates (Bonenfant et al., 2004).

Not only do young children strongly prefer peers of their own sex, they also spend relatively little time with only peers of the other sex. Over half of all young children's peer interactions involve play with same-sex peers, about 30% involves play with both a boy and a girl, and less than 10% involves play exclusively with other-sex peers (Fabes, 1994).

Preference for same-sex play partners escalates over childhood. In one illustrative study, the ratio of play with same versus other-sex peers was 3 to 1 in preschoolers, but 11 to 1 in 6 ½-year-olds (Maccoby & Jacklin, 1987). Throughout childhood, boys and girls prefer same-sex friends and have more positive interactions with them than with other-sex friends (Vandell et al., 2006). Play with other-sex friends decreases through childhood (Smith et al., 2001). For example, by middle childhood, only about 15% of children have other-sex friends (Kovacs et al., 1996).

Children's preferences for same-sex play partners are dramatic. For many characteristics, a person's sex accounts for a relatively small percent of the variation. But, sex of a play partner is predicted almost completely by sex of the target child, accounting for 70%–80% of the variance, equivalent to a difference (*d*) of 3 to 4 standard deviations (Martin & Fabes, 2001). This is illustrated in Figure 14.1 with observational data

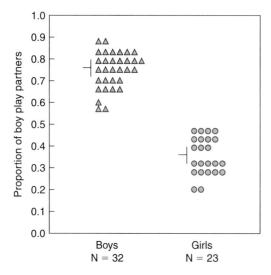

Figure 14.1. Distribution of proportion of boy play partners by sex of child. △=1 boy; ○ = 1 girl. Horizontal line = means; vertical line = standard deviations.

from preschool and kindergarten children. Boys and girls do not overlap in the proportion of their play with boy partners. The boy with the lowest level of play with boy playmates still played with boys more than the girl with the highest level of play with boys; similar but reverse patterns were found for play with girls (Martin et al., 2006, unpublished data).

Interestingly, same-sex play partner preferences are child-driven rather than adult-driven. The strongest sex segregation occurs in settings where children make their own choices. Same-sex peer play is strongest when activities are unstructured and adults are not immediately present or involved in children's play (Thorne, 2001). Play with other-sex peers is more likely to occur when adults are in the vicinity, especially for girls playing with boys (Fabes et al., 2003b). Moreover, these preferences are not easily changed by adults. For example, when preschool teachers reinforced play with other-sex peers, such play increased while the contingency was in effect, but play quickly became segregated when reinforcement was discontinued (Serbin et al., 1977).

During adolescence, sex-based peer preferences begin to change. Young adolescents congregate in small cliques of same-sex peers and have same-sex friends (Bukowski et al., 1999). Although same-sex preferences are still obvious among mid-adolescents (15–16 years), heterosexual dating and other-sex re-

lationships emerge (Sippola, 1999). Even so, girls (but not boys) report feeling more comfortable with same- than with other-sex peers (Lundy et al., 1998). Longitudinal data across grades 9 to 11 show that children's same-sex peer networks remain about the same but their other-sex peer networks increase in size (Richards et al., 1998).

Play Styles: How Do Boys and Girls Play?

Boys' and girls' play styles are characterized by different behaviors and patterns of social interaction, beyond their toys and partners (reviewed in Leaper, 1994). Boys' play tends to be unstructured, more peer- than adult-directed, and guided by the peer group, with boys generating their own rules and standards for appropriate behavior (Carpenter et al., 1986; Smith & Inder, 1993). It is no surprise, therefore, that boys' play tends to be rougher and more active than girls' play, more often involving physical contact, fighting, and taunting (Maccoby, 1998). Indeed, boys are more likely than girls to engage in rough-and-tumble play, involving physical activities characterized as playful and joyous, and to participate in large motor activities (e.g., running, jumping, Fabes et al., 2003b). Boys tend to play more than do girls in large groups characterized by competition and the establishment and maintenance of dominance hierarchies (Maccoby & Jacklin, 1987). Thus, boys' play is characterized as active, dominance-oriented, and physically-assertive.

In contrast, girls' play is structured and adult-oriented. Girls' play groups more than boys' are likely to be near teachers (Fabes et al., 2003b; Martin & Fabes, 2001) and girls' interactions tend to be adult-oriented and adult-structured (Smith & Inder, 1993). Girls tend to interact in dyads, rather than large groups (Fabes et al., 2003a), which is important because dyadic play is more likely than large-group play to elicit behaviors that are sensitive to peers' needs (Maccoby, 1998). Girls are more likely than boys to emphasize cooperation and verbal interaction among play partners and to use enabling forms of communication that promote group harmony. In contrast to boys, girls display dominance and leadership using verbal means, such as negotiation (Maccoby, 1990). Furthermore, girls often play quietly in activities that require verbal interaction (e.g., playing house). Thus, girls' play is characterized as quiet, verbal, and governed by adult-based rules designed to maintain social harmony.

These sex differences in play styles emerge early in childhood and are apparent by the time children enter preschool. Just as the preschool years mark increasing segregation of boys and girls, they also mark increasing differentiation in boys' and girls' play behaviors (Maccoby & Jacklin, 1987; Maccoby, 1998). Moreover, the divergence in boys' and girls' play styles is influenced by the amount of time that children spend in same-sex play. Longitudinal data show that the more time that preschool children spent in same-sex peer play during the fall, the more sex-differentiated their patterns of behavior became the following spring, even after controlling for children's initial individual differences to engage in sex-typical ways. Thus, as boys play with other boys and girls play with other girls, they are repeatedly exposed to the play styles and interaction patterns that characterize their own sex, thereby strengthening the sex-specific patterns (Martin & Fabes, 2001).

Sex-differentiated play style also characterizes other species. From rats to primates, play fighting or rough-and-tumble play is much more common in males than in females, peaking in frequency in the juvenile period (reviewed in Beatty, 1992; Wallen, 2005).

THE SIGNIFICANCE OF SEX DIFFERENCES IN PLAY

Sex differences in children's play and activity interests are associated with sex differences in other behaviors concurrently and in the future. Some of these links reflect the direct effects of play on other behavior, whereas others may reflect the operation of a common yet unidentified third factor. We focus here on links between childhood play and other psychological characteristics, but it seems likely that play also has consequences for physical health.

Consequences of Sex-Typed Toy and Activity Preferences

Sex differences in children's toy and activity preferences have received much attention for their association with sexual orientation and cognitive abilities. The causal nature of the play-ability associations has been assumed in discussions of interventions to enhance girls' spatial ability through modification of their toy play.

Sexual Orientation

Individuals with homosexual orientation in adulthood are more likely than those with heterosexual orientation to have shown sex-atypical childhood toy and playmate choices, with this effect larger for males than for females (Bailey & Zucker, 1995). Most evidence is based on retrospective reports, but one prospective study showed that boys who were extremely "feminine" in childhood (e.g., dressing in feminine clothing, preferring dolls to trucks, playing with girls, and even preferring to be girls) were very likely to become homosexual adults (Green, 1987).

Cognitive Abilities

A popular explanation for sex differences in cognitive abilities involves sex differences in childhood toy play. In particular, high spatial abilities of boys and men compared to girls and women are often considered to result directly from boys' experiences with toys that encourage manipulation and exploration of the environment, so that sex differences in spatial abilities would be eliminated if girls were encouraged to play more with boys' toys.

Evidence supports a weak-to-moderate link between spatial ability and aspects of sex-typed activities (e.g., Newcombe et al., 1983), although there is some variability and inconsistency that likely reflects methodological and conceptual issues (Baenninger & Newcombe, 1989; Voyer et al., 2000). These associations are not evidence of causation: play with male-typical toys/activities might enhance spatial ability or instead reflect that ability (i.e., children with high spatial ability are attracted to toys that allow spatial activities). In fact, some longitudinal data suggest that the causal path is from abilities to activities rather than the reverse (Newcombe & Dubas, 1992). Therefore, it is important to note some direct evidence for the beneficial effect of experiences on spatial ability from experimental studies (reviewed by Baenninger & Newcombe, 1989).

Thus, sex differences in spatial abilities may partly reflect boys' and girls' differential engagement with toys and activities that facilitate the development of those abilities. Nevertheless, caution is necessary before concluding that girls' spatial abilities can be improved simply by encouraging them to play with boys' toys: there have been no studies showing the long-term cognitive effects of spatial training, there is limited generalizability of training, and sex differences in spatial effects of practice are eliminated only when everyone scores well. Further, there may be a cost to encouraging girls to play more with boys' toys, because they typically play some with boys' toys, time use is finite, and there may be benefits to playing with girls' toys.

Consequences of Sex-Segregated Play

Playing with boys provides different opportunities and experiences than does playing with girls. Because children vary in the extent to which they show sex-segregated play, they also vary in the consequences of this play. As shown in Figure 14.2 (for the sample described earlier), the proportion of same-sex peer play in both sexes varies from .30 to .80 (Martin et al., 2006, unpublished data). And the more a child is exposed to same-sex peers, the more the child will be affected by these experiences, although these effects depends on the child's characteristics (Fabes et al., 1997; Fabes et al., 2003a).

For children low in self-control, play with same-sex peers enhanced social competence for girls but lowered social competence for boys, suggesting that playing with other boys enhances dysregulated tendencies for those who already have a difficult time regulating themselves, but playing with other girls enhances the ability to self-regulate for girls who have

difficulty doing so. Relatedly, young children's self-control moderated the relation between same-sex play and academic readiness for kindergarten, with boys high in self-control and girls low in self-control benefiting most from same-sex play. These findings may reflect sex differences in peer groups' self-regulation (more in girls' groups than boys' groups), with differential effects on children who vary in levels of self-control. Importantly, these effects are not a function of general sociability (Fabes et al., 1997).

Thus, the experiences that result from segregated peer interactions likely contribute to development in both positive and negative ways, which extend beyond the individual differences that lead children to initially select themselves into same-sex peer play. Experiences gained within boys' and girls' peer groups foster different behavioral norms and interaction styles, which have the effect over time and exposure of promoting the development of different skills, attitudes, motives, interests, and behaviors.

Sex-differentiated early play experiences have consequences for later behavior in non-human species too. The absence of rough play in male monkeys is associated with adjustment problems (Wallen, 2005). The sex composition of monkeys' rearing groups affects aspects of adult sexual behavior; for example, males reared only with same-sex others display less mounting behavior than males reared in mixed-sex groups, but the reverse effect is observed in females (Wallen, 1996).

Thus, same-sex peer groups and their activities represent a powerful context for socialization. The research described above illustrates the potential of this work to explain development across species, with particular implications for aspects of human physical and mental health.

Summary: The Nature and Consequences of Sex Differentiated Play

Some sex differences in toy preferences are obvious by age 2 and become marked in the following few years. Preferences for same-sex peers appear by age 3, and become pronounced in middle childhood, with very little play with other-sex peers. For all aspects of play, there are early sex differences in a few domains, and the differences grow in size and scope through childhood and into adolescence. Sex-differentiated play patterns are dynamically interrelated: the more chil-

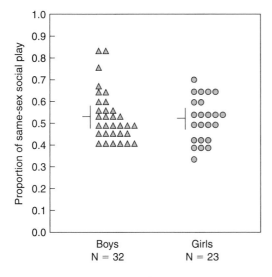

Figure 14.2. Distribution of proportion of same-sex social play by sex of child.

dren play with same-sex peers, the more sex-differentiated their toy choices and play styles become, and the more sex-differentiated their play styles and toy choices, the more likely they are to attract and maintain same-sex peer interactions.

The consequences of children's sex-typed play extend well beyond play itself. The largest effects appear to come from children's segregation into girls' and boys' groups, although there are some effects for toy play. The different socialization experiences of girls and boys may play a role in many of the sex differences discussed elsewhere in this book. It would be interesting to examine, for example, the ways in which early sex-differentiated play patterns affect the development of sex differences in response to stress, affiliation, and eating behaviors.

THE CAUSES OF SEX DIFFERENCES IN PLAY

Because sex differences in play represent one of the largest psychological sex differences, understanding their origins will likely help to understand the origins of sex differences in other characteristics. Theoretical explanations of sex differences in play parallel those invoked for most sex differences, involving influences of sex hormones and socialization. An important additional theoretical perspective on children's play— and gender-related psychological development in general—is provided by cognitive theories, which emphasize children's active construction of their world through their thoughts about and use of gender-related information. This perspective could also be usefully extended to other characteristics that show sex differences.

Hormonal Theories of Sex Differences in Play

Studies in a variety of species clearly show how sex hormones present during sensitive developmental periods induce sex-differentiated sexual, social, and cognitive behaviors and their underlying neural substrates (reviewed in Becker et al., 2002; Ryan & Vandenbergh, 2002; Wallen, 2005). Hormones affect aspects of juvenile play; for example, rough play is reduced in male rats deprived of testosterone, and increased in female monkeys exposed to high prenatal androgen (Beatty, 1992; Wallen, 2005). A key question concerns the generalizability of these findings to human beings, particularly the extent to which prenatal sex hormones shape sex differences in childhood play.

It is, of course, not possible to manipulate hormones in people, but much has been learned from children whose prenatal hormones are atypical for their sex as a result of disorders of sex development, particularly congenital adrenal hyperplasia (CAH), a genetic disease in which the fetus is exposed to high levels of androgens beginning early in gestation. Females with CAH provide an excellent opportunity to examine the behavioral effects of prenatal androgens because they are reared as females but exposed to high levels of sex-atypical hormones during prenatal development; their postnatal development is generally sex-typical after they are diagnosed at birth, and treated medically to reduce androgen excess, and surgically to feminize their genitalia.

Studies of females with CAH indicate that early androgen exposure has a large effect on sex-differentiated toy play and activity interests, with findings replicated across labs, methods, and countries (reviewed in Meyer-Bahlburg, 2001; Berenbaum, 2004). Girls with CAH play much more with boys' toys than do their unaffected sisters or other controls, and interest in boy-typical activities continues into adolescence. Paralleling the increased preference for male-typical activities is reduced preference for female-typical activities.

Differences between CAH and unaffected girls in toy play and activities are large, with means for girls with CAH generally between those for typical boys and girls. A typical difference is illustrated in Table 14.2 with data from a longitudinal study of boys and

Table 14.2. Toy Chosen to Keep by Girls and Boys With and Without CAH

	Control Girls	Girls with CAH	Control Boys	Boys with CAH
% who chose a transportation toy at any session	4%	43%	74%	78%
Average toy choice (SD) (1: feminine; 5: masculine)	1.9 (1.0)	3.1 (1.4)	4.2 (1.1)	4.3 (1.1)

girls with CAH and their unaffected siblings (summarized in Berenbaum, 2004; Berenbaum & Bryk, 2007). When choosing a toy to keep, girls with CAH were more likely than their sisters without CAH to pick a transportation toy; $d = 1.0$.

Congenital adrenal hyperplasia is not a perfect experiment for testing the behavioral effects of prenatal androgens because it is a disease that causes virilized genitalia. Recent work testing alternative explanations of behavioral changes (e.g., parent responses to the girls' genitalia, postnatal androgen) show that masculinized toy and activity play in girls with CAH results directly from prenatal androgen. Play with boys' toys is related to the degree of prenatal androgen excess inferred from genetic defect and other indicators of disease severity (Berenbaum et al., 2000; Nordenström et al., 2002). There is little evidence that parents socialize girls with CAH in a masculine way. For example, the amount of time that girls with CAH played with boys' toys was not increased when parents were present (Nordenström et al., 2002), and parents were observed to encourage girls with CAH to play with girls' toys (Pasterski et al., 2005).

Evidence from other clinical conditions converges with that from CAH. Individuals with a Y-chromosome and male-typical prenatal androgen exposure reared as girls because they lack a penis show boy-typical childhood activity preferences (reviewed in Meyer-Bahlburg, 2005; Hughes et al., 2006).

Recent work has examined the generalizability of results obtained in clinical populations. Fetal hormones in typical samples have been measured indirectly from amniotic fluid, mother's blood, or markers such as sharing a uterus with an opposite-sex fetus (parallelling studies in non-human species showing behavioral and physical masculinization in females who gestate between two males vs. two females; Ryan & Vandenbergh, 2002) (for review of methods and findings see Cohen-Bendahan et al., 2005). Results from these studies are mixed. Play behavior in typical girls at age 3½ years has been found to relate to testosterone in their mother's serum during pregnancy (Hines et al., 2002), but because the placenta generally protects the fetus against masculinizing effects of androgens, the association most likely reflects genetic effects, that is, the transmission of genes that affect testosterone levels which, in turn, affect activity interests. Other studies have failed to find associations between child toy and activity preferences and prenatal androgen determined from amniocentesis (Grimshaw et al., 1995; Knickmeyer et al., 2005) or gestating with an opposite-sex co-twin (Elizabeth & Green, 1984; Henderson & Berenbaum, 1997; Rodgers et al., 1998). It is unclear whether these findings reflect a lack of association between testosterone and activity interests within the normal range or methodological issues (discussed in Cohen-Bendahan et al., 2005).

There has been little study of hormonal influences on other aspects of sex-differentiated play, such as play partners and play styles. Girls with CAH report that they are more likely than control girls to prefer boy playmates (Hines & Kaufman, 1994; Berenbaum & Snyder, 1995; Servin et al., 2003), but peer play has not been directly observed. Interestingly, differences between girls with and without CAH are smaller for playmate preference than for toy play, despite the fact that the sex differences are much larger for the former than the latter. This reflects findings that less than half of girls with CAH report preference for boy playmates but almost all prefer boys' toys. In light of evidence from typical children described above about limited play with other-sex peers and the impact of same-sex peer groups, it is important to observe girls with CAH playing with peers to see where they "fit" in the distribution of same- vs. other-sex peer play, and whether they are affected by peer groups in the same ways as typical girls. Girls with CAH were found not to be significantly different from their sisters in the only study of rough play, which involved observation of girls playing with a friend who they brought to the testing situation (Hines & Kaufman, 1994). It is unclear whether androgen has less effect on rough play in people than in other primates or whether female-typical levels of rough play in girls with CAH reflect reduced opportunity (rather than desire) to engage in rough play related to less time spent with boys.

Overall, then, there is good evidence that prenatal androgens influence some aspects of childhood play. Effects are larger for toy play and activity interests than for play styles and partners. There is clearer evidence that prenatal androgens produce differences between the sexes than variations within sex.

Socialization Theories of Sex Differences in Play

Broadly defined, socialization is the process by which individuals learn about and internalize social norms. Socialization is not merely imposed on individuals, but reflects a complex transactional process and effects of many socializing agents, including parents, other adults, peers, and broad community influences, such as electronic media. Due to space limitations, we focus on two of the most immediate socializing agents in early childhood, parents and peers.

Parents as Socializing Agents of Sex-typed Play

In 1966, Mischel proposed that gender development could be explained by principles of social learning theory (Mischel, 1966). Children's gendered behavior was seen to be shaped by contingencies provided by parents and other socializing agents. Subsequent versions acknowledge the role of specific cognitive processes involved in learning about gender such as attention, memory, and motivation (Bandura, 1986). Parents are hypothesized to socialize children's sex–typed activities and behavior through three mechanisms: (a) direct reinforcement, (b) provision of different opportunities for boys and girls to engage in certain types of behavior, and (c) modeling.

With regard to direct reinforcement, parents are generally more involved with, and give more positive responses to, children when they are playing with toys typical for their sex than those that are typical for the other sex (Langlois & Downs, 1980; Roopnarine, 1986; Caldera et al., 1989; Fagot & Hagan, 1991). The magnitudes of these effects vary, however, by several factors, including child sex, parent sex, and parent attitudes. Both mothers and fathers with traditional attitudes towards family gender roles are more likely than those with egalitarian attitudes to encourage sex-typed play (Fagot, 1995). Parents reinforce sex-appropriate play more in sons than in daughters (Leaper, 2000), with fathers more likely than mothers to do so (Siegal, 1987). This may reflect the higher social status afforded males, so that fathers are more likely than mothers to emphasize gender roles, especially when interacting with sons.

But, parents do not work on a blank slate. Children have a significant amount of input into their own socialization through the way they behave. For example, preschool children instructed to initiate play with an unfamiliar adult elicited different behaviors depending on the adult's sex: children of both sexes were more likely to initiate ball play with a man than with a woman, but to ask for help more often from a woman than a man (Fagot, 1984). Thus, children are not just passive recipients of parental socialization, but active players in socializing themselves.

The second mechanism by which parents socialize children's sex-related play is by channeling girls and boys towards different activities. Even male and female infants have different environments: boys' rooms are significantly more likely than are girls' rooms to have toy vehicles, spatial toys, sports equipment, and toy animals, whereas girls' rooms are significantly more likely than are boys' rooms to have dolls and floral furnishings (Rheingold & Cook, 1975). Thus, it seems reasonable to suggest that children become exposed at an early age to sex-typed toys, develop familiarity and experience with these toys, and then maintain their preferences through parents' direct reinforcement. But, this proposal is difficult to confirm as there has been little longitudinal research on the trajectories of children's sex-typed toy preferences and how those are influenced by parental practices.

The third mechanism by which parental socialization affects children's sex-typed play activities is modeling (Bandura, 1986). When children observe a parent engaging in an activity, they are hypothesized to extract the rules of the activity, and generate new behaviors that conform to the same structures and rules (Perry & Bussey, 1979). Children are most likely to imitate sex-typed behavior from multiple models of the same-sex (Bussey & Perry, 1982) as compared to modeling a single person.

Parental socialization of gendered activities is more complex and nuanced than suggested by traditional learning theories. Evidence suggests that parents influence children's interests beyond the mechanisms described above, including provision of resources and support, and through their beliefs about the abilities of males and females in general, and of their own children (Eccles, 1993). Parents' beliefs relate to children's interests, ability self-concepts, and values about those interests (Eccles et al., 1990). Further, parents' beliefs about some activities (such as sports) appear to set the stage for later development in two ways. First, they shape children's early motivation for the activities, which may affect children's feelings of competence about those activities. Second, parents provide opportunities for children to engage in the activities and thus improve their competence (Fredricks & Eccles, 2005).

Further, socialization depends on family context (McHale et al., 2003), as illustrated by data on gender socialization within families. Children in European-

American families engaged most in sex-typed activities when they had an opposite-sex sibling and parents with traditional gender-role attitudes (McHale et al., 1999). Mexican-American parents who identified with Mexican culture provided stronger gender socialization to their children than did those who identified with Anglo culture, likely reflecting cultural differences in gender roles (McHale et al., 2005).

In sum, evidence suggests that parents socialize children's sex-typed play and related interests through reinforcement, provision and channeling of opportunities, modeling, and attitudes. Although this process is bidirectional and transactional, socialization theories propose that effects are initially driven by parents' responses to the child's sex. But, socialization theories alone are insufficient to explain children's sex-typed play, given evidence for effects of prenatal androgens described above, and cognitive contributions discussed below. Further, parents are not the only socialization agents in children's lives: there is increasing evidence for the impact of other social forces (Ruble et al., 2006), especially peers.

Peers as Socializing Agents of Sex-typed Play

A challenge for understanding peer socialization comes from the fact that children are drawn to others who are like them. Children's selection of peers affects how they are, in turn, influenced by those peers (Jaccard et al., 2005). Friends are chosen for similarity in values, personality dynamics, interests, and attitudes, and these similarities reinforce or discourage behaviors. A child with an initial set of values and characteristics that predispose him or her toward a certain behavior might engage in that behavior regardless of his or her peers. If peers are selected for similar values and characteristics, it is difficult to determine the relative contribution of the child vs. the peer group (Berndt, 1996). When such selection effects are controlled, however, peers have still been shown to have an effect on sex-typed play (e.g., Martin & Fabes, 2001).

Most research on peer influence has focused on older children and adolescents, but recent studies confirm these effects in young children. For example, preschool children's exposure to peers who were high in externalizing behavior predicted externalizing problem behavior a semester later (Hanish et al., 2005). Similarly, preschoolers exposed to prosocial peers evidenced more positive social interactions later in the year and were more prosocial one year later than children not exposed to those peers (Fabes & Martin, 2005). In both studies, there were sex differences, with effects generally stronger for girls than for boys, suggesting that young girls and boys are differentially sensitive to peer influences. Boys' relative insensitivity to peer exposure effects may reflect the difficulty of altering boy-typical behaviors (e.g., aggression, low prosociality). Because active and competitive play styles characterize boys' groups and are normative for young boys (Fabes et al., 2003b), and boys are particularly sensitive to what constitutes sex-typical behavior, there may be little incentive for them to change behavior (Fagot & Leinbach, 1983). Girls, however, are sensitive to both normative and non-normative behaviors and activities, so may be more susceptible than boys to peer effects.

We still have a lot to learn about the specific processes through which peers socialize gender-related play. Certainly, modeling, reinforcement, extinction, and other forms of behaviorally contingent peer responses help shape and guide such behaviors (Fagot, 1985; Gifford-Smith et al., 2005), but it is likely that children contribute to their own socialization of play behavior and activities through their own biological predispositions and social cognitive processes (Martin et al., 1999; Ruble et al., 2006).

Cognitive Theories of Sex Differences in Play

The role of children's cognitive processes in the development of sex-typed play was first described by Kohlberg who emphasized children's active participation in their own socialization (Kohlberg, 1966). As children become aware of their sex, and their membership in a group of people of similar sex, gender-related information becomes more salient, and children become motivated to actively construct the meaning of gender categories and align their behavior with those categories. Kohlberg revolutionized the view of gender development by focusing on self-socialization, that is, how children seek out and learn about gender on their own.

Work over the past 40 years has elaborated Kohlberg's ideas and produced other cognitive approaches to gender development (Ruble et al., 2006). Gender Schema Theory (GST) represents the most influential of these cognitive approaches. Central to GST is the notion that children are active participants in their own socialization because they are motivated to be like others of their own sex, with children forming cognitive constructions or networks of associations about the sexes that influence their behavior and thinking (Bem, 1981; Martin & Halverson, 1981). These *gender schemas* are presumed to direct children's attention, influence how information is interpreted, organized, and remembered, and guide behavior with objects and people. Specifically, children are expected to pay selective attention to and remember sex-typed information and to show biases towards members of their own group (for review, see Martin et al., 2002). Gender schemas are hypothesized to develop from an interaction of innate tendencies to categorize and the functional significance of gender.

How do gender schemas lead to self-socialization? As children develop a sense of their own sex, they are motivated to learn about their own sex and what members of their sex do, and then to apply this knowledge to their own behavior so that their behavior is *schema consistent*. Imagine a boy who is shown toys he has never seen before; he is told that a "scople" is a toy that lots of boys like and that a "fangle" is a favorite of girls, and is then left to play with the toys. A young boy will typically pick up, examine, and manipulate the scople, but ignore the fangle (Bradbart et al., 1986). The boy's attention, exploration, and interest has been directed by his schemas: "boys like scoples and girls like fangles, I am a boy, so I will probably like the scople and not the fangle." There is no external pressure to adhere to what he was told about these toys; the boy himself decides how to direct his attention and behavior.

Many studies confirm the power of gender schemas to influence behavior and thinking, including children's toy play (for review, see Martin & Dinella, 2002). Investigations of self-socialization involving toys cannot include real toys because children may have differential exposure to sex-typed toys and stereotypes about them. For that reason, studies have included novel toys that are given labels providing gender information. Consider two illustrative studies. In one (Bradbart & Endsley, 1983), children were shown six novel toys, two labeled as toys that boys like, two that girls like, and two that both sexes like, and each toy was named. Children were encouraged to play with and ask questions about the toys. Consistent with GST, children touched same-sex labeled toys most and other-sex labeled toys least, with both-sex labeled toys in between. In another study (Masters et al., 1979),

children were observed playing with novel toys after demonstrations by male or female models and after toys were given gender labels. Play was affected by gender labels, but not by sex of models.

Just as young children guide their behavior into schema consistent patterns, older children also try harder on games or tasks that they think are appropriate for their own sex. In one study (Montemayor, 1974), children where shown a novel game, and some children were told that this was a game for boys ("like basketball"), some were told it was a game for girls, and some were given no information. Both girls and boys performed better on the game and liked it more when it was labeled for their own sex rather than when it was labeled for the other sex. Similar results have been found using even subtle ability labels (e.g., "this is a test to see how good you would be at mechanics or operating machinery") (Hargreaves et al., 1985). Although much evidence demonstrates effects of gender labels on motivation, not all studies confirm these patterns: in some cases only boys are influenced by labels, and in one study, children did not accept experimental labels for the novel game so no labeling effects were found (for review, see Martin & Dinella, 2002). Ability labels are more effective with older children, whereas category labels are more effective with younger children (Miller & Ruble, 2006).

Gender schemas serve not only to affect children's interactions with toys (reducing interactions with toys that they believe are not "for them" and encouraging interactions with toys that are "for them"), but also to influence children's skill development by reducing information garnered about particular toys. Children pay less attention to and later remember less about how to interact with particular objects that were labeled for the other sex (Bradbart et al., 1986). Even incentives do not improve memory about other-sex toys, suggesting that children fail to attend and learn relevant information when it is first presented.

Gender schemas affect not just toys and activities, but children's choices about play partners. Children use gender schemas to infer whether they are likely to enjoy interacting with unfamiliar children. Children often prefer to play with children of their own sex rather than their own age. When children are given information about others' sex and interests, young children often use only sex of the child to make decisions about play partners, whereas older children and adults are likely to take interests into account (reviewed in Ruble et al., 2006).

Both adults and children assign stereotypic qualities to others based on their sex, and they use sex as a way to generalize new characteristics to others (Martin, 2000). For example, a child who is told about a girl who has "estro in her blood" is likely to infer that estro is a quality of other girls, and not of other boys (Gelman et al., 1986). Preschool children make assumptions about shared interests among members of the same group, even when there is no relevant information upon which to make these assumptions (Martin et al., 1995). In naturalistic studies of observed play behavior, children's beliefs about shared interests with same-sex peers correlate with their tendencies to play with same-sex peers (Martin et al., 2005).

The novel toy studies provide evidence that gender schemas influence children's exploration, attention, memory, and motivation toward objects and people. Whether they function this way in more typical circumstances is difficult to answer definitively. However, to the extent that they do, they will have both short- and long-term effects. Children who are motivated to adhere to gender schemas will avoid and forget information about toys and activities that they believe are not for their own sex. They will be less likely to play with other-sex peers because they will assume that these children do not share their interests. Over time, children who are susceptible to these influences are unlikely to develop a full range of skills and abilities because they will not have in-depth information or scripts to carry out other-sex activities. A cycle emerges: children avoid the activity because they think it is not appropriate for them, which leads to heightened avoidance as they then feel (and may actually be) less competent to engage in these activities (Martin & Dinella, 2002). This cycle can have serious consequences for performance in sex-related fields. For example, girls may drop out of high-level math and science classes because they think they are "not for me" (Nosek et al., 2002).

Summary: Causes of Sex Differences in Childhood Play

All three primary causal explanations for the development of sex-differentiated play have received some empirical support. Although early sex hormones, parent and peer socialization, and gender schemas have often been pitted against each other, these influences almost certainly act together, and the key question concerns how that happens.

There is good evidence from non-human primates for combined effects of hormones and social experience. Behavioral sex differences in monkeys result from hormonally influenced predispositions to engage in certain behaviors, but the ultimate expression is shaped by the social environment in which the animal develops (Wallen, 1996).

Children come into this world with certain predispositions that are manifested and exaggerated or suppressed by the environment in which they are reared, and those with sex-atypical predispositions provide a unique opportunity to examine causal influences on the development of sex-related play, as well as many of the other characteristics discussed in this book. Studies of girls with CAH, for example, might help us to understand more about the causes of sex-segregation and the nature of parent socialization. Do girls with CAH play with girls who share their identity, with boys who share their interests, or with children who share their play style or strategy for influencing others (which have not yet been studied in CAH)? Do parent attitudes affect the interests of girls with CAH as much as they do typical girls?

CONCLUSIONS

Sex differences in childhood play are important for many reasons: they are large, they lead to sex differences in other characteristics (including cognition and adjustment), and they reflect the joint effects of biological predispositions, the social world, and children's constructions of that world.

These differences also have indirect long-term consequences. Children's environments are changed as a result of their play, and this, in turn, affects later opportunities. This means that the lives of boys and girls are differently channeled, constrained, or expanded as a result of early differences. For these reasons, further study of sex differences in play patterns provides both a model for understanding sex differences in other characteristics and highlights the importance of assessing the long-term consequences of early sex differences. It might be worthwhile to consider, for example, the ways in which the different play styles of young boys and girls promote adult sex differences in affiliation or the ways in which sex differences in interaction styles and in cognitive schemas influence the perception and reporting of pain. Children's activities, their play partners, and the playstyles they exhibit are remarkably important for the breadth and depth of influence they exert across the life span.

Acknowledgments

Preparation of this chapter and our own work reported here were supported in part by NIH grants HD19644 and HD044398 (to Sheri Berenbaum) and HD45816 (to Carol Martin, Richard Fabes, and Laura Hanish). We thank Stephanie Barbu for telling us about some of the research on sex segregation in nonhuman species.

References

Alexander GM, Hines M. (2002). Sex differences in response to children's toys in nonhuman primates (*Cercopithecus aethiops sabaeus*). *Evolution and Human Behavior*, 23:467–479.

Baenninger M, Newcombe N. (1989). The role of experience in spatial test performance: A meta-anaylsis. *Sex Roles*, 20:327–344.

Bailey JM, Zucker KJ. (1995). Childhood sex-typed behavior and sexual orientation: A conceptual and quantitative review. *Dev Psychol*, 31:43–55.

Bailey JM, Bechtold KT, Berenbaum SA. (2002). Who are tomboys and why should we study them? *Arch Sex Behav*, 31:333–341.

Bandura A. (1977). *Social learning theory*. Englewood Cliffs: Prentice Hall.

Bandura A. (1986). *Social foundations of thought and action: A social cognitive theory*. Englewood Cliffs: Prentice Hall.

Barbu S. (2006). Ethological and comparative perspectives on gender development. Paper presented at the Second Gender Development Research Conference. San Francisco.

Beatty WW. (1992). Gonadal hormones and sex differences in nonreproductive behaviors. In Gerall AA, Moltz H, Ward IL, (Eds.), *Handbook of behavioral neurobiology*, Vol 11, Sexual differentiation. (pp. 85–128). New York: Plenum.

Becker JB, Breedlove SM, Crews D, McCarthy MM, (Eds). (2002). *Behavioral endocrinology*, 2nd Edition. Cambridge, MA: MIT Press.

Bem SL. (1981). Gender schema theory: A cognitive account of sex typing. *Psychol Rev*, 88:354–364.

Berenbaum SA. (2004). Androgen and behavior: Implications for the treatment of children with disorders of sexual differentiation. In Pescovitz OH, Eugster EA, (Eds.), *Pediatric endocrinology: Mechanisms, manifestations, and management* (pp. 275–284). Philadelphia: Lippincott Williams & Wilkins.

Berenbaum SA, Snyder E. (1995). Early hormonal influences on childhood sex-typed activity and playmate preferences: Implications for the development of sexual orientation. *Dev Psychol*, 31:31–42.

Berenbaum SA, Bryk KK. (2007). Biological contributors to gendered occupational outcome: Prenatal androgen effects on predictors of outcome. In Watt HMG, Eccles JS (Eds.), *Explaining gendered occupational outcomes: Examining individual and social explanations through school and beyond* (in press). Washington, D.C.: APA Books.

Berenbaum SA, Duck SC, Bryk K. (2000). Behavioral effects of prenatal versus postnatal androgen excess in children with 21-hydroxylase-deficient congenital adrenal hyperplasia. *J Clin Endo Metab*, 85:727–733.

Berndt TJ. (1996). Transitions in friendship and friends' influence. In Graber J, Brooks-Gunn J, Petersen AC, (Eds.), *Transitions through adolescence: Interpersonal dimensions and context* (pp. 57–84). Mahwah, NJ: Erlbaum.

Bernstein IS, Judge PG, Ruehlmann TE. (1993). Sex differences in adolescent rhesus monkey (Macaca mulatta) behavior. *Am J Primatol*, 31:197–210.

Blakemore JEO, Centers RE. (2005). Characteristics of boys' and girls' toys. *Sex Roles*, 53:619–633.

Bonenfant C, Loe LE, Mysterud A, Langvatn R, Stenseth NC, Gaillard J-M, Klein F. (2004). Multiple causes of sexual segregation in European red deer: Enlightenments from varying breeding phenology at high and low latitude. *Proc Biol Sci*, 271:883–892.

Bradbard MR, Endsley RC. (1983). The effects of sex-typed labeling on preschool children's information-seeking and retention. *Sex Roles*, 9:247–260.

Bradbard MR, Martin CL, Endsley RC, Halverson CF. (1986). Influence of sex stereotypes on children's exploration and memory: A competence versus performance distinction. *Dev Psychol*, 22:481–486.

Bukowski WH, Gauze C, Hoza B, Newcomb AF. (1993). Differences and consistency between same-sex and other-sex peer relationships during early adolescence. *Dev Psychol*, 29:255–263.

Bukowski WM, Sippola LK, Hoza B. (1999). Same and other: Interdependency between participation in same- and other-sex friendships. *J Youth Adolesc*, 28:439–459.

Bussey K, Perry DG. (1982). Same-sex imitation: The avoidance of cross-sex models or the acceptance of same-sex models? *Sex Roles*, 8:773–784.

Caldera YM, Huston AC, O'Brien M. (1989). Social interactions and play patterns of parents and toddlers with feminine, masculine, and neutral toys. *Child Development*, 60:70–76.

Campbell A, Shirley L. (2002). Sex-typed preferences in three domains: Do two-year-olds need cognitive variables? *Br J Psychol*, 93:203–217.

Caro TM. (1981). Sex differences in the termination of social play in cats. *Anim Behav*, 29:271–279.

Carpenter CJ, Huston AC, Holt W. (1986). Modification of preschool sex-typed behaviors by participation in adult-structured activities. *Sex Roles*, 14:603–615.

Cohen J. (1988). *Statistical power analysis for the behavioral sciences*, 2nd Edition. New York: Academic Press.

Cohen-Bendahan CCC, van de Beek C, Berenbaum SA. (2005). Prenatal sex hormone effects on child and adult sex-typed behavior: Methods and findings. *Neurosci Biobehav Rev*, 29:353–384.

Eccles JS. (1993). School and family effects of the ontogeny of children's interests, self-perception, and activity choice. In Jacobs J, (Ed.), Nebraska Symposium on Motivation, 1992: *Developmental perspectives on motivation* (pp 145–203). Lincoln, NE: University of Nebraska Press.

Eccles JS, Jacobs JE, Harold RD. (1990). Gender role stereotypes, expectancy effects, and parents' socialization of gender differences. *J Soc Issues*, 46:183–201.

Elizabeth PH, Green R. (1984). Childhood sex-role behaviors: Similarities and differences in twins. *Acta Geneticae Medicae et Gemellologiae: Twin Research* 33:173–179.

Etaugh C, Liss MB. (1992). Home, school, and playroom: Training grounds for adult gender roles. *Sex Roles*, 26:129–147.

Fabes RA. (1994). Physiological, emotional, and behavioral correlates of gender segregation. In Leaper C, (Ed.), *Childhood gender segregation: Causes and consequences. New directions for child development* (pp. 19–34). San Francisco: Jossey-Bass.

Fabes RA, Martin CL. (2005, May). Beyond acceptance and rejection: Understanding the role of peers in early development and adjustment. Paper presented at the University of Rome.

Fabes RA, Hanish LD, Martin CL. (2003a). Children at play: The role of peers in understanding the effects of childcare. *Child Dev*, 74:1039–1043.

Fabes RA, Martin CL, Hanish LD. (2003b). Qualities of young children's same-, other-, and mixed-sex play. *Child Dev*, 74:921–932.

Fabes RA, Shepard AS, Guthrie IK, Martin CL. (1997). Roles of temperamental arousal and gender segregated play in young children's social adjustment. *Dev Psychol*, 33:693–702.

Fagot BI. (1984). The child's expectations of differences in adult male and female interactions. *Sex Roles*, 11: 593–600.

Fagot BI. (1985). Beyond the reinforcement principle: Another step toward understanding sex role development. *Dev Psychol*, 21:1097–1104.

Fagot BI. (1995). Parenting boys and girls. In Marc HB, (Ed.), *Handbook of parenting*, Vol. 1: Children and parenting. (pp. 163–183): Mahwah, NJ: Erlbaum.

Fagot BI, Leinbach MD. (1983). Play styles in early childhood: Social consequences for boys and girls. In Liss MB, (Ed.), *Social and cognitive skills: Sex roles and children's play* (pp. 93–116). New York: Academic Press.

Fagot BI, Hagan R. (1991). Observations of parent reactions to sex-stereotyped behaviors: Age and sex effects. *Child Dev*, 62:617–628.

Fagot BI, Leinbach MD, Hagan R. (1986), Gender labeling and the adoption of sex-typed behaviors. *Dev Psychol*, 22:440–443.

Fredricks JA, Eccles JS. (2005). Family socialization, gender, and sport motivation and involvement. *J Sport Exercise Psychol*, 27:3–31.

Gelman SA, Collman P, Maccoby EE. (1986). Inferring properties from categories versus inferring categories from properties: The case of gender. *Child Dev*, 57:396–404.

Gifford-Smith M, Dodge KA, Dishion TJ, McCord J. (2005). Peer influence in children and adolescents: Crossing the bridge from developmental to intervention science. *J Abnorm Child Psychol*, 33:255–265.

Green R. (1987). *The "sissy boy syndrome" and the development of homosexuality*. New Haven, CT: Yale University Press.

Grimshaw GM, Sitarenios G, Finegan JA. (1995). Mental rotation at 7 years: Relations with prenatal testosterone levels and spatial play experience. *Brain Cogn*, 29:85–100.

Hanish LD, Martin CL, Fabes RA, Leonard S, Herzog M. (2005). Exposure to externalizing peers in early childhood: Homophily and peer contagion processes. *J Abnorm Child Psychol*, 33:267–281.

Hargreaves DJ, Bates HM, Foot JM. (1985). Sex-typed labelling affects task performance. *Br J Soc Psychol*, 24:153–155.

Hassett JM, Siebert ER, Wallen K. (2004). Sexually differentiated toy preferences in rhesus monkeys [Abstract]. *Horm Behav*, 46:91.

Henderson BA, Berenbaum SA. (1997). Sex-typed play in opposite-sex twins. *Dev Psychobiol*, 31:115–123.

Hines M, Kaufman F. (1994). Androgen and the development of human sex-typical behavior: Rough-and-tumble play and sex of preferred playmates in children with congenital adrenal hyperplasia (CAH). *Child Dev*, 65:1042–1053.

Hines M, Golombok S, Rust J, Johnston KJ, Golding J, Avon Longitudinal Study of Parents and Children Study Team. (2002). Testosterone during pregnancy and gender role behavior of preschool children: A longitudinal, population study. *Child Dev*, 73:1678–1687.

Hughes IA, Houk C, Ahmed F, Lee PA, LWPES/ESPE Consensus Group. (2006). Consensus statement on management of intersex disorders. *Arch Dis Childhood*, 91:554–563.

Huston AC, Wright JC, Marquis J, Green SB. (1999). How young children spend their time: Television and other activities. *Dev Psychol*, 35:921–925.

Jaccard J, Blanton H, Dodge T. (2005). Peer influences on risk behavior: An analysis of the effects of a close friend. *Dev Psychol*, 41:135–147.

Knickmeyer RC, Wheelwright S, Taylor K, Raggatt P, Hackett G, Baron-Cohen S. (2005). Gender-typed play and amniotic testosterone. *Dev Psychol*, 41: 517–528.

Kohlberg LA. (1966). A cognitive-developmental analysis of children's sex role concepts and attitudes. In Maccoby EE (Ed.), *The development of sex differences,* (pp. 82–173). Stanford: Stanford University Press.

Kovacs DM, Parker JG, Hoffman LW. (1996). Behavioral, affective, and social correlates of involvement in cross-sex friendship in elementary school. *Child Dev,* 67:2269–2286.

LaFreniere PJ, Strayer FF, Gauthier R (1984) The emergence of same-sex affiliative preference among preschool peers: A developmental/ethological perspective. *Child Dev* 55:1958–1965.

Langlois JH, Downs AC. (1980). Mothers, fathers, and peers as socialization agents of sex-typed play behaviors in young children. *Child Dev,* 51:1237–1247.

Leaper C. (1994). Exploring the consequences of gender segregation on social relationships. In Leaper C (Ed.), *Childhood gender segregation: Causes and consequences,* (pp. 67–86). San Francisco: Jossey-Bass.

Leaper C. (2000). The social construction and socialization of gender during development. In Miller PH, Scholnick EK (Eds.), *Toward a feminist developmental psychology* (pp. 127–152). New York: Routledge.

Lundy BL, Field T, McBride C, Field T, Largie S. (1998). Same-sex and opposite-sex best friend interactions among high school juniors and seniors. *Adolescence,* 33:279–290.

Maccoby EE. (1990). Gender and relationships: A developmental account. *Am Psychol,* 45:513–520.

Maccoby EE. (1998). *The two sexes: Growing up apart, coming together.* Cambridge, MA: Harvard University Press.

Maccoby EE, Jacklin CN. (1987). Gender segregation in childhood. In Reese HW, (Ed.), *Advances in child development and behavior,* (pp. 239–287). New York: Academic Press.

Martin CL (2000) Cognitive theories of gender development. In Eckes T, Trautner HM (Eds.), *The developmental social psychology of gender* (pp. 91–121). Mahwah, NJ: Erlbaum.

Martin CL, Halverson. CF (1981). A schematic processing model of sex typing and stereotyping in children. *Child Dev,* 52:1119–1134.

Martin CL, Fabes RA. (2001). The stability and consequences of young children's same-sex peer interactions. *Dev Psychol,* 37:431–446.

Martin CL, Dinella L (2002) Children's gender cognitions, the social environment, and sex differences in the cognitive domain. In McGillicuddy-De Lisi A, De Lisi R (Eds.), *Biology, society, and behavior: The development of sex differences in cognition* (pp. 207–239). Westport, CO: Ablex.

Martin CL, Eisenbud L, Rose H. (1995). Children's gender-based reasoning about toys. *Child Dev,* 66:1453–1471.

Martin CL, Ruble DN, Szkrybalo J. (2002). Cognitive theories of early gender development. *Psychol Bull,* 128:903–933.

Martin CL, Fabes RA, Evans SM, Wyman H. (1999). Social cognition on the playground: children's beliefs about playing with girls versus boys and their relations to sex segregated play. *J Social Personal Relationships,* 16:751–771.

Martin CL, Fabes RA, Hanish L, Hollenstein T. (2005). Social dynamics in the preschool. *Dev Rev,* 25:299–327.

Masters JC, Ford ME, Arend R, Grotevant HD, Clark LV. (1979). Modeling and labeling as integrated determinants of children's sex-typed imitative behavior. *Child Dev,* 50:364–371.

McHale SM, Crouter AC, Tucker CJ. (1999). Family context and gender role socialization in middle childhood: Comparing girls to boys and sisters to brothers. *Child Dev,* 70:990–1004.

McHale SM, Crouter AC, Whiteman SD, (2003). The family contexts of gender development in childhood and adolescence. *Social Dev,* 12:125–148.

McHale SM, Kim J, Whiteman S, Crouter AC. (2004a). Links between sex-typed time use in middle-childhood and gender development in early adolescence. *Dev Psychol,* 40:868–881.

McHale SM, Shanahan L, Updegraff KA, Crouter AC, Booth A. (2004b). Developmental and individual differences in girls' sex-typed activities in middle childhood and adolescence. *Child Dev,* 75:1575–1593.

McHale SM, Updegraff KA, Shanahan L, Crouter AC, Killoren SE. (2005). Siblings' differential treatment in Mexican American families. *J Marriage Fam,* 67:1259–1274.

Meaney MJ, Stewart J. (1981). A descriptive study of social development in the rat (*Rattus norvegicus*). *Anim Behav,* 29:34–45.

Meyer-Bahlburg HFL. (2001). Gender and sexuality in congenital adrenal hyperplasia. *Endocrinol Metab Clin North Am,* 30:155–171.

Meyer-Bahlburg HFL. (2005). Gender identity outcome in female-raised 46,XY persons with penile agenesis, cloacal exstrophy of the bladder, or penile ablation. *Arch Sex Behav,* 34:423–438.

Miller C, Ruble DN. (2006, April). Children's reactions to gender stereotypes: Developmental predictions. Paper presented at Second Gender Development Research Conference. San Francisco.

Mischel W. (1966). A social learning view of sex differences in behavior. In Maccoby E, (Ed.), *The development of sex differences* (pp. 56–81). Stanford: Stanford University Press.

Montemayor R. (1974). Children's performance in a game and their attraction to it as a function of sex-typed labels. *Child Dev,* 45:152–156.

Newcombe N, Dubas JS. (1992). A longitudinal study of predictors of spatial ability in adolescent females. *Child Dev,* 63:37–46.

Newcombe N, Bandura MM, Taylor DG. (1983). Sex differences in spatial ability and spatial activities. *Sex Roles,* 9:377–386.

Nordenström A, Servin A, Bohlin G, Larsson A, Wedell A. (2002). Sex-typed toy play behavior correlates with the degree of prenatal androgen exposure assessed by CYP21 genotype in girls with congenital adrenal hyperplasia. *J Clin Endo Metab*, 87:5119–5124.

Nosek BA, Banaji MR, Greenwald AG. (2002). Math = male, me = female, therefore math does not equal me. *J Pers Soc Psychol*, 83:44–59.

Omark DR, Omark M, Edelman M. (1975). Formation of dominance hierarchies in young children. In Williams TR (Ed.), *Psychological anthropology*, (pp. 133–156). The Hague: Mouton.

Pasterski VL, Geffner ME, Brain C, Hindmarsh P, Brook C, Hines M. (2005). Prenatal hormones and postnatal socialization by parents as determinants of male-typical toy play in girls with congenital adrenal hyperplasia. *Child Dev*, 76:264–278.

Perry DG, Bussey K. (1979). The social learning theory of sex differences: Imitation is alive and well. *J Pers Soc Psychol*, 37:1699–1712.

Rheingold HL, Cook KV. (1975). The contents of boys' and girls' rooms as an index of parent's behavior. *Child Dev*, 46:459–463.

Richards M, Crowe P, Larson R, Swarr A. (1998). Developmental patterns and gender differences in the experience of peer companionship during adolescence. *Child Dev*, 69:154–163.

Rodgers CS, Fagot BI, Winebarger A. (1998). Gender-typed toy play in dizygotic twins: A test of hormone transfer theory. *Sex Roles*, 39:173–184.

Roopnarine JL. (1986). Mothers' and fathers' behaviors toward the toy play of their infant sons and daughters. *Sex Roles*, 14:59–68.

Ruble DN, Martin CL, Berenbaum SA. (2006). Gender development. In Eisenberg N, (Ed.), *Handbook of child psychology*. Volume 3. Social, emotional, and personality development, 6th Edition (pp. 858–932). New York: Wiley.

Ryan BC, Vandenbergh JG. (2002). Intrauterine position effects. *Neurosci Biobehav Rev*, 26:665–678.

Sandberg DE, Meyer-Bahlburg HFL, Ehrhardt AA, Yager TJ. (1993). The prevalence of gender-atypical behavior in elementary school children. *J Am Acad Child Psychiatry*, 32:306–314.

Serbin LA, Tonick IJ, Sternglanz SH. (1977). Shaping cooperative cross-sex play. *Child Dev*, 48:924–929.

Serbin LA, Moller LC, Gulko J, Powlishta KK, Colbourne KA. (1994). The emergence of sex segregation in toddler playgroups. In Leaper C, (Ed.), *The development of gender and relationships*, (pp. 7–18). San Francisco: Jossey-Bass.

Servin A, Nordenström A, Larsson A, Bohlin G. (2003). Prenatal androgens and gender-typed behavior: A study of girls with mild and severe forms of congenital adrenal hyperplasia. *Dev Psychol*, 39:440–450.

Siegal M. (1987). Are sons and daughters treated more differently by fathers than by mothers? *Dev Rev*, 7: 183–209.

Sippola LK. (1999). Getting to know the "other": The characteristics and developmental significance of other-sex relationships in adolescence. *J Youth Adolesc*, 28:407–418.

Smith AB, Inder PM. (1993). Social interaction in same and cross gender pre-school peer groups: A participant observation study. *Educ Psychol*, 13:29–42.

Smith RB, Davidson J, Ball P. (2001). Age-related variations and sex differences in gender cleavage during middle childhood. *Personal Relationships*, 8: 153–165.

Thorne B. (2001). Girls and boys together, but mostly apart: Gender arrangement in elementary school. In Satow R, (Ed.), *Gender and social life*, (pp. 152–166). New York: Wiley.

Vandell DL, Nenide L, Van Winkle SJ. (2006). Peer relationships in early childhood. In McCartney K, Phillips D, (Eds.) *Handbook of early childhood development*, (pp. 455–470). New York: Blackwell.

Voyer D, Nolan CL, Voyer S. (2000). The relation between experience and spatial performance in men and women. *Sex Roles*, 43:891–915.

Wallen K. (1996). Nature needs nurture: The interaction of hormonal and social influences on the development of behavioral sex differences in rhesus monkeys. *Horm Behav*, 30:364–378.

Wallen K. (2005). Hormonal influences on sexually differentiated behavior in nonhuman primates. *Frontiers Neuroendocrinol*, 26:7–26.

Zucker KJ, Bradley SJ. (1995). *Gender identity disorder and psychosexual problems in children and adolescents*. New York: Guilford.

Chapter 15

Sex Differences in the Neurocognition of Language

Michael T. Ullman, Robbin A. Miranda, and Michelle L. Travers

Language is often studied under the assumption that it is similarly computed in all native speakers. However, increasing evidence suggests that in fact a variety of individual and group-related factors affect the biological, psychological, and computational basis—that is, the neurocognition—of language (Ullman, 2004, in press). One of the most important such factors appears to be sex. Here we examine evidence pertaining to the existence of possible sex differences in the neurocognition of language. We first discuss evidence and explanatory hypotheses related to sex differences in performance on language-related tasks, and then those related to sex differences in the neural bases of language. Next we present a novel theoretical perspective on sex differences in the neurocognition of language and memory. Finally, we summarize and discuss implications.

SEX DIFFERENCES IN PERFORMANCE ON LANGUAGE-RELATED TASKS

Sex differences in performance have been observed in a wide range of tasks involving language. In most, but not all of these tasks women tend to outperform men. Women have been found to show better performance than men in episodic memory tasks (remembering a given set of stimuli) for a wide range of verbal item types, including words (Kramer et al., 1988; Trahan & Quintana, 1990; Herlitz et al., 1997; Kramer et al., 1997; Kimura, 1999; Maitland et al., 2004), digits (Kimura, 1999) and paragraph content (Kimura, 1999). Women have also shown superior performance at episodic memory tasks involving nameable items such as landmarks (Galea & Kimura, 1993; Saucier et al., 2003) and real objects (Silverman and Eals, 1992; Herlitz et al., 1999; Levy et al., 2005).

A female advantage has also been observed when subjects are asked to list as many synonyms as possible for a given word (Herlitz et al., 1999), and in verbal fluency tasks, in which subjects must produce as many words as possible of a certain type (e.g., animals, or words beginning with the letter "c") in a limited time period (Kimura & Harshman, 1984; Herlitz et al., 1997; Herlitz et al., 1999; Kimura, 1999; Loonstra et al., 2001; Larsson et al., 2003; Maitland et al., 2004). However, verbal analogy tasks (e.g., sailor is to navy as soldier is to gun, cap, hill, or army) seem to yield either no sex difference (Gur et al., 2000) or better performance among men than women (Lim, 1994).

The general female advantage at language-related tasks appears to begin quite early. In one study, among 16- to 24-month old infants, girls demonstrated larger vocabularies than boys, with this sex difference not being explained by how much mothers speak to their children (Huttenlocher et al., 1991). In a study of somewhat older children, who ranged in age from 2 to 4, girls used longer and more complex utterances than boys (Horgan, 1975). The female advantage appears to persist into elementary school. For example, in one study girls in grades 3 to 8 scored higher than boys on tests of reading comprehension and spelling (Martin & Hoover, 1987).

However, sex differences in language abilities in children have not always been observed. For example, while sex differences in vocabulary growth have been found consistently in children less than two years of age, they have not been reliably observed after that age (see Huttenlocher et al., 1991). Although these sex differences are subtle and difficult to observe experimentally, it is nevertheless possible that such female advantages continue even after this age. A recent study supports this view (Walenski et al., under review). Typically developing age-matched boys and girls (in addition to children with autism, not discussed here) with a mean age of 10 were asked to name pictures of objects as quickly and accurately as possible. No sex differences were observed in mean accuracy or mean response time. However, it was hypothesized that sex differences might be obscured by normal performance or ceiling effects on easier items, such as higher frequency words. Higher and lower frequency items were therefore examined separately. Indeed, girls were faster than boys at object naming, but only among low frequency items. No sex differences at low frequency were observed in accuracy, a measure that is more susceptible to ceiling effects than is response time. These findings suggest that sex differences may indeed be found even when those differences are not initially observed with standard measures and analyses.

Evidence also suggests sex differences in strategies that may be related to language. For instance, in episodic memory tasks women and girls tend to recall words in clusters of meaningful categories (Cox & Waters, 1986; Kramer et al., 1988; Kramer et al., 1997; Kimura, 1999), while men tend to recall words in the order in which they were presented (Kramer et al., 1988; Kimura, 1999). In addition, in both rats and humans, females rely more than males on landmarks during navigation, while males tend to rely more on geometric cues (Williams et al., 1990; Bever, 1992; Sandstrom et al., 1998; Saucier et al., 2002).

The apparent female advantage at many language-related tasks has led to the widely-accepted hypothesis that females have an advantage over males in processing verbal information, while males have an advantage over females at visuospatial processing (Kimura, 1996, 1999; Lewin et al., 2001; Sherwin, 2003). On this view, females' superior memory for non-verbal stimuli, such as faces and objects, and their reliance on landmarks during spatial navigation tasks, results from their ability to internally verbalize these stimuli (Kimura, 1999; Lewin et al., 2001; Saucier et al., 2003).

However, a verbal/spatial distinction does not easily account for certain data, such as reports of a female advantage in memory for object locations (Silverman & Eals, 1992; Eals & Silverman, 1994; James & Kimura, 1997; McBurney et al., 1997; Barnfield, 1999; Alexander et al., 2002), novel (as opposed to famous and thus already-named) faces (Lewin et al., 2001; Herlitz & Yonker, 2002; Lewin & Herlitz, 2002; Yonker et al., 2003; Maitland et al., 2004; Guillem & Mograss, 2005), and complex abstract patterns (in both girls and women) (McGivern et al., 1997) (but see Herlitz et al., 1999). Women have also been found to recognize familiar melodies more rapidly than men, irrespective of whether the melodies were associated with lyrics (Miranda & Ullman, under review). Below we discuss a novel explanatory hypothesis that attempts to account for this pattern of data.

SEX DIFFERENCES IN THE NEURAL
BASES OF LANGUAGE

A substantial portion of the literature examining potential sex differences in the neural bases of language has focused on the issue of lateralization. In particular, a number of studies have suggested that language is more left-lateralized in males than females—that is, that males depend particularly on the left-hemisphere of the brain for language, whereas in females the brain bases of language are more bilaterally distributed.

Kansaku, Yamaura and Kitazawa (2000) performed functional Magnetic Resonance Imaging (fMRI) on healthy (cognitively unimpaired) right-handed adult male and female subjects during three sets of tasks: listening to a story, with silence as the baseline control condition; listening to a story, with the story played in reverse as the control condition; and listening to randomly ordered one second segments of a story, as compared to each segment played backwards.

In the two story-listening tasks compared to their respective control conditions, male subjects showed left lateralized fMRI activation in the lateral temporal lobes, particularly in the middle temporal gyri (both tasks), but also in the superior temporal gyrus (listening compared to reverse), as well as in the inferior frontal gyrus (both tasks, but only approaching significance in listening compared to silence). Females instead showed bilateral distributions of activation in these regions. Additionally, both sexes showed left lateralized activation in temporo-parietal regions (supramarginal and angular gyri). In the third contrast, in which randomly ordered speech segments were presented, no lateralization differences were observed in either sex.

Similarly, Phillips et al. (2000) asked healthy right-handed men and women to passively listen to a simple narrative, as well as the same narrative played backwards as the control condition. The investigators reported that the men showed greater left lateralized fMRI activation than the women in the posterior superior temporal gyrus, the anterior superior temporal gyrus, and the middle superior temporal sulcus.

Greater left lateralization in males than females has also been found in tasks involving phonological processing. Shaywitz et al. (1995) (results also reported in Pugh et al., 1996) observed greater fMRI left lateralization among right-handed males than females in the inferior frontal gyrus (centered on Brodmann's

Areas (BA) 44 and 45) in a rhyme-judgment task (to decide whether two visually presented nonsense words rhyme), as compared to a case-judgment task (decide whether two visually presented strings of consonants have the same pattern of upper and lower case letters).

Jaeger et al. (1998) carried out Positron Emission Tomography (PET) scanning while right-handed men and women performed several tasks: reading verb stems (e.g., walk); reading novel (that is, nonsense) verb stems (e.g., brep); producing past-tense forms visually-presented regular verb stems of regular verbs (e.g., jump-jumped); producing the past-tenses of irregular verbs (e.g., build-built); and producing the past tenses of novel verb stems (e.g., plag-plagged). Although the two sexes showed similar activation patterns, women were less left-lateralized than men, showing greater activation in the right hemisphere in several areas, including the right temporal pole (in reading novel stems, and in producing all three kinds of past-tense forms), the right inferior frontal gyrus (BA 45/47, in the three past-tense tasks), and the right pre-central gyrus (BA 6/4, again in the three past-tense tasks).Vikingstad, George, Johnson, and Cao (2000) asked right-handed men and women to silently name pictures of objects, as well as to silently generate verbs related to visually presented nouns (e.g., *eat* for *cake*). In comparison to control conditions (viewing nonsense drawings for picture naming, and viewing slashes for verb generation), males showed greater left lateralization than women in an inferior parietal-superior temporal region in picture naming, and in an inferior frontal-middle frontal region in verb generation. Baxter et al. (2003) examined functional fMRI activation patterns in right-handed men and women while they performed a semantic decision task, in which subjects had to determine whether or not word pairs consisted of a superordinate category with a subordinate category examplar (e. g., *beverage-milk* is a correct pairing while *vehicle-carrot* is an incorrect pairing). Compared to rest (i.e., compared to activation when no stimuli were being presented), males showed greater activation than females in the left inferior frontal gyrus, while females showed greater activation than males in the right temporal lobe.

These neuroimaging studies showing greater left lateralization in language use in males than females seem to support similar claims made on the basis of neurological evidence (McGlone, 1977; Inglis & Lawson, 1981). For example, McGlone (1977) found that language deficits were more than three times as likely to occur in males than females following left-hemisphere adult-onset focal lesions. In contrast, right-hemisphere lesions led to language impairments only in females. Frith and Vargha-Khadem (2001) reported that among 6 to 19 year old children with unilateral left or right side damage, boys showed impairments in reading text and at spelling familiar and unfamiliar words only following left-side damage, whereas girls showed no significant impairments following lesions to either side.

In a study of the recovery of language function, Pizzamiglio, Mammucari and Razzano (1985) gave right-handed male and female non-fluent, fluent, and global aphasics with adult-onset left-hemisphere lesions a variety of language tests both before and after three months of language therapy. Although no differences in language impairments were observed at initial testing, a specific sex difference was found in the degree of recovery: females showed better recovery than males, but only among the global aphasics, and only on three tests (phonemic discrimination, semantic discrimination, and syntactic comprehension). The authors suggest that this pattern can be accounted for by a more bilateral representation of language in females than in males.

However, numerous other studies have failed to find greater left language lateralization in males. Many studies of brain-damaged patients have found evidence for greater functional asymmetry in males to be either transitory, not statistically significant, or unreplicable, particularly when the higher incidence of men suffering from strokes is taken into account (for discussion, see McGlone, 1977; Pizzamiglio et al., 1985).

Sommer, Aleman, Bouma and Kahn (2004) examined previous neuroimaging studies that had probed sex differences in language lateralization. In their list of such studies (Table 1 in Sommer et al., 2004), only the neuroimaging tasks described above showed greater left lateralization in males. In contrast, 21 tasks did *not* show this pattern.[1] For example, Frost et al (1999) tested healthy right-handed men and women on a semantic-monitoring task (respond to spoken names of animals that are both found in the United States and used by humans) and a tone-monitoring task as a control condition (respond to sequences containing two high tones). In this task contrast both sexes showed strong left lateralization patterns of fMRI activation, with no sex differences in lateralization in any region of interest. Sommer et al. (2004) also

performed a meta-analysis on 14 studies (those with enough information to enter into the meta-analysis), and found no statistically significant sex differences in language lateralization.

In response to these apparently inconsistent findings, the possibility has been raised that sex differences in language lateralization may be task-dependent. For example, in their meta-analysis, Sommer et al. (2004) also examined whether sex differences might vary with between word production tasks and receptive language tasks. However, they found no differences between the two types of tasks with respect to sex differences in lateralization.

Shaywitz et al. (1995) suggested that sex differences in language lateralization may be specific to phonological processing. In addition to explaining their own results, this observation does indeed seem to account for a substantial portion of subsequent findings. Jaeger et al. reported that women showed greater right-hemisphere activation than men while reading novel verb stems and while producing novel past-tense forms. Because Frith and Vargha-Khadem (2001) found that left-side damage impaired spelling unfamiliar as well as familiar words in boys but not girls, they suggest that their results are also consistent with the Shaywitz et al. hypothesis that phonological processes (assumed to be involved in spelling unfamiliar words) are more left lateralized in males than females, even in children. Moreover, none of the 21 neuroimaging studies that failed to show lateralization (see above) [specifically tapped phonological processing. Indeed, although the left-lateralization patterns observed for picture naming and verb generation by Vikingstad et al. (2000) and for semantic decision by Baxter et al. (2003) were found in tasks that do not specifically tap phonological processing, these results do not appear to be reliable. Thus lateralization was not observed in any of the other five verb generation tasks, nine semantic decision tasks, or other single-word processing tasks listed by Sommer et al. (2004). Additionally, the effect size assigned by Sommer et al. to the sex difference in Vikingstad et al. was the smallest effect size of all studies listed by Sommer et al. (no effect size was assigned to Baxter et al. due to insufficient data).

However, the hypothesis that sex differences in language lateralization are specific to phonological processing fails to explain the left lateralization observed among males in both of the story listening tasks (Kansaku et al., 2000; Phillips et al., 2000), which had among the largest effect sizes assigned by Sommer et al. (indeed, the effect sizes for these two studies may have been even larger; see Kitazawa & Kansaku, 2005). A restriction of left-lateralization to phonological processes is also inconsistent with the results from the past-tense generation study (Jaeger et al., 1998), in which a sex difference in lateralization was found for the past-tense generation of real as well as novel forms (note that Sommer et al. assigned no effect size to this study due to insufficient data).

Kansaku et al. (2000) instead suggest that sex differences in language lateralization may be specific to the "global semantic structure" of narratives. Although this could account for their findings and those of Phillips et al. (2000), as well as the general lack of sex differences in lateralization for non-narrative tasks such as verbal fluency or semantic decision, it does not explain the pattern of left lateralization observed in phonological processing and past-tense generation tasks (Shaywitz et al., 1995; Jaeger et al., 1998).

In a review of the neuroimaging literature, Kansaku and Kitazawa (2001) (also see Kitazawa & Kansaku, 2005) suggest that sex differences in language lateralization can be characterized as occurring during tasks that involve passive listening to stories with global narrative structure (Kansaku et al., 2000; Phillips et al., 2000) and during single-word processing tasks when these involve novel words (Shaywitz et al., 1995; Jaeger et al., 1998), but not real words. This characterization does indeed seem to capture a large portion of the variability found across neuroimaging studies, although it does not seem to explain the lateralization observed in the production of real past-tense forms (Jaeger et al., 1998).

Kansaku and Kitazawa further argue that the lateralization sex differences observed in tasks with global narrative structures may be explained, at least in part, by time demands relative to interhemispheric conduction delays. Specifically, they suggest that processing these global structures is slow (in the order of seconds), allowing for the use of both hemispheres, whereas faster processes may be restricted to a single hemisphere. Moreover, they argue that this bihemispheric reliance should be particularly prevalent among women, given evidence that the size of the isthmus of the corpus callosum, which may contain commissural fibers from posterior language areas, may be larger in women relative to the total area of the corpus callosum. However, even if the various assump-

tions made by this hypothesis held true, it would not explain lateralization sex differences observed in tasks not involving global narrative structures, such as phonological processing and past-tense production tasks.

Not all research examining sex differences in the brain bases of language has focused on lateralization. Kimura (1983) examined 49 male and 32 female patients with adult-onset unilateral left hemisphere lesions restricted to either anterior or posterior regions. Although aphasia occurred in similar proportions in the males with anterior and posterior lesions (40% and 41%, respectively), and in the females with anterior lesions (62%), it was significantly less common in the females with posterior lesions (11%).

Kimura (1993) reported that among 108 patients (apparently a somewhat larger superset of the same patients that were reported in the 1983 study), left anterior lesions led to aphasia in 28% of males but 64% of females ($P<.04$), whereas left posterior lesions led to the opposite pattern, with aphasia in only 13% of females but 41% of males ($P<.01$). Moreover, among the posterior-lesioned patients with posteri lesions, temporal-lobe damage was equally likely to lead to aphasia in males and females (33% and 22% respectively; difference not significant), whereas parietal damage led to aphasia in men (67%), but not in women (0%; $P<.01$) (Kimura, 1993). On the basis of these data, Kimura argued that anterior pathology is more likely to lead to aphasia in women than men, whereas posterior pathology, in particular in parietal cortex, is more likely to lead to aphasia in men than women, suggesting that left parietal cortex is particularly important for language function in men, whereas left anterior regions are especially important for language in women (Kimura, 1993, 1999).

However, the neuroimaging results reported thus far do not seem consistent with this hypothesis. For example, Shaywitz et al. (1995) found higher levels of activation among men than women (14.3 vs. 8.9) in the left inferior frontal gyrus, although direct comparisons between the sexes were not reported. Similarly, Kansaku et al. (2000) report higher median volumes of activation among males than females (4.3 vs. 2.5) during story listening as compared to reverse. Moreover, the direct comparisons between the sexes in Jaeger et al. (1998) indicate that no regions in the left hemisphere were more active in one sex than the other. Additional studies specifically focused on testing Kimura's hypothesis may further clarify this issue.

SEX DIFFERENCES IN
DECLARATIVE MEMORY

A recently proposed explanatory account of neuro-cognitive sex differences in language and memory posits that females tend to have an advantage over males at storing and/or retrieving knowledge in the declarative memory brain system (Ullman et al., 2002; Ullman, 2004, 2005; Hartshorne & Ullman, 2006).

This memory system underlies the learning, representation, and use of knowledge about facts ("semantic knowledge") and events ("episodic knowledge") (Mishkin et al., 1984; Schacter & Tulving, 1994; Squire & Knowlton, 2000; Eichenbaum & Cohen, 2001), and has been implicated in the knowledge of stored words ("lexical knowledge"), including both word forms and meanings (Ullman et al., 1997; Ullman, 2001b, 2004, In Press).

The declarative memory system subserves spatial as well as verbal memory (Eichenbaum & Cohen, 2001; Egan et al., 2003; Ullman, 2004), and is closely related to the ventral stream or "what" pathway, which underlies visual object recognition (Norman, 2002; Ullman, 2004). The system may be particularly important for learning idiosyncratic information, specifically arbitrary relations (e.g., that fact that Ouagadougou is the capital of Burkina Faso) (Schacter & Tulving, 1994; Squire & Knowlton, 2000; Eichenbaum & Cohen, 2001). Knowledge is learned very rapidly in declarative memory, with as little as a single exposure to the stimulus being necessary for retention, although multiple exposures greatly improve the recognition and retrieval of the relevant information (Marche, 1999; Van Strien et al., 2005). Finally, knowledge learned in declarative memory is at least partly (but not completely, Chun, 2000) explicit, that is, available to conscious awareness.

The declarative memory system is subserved by medial temporal lobe structures, in particular the hippocampus and the parahippocampal gyrus, which are connected extensively with temporal and parietal neocortical regions (Suzuki & Amaral, 1994). The medial temporal structures are involved in the consolidation, recognition and retrieval of new memories (Mishkin et al., 1984; Schacter & Tulving, 1994; Squire & Knowlton, 2000; Eichenbaum & Cohen, 2001).

Eventually, memories seem to become at least partly independent of medial temporal structures (but see Nadel & Moscovitch, 1997; Rekkas & Constable, 2005) and dependent on neocortical regions, particularly in the temporal lobes (Squire & Alvarez, 1995; Squire & Zola, 1996; Hodges & Patterson, 1997; Martin et al., 2000).

Other brain structures also play a role in declarative memory. Portions of ventro-lateral prefrontal cortex (corresponding largely to BA 45/47) seem to play a role in the retrieval of declarative memories, while parts of the right cerebellum may underlie searching for this knowledge (Desmond & Fiez, 1998; Wagner et al., 1998; Buckner & Wheeler, 2001). Note that we use the term "declarative memory system" to refer to the *entire* system involved in the learning and use of the relevant knowledge (Eichenbaum, 2000), not just to those structures or mechanisms underlying memory consolidation.

The declarative memory system has been intensively studied not only from functional and neuroanatomical perspectives, but also at physiological, cellular, endocrine, molecular, and genetic levels, in both animals and humans (Curran, 2000; Eichenbaum & Cohen, 2001; Lynch, 2002; Ullman, 2004).

Memory-related modifications in the hippocampus pertaining to synaptic transmission occur in two stages, early-phase and late-phase, long-term potentiation (LTP) (Kandel, 2001). The protein brain derived neurotrophic factor (BDNF) plays an important role in both of these phases (Lu & Gottschalk, 2000; Poo, 2001; Egan et al., 2003). The gene for BDNF has also been shown to play a role in declarative memory. For example, individuals with the *val* as opposed to the *met* allele of the V66M single nucleotide polymorphism in the BDNF gene have better recognition in both language and non-language episodic memory tasks, as well as increased hippocampal activation during this recognition, and larger hippocampal grey matter volumes (Egan et al., 2003; Hariri et al., 2003; Pezawas et al., 2004). Additionally, the neurotransmitter acetylcholine seems to play an important role in declarative memory and hippocampal and parahippocampal function (Packard, 1998; Massey et al., 2001; Freo et al., 2002; Schon et al., 2005).

A large amount of evidence indicates that estrogens affect declarative memory and (para)hippocampal function (Sherwin, 1988; Phillips & Sherwin, 1992). Studies have shown that estrogens can enhance performance on a variety of declarative memory tasks in women (Sherwin, 1998; Maki and Resnick, 2000) as well as men (Kampen & Sherwin, 1996; Miles et al., 1998). For example, higher levels of estrogens in the menstrual cycle or through hormone replacement therapy have been found to lead to improved verbal fluency (Hampson, 1990; Maki et al., 2002) and better episodic memory for words and names (Robinson et al., 1994; Resnick et al., 1998), paragraph content (Kampen & Sherwin, 1994), and complex abstract figures (Resnick et al., 1997; Resnick et al., 1998).

In surgically menopausal women, estrogen replacement therapy can prevent the decline of both paragraph recall and paired-associate memory, compared to women who have not received estrogen treatment (Sherwin & Phillips, 1990; Sherwin & Tulandi, 1996). During both verbal (word lists) and visual (abstract figures) episodic memory tasks, hormone replacement therapy in healthy postmenopausal women has been found to lead to changes in activation in medial temporal lobe (hippocampal and parahippocampal) and neocortical temporal lobe regions (Resnick et al., 1998; Maki & Resnick, 2000). Additionally, women with Turner's syndrome, who do not produce estrogen, have impaired verbal memory (which improves with estrogen therapy Ross et al., 2000) and smaller hippocampi, as compared to control subjects (Murphy et al., 1993).

The biological mechanisms underlying these estrogen effects have also been quite well-studied. Numerous experiments have shown that estrogens strengthen the cellular and molecular correlates of long-term hippocampal learning (McEwen et al., 1998; Woolley & Schwartzkroin, 1998). For example, estrogen treatment of ovariectomized rats increases dendritic spine density in hippocampal pyramidal neurons (Woolley, 1999; McEwen et al., 2001; Sherwin, 2003) and induces the formation of new synaptic connections within the hippocampus (McEwen, 1999; Woolley, 1999).

Additionally, studies have begun to reveal the molecular mechanisms that underlie the physiological and functional effects of estrogens. Intriguingly, these effects appear to be modulated, at least in part, by acetylcholine (Simpkins et al., 1997; Packard, 1998; Shughrue et al., 2000) and/or BDNF (Simpkins et al., 1997; Murphy et al., 1998; Woolley, 1999; Scharfman & MacLusky, 2005).

Several lines of evidence support the hypothesis that women tend to have an advantage over men at declarative memory, across both language and non-language domains. (It is important to emphasize that, like other hypotheses of brain and behavioral sex differences, this particular hypothesis does not posit absolute sex differences, but rather probabilistic ones, likely with substantial overlap between the sexes.) Moreover, the data suggest that one particular brain region within the declarative memory system plays an especially important role in these sex differences—that is, the medial temporal lobe, in particular the hippocampus and the parahippocampal gyrus.

First, the types of language and non-language tasks described above on which females typically demonstrate a performance advantage have been shown to depend on declarative memory, both in neuroimaging experiments and in lesion studies of brain-damaged patients (Zola-Morgan et al., 1986; Gabrieli et al., 1988; Schacter & Tulving, 1994; Boller & Grafman, 1995; Brewer et al., 1998; Postle & Corkin, 1998; Wagner et al., 1998; Squire & Knowlton, 2000; Eichenbaum & Cohen, 2001; Ullman, 2004). Moreover, evidence specifically links these female-advantaged language and non-language tasks to the hippocampus and parahippocampal gyrus.

Episodic memory tasks are strongly associated with both of these medial temporal lobe structures. Evidence suggests that both structures underlie the learning phase of both verbal (Alkire et al., 1998; Fernandez et al., 1998; Wagner et al., 1998; Henke et al., 1999; Otten et al., 2001; Strange et al., 2002; Eldridge et al., 2005; Meltzer & Constable, 2005; Powell et al., 2005; Prince et al., 2005; Uncapher & Rugg, 2005) and non-verbal stimuli (e.g., unknown faces or visual routes) (Maguire et al., 1996; Brewer et al., 1998; Bernard et al., 2004; Powell et al., 2005). Following the learning phase, the hippocampus and the parahippocampal cortex also subserve the recognition of both verbal (Eldridge et al., 2000; Wheeler & Buckner, 2004; Yonelinas et al., 2005) and non-verbal (Cansino et al., 2002; Montaldi et al., 2006) stimuli (for a review see Henson, 2005), as well as the recall of verbal stimuli (Heckers et al., 2002; Meltzer & Constable, 2005).

Consistent with a role for these structures in previously observed sex differences, the hippocampus and parahippocampal gyrus have also been implicated in the retrieval and recognition of long-term verbal and non-verbal memories, including in verbal fluency tasks (Pihlajamaki et al., 2000; Vitali et al., 2005), the recall of topographic routes (as far back as 11 years) (Maguire et al., 1997; Nunn et al., 2000), the recognition of famous faces (even for faces that were famous as far back as the 1940s) (Bernard et al., 2004), and the recognition of famous faces together with the recall of their names (Haist et al., 2001; Elfgren et al., 2006).

Second, estrogens constitute a plausible biological substrate for declarative memory-dependent sex differences. As discussed previously, estrogens have been found to enhance performance at many tasks that depend on declarative memory, including the verbal fluency and language and non-language episodic memory tasks that show a female performance advantage. As we have seen, these estrogen-related performance enhancements are linked to the hippocampus and parahippocampal cortex.

Moreover, the gene for BDNF, whose regulation may be modulated by estradiol (Scharfman & MacLusky, 2005), has been found to affect hippocampal function and anatomy, as well as performance in both language and non-language episodic memory tasks (see above). Thus, given that even prepubertal girls, let alone older girls and pre-menopausal women, have higher estrogen levels than age-matched boys and men (Klein et al., 1994; Cutler Jr., 1997; Klein et al., 1998; Wilson et al., 1998; Ikegami et al., 2001; Bay et al., 2004), these estrogen and BDNF effects on declarative memory and medial temporal lobe structures provide specific plausible biological mechanisms for the posited sex differences.

Third, anatomical and related functional sex differences also seem to support the hypothesis of a female advantage at declarative memory. For example, the hippocampus develops at a faster rate, in comparison to the rest of the brain, in girls than in boys between the ages of one and 16 (Pfluger et al., 1999). In contrast, a study of 18 to 42 year old men and women found that the volume of the hippocampus correlated negatively with age in men, but not in women (Pruessner et al., 2001). Perhaps reflecting this male decrease in hippocampal volume, verbal episodic memory seems to decline in men, but not women between the ages of 16 and 47 (Kramer et al., 2003).

Fourth, recent evidence suggests that females not only have superior declarative memory functionality as compared to men, but that this advantage leads to differences in how the two sexes actually represent and process aspects of language. All people learning a language must memorize arbitrary word-specific knowledge, such as the sound pattern /cat/, what this sound pattern refers to, or the fact that the past-tense of 'dig' is the irregular form 'dug.' As discussed above, evidence suggests that this lexical knowledge is memorized in declarative memory (Ullman et al., 1997; Ullman, 2001b, 2004, in press).

However, language does not consist only of individual words. We also combine words and other basic elements such as phonemes in rule-governed ways to produce more complex linguistic forms, such as new or novel words (e.g., combining phonological elements to form /blep/), morphologically complex words (e.g., regular past-tense forms such as 'walk' + '-ed'), and phrases and sentences (e.g., 'Clementina likes obstreperous pachyderms').

Evidence suggests that this grammatical rule-governed composition of complex forms depends on the procedural memory system, a distinct memory system that seems to be specialized for rules and sequences (Ullman et al., 1997; Ullman, 2001b, 2004, 2006). This system depends particularly on frontal/basal-ganglia circuits (Schacter & Tulving, 1994; Squire & Knowlton, 2000; Eichenbaum & Cohen, 2001; Ullman, 2004, 2006), particularly in the left hemisphere (De Renzi, 1989; Haaland & Harrington, 1996; Heilman et al., 1997; Haaland et al., 2000). Within frontal cortex, premotor regions and BA 44 appear to play especially important roles in procedural memory function (Ullman, 2004, 2006).

Crucially, complex linguistic forms can in principle not only be composed by the grammatical system in procedural memory (e.g., 'walk' + '-ed'), but also stored as chunks in lexical/declarative memory (e.g., 'walked'). If females have superior declarative memory abilities as compared to males, we might expect females to be more likely to rely on stored complex forms, while men depend more on rule-based composition.

The evidence supports this prediction (Steinhauer & Ullman, 2002; Ullman et al., 2002; Ullman & Estabrooke, 2004; Hartshorne & Ullman, 2006; Prado & Ullman, Under Review; Ullman et al., Under Revision-b; Ullman et al., Under Revision-a).

For example, psycholinguistic evidence suggests that cognitively unimpaired women tend to rely on regular past-tense forms retrieved as whole forms from memory (e.g., 'walked'), while men tend to compose them from their parts (e.g., 'walk' + '-ed') (Prado & Ullman, Under Review; Ullman et al., Under Revision-b; Ullman et al., Under Revision-a). This increased female reliance on memorized complex forms can also explain the finding that in Parkinson's disease, which affects the frontal/basal-ganglia circuits of the procedural memory system, higher levels of basal ganglia degeneration (as reflected by higher levels of hypokinesia) lead to worse performance on producing regular past-tenses among men but not women (Ullman & Estabrooke, 2004; Estabrooke & Ullman, in preparation).

An increased female reliance on stored complex forms seems to be found even in young children. Hartshorne and Ullman (2006) examined over-regularizations (e.g., 'blowed') in children of about ages 2 to 5. They had predicted that girls would over-regularize *less* than boys, since girls' superior lexical/declarative memory abilities would be expected give them an advantage at retrieving correct irregular past-tense forms (e.g., 'blew'), thus reducing the degree to which they would have to resort to the grammatical/procedural system in composing rule-governed over-regularizations (e.g., 'blow' + '-ed').

To their surprise, and contrary to their predictions, Hartshorne and Ullman found that girls over-regularized more than three times the rate of boys (means of 5.7% vs. 1.8%). Further analyses revealed the probable explanation. If girls are more likely than boys to memorize regular past-tense forms (e.g., 'flowed,' 'rowed,' 'stowed'), then these memorized forms may encourage the analogy-based formation of over-regularizations within lexical memory.

Indeed, Hartshorne and Ullman found that among girls, irregular verbs whose over-regularizations were phonologically similar to (e.g., rhymed with) a larger number of regulars were over-regularized more than those irregular verbs with fewer phonologically similar regulars. For example, if 'blowed' rhymes with more regulars than 'digged,' girls would produce 'blowed' at a higher rate than 'digged.' In contrast, the boys showed no such correlation, suggesting that they did not memorize regular past-tense forms, and their over-regularizations were computed in the rule-governed grammatical system rather than in lexical/declarative memory.

An increased female dependence on declarative memory in the use of complex forms may also help to explain the pattern of sex differences observed in the neural bases of language. If females rely more than males on declarative memory for complex forms, then females should show increased activation during the use of such forms in declarative memory brain structures, as compared to males, who in turn should show increased activation in procedural memory brain structures. In contrast, tasks that are expected to depend on lexical/declarative memory in both sexes, such as single-word lexical and semantic processing tasks, should elicit either no sex differences at all in brain activation, or perhaps activation differences only within the declarative memory system due to the two sex's differential abilities within this system.

Unfortunately, the extant data on sex differences in the neural bases of language is somewhat difficult to interpret with respect to these predictions, since it is focused on laterality rather than on sex differences in the use of specific brain structures. Nevertheless, the data do shed some light on the hypothesis. As we have seen, the only reliable sex differences seem to be found in tasks involving sentences (Kansaku et al., 2000; Phillips et al., 2000), inflected forms (Jaeger et al., 1998), and novel words (Shaywitz et al., 1995; Jaeger et al., 1998). All of these involve complex forms, leading to the prediction of sex differences in the neural bases of these forms: while males should tend to compose novel words (Shaywitz et al., 1995; Jaeger et al., 1998), regularly inflected forms (Jaeger et al., 1998)[2], and phrases and sentences (Kansaku et al., 2000; Phillips et al., 2000) in the grammatical/procedural system, females should be more likely to retrieve them from lexical/declarative memory, or to compute them by analogy in this system (e.g., for novel forms). In contrast, we have seen that single-word lexical and semantic tasks such as verb generation, verbal fluency and semantic decision yielded no reliable sex differences, as would be expected since these tasks should rely on lexical/declarative memory in both sexes.

Moreover, despite the difficulty in interpreting data focused on laterality, the specific patterns of activation reported by studies of complex forms seem to be consistent with a differential male/female reliance on declarative and procedural memory. In the one study that reported direct male/female differences in activation, females showed increased activation in declarative memory brain structures as compared to men—that is, in temporal cortex and BA 45/47 (Jaeger et al., 1998). Greater female than male activation was also found in right BA 6/4; however, given the predominance of left hemisphere structures in grammatical/procedural functions, particularly among right-handers (De Renzi, 1989; Haaland & Harrington, 1996; Heilman et al., 1997; Haaland et al., 2000; Ullman, 2004; Moffa et al., 2005), it seems unlikely that this activation reflects grammatical/procedural processing. In contrast, as we have seen, Shaywitz et al. (1995) and Kansaku et al (2000) found higher levels of activation among men than women in the left (but not right) inferior frontal gyrus, although activation was not compared directly between the sexes.

Methodologies other than fMRI and PET neuroimaging also suggest a greater reliance of females on declarative memory and males on procedural memory in the processing of complex forms. In an Event-Related Potential (ERP) study of inflectional morphology and syntax, violations of both regular morphology (e.g., 'Yesterday John *walk* over there' vs. 'Yesterday John *walked* over there') and syntax (e.g., 'The scientist criticized Max's *of* proof the theorem' vs. 'The scientist criticized Max's proof *of* the theorem') elicited Left Anterior Negativities in males, but not in females (Steinhauer & Ullman, 2002; Ullman et al., 2002).

These negativities have been linked to automatic grammatical processing and procedural memory (Ullman, 2001a, b). In females, these violations instead elicited only posterior negativities that resembled N400s, which have been tied to lexical and declarative memory (Ullman, 2001a, b). Purely lexical-semantic violations (e.g., 'I had my coffee with milk and *concrete*' vs. 'I had my coffee with milk and *sugar*'), and violations of irregular morphology (e.g., 'Yesterday I *dig* a hole' vs. 'Yesterday I *dug* a hole'), yielded N400s in both sexes. Interestingly, the N400s elicited by the lexical-semantic violations were larger (higher amplitude) in the females than the males, suggesting a greater lexical-semantic expectation among the females (i.e., females being more likely to expect an appropriate word), as might be expected if females have superior lexical/declarative abilities.

However, not all evidence suggests a female advantage at declarative memory. For example, sex differences have not always been reported in episodic memory tests, such as in tests for unrelated word pairs (Trahan & Quintana, 1990), pictures of common objects (Alexander et al., 2002), and common physical objects (Cherney & Ryalls, 1999). Such null effects could evidently be due to many factors, including experimental or statistically related factors, such as ceiling effects or inappropriate measures, tasks, or items. For example, Cherney and Ryalls (1999) found a female episodic memory advantage for female-oriented objects (e.g., lipstick), a male advantage for male-oriented objects (e.g., necktie), but no sex difference over both conditions. However, it is not particularly surprising that each sex would tend to better remember items that they are more interested in and are more familiar with, and thus that no sex difference would be found over both conditions. Indeed, another study that examined episodic memory for pictures of

such objects found a female advantage for female-oriented and neutral objects, as well as for complex abstract patterns, but no sex differences for male-oriented objects (McGivern et al., 1997). Interestingly, all three of the null-effect studies examined episodic memory for verbal or verbalizable material. Thus, these findings are no more problematic for the female declarative-advantage hypothesis than for the female verbal-advantage hypotheses.

The lack of sex differences in some of episodic memory studies could also be due to more substantive issues than experimental or statistical problems. For example, a male advantage in certain aspects of visuospatial processing (McKeever, 1986; Herlitz et al., 1999; Lewin et al., 2001; Saucier et al., 2002) might help to explain a lack of sex differences in tasks involving visuospatial stimuli or knowledge (Cherney & Ryalls, 1999; Herlitz et al., 1999; Lewin et al., 2001; Alexander et al., 2002), since a male visuospatial advantage on these tasks could outweigh a competing female declarative memory advantage. In fact, the only episodic memory studies we are aware of that showed a reliable *male* advantage involved visuospatial processing, with men being significantly better than women at recalling which cube faces were black in complex three-dimensional cube designs (Lewin et al., 2001).

One intriguing possibility is that while females tend to show an advantage over males at declarative memory, males may tend to show an advantage over females at procedural memory. Such a male advantage at procedural memory could be explained, at least in part, by animal and human studies suggesting that the declarative and procedural memory systems interact competitively (Packard & Knowlton, 2002; Poldrack & Packard, 2003; Ullman, 2004).

This leads to a "see-saw effect" (Ullman, 2004), such that a dysfunction of one system can enhance learning in the other, or that learning in one system may depress the functionality of the other. The see-saw effect may be explained by a number of factors (Ullman, 2004), including direct anatomical projections between the two systems (Sorensen & Witter, 1983), and a role for acetylcholine, which may not only enhance declarative memory (see above), but might also play an inhibitory role in brain structures underlying procedural memory (Calabresi et al., 2000). Estrogen may also contribute to the see-saw effect, perhaps via the modulation of acetylcholine (Ullman, 2004).

The possibility of a male advantage at procedural memory is much less well studied than the hypothesized female advantage at declarative memory. Nevertheless, such a male advantage may help explain certain previously observed patterns of data. For example, boys and men show better performance than girls and women at tasks such as aimed throwing and catching (Watson & Kimura, 1991; Kimura, 1999) that are likely to depend on the this memory system.

Similarly, mental rotation, which shows a large male advantage (Kimura, 1999; Halpern, 2000), depends at least in part on procedural memory brain structures (Ullman & Pierpont, 2005). A male advantage at procedural memory could also help explain sex differences in the relative reliance on declarative and procedural memory in the processing of complex linguistic forms. On this view these neurocognitive sex differences may be due not only to a female advantage at declarative memory, but also to a greater propensity for males to use procedural memory.

A male advantage at procedural memory may also account for sex differences in the neuroanatomy of brain structures that are important for procedural memory. For example, Blanton et al. (2004) found that among children ages 6 to 17, the white matter volume of the left (but not right) inferior frontal gyrus showed a significant positive correlation with age among boys, whereas no correlation was observed among girls. Additionally, the left (but not right) inferior frontal gyrus was significantly larger in boys than girls, even after correcting for total cerebral volume.

However, it is not yet clear whether or how other data may be accounted for by a male advantage at procedural memory. In particular, a female performance advantage has been reported in certain motor-related tasks, such as in Pegboard tasks (moving small pegs in holes) or at reproducing (relatively common) hand postures (Ingram, 1975; Kimura, 1999). In at least some cases these findings may not be inconsistent with a male advantage at procedural memory. Performance at the Pegboard or similar complex tasks involving movement are typically examined prior to substantial (presumably procedural) learning, and thus may not tap this system. Moreover, the female advantage at reproducing hand postures might be explained by a female declarative memory advantage for these postures. Further studies specifically testing a male advantage at procedural memory should further elucidate this hypothesis.

SUMMARY AND DISCUSSION

In this chapter we have reviewed the literature examining sex differences both in the performance of language-related tasks and in the neural bases of language. The behavioral evidence suggests that both girls and women show an advantage over boys and men at a variety of language-related tasks. Evidence suggesting that the female advantage extends to similar tasks that are unlikely to involve language makes it difficult to conclude that these sex differences can be best characterized as a female advantage at verbal processing.

The neural evidence, which is strongly focused on the issue of lateralization, is somewhat controversial. Although a number of studies suggest greater left-lateralization of language among males than females, other studies have found no sex differences in language lateralization. It has been suggested that these apparent inconsistencies may be due to sex differences in lateralization being found only for certain kinds of tasks or processes. Indeed, previous hypotheses along these lines, such as those proposed by Shaywitz et al. (1995) and Kansaku and Kitazawa (2001), seem to explain a portion of the lateralization data. However, these hypotheses also leave other neural evidence unaccounted for. Moreover, just as the hypothesis that females have an advantage at verbal processing is not targeted at and does not easily explain the neural data, so these accounts of sex differences in lateralization do not easily explain the behavioral data.

We suggest that the full range of neurocognitive data may perhaps be better explained by the hypothesis that females have an advantage over males at declarative memory. This brain system, which underlies the learning and use of knowledge across both verbal and spatial domains, is rooted in medial temporal lobe structures, although other brain structures also play important roles. Estrogens modulate declarative memory functionality, perhaps primarily through the action of acetylcholine and/or the protein BDNF. A female advantage at declarative memory can help explain a wide range of data, including better female performance at various language and non-language tasks, and neurocognitive evidence suggesting that women depend more on lexical/declarative memory for the processing of complex linguistic forms, while men tend to rely more on the rule-governed combination of these forms in the grammatical/procedural system. We also briefly discussed the possibility that certain patterns of data might be at least partly explained by a male advantage at procedural memory, which would co-occur with the posited female advantage at declarative memory.

Despite a range of evidence supporting the hypothesized sex differences in one or both memory systems, it is important to emphasize that only a few studies have been designed to directly test and potentially falsify these hypothesized differences. Indeed, few studies of sex differences in the brain bases of language have examined issues other than lateralization. It is also important to point out that whereas substantial data seems to support a female advantage at declarative memory, much less evidence seems relevant to the more speculative hypothesis that males show an advantage at procedural memory, which would thus benefit particularly from direct testing.

The posited sex differences in memory systems are quite appealing in ways that seem to be lacking in other explanatory accounts of sex differences in language. Most importantly, this perspective attempts to integrate and account for a wide range of types of data, across language and non-language domains, from different methodologies in both animals and humans, across different neurocognitive levels, from behavior to anatomy and even to hormones, proteins and genes. Thus this theoretical account seems to have substantially more explanatory power than other accounts. Additionally, because the sex differences in language are posited to depend on sex differences in independently studied memory systems, one can make predictions about sex differences in language based on *independent* knowledge of these memory systems—predictions that would be difficult to make based on the more circumscribed study of language alone.

Finally, the hypothesized sex differences may have interesting and potentially important implications. For example, such differences may help to explain sex differences in the incidence of various brain and behavioral disorders. If females rely more than males on declarative memory and less on procedural memory in the processing of complex forms, one might expect that a dysfunction of declarative memory may be more evident among females, simply because they rely more on that system. This in turn may lead to greater detection of the disorder among females, and thus to a higher reported female incidence. Such a pattern would be even more striking if the female advantage at declarative memory also resulted in an increased female reliance on this system for domains other than language, such as navigation, in which females depend more than males on memorized landmarks. Indeed, Alzheimer's disease, which primarily affects declarative memory brain structures, seems to have a higher incidence among women than men, at least among older patients (Amaducci & Lippi, 1991; Miech et al., 2002).

In contrast, one might expect that a dysfunction of procedural memory should be more evident among males if they depend more on this system than females, and thus a higher male incidence should be reported in such cases. Indeed, Parkinson's disease, which primarily affects procedural memory system structures, seems to have a higher incidence among men (Amaducci & Lippi, 1991). Likewise, a number of developmental disorders that are associated with abnormalities of procedural memory structures, such as Specific Language Impairment (Ullman & Pierpont, 2005), dyslexia (Bonin et al., 2006), and autism (Walenski et al., 2006), seem to have a higher incidence among boys than girls (Johnston et al., 1981; Ludlow & Cooper, 1983; Robinson, 1987; Tallal et al., 1989; Wolff & Melngailis, 1994; Tomblin, 1996; Lord & Spence, 2006).

Thus it may be that sex differences in the incidence of these disorders may be explained, at least in part—we are *not* claiming that they fully explain such differences—by sex differences in the *detection* of these disorders, which may in turn be largely due to differences between males and females in their relative reliance on the two memory systems.

In sum, previous evidence suggests the existence of both behavioral and neural sex differences in language. We have suggested that this pattern of data, as well as a range of other evidence, can be explained by a female advantage at declarative memory, perhaps accompanied by a male advantage at procedural memory. This perspective, which makes clear testable predictions and has potentially important implications, may constitute a useful paradigm for the study of sex differences in language and cognition.

Notes

1. Sommer et al. (2004) listed 22 tasks as showing no sex differences in language lateralization (Table 1 in Sommer et al.). We did not include three of these studies in our count (22−3 = 19): like Sommer et al. in their meta-analysis, we excluded Frost et al. (1999) because that study examines the same subjects as Springer et al.

(1999), and Vingerhoets and Stroobant (1999) because data were not reported separately for the spatial and language tasks. Additionally, we excluded Billingsley, McAndrews, Crawley, and Mikulis (2001) because they report sex differences over both healthy *and* brain-damaged patients. Moreover, examination of the original studies revealed that two tasks listed by Sommer et al. as showing sex differences in lateralization in fact did not (Schlosser et al., 1998; Gur et al., 2000), yielding a count of 21 tasks (19 + 2 = 21). Finally, note that we did not consider the left lateralization reported by Rossell, Bullmore, Williams, and David (2002) because, unlike all other tasks examined, the stimuli in this study were presented to one or the other visual hemifield.

2. Although Jaeger et al. (1998) reported that the production of irregular past-tense forms also showed sex differences in activation, these activation sex differences were substantially smaller (287 voxels across right temporal and frontal cortex) than those found for the production of regular or novel past-tenses (798 and 570 voxels, respectively). Thus the sex differences in activation for irregular past-tenses seem to be less reliable than those found for regular and novel forms.

Acknowledgments

This chapter was written with support for MTU from NIH R01 HD049347 and NIH R03 HD050671, and for RAM from an NSF Graduate Research Fellowship. We thank Cristina Dye, Elizabeth Hampson and Kathryn Sandberg for helpful comments.

References

Alexander GM, Packard MG, Peterson BS. (2002). Sex and spatial position effects on object location memory following intentional learning of object identities. *Neuropsychologia*, 40:1516–1522.

Alkire MT, Haier RJ, Fallon JH, Cahill L. (1998). Hippocampal, but not amygdala, activity at encoding correlates with long-term, free recall of nonemotional information. *Proceedings of the National Academy of Sciences of the United States of America* 95:14506–14510.

Amaducci L, Lippi A. (1991). The epidemiology of dementia, Alzheimer's disease and Parkinson's disease. In Boller F, Grafman J (Eds.), *Handbook of neuropsychology*, (pp. 3–13). New York: Elsevier Science Publishers B. V.

Barnfield A. (1999). Development of sex differences in spatial memory. *Perceptual and Motor Skills*, 89: 339–350.

Baxter LC, Saykin AJ, Flashman LA, Johnson SC, Guerin SJ, Babcock DR, Wishart HA. (2003). Sex differences in semantic language processing: a functional MRI study. *Brain Lang*, 84:264–272.

Bay K, Andersson A-M, Skakkebaek NE. (2004). Estradiol levels in prepubertal boys and girls—analytical challenges. *Int J Androl*, 27:266–273.

Bernard FA, Bullmore ET, Graham KS, Thompson SA, Hodges JR, Fletcher PC. (2004). The hippocampal region is involved in successful recognition of both remote and recent famous faces. *NeuroImage*, 22:1704–1714.

Bever TG (1992). The logical and extrinsic sources of modularity. In Gunnar M, Maratsos M (Eds.), *Modularity and constraints in language and cognition* (pp. 179–212). London: Lawrence Erlbaum.

Billingsley RL, McAndrews MP, Crawley AP, Mikulis DJ. (2001). Functional MRI of phonological and semantic processing in temporal lobe epilepsy. *Brain*, 124:1218–1227.

Blanton RE, Levitt JG, Peterson JR, Fadale D, Sporty ML, Lee M, et al. (2004). Gender differences in the left inferior frontal gyrus in normal children. *NeuroImage*, 22:626–636.

Boller F, Grafman J (Eds). (1995). *Handbook of neuropsychology*. New York: Elsevier.

Bonin CJ, Hartshorne JK, Ullman M. (2006). The procedural deficit hypothesis of dyslexia. In: The 25th Rodin Remediation Academy Conference. Washington DC: Georgetown University.

Brewer JB, Zhao Z, Desmond JE, Glover GH, Gabrieli JD. (1998.) Making memories: Brain activity that predicts how well visual experience will be remembered. *Science*, 281:1185–1187.

Buckner RL, Wheeler ME. (2001). The cognitive neuroscience of remembering. *Nature Review Neuroscience*, 2:624–634.

Calabresi P, Centonze D, Gubellini P, Pisani A, Bernardi G. (2000). Acetylcholine-mediated modulation of striatal function. *Trends in Neurosciences*, 23:120–126.

Cansino S, Maquet P, Dolan RJ, Rugg MD. (2002). Brain activity underlying encoding and retrieval of source memory. *Cerebral Cortex*, 12:1048–1056.

Cherney ID, Ryalls BO. (1999). Gender-linked differences in the incidental memory of children and adults. *Journal of Experimental Child Psychology*, 72:305–328.

Chun MM. (2000). Contextual cueing of visual attention. *Trends in Cognitive Sciences*, 4:170–178.

Cox D, Waters HS. (1986). Sex differences in the use of organization strategies: a developmental analysis. *Journal of Experimental Child Psychology*, 41: 18–37.

Curran HV. (2000). Psychopharmacological approaches to human memory. In Gazzaniga MS. (Ed.), *The new cognitive neurosciences*. (pp 797–804). Cambridge, MA: MIT Press.

Cutler GB. Jr. (1997). The role of estrogen in bone growth and maturation during childhood and adolescence. *The Journal of Steroid Biochemistry and Molecular Biology*, 61:141–144.

De Renzi E. (1989). Apraxia. In Boller F, Grafman J, (Eds.), *Handbook of Neuropsychology*, (pp. 245–263). New York: Elsevier Science Publishers B.V.

Desmond JE, Fiez JA. (1998). Neuroimaging studies of the cerebellum: language, learning, and memory. *Trends in Cognitive Sciences*, 2:355–362.

Eals M, Silverman I. (1994). The Hunter-Gatherer theory of spatial sex differences: Proximate factors mediating the female advantage in recall of object arrays. *Ethology and Sociobiology*, 15:95–105.

Egan MF, Kojima M, Callicott JH, Goldberg TE, Kolachana BS, Bertolino A, et al. (2003) The BDNF va166met polymorphism affects activity-dependent secretion of BDNF and human memory and hippocampal function. *Cell*, 112:257–269.

Eichenbaum H. (2000). A cortical-hippocampal system for declarative memory. *Nature Reviews Neuroscience*, 1:41–50.

Eichenbaum H, Cohen NJ. (2001). From conditioning to conscious recollection: Memory systems of the brain. New York: Oxford University Press.

Eldridge LL, Knowlton BJ, Furmanski CS, Bookheimer SY, Engel SA. (2000). Remembering episodes: A selective role for the hippocampus during retrieval. *Nature Neuroscience*, 3:1149–1152.

Eldridge LL, Engel SA, Zeineh MM, Bookheimer SY, Knowlton BJ. (2005). A Dissociation of encoding and retrieval processes in the human hippocampus. *Journal of Neuroscience*, 25:3280–3286.

Elfgren C, van Westen D, Passant U, Larsson E-M, Mannfolk P, Fransson P. (2006). fMRI activity in the medial temporal lobe during famous face processing. *Neuroimage*, 30:609–616.

Estabrooke IV, Ullman MT. (in preparation). Sex differences in the production of the English past tense: Evidence from patients with Parkinson's disease.

Fernandez G, Weyerts H, Schrader-Bolsche M, Tendolkar I, Smid HG, Tempelmann C, et al. (1998). Successful verbal encoding into episodic memory engages the posterior hippocampus: A parametrically analyzed functional magnetic resonance imaging study. *J Neurosci*, 18:1841–1847.

Freo U, Pizzolato G, Dam M, Ori C, Battistin L. (2002). A short review of cognitive and functional neuroimaging studies of cholinergic drugs: Implications for therapeutic potentials. *Journal of Neural Transmission*, 109:857–870.

Frith U, Vargha-Khadem F. (2001). Are there sex differences in the brain basis of literacy related skills? Evidence from reading and spelling impairments after early unilateral brain damage. *Neuropsychologia*, 39:1485–1488.

Frost JA, Binder JR, Springer JA, Hammeke TA, Bellgowan PS, Rao SM, Cox RW. (1999). Language processing is strongly left lateralized in both sexes: Evidence from functional MRI. *Brain*, 122:199–208.

Gabrieli JDE, Cohen NJ, Corkin S. (1988). The impaired learning of semantic knowledge following bilateral medial temporal-lobe resection. *Brain and Cognition*, 7:157–177.

Galea LAM, Kimura D. (1993). Sex differences in route-learning. *Personality and Individual Differences*, 14:53–65.

Guillem F, Mograss M. (2005). Gender differences in memory processing: evidence from event-related potentials to faces. *Brain and Cognition*, 57:84–92.

Gur RC, Alsop D, Glahn D, Petty R, Swanson CL, Maldjian JA, et al. (2000). An fMRI study of sex differences in regional activation to a verbal and a spatial task. *Brain and Language*, 74:157–170.

Haaland K, Harrington D, Knight R. (2000). Neural representations of skilled movement. *Brain*, 123:2306–2313.

Haaland KY, Harrington DL. (1996). Hemispheric asymmetry of movement. *Current Opinion in Neurobiology*, 6:796–800.

Haist F, Gore JB, Mao H. (2001). Consolidation of human memory over decades revealed by functional magnetic resonance imaging. *Nature Neuroscience*, 4:1139–1145.

Halpern DF. (2000). *Sex differences in cognitive abilities*, 3rd Edition. Mahwah, NJ: Lawrence Erlbaum Associates.

Hampson E. (1990). Variations in sex-related cognitive abilities across the menstrual cycle. *Brain and Cognition*, 14:26–43.

Hariri AR, Goldberg TE, Mattay VS, Kolachana BS, Callicott JH, Egan MF, Weinberger DR. (2003). Brain-derived neurotrophic factor va166met polymorphism affects human memory-related hippocampal activity and predicts memory performance. *Journal of Neuroscience*, 23:6690–6694.

Hartshorne JK, Ullman MT. (2006). Why girls say 'holded' more than boys. *Developmental Science*, 9:21–32.

Heckers S, Weiss AP, Alpert NM, Schacter DL. (2002). Hippocampal and brain stem activation during word retrieval and after repeated and semantic encoding. *Cerebral Cortex*, 12:900–907.

Heilman KM, Watson RT, Rothi LG. (1997). Disorders of skilled movements: Limb apraxia. In Feinberg TE, Farah MJ, (Eds.), *Behavioral neurology and neuropsychology* (pp. 227–235). New York: McGraw-Hill.

Henke K, Weber B, Kneifel S, Wieser HG, Buck A. (1999). Human hippocampus associates information in memory. *Proceedings of the National Academy of Sciences of the United States of America*, 96:5884–5889.

Henson R. (2005). A mini-review of fMRI studies of human medial temporal lobe activity associated with recognition memory. *Q J Exp Physiol*, 58(B):340–360.

Herlitz A, Yonker JE. (2002). Sex differences in episodic memory: the influence of intelligence. *Journal of Clinical and Experimental Neuropsychology*, 24:107–114.

Herlitz A, Nilsson LG, Backman L. (1997). Gender differences in episodic memory. *Memory and Cognition*, 25:801–811.

Herlitz A, Airaksinen E, Nordstrom E. (1999). Sex differences in episodic memory: The impact of verbal and visuospatial ability. *Neuropsychology*, 13:590–597.

Hodges JR, Patterson K. (1997). Semantic memory disorders. *Trends in Cognitive Sciences*, 1:68–72.

Horgan DM. (1975). Language development. In: *Neuroscience*. Ann Arbor: University of Michigan.

Huttenlocher J, Haight W, Bryk A, Seltzer M, Lyons T. (1991). Early vocabulary growth: Relation to language input and gender. *Developmental Psychology*, 27:236–248.

Ikegami S, Moriwake T, Tanaka H, Inoue M, Kubo T, Suzuki S, Kanzaki S, Seino Y. (2001). An ultrasensitive assay revealed age-related changes in serum oestradiol at low concentrations in both sexes from infancy to puberty. *Clin Endocrinol*, (Oxf) 55:789–795.

Inglis J, Lawson JS. (1981). Sex differences in the effects of unilateral brain damage on intelligence. *Science*, 212:693–695.

Ingram D. (1975). Motor asymmetries in young children. *Neuropsychologia*, 13:95–102.

Jaeger JJ, Lockwood AH, Van Valin RD, Jr., Kemmerer DL, Murphy BW, Wack DS. (1998). Sex differences in brain regions activated by grammatical and reading tasks. *NeuroReport*, 9:2803–2807.

James TW, Kimura D. (1997). Sex differences in remembering the locations of objects in an array: Location-shifts versus location-exchanges. *Evolution and Human Behavior*, 18:155–163.

Johnston RB, Stark RE, Mellits ED, Tallal P. (1981). Neurological status of language-impaired and normal children. *Annals of Neurology*, 10:159–163.

Kampen DL, Sherwin BB. (1994). Estrogen use and verbal memory in healthy postmenopausal women. *Obstetrics & Gynecology*, 83:979–983.

Kampen DL, Sherwin BB. (1996). Estradiol is related to visual memory in healthy young men. *Behavioral Neuroscience*, 110:613–617.

Kandel ER. (2001). The molecular biology of memory storage: A dialogue between genes and synapses. *Science*, 294:1030–1038.

Kansaku K, Kitazawa S. (2001). Imaging studies on sex differences in the lateralization of language. *Neuroscience Research*, 41:333–337.

Kansaku K, Yamaura A, Kitazawa S. (2000). Sex differences in lateralization revealed in the posterior language areas. *Cerebral Cortex*, 10:866–872.

Kimura D. (1983). Sex differences in cerebral organization for speech and praxic functions. *Canadian Journal of Psychology*, 37:19–35.

Kimura D. (1993). *Neuromotor mechanisms in human communication*. New York, Oxford: Oxford University Press, Clarendon Press.

Kimura D. (1996). Sex, sexual orientation and sex hormones influence human cognitive function. *Current Opinion in Neurobiology*, 6:259–263.

Kimura D. (1999). *Sex and cognition*. Cambridge, MA: The MIT Press.

Kimura D, Harshman RA. (1984). Sex differences in brain organization for verbal and non-verbal functions. *Progress in Brain Research*, 61:423–441.

Kitazawa S, Kansaku K. (2005). Sex difference in language lateralization may be task-dependent. *Brain*, 128:E30; author reply E31.

Klein K, Baron J, Colli M, McDonnell D, Cutler G. (1994). Estrogen levels in childhood determined by an ultrasensitive recombinant cell bioassay. *Journal of Clinical Investigation*, 94:2475–2480.

Klein KO, Baron J, Barnes KM, Pescovitz OH, Cutler GB. (1998). Use of an ultrasensitive recombinant cell bioassay to determine estrogen levels in girls with precocious puberty treated with a luteinizing hormone-releasing hormone agonist. *Journal of Clinical Endocrinology and Metabolism*, 83:2387–2389.

Kramer J, Yaffe K, Lengenfelder J, Delis D. (2003). Age and gender interactions on verbal memory performance. *Journal of the International Neuropsychological Society*, 9:97–102.

Kramer JH, Delis DC, Daniel M. (1988). Sex differences in verbal learning. *Journal of Clinical Psychology*, 44:907–915.

Kramer JH, Delis DC, Kaplan E, O'Donnell L, Prifitera A. (1997). Developmental sex differences in verbal learning. *Neuropsychology*, 11:577–584.

Larsson M, Lovden M, Nilsson LG. (2003). Sex differences in recollective experience for olfactory and verbal information. *Acta Psychologica*, 112:89–103.

Levy LJ, Astur RS, Frick KM. (2005). Men and women differ in object memory but not performance of a virtual radial maze. *Behavioral Neuroscience*, 119:853–862.

Lewin C, Herlitz A. (2002). Sex differences in face recognition—Women's faces make the difference. *Brain and Cognition*, 50:121–128.

Lewin C, Wolgers G, Herlitz A. (2001). Sex differences favoring women in verbal but not in visuospatial episodic memory. *Neuropsychology*, 15:165–173.

Lim TK. (1994). Gender-related differences in intelligence: Application of confirmatory factor analysis. *Intelligence*, 19:179–192.

Loonstra A, Tarlow A, Sellers A. (2001). COWAT meta-norms across age, education, and gender. *Applied Neuropsychology*, 8:161–166.

Lord C, Spence SJ. (2006). Autism spectrum disorders: phenotype and diagnosis. In Moldin SO, Rubenstein JLR, (Eds.), *Understanding autism: From basic neuroscience to treatment* (pp 1–23). Boca Raton, FL: CRC Press.

Lu B, Gottschalk W. (2000). Modulation of hippocampal synaptic transmission and plasticity by neurotrophins. *Progress in Brain Research*, 128:231–241.

Ludlow CL, Cooper JA. (1983). *Genetic aspects of speech and language disorders*. New York: Academic Press.

Lynch G. (2002.) Memory enhancement: The search for mechanism-based drugs. *Nature Neuroscience*, 5:1035–1038.

Maguire EA, Frackowiak RS, Frith CD. (1996). Learning to find your way: A role for the human hippocampal formation. *Proceedings of the Royal Society of London Series B Biological Sciences* 263:1745–1750.

Maguire EA, Frackowiak RS, Frith CD. (1997). Recalling routes around London: Activation of the right hippocampus in taxi drivers. *Journal of Neuroscience,* 17:7103–7110.

Maitland SB, Herlitz A, Nyberg L, Backman L, Nilsson LG. (2004). Selective sex differences in declarative memory. *Memory and Cognition,* 32:1160–1169.

Maki PM, Resnick SM. (2000). Longitudinal effects of estrogen replacement therapy on PET cerebral blood flow and cognition. *Neurobiology of Aging,* 21:373–383.

Maki PM, Rich JB, Rosenbaum RS. (2002). Implicit memory varies across the menstrual cycle: Estrogen effects in young women. *Neuropsychologia,* 40:518–529.

Marche TA. (1999). Memory strength affects reporting of misinformation. *Journal of Experimental Child Psychology,* 73:45–71.

Martin A, Ungerleider LG, Haxby JV. (2000). Category specificity and the brain: The sensory/motor model of semantic representations of objects. In Gazzaniga MS, (Ed.), *The cognitive neurosciences* (pp. 1023–1036). Cambridge, MA: The MIT Press.

Martin DJ, Hoover HD. (1987). Sex differences in educational achievement: A longitudnal study. *Journal of Early Adolescence,* 7:65–83.

Massey PV, Bhabra G, Cho K, Brown MW, Bashir ZI. (2001). Activation of muscarinic receptors induces protein synthesis-dependent long-lasting depression in the perirhinal cortex. *European Journal of Neuroscience,* 14:145–152.

McBurney DH, Gaulin SJC, Devineni T, Adams C. (1997). Superior spatial memory of women: Stronger evidence for the gathering hypothesis. *Evolution and Human Behavior,* 18:165–174.

McEwen B, Akama K, Alves S, Brake WG, Bulloch K, Lee S, et al. (2001). Tracking the estrogen receptor in neurons: Implications for estrogen-induced synapse formation. *Proceedings of the National Academy of Science* 98:7093–7100.

McEwen BS. (1999). Clinical review 108: The molecular and neuroanatomical basis for estrogen effects in the central nervous system. *Journal of Clinical Endocrinology and Metabolism,* 84:1790–1797.

McEwen BS, Alves SE, Bulloch K, Weiland NG. (1998). Clinically relevant basic science studies of gender differences and sex hormone effects. *Psychopharmacology Bulletin,* 34:251–259.

McGivern RF, Huston JP, Byrd D, King T, Siegle GJ, Reilly J. (1997). Sex differences in visual recognition memory: Support for a sex-related difference in attention in adults and children. *Brain and Cognition,* 34:323–336.

McGlone J. (1977). Sex differences in the cerebral organization of verbal functions in patients with unilateral brain lesions. *Brain,* 100:775–793.

McKeever WF. (1986). The influences of handedness, sex, familial sinistrality and androgyny on language laterality, verbal ability, and spatial ability. *Cortex,* 22:521–537.

Meltzer JA, Constable RT. (2005). Activation of human hippocampal formation reflects success in both encoding and cued recall of paired associates. *NeuroImage,* 24:384–397.

Miech R, Breitner J, Zandi P, Khachaturian A, Anthony J, Mayer L. (2002). Incidence of AD may decline in the early 90s for men, later for women: The Cache County study. *Neurology,* 58:209–218.

Miles C, Green R, Sanders G, Hines M. (1998). Estrogen and memory in a transsexual population. *Hormones and Behavior,* 34:199–208.

Miranda RA, Ullman MT. (under review). Sex differences in music: A female advantage in the recognition of familiar melodies. *Memory and Cognition.*

Mishkin M, Malamut B, Bachevalier J. (1984). Memories and habits: Two neural systems. In Lynch G, McGaugh JL, Weinburger NW, (Eds.),*Neurobiology of learning and memory* (pp. 65–77). New York: Guilford Press.

Moffa M, Lee S, Ullman MT. (2005). Left-handedness, procedural memory and grammar. *Journal of Cognitive Neuroscience,* Supplement:127.

Montaldi D, Spencer TJ, Roberts N, Mayes AR. (2006). The neural system that mediates familiarity memory. *Hippocampus,* 16:504–520.

Murphy DD, Cole NB, Segal M. (1998). Brain-derived neurotrophic factor mediates estradiol-induced dendritic spine formation in hippocampal neurons. *Proceedings of the National Academy of Sciences, USA,* 95:11412–11417.

Murphy DG, De Carli C, Daly E, Haxby JV, Allen G, White BJ, McIntosh AR, et al. (1993). X-chromosome effects on female brain: A magnetic resonance imaging study of Turner's syndrome. *Lancet,* 342:1197–1200.

Nadel L, Moscovitch M. (1997). Memory consolidation, retrograde amnesia and the hippocampal complex. *Current Opinion in Neurobiology,* 7:217–227.

Norman J. (2002). Two visual systems and two theories of perception: An attempt to reconcile the constructive and ecological approaches. *Behavioral and Brain Sciences,* 25:73–96.

Nunn JA, Wilkinson I, Spencer T, Khiami R, Griffiths PD, Mayes A (2000) Both long- and short-term topographical memory recall produces activation of the medial temporal lobe: A functional magnetic resonance study. *Proceedings of the International Society of Magnetic Resonance in Medicine* 8:909.

Otten LJ, Henson RN, Rugg MD. (2001). Depth of processing effects on neural correlates of memory encoding: Relationship between findings from across- and within-task comparisons. *Brain,* 124: 399–412.

Packard MG. (1998). Posttraining estrogen and memory modulation. *Hormones and Behavior,* 34:126–139.

Packard MG, Knowlton BJ. (2002). Learning and memory functions of the basal ganglia. *Annual Review of Neuroscience*, 25:563–593.

Pezawas L, Verchinski BA, Mattay VS, Callicott JH, Kolachana BS, Straub RE, et al. (2004). The brain-derived neurotrophic factor va166met polymorphism and variation in human cortical morphology. *Journal of Neuroscience*, 24:10099–10102.

Pfluger T, Weil S, Weis S, Vollmar C, Heiss D, Egger J, Scheck R, Hahn K. (1999). Normative volumetric data of the developing hippocampus in children based on magnetic resonance imaging. *Epilepsia*, 40:414–423.

Phillips MD, Lurito JT, Dzemidzic M, Lowe MJ, Wang Y, Mathews VP. (2000). Gender based differences in temporal lobe activation demonstrated using a novel passive listening paradigm. *NeuroImage*, 11:S352.

Phillips SM, Sherwin BB, (1992), Effects of estrogen on memory function in surgically menopausal women. *Psychoneuroendocrinology*, 17:485–495.

Pihlajamaki M, Tanila H, Hanninen T, Kononen M, Laakso M, Partanen K, et al. (2000). Verbal fluency activates the left medical temporal lobe: A functional magnetic resonance imaging study. *Annals of Neurology*, 47:470–476.

Pizzamiglio L, Mammucari A, Razzano C. (1985). Evidence for sex differences in brain organization in recovery in aphasia. *Brain Lang*, 25:213–223.

Poldrack RA, Packard MG. (2003). Competition among multiple memory systems: Converging evidence from animal and human brain studies. *Neuropsychologia*, 41:245–251.

Poo M-M. (2001). Neurotrophins as synaptic modulators. *Nature Reviews Neuroscience*, 2:24–32.

Postle BR, Corkin S. (1998). Impaired word-stem completion priming but intact perceptual identification priming with novel words: Evidence from the amnesic patient H.M. *Neuropsychologia*, 15:421–440.

Powell HWR, Koepp MJ, Symms MR, Boulby PA, Salek-Haddadi A, Thompson PJ, et al. (2005). Material-specific lateralization of memory encoding in the medial temporal lobe: Blocked versus event-related design. *NeuroImage*, 27:231–239.

Prado E, Ullman MT. (under review). Can imageability help us draw the line between storage and composition? *Journal of Experimental Psychology: Language, Memory, and Cognition*.

Prince SE, Daselaar SM, Cabeza R. (2005). Neural correlates of relational memory: successful encoding and retrieval of semantic and perceptual associations. *The Journal of Neuroscience*, 25:1203–1210.

Pruessner JC, Collins DL, Pruessner M, Evans AC. (2001). Age and gender predict volume decline in the anterior and posterior hippocampus in early adulthood. *Journal of Neuroscience*, 21:194–200.

Pugh KR, Shaywitz BA, Shaywitz SE, Constable T, Skudlarski P, Fulbright RK, et al. (1996). Cerebral organization of component processes in reading. *Brain*, 119:1221–1238.

Rekkas PV, Constable RT. (2005). Evidence that autobiographic memory retrieval does not become independent of the hippocampus: An fMRI study contrasting very recent with remote events. *Journal of Cognitive Neuroscience*, 17:1950–1961.

Resnick S, Maki P, Golski S, Kraut M, Zonderman A. (1998). Effects of estrogen replacement therapy on PET cerebral blood flow and neuropsychological performance. *Hormones and Behavior*, 34:171–182.

Resnick SM, Metter EJ, Zonderman AB. (1997). Estrogen replacement therapy and longitudinal decline in visual memory. A possible protective effect? *Neurology*, 49:1491–1497.

Robinson D, Friedman L, Marcus R, Tinklenberg JR, Yesavage JA. (1994). Estrogen replacement therapy and memory in older women. *Journal of the American Geriatrics Society*, 42:919–922.

Robinson R (1987) The causes of language disorder: Introduction and overview. In: *Proceedings of the First International Symposium on Specific Speech and Language Disorders in Children*, pp 1–19. London: Association for All Speech Impaired Children.

Ross JL, Roeltgen D, Feuillan P, Kushner H, Cutler GB, Jr. (2000). Use of estrogen in young girls with Turner syndrome: Effects on memory. *Neurology*, 54:164–170.

Rossell SL, Bullmore ET, Williams SCR, David AS. (2002). Sex differences in functional brain activation during a lexical visual field task. *Brain and Language*, 80:97–105.

Sandstrom NJ, Kaufman J, Huettel SA. (1998). Males and females use different distal cues in a virtual environment navigation task. *Cognitive Brain Research*, 6:351–360.

Saucier D, Bowman M, Elias L. (2003). Sex differences in the effect of articulatory or spatial dual-task interference during navigation. *Brain and Cognition*, 53:346–350.

Saucier D, Green S, Leason J, MacFadden A, Bell S, Elias LJ. (2002). Are sex differences caused by sexually dimorphic strategies or by differences in the ability to use the strategies? *Behavioral Neuroscience*, 116:403–410.

Schacter DL, Tulving E (Eds.). (1994). Memory systems 1994. Cambridge, MA: The MIT Press.

Scharfman HE, MacLusky NJ. (2005). Similarities between actions of estrogen and BDNF in the hippocampus: coincidence or clue? *Trends in Neurosciences*, 28.

Schlosser R, Hutchinson M, Joseffer S, Rusinek H, Saarimaki A, Stevenson J, et al. (1998). Functional magnetic resonance imaging of human brain activity in a verbal fluency task. *Journal of Neurology, Neurosurgery, and Psychiatry*, 64:492–498.

Schon K, Atri A, Hasselmo ME, Tricarico MD, LoPresti ML, Stern CE. (2005). Scopolamine reduces persistent activity related to long-term encoding in the parahippocampal gyrus during delayed matching in humans. *Journal of Neuroscience*, 25:9112–9123.

Shaywitz BA, Shaywitz SE, Pugh KR, Constable RT, Skudlarski P, Fulbright RK, et al. (1995). Sex differences in the functional organization of the brain for language. *Nature*, 373:607–609.

Sherwin BB. (1988). Estrogen and/or androgen replacement therapy and cognitive functioning in surgically menopausal women. *Psychoneuroendocrinology*, 13: 345–357.

Sherwin BB. (1998). Estrogen and cognitive functioning in women. *Proceedings of the Society for Experimental Biology and Medicine* 217:17–22.

Sherwin BB. (2003). Estrogen and cognitive functioning in women. *Endocr Rev*, 24:133–151.

Sherwin BB, Phillips S. (1990). Estrogen and cognitive functioning in surgically menopausal women. *Annals New York Academy of Science*, 592:474–475.

Sherwin BB, Tulandi T. (1996). "Add-Back" estrogen reverses cognitive deficits induced by a gonadotrophin-releasing hormone agonist in women with leiomyomata uteri. *J Clin Endocrinol Metab*, 81: 2545–2549.

Shughrue PJ, Scrimo PJ, Merchenthaler I. (2000). Estrogen binding and estrogen receptor characterization (ERalpha and ERbeta) in the cholinergic neurons of the rat basal forebrain. *Neuroscience*, 96:41–49.

Silverman I, Eals M (1992) Sex differences in spatial abilities: Evolutionary theory and data. In Barkow J, Cosmides L, Tooby J (Eds.). *The adapted mind: Evolutionary psychology and the generation of culture*, New York: Oxford University Press.

Simpkins JW, Green PS, Gridley KE, Singh M, de Fiebre NC, Rajakumar G. (1997). Role of estrogen replacement therapy in memory enhancement and the prevention of neuronal loss associated with Alzheimer's disease. *American Journal of Medicine*, 103: 19S–25S.

Sommer IE, Aleman A, Bouma A, Kahn RS. (2004). Do women really have more bilateral language representation than men? A meta-analysis of functional imaging studies. *Brain*, 127:1845–1852.

Sorensen KE, Witter MP. (1983). Entorhinal efferents reach the caudato-putamen. *Neuroscience Letters*, 35:259–264.

Springer JA, Binder JR, Hammeke TA, Swanson SJ, Frost JA, Bellgowan PS, et al. (1999). Language dominance in neurologically normal and epilepsy subjects: A functional MRI study. *Brain*, 122:2033–2046.

Squire LR, Alvarez P. (1995). Retrograde amnesia and memory consolidation: a neurobiological perspective. *Current Opinion in Neurobiology*, 5:169–177.

Squire LR, Zola SM. (1996). Structure and function of declarative and nondeclarative memory systems. *Proceedings of the National Academy of Science USA*, 93:13515–13522.

Squire LR, Knowlton BJ. (2000). The medial temporal lobe, the hippocampus, and the memory systems of the brain. In Gazzaniga MS (Ed.), *The new cognitive neurosciences* (pp. 765–780). Cambridge, MA: MIT Press.

Steinhauer K, Ullman MT. (2002). Consecutive ERP effects of morph-phonology and morpho-syntax. *Brain and Language*, 83:62–65.

Strange BA, Otten LJ, Josephs O, Rugg MD, Dolan RJ. (2002). Dissociable human perirhinal, hippocampal, and parahippocampal roles during verbal encoding. *J Neurosci*, 22:523–528.

Suzuki WA, Amaral DG. (1994). Perirhinal and parahippocampal cortices of the macaque monkey: Cortical afferants. *Journal of Comparative Neurology*, 350:497–533.

Tallal P, Ross R, Curtiss S. (1989). Unexpected sex-ratios in families of language/learning-impaired children. 987–998.

Tomblin JB. (1996). Genetic and environmental contributions to the risk for specific language impairment. In Rice ML (Ed.), *Toward a genetics of language* (pp. 191–210). Mahwah, NJ: Lawrence Erlbaum Associates.

Trahan DE, Quintana JW. (1990). Analysis of gender effects upon verbal and visual memory performance in adults. *Archives of Clinical Neuropsychology*, 5:325–334.

Ullman MT. (2001a). The neural basis of lexicon and grammar in first and second language: The declarative/procedural model. *Bilingualism: Language and Cognition*, 4:105–122.

Ullman MT. (2001b). A neurocognitive perspective on language: The declarative/procedural model. *Nature Reviews Neuroscience*, 2:717–726.

Ullman MT. (2004). Contributions of memory circuits to language: The declarative/procedural model. *Cognition*, 92:231–270.

Ullman MT. (2005). A cognitive neuroscience perspective on second language acquisition: The declarative/procedural model. In Sanz C (Ed.), *Mind and context in adult second language acquisition: methods, theory and practice* (pp. 141–178). Washington, DC: Georgetown University Press.

Ullman MT. (2006). Is Broca's area part of a basal ganglia thalamocortical circuit? *Cortex*, 42:480–485.

Ullman MT. (in press). The biocognition of the mental lexicon. In Gaskell MG, (Ed.). *The Oxford handbook of psycholinguistics*. Oxford, UK: Oxford University Press.

Ullman MT, Estabrooke IV. (2004). Grammar, tools and sex. *Journal of Cognitive Neuroscience*, Supplement:67.

Ullman MT, Pierpont EI. (2005). Specific language impairment is not specific to language: the procedural deficit hypothesis. *Cortex*, 41:399–433.

Ullman MT, Walenski M, Prado EL, Ozawa K, Steinhauer K. (under revision-a). The compositionality and storage of inflected forms: Evidence from working memory effects. *Cognition*.

Ullman MT, Maloof CJ, Hartshorne JK, Estabrooke IV, Brovetto C, Walenski M (under revision-b). Sex, regularity, frequency and consistency: A study of factors predicting the storage of inflected forms.

Ullman MT, Corkin S, Coppola M, Hickok G, Growdon JH, Koroshetz WJ, Pinker S. (1997). A neural dissociation within language: Evidence that the mental dictionary is part of declarative memory, and that grammatical rules are processed by the procedural system. *Journal of Cognitive Neuroscience*, 9:266–276.

Ullman MT, Estabrooke IV, Steinhauer K, Brovetto C, Pancheva R, Ozawa K, et al. (2002). Sex differences in the neurocognition of language. *Brain and Language*, 83:141–143.

Uncapher MR, Rugg MD. (2005). Encoding and the durability of episodic memory: A functional magnetic resonance imaging study. *The Journal of Neuroscience*, 25:7260–7267.

Van Strien JW, Hagenbeek RE, Stam CJ, Rombouts SARB, Barkhof F. (2005). Changes in brain electrical activity during extended continuous word recognition. *Neuroimage*, 26.

Vikingstad EM, George KP, Johnson AF, Cao Y. (2000). Cortical language lateralization in right handed normal subjects using functional magnetic resonance imaging. *Journal of the Neurological Sciences*, 175:17–27.

Vingerhoets G, Stroobant N. (1999). Lateralization of cerebral blood flow velocity changes during cognitive tasks: A simultaneous bilateral transcranial Doppler study. *Stroke*, 30:2152–2158.

Vitali P, Abutalebi J, Tettamanti M, Rowe J, Scifo P, Fazio F, Cappa SF, Perani D. (2005). Generating animal and tool names: An fMRI study of effective connectivity. *Brain and Language*, 93:32–45.

Wagner AD, Schacter DL, Rotte M, Koutstaal W, Maril A, Dale AM, et al. (1998). Building memories: Remembering and forgetting of verbal experiences as predicted by brain activity. *Science*, 281:1188–1191.

Walenski M, Tager-Flusberg H, Ullman MT. (2006). Language in autism. In Moldin SO, Rubenstein JLR (Eds.), *Understanding autism: From basic neuroscience to treatment* (pp. 175–203). Boca Raton, FL: Taylor and Francis Books.

Walenski M, Mostofsky SH, Larson JCG, Ullman MT. (under review). Enhanced picture naming in autism. *Journal of Autism and Developmental Disorders*.

Watson NV, Kimura D. (1991). Nontrivial sex differences in throwing and intercepting: Relation to psychometrically-defined spatial functions. *Personality and Individual Differences*, 12:375–385.

Wheeler ME, Buckner RL. (2004). Functional-anatomic correlates of remembering and knowing. *NeuroImage*, 21:1337–1349.

Williams CL, Barnett AM, Meck WH. (1990). Organizational effects of early gonadal secretions on sexual differentiation in spatial memory. *Behavioral Neuroscience*, 104:84–97.

Wilson JD, Foster DW, Kronenberg HM, Larsen PR (Eds.). (1998). Williams textbook of endocrinology, 9th Edition. Philadelphia, PA: W.B. Saunders Company.

Wolff P, Melngailis I. (1994.) Family patterns of developmental dyslexia: Clinical findings. *Am J Med Genet*, 54:122–131.

Woolley CS. (1999). Effects of estrogen in the CNS. *Current Opinion in Neurobiology*, 9:349–354.

Woolley CS, Schwartzkroin PA. (1998). Hormonal effects on the brain. *Epilepsia*,39:S2–S8.

Yonelinas AP, Otten LJ, Shaw KN, Rugg MD. (2005). Separating the brain regions involved in recollection and familiarity in recognition memory. *Journal of Neuroscience*, 25:3002–3008.

Yonker JE, Eriksson E, Nilsson LG, Herlitz A. (2003). Sex differences in episodic memory: Minimal influence of estradiol. *Brain Cogn*, 52:231–238.

Zola-Morgan S, Squire LR, Amaral DG. (1986). Human amnesia and the medial temporal region: Enduring memory impairment following a bilateral lesion limited to field CA1 of the hippocampus. *J Neurosci*, 6:2950–2967.

Chapter 16

Endocrine Contributions to Sex Differences in Visuospatial Perception and Cognition

Elizabeth Hampson

In the past 25 years, studies of non-human species have shown that reproductive steroids, especially estradiol and testosterone, can alter patterns of neural development in some parts of the brain during early life (Breedlove & Hampson, 2002), and exert a wide range of effects on neurochemistry and the microstructure of synapses in the adult brain (McEwen & Alves, 1999). Sex is therefore a significant variable for many aspects of brain function. This is likely to be true in humans as well, even though it is hard to study the human brain at the cellular or molecular level. The occurrence of sex differences in several areas of perception and cognition suggests that these processes could be among the functions modulated by sex and sex-related metabolic differences. In this chapter, we will concentrate on one particular perceptual and cognitive domain where sex differences have been reliably identified: visual-spatial abilities. This area of cognition has been the most extensively studied, both with respect to sex differences per se and with respect to the endocrine regulation of those differences. It can

serve as a potential model for investigations in other cognitive domains.

Spatial abilities are a diverse set of evolved abilities that are controlled by a large array of different brain systems. They serve a range of adaptive functions related to the perception or cognitive understanding of the spatial environment—they allow us to encode the spatial positions of our own bodies; the positions of objects in the environment, near or far; they allow us to anticipate the results of movement on the part of other objects or of our bodies in relation to external objects; and to use our acquired spatial knowledge of our environment for everyday tasks like navigation or way-finding.

HISTORICAL OVERVIEW

Sex differences in perception and cognition were first reported over 100 years ago. For example, Nichols (1885) found that men perceived color pigments at

311

lower degrees of saturation than women did. Such observations were treated as scientific curiosities. In the early 1900s, the field of psychology emerged, and with it, the mental testing movement began. This was an effort to identify and measure the fundamental mental processes that comprise the mind. In retrospect, this was naïve. But one useful by-product of the work was the identification of sex differences in many new domains, ranging from achievement on reading comprehension tests to the ability to visualize moving objects in one's mind.

Maccoby and Jacklin (1974) summarized data from the first half of the twentieth century in their landmark review of sex differences in human cognition and behavior. Many of the findings could be summarized only at the descriptive level, i.e., as a difference in performance on a particular type of experimental task without understanding the exact components of cognition that are the latent sources of the surface sex difference. Though some progress has been made, we still lack a deep understanding of many of the sex differences recognized today. In particular, little effort has been made to interpret the early findings in light of advances in cognitive neuroscience, which has greatly deepened our understanding of how the brain controls spatial processes.

One achievement of the mental testing movement was the development of standardized IQ tests, which are still widely used in education and the mental health professions. Studies of intelligence and its measurement showed no evidence of a sex difference in IQ—men and women scored equally on tests of general intelligence (Maccoby & Jacklin, 1974; Matarazzo, 1972). The consensus today, therefore, is that sex differences in cognition are not related to IQ, but are tied to more fundamental and domain-specific cognitive processes. Arriving at a description of the precise functions that are sexually differentiated, understanding which events bring about the sexual differentiation, and grasping the broad theoretical context for these effects, are key issues driving sex differences research today.

Studies of causes began in the 1960s and 70s from a strong environmentalist perspective—it was tacitly assumed that all sex differences in human cognition or behavior must be based on learning derived from the psychosocial or cultural environment. We now recognize that this is an over-simplified view, one that neglects the role of our evolved heritage. One of the most fascinating trends to emerge in the past 25 years is the increasing recognition that endocrine factors might contribute to certain cognitive differences, particularly those differences that equip males and females for their respective roles in reproduction. Recent studies have changed our thinking about cognitive differences in fundamental ways. They have suggested, for instance, that interactionist models of cognitive sex differences are more viable than strict environmental models which attribute sex differences solely to culture, experience, or domain-general learning. They suggest that at least some cognitive sex differences are not static quantities but dynamic entities that can change in magnitude with the reproductive state of individuals. In some cases, cognitive sex differences can disappear altogether when the 'right' endocrine conditions are met.

WHAT IS A SEX DIFFERENCE?

At the simplest level, sex differences in cognition are statistical differences between the two biological sexes. As a group, either men or women reliably achieve a higher average score on a particular test, or there are other differences in the frequency distribution at the population level. For example, it is not unusual for the variance in the scores to be higher in males than in females, a phenomenon that can lead to overrepresentation of males among those individuals obtaining the highest and the lowest scores on a test. Differences are visible in *group* averages; individual men or women do not predictably achieve a higher score than a random member of the other sex.

It is essential to understand that on most cognitive tests, sex is only one of a large number of factors that contribute to performance. Therefore, if we wanted to accurately predict an *individual's* score on a cognitive test we need to go beyond sex: we would need to take into consideration factors like general intelligence, experience with this or similar functions in the life history of the individual, metabolic factors, motivational variables, and many other variables. Sex typically accounts for less than 15% of the variance on its own. Therefore, there is a wide range of variability *within* each sex, and biological sex is a modulator but is not a determinant of cognitive performance.

ACTIVATIONAL EFFECTS OF OVARIAN STEROIDS ON SPATIAL PERCEPTION AND VISUALIZATION

In the 1980s, studies began to suggest that reproductive hormones might influence spatial processes through activational effects in the CNS. This implies the changes in spatial perception are reversible and dependent on the short-term hormone environment. The main hormone implicated has been estradiol. To date, most studies have not found significant correlations with progesterone, the other major steroid secreted by the ovaries. This could mean that progesterone is not important for spatial cognition, but it could also signify that the proper spatial functions have not been investigated yet. Sex steroids might also be important in spatial cognition in men, and we will address this possibility later in the chapter.

Much of the available data on estradiol comes from studies of the menstrual cycle (MC). This evidence has been supported by studies of oral contraceptive use, and even transsexual men being treated with estrogens for sex re-assignment. The ideal method to investigate the effects of estradiol on cognition would be a true experiment in which participants were randomly assigned to treatment groups, estradiol concentrations were systematically manipulated, and the outcomes at different dosage levels were observed. However, except under rare circumstances, disrupting reproductive hormones in humans is not ethically permitted. Hormones may only be purposively administered or suppressed as part of standard medical treatments. This constrains the research designs that are possible in human studies.

When they were first reported, the possibility of activational effects of estrogens on high-level components of cognition was surprising at multiple levels including the mechanistic one, because it was believed that estrogen receptors did not exist outside the hypothalamic-pituitary axis. However, effects in limbic and cortical brain areas make sense when you consider that hormones evolved to influence the CNS in ways that promote reproductive success. This might include sharpening the salience of sex-related cues when it's beneficial to attend to them (e.g., Penton-Voak et al, 1999) or down-regulating behaviors that could potentially interfere with optimal reproductive success. One important outcome of studies to date is the realization that the effects of estrogens on perception and cognition are not unidirectional. It is possible to see either positive or negative effects of increased estrogen levels depending on the exact spatial function being investigated.

In the 1980s, the first studies suggested that high levels of estradiol, such as those at the preovulatory or midluteal stages of the menstrual cycle, were associated with modest decreases in accuracy on tests of spatial perception. Performance was found to improve during menses when estradiol levels are decreased. Some of the earliest data came from our lab: we found that accuracy varied on a simple test of spatial perception (Fig. 16.1a), where a bar was presented at various orientations and had to be set to the true vertical on each trial. Women's estimates were the most accurate at menses, when estradiol is lowest, and showed increased error during high estrogen stages of the cycle (e.g., Fig. 16.1b; Hampson & Kimura, 1988). This was of interest because previous studies had revealed a sex difference in accuracy on the task, on the order of 2 or 3 degrees. Our data suggested that hormones could be involved in generating the sex difference.

Changes across the MC were subsequently reported on other tests of spatial perception, including rather exotic ones like judgments of symmetry (Oinonen, 2003). McCourt et al. (1997), for example, found that the perceived location of the visual midline varied over the MC on a spatial bisection task. Horizontal displacement error was greatest during the luteal phase, when estradiol and progesterone are elevated. Akar et al. (2005), using short-wavelength automated perimetry, found a small reduction in sensitivity to visual targets situated in the left hemifield when women were tested during the luteal phase of the cycle. Sex differences in the response of primary visual cortex to red or blue light have been reported (e.g., Cowan et al., 2000). It is important to appreciate that while accuracy did vary, the scores in these studies were always in the normal not clinical range. Nevertheless, the fact that performance changed over the MC suggested that something might be happening at very basic levels of visual perception.

Around 1990, it was discovered that the MC effect could also be identified on tests of spatial *visualization*. These are tests where accurate performance depends on the ability to form a mental representation of the movements of objects or their component parts. Stimuli are often presented in the form of diagrams or

A

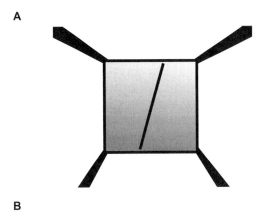

B

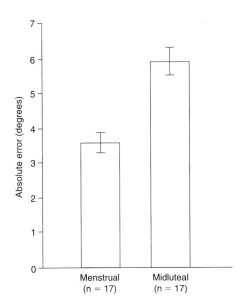

Figure 16.1. (A) A view inside the Rod and Frame apparatus. On a typical trial, both the rod and the surrounding frame are tilted, but to differing degrees, relative to the true upright. The rod is to be set to true vertical on each trial. (B) Women showed greater displacement error when tested during the luteal phase of the menstrual cycle (Hampson and Kimura, 1988).

on a computer screen. Figure 16.2a shows a sample item from one test widely used by psychologists to assess spatial visualization in the laboratory. Each item requires the subject to decide what a target figure would look like when seen from other vantage points. Psychometric studies have confirmed that spatial visualization is a related but separable ability from the types of spatial perception described above (Voyer

et al., 1995). In the example in Figure 16.2, we say the test requires 'mental rotation' because, in order to arrive at the correct answer, you must visualize a rotation of the object in your mind. Earlier studies that presented stimuli in pairs, where subjects were asked to judge whether the two figures were the same or different, found the response times varied in direct proportion to the angle of rotation (Shepard & Metzler, 1971, Fig. 16.2b) so that response times were longer to pairs of stimuli where the figure had to travel through a longer trajectory. This was taken as evidence that people engage in some type of analog rotation process when performing the task.

In 1990, we described a MC effect on a spatial visualization task in which objects shown as flat patterns had to be mentally "folded" into three-dimensional objects (Hampson, 1990a). The preovulatory peak in estradiol was associated with reduced scores on the visualization test, but not on several control tasks that tapped other cognitive functions. In favor of estradiol being the hormone driving the effect, there was a significant correlation between serum estradiol and the visualization scores, accounting for 18% of the variance. There was no correlation with other candidate hormones, including serum LH, FSH, or progesterone. We found a decline in spatial scores only when estradiol reached very high levels, consistent with the preovulatory peak. This suggested to us that any effect on visualization might only occur at the highest estrogen stages of the cycle.

In the last 10 years, the MC effect has been replicated by other labs on the same test (e.g., Phillips & Silverman, 1997) and on other visualization tests. Most studies have focused on the midluteal phase to study the effects of high estradiol, because the preovulatory peak is difficult to target accurately (see Chapter 4). Because mental rotation tests elicit a large sex difference and so hypothetically might have greater scope for revealing a hormonal effect, many studies have employed tests of mental rotation. Better performance at menses on the test in Figure 2a or on equivalent mental rotation tests, and a decline in scores during the middle of the luteal phase has been demonstrated in about a dozen studies (e.g., Hausmann et al., 2000; Maki et al., 2002; McCormick & Teillon, 2001; Moody, 1997; Phillips & Silverman, 1997; Saucier & Kimura, 1998; Silverman & Phillips, 1993; but for an exception see Epting & Overman, 1998).

Mental rotation is of additional relevance because it has been implicated as a fundamental process in

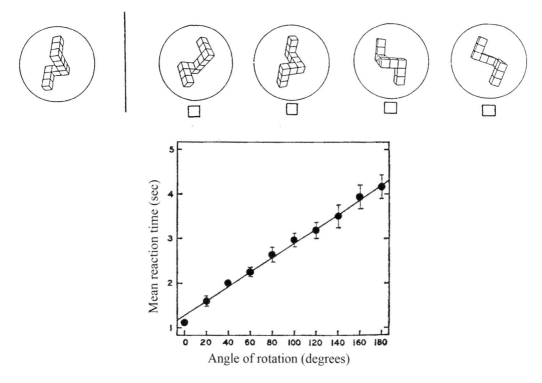

Figure 16.2. (A) A sample item from the Vandenberg and Kuse (1978) mental rotations test. The task is to identify which of the figures on the right are rotated versions of the target figure shown on the left. (B). Studies have shown a correlation between reaction times on mental rotation tests and the angular disparity between the two figures that must be compared. Data are adapted from Shepard and Metzler (1971).

both object identification and in spatial navigation in external environments. As one example, Silverman et al. (2000) found that mental rotation was a good predictor of the ability to maintain orientation in a wooded terrain. Mental rotation scores, but not general intelligence or a Piagetian water-level test, predicted the ability to maintain correct orientation and to find the most direct route out of the woods after being led along a circuitous series of twists and turns.

Studies by Hausmann et al. (2000) and Maki et al. (2002) exemplify recent work using tests of mental rotation to study the MC effect. Both labs found more accurate rotations during the menstrual phase and reduced accuracy during the luteal phase. Both used within-subjects designs. Both studies also demonstrated a substantial negative correlation with serum estradiol (Hausmann: partial correlations of −0.48 and −0.70 for the two test sessions, respectively; Maki et al: $r = -0.51$), but no significant correlation between mental rotation scores and progesterone. Because women were tested during menses and during the luteal phase (when

progesterone is normally secreted at high concentrations), the range in progesterone levels was maximized in these studies. Still, no correlation between spatial scores and progesterone was found. Maki did find *positive* correlations between circulating estradiol and scores on verbal fluency tests, a pattern opposite to that seen for spatial visualization. This speaks to the selectivity of the effects. The spatial effect does not automatically generalize to other domains of cognitive functioning. If the association between visualization and phase of the MC is really due to an effect of estradiol, similar effects ought to be found in women taking oral contraceptives (OCs).

Oral contraceptives provide ethinyl estradiol plus a synthetic progestin, while suppressing the body's endogenous production of ovarian steroids. Several studies have, in fact, found an effect of OC use on spatial visualization, using tests of mental rotation or other measures (e.g., Silverman and Phillips, 1993; Hampson & Szekeley, unpublished observations). In our own work, we found improvement in mental rotation during weeks when women were off their contraceptives and a mild decrease in visualization scores when the contraceptives were resumed. However, the relationships have not been replicated in all studies (e.g., Hampson, 1990b; McCormick & Teillon, 2001). The effect in contraceptive users appears to be weaker than in naturally cycling women. This might reflect the low levels of ethinyl estradiol contained in contemporary OCs. The concentrations may not be sufficient to generate a full-fledged MC effect.

Besides their use in contraception, OCs can be used, in combination with anti-androgens, to stimulate the development of female secondary sex characteristics in men who desire a gender change. Spatial visualization has been studied, as have several other cognitive functions, before and after treatment with cross-sex hormones in male-to-female transsexuals. While there are reports of diminished spatial scores after 3 months of treatment with estradiol (Van Goozen et al., 1995), here too, the results have proved less reliable than in studies of the MC (Haraldsen et al., 2005; Slabbekoorn et al., 1999). It is possible that the effects are weak or that insensitive tests have been used to assess visualization, or that the brain areas underlying spatial functions, once organized by androgens, are resistant to the effects of estrogens on performance.

ACTIVATIONAL EFFECTS OF OVARIAN HORMONES ON SPATIAL MEMORY

The literature we've just reviewed has grown up simultaneously with an entirely different body of literature devoted to memory, and how various forms of memory might be influenced by hormones. Though object positions or configurations are among the things we need to remember or keep track of in everyday life, the ability to remember spatial information has taken a backseat relative to studies focusing on verbal stimuli.

Spatial memory involves the encoding, storage, and retrieval of information about spatial layouts. Like spatial abilities in general, there are multiple varieties of spatial memory controlled by different brain systems. Not all forms of spatial memory are sexually differentiated. Of those that are, men show a selective advantage for fine-grained metric positional reconstruction, where absolute spatial coordinates are emphasized (Postma et al., 1999). Importantly, there are also components of spatial memory where females

show a performance advantage. These include the ability to accurately remember *relative* object positions (the whereabouts of objects in relation to other nearby objects without regard to metric distances) (Silverman & Eals, 1992; James & Kimura, 1997) and, tentatively, a female advantage in spatial working memory (Duff & Hampson, 2001).

Many studies have investigated memory in postmenopausal women treated with hormone replacement therapy (HRT). Some studies have suggested positive effects of HRT on episodic memory, the form of memory involved in our day-to-day recall of events. Little can be said about *spatial* memory on the basis of these studies because suitable memory tests have seldom been included. So far, effects have been found almost entirely on tests emphasizing the recall of verbal material, such as word lists or stories. Because there are differences in how the brain encodes verbal and spatial stimuli, it is risky to generalize to the spatial context in the absence of empirical data.

Estradiol is only one of several estrogens that are present in standard HRT. Therefore, another problem is the inability to attribute the effects to estradiol per se. However, it is likely that estradiol is, in fact, the operative hormone because animal studies have shown that estradiol has trophic effects in the hippocampus (Woolley & McEwen, 1992) and basal forebrain, structures important in episodic memory in humans and other primates. In favor of estradiol being the active constituent of HRT, a few small-scale clinical trials have used standardized clinical tests to evaluate episodic memory in young surgically menopausal women treated with estradiol following oophorectomy (Phillips & Sherwin, 1992; Sherwin, 1988). Small but significant effects on episodic memory, particularly memory for verbal stimuli, were found.

To summarize the current state of the literature, either positive or no effects of HRT on episodic memory have been observed in aging women (for reviews, see Hogervorst et al., 2000; LeBlanc et al., 2001). Observational studies have been criticized because the women electing to use HRT could be healthier, better educated, or more health-conscious (the "healthy user bias") conferring a memory advantage independent of HRT use. Although data pertaining directly to spatial memory are lacking, physiologically we would expect spatial memory tests that depend heavily on the integrity of the hippocampus to be favorably influenced by estrogen, based on the animal data cited above (*c.f.*, Resnick et al., 1998).

A positive effect of estradiol on episodic memory is different from the findings for spatial perception and visualization. However, episodic memory depends on other neural systems, and an important lesson we have learned is that estradiol's effects on elements of cognition are not unidimensional. A hormone can have either positive, negative, or no effects on performance depending on the exact information processing demands intrinsic to a task and, consequently, on which neural systems are recruited.

Another form of memory important in humans and other primates is working memory. A form of short-term memory, working memory is invoked when you actively "hold" information in mind over short intervals. This form of memory shows significant decline with aging. Figure 16.3a shows a spatial working memory task (the SPWM) that we've devised in our research and on which we've found positive effects of estrogens. It is modeled after a test used in studies of non-human primates (Passingham, 1985). In the monkey work, animals searched for peanuts hidden behind each of a set of 25 hinged doors. The object was to retrieve each peanut without missing any or going back to already searched locations, which were considered working memory (WM) errors. Passingham found that lesions of prefrontal cortex (PFC) greatly impaired performance on the task. This is in agreement with lesion studies and imaging studies in humans which also show that the PFC, especially the dorsolateral PFC, is intimately involved in WM and especially in *spatial* working memory (Owen et al., 1990; McCarthy et al., 1994).

In our task, people have to find, not peanuts, but pairs of colored dots hidden behind the hinged doors. They do this by opening two doors at a time, until they've found all 10 matching pairs. A WM error is committed whenever they go back to previously searched locations (for details see Duff and Hampson, 2000). The SPWM task is interesting because it shows a robust sex difference in favor of women, despite being a spatial task. In three separate experiments (Duff & Hampson, 2001), we found that women consistently made fewer WM errors than men, and the effect size ($d = 0.6-0.8$) was moderate to large by Cohen's criteria (Cohen, 1988). It is unusual to see a sex difference that favors women on a spatial task, though sex differences in favor of men have been documented on many tests of spatial perception and especially, on tests of spatial visualization (Voyer et al., 1995). Our work suggests the sex difference may reflect the WM demands inherent in the SPWM. In favor of this interpretation, we also found a female advantage on a parallel verbal WM task (Duff & Hampson, 2001). Therefore, in contrast to spatial perception or visualization, the sex difference on the SPWM is in the opposite direction. Preliminary evidence suggests the role of estrogens on the SPWM might also be the opposite, i.e., increases in estrogens might have a *facilitative* effect on performance.

One piece of evidence comes from postmenopausal women using hormone replacement therapy (Duff & Hampson, 2000). We tested three groups of healthy postmenopausal women, about 100 women in all, on a short form of the SPWM (as well as a set of other cognitive tests). The number of WM errors was recorded. All the women were postmenopausal and were either on estrogens only, estrogens plus a progestin, or not on hormone replacement at the time they were tested. Though the groups were matched in SES, education, and a great range of other variables, the women in the treatment groups, who were receiving estrogens, made significantly fewer WM errors than women who were not on replacement therapy (Figure 16.3b).

Women in the non-HRT group committed almost 40% more errors than women in the E + P group, suggesting the effect on WM is potentially quite large. In favor of the possibility that it is the WM element of the task that is driving this pattern, we found a similar effect on a verbal WM task, digit ordering, a task that has been shown in PET imaging studies to substantially activate the PFC (Petrides et al., 1993). Physiological work has suggested the PFC might be a significant site of estrogen activity in the primate brain (reviewed in Duff & Hampson, 2000), providing potential insight into how HRT could accomplish its effect on spatial working memory.

Recent studies of postmenopausal women treated with estrogens (Keenan et al., 2001; Krug et al., 2006), studies of the menstrual cycle (Rosenberg & Park, 2002; Hampson & Moffat, 2004), and work in other primates using the delayed response task (Rapp et al., 2003) support the possibility of a positive effect of estradiol on the PFC and spatial working memory. However, these studies must be regarded as preliminary only because of the small sample sizes in most of the studies or other methodological limitations. Confirmatory work is needed. At the anatomical level, Shaywitz et al. (1999), in a fMRI study, observed changes in activation in the frontal cortex during a working memory task when women were treated

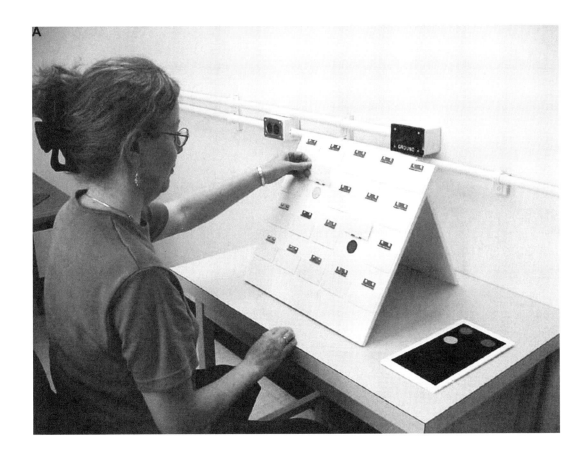

B

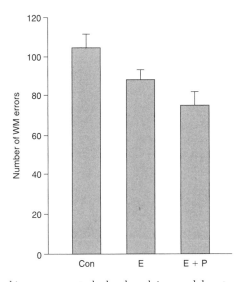

Figure 16.3. (A) A spatial working memory task developed in our laboratory (for details, see Duff and Hampson, 2001). (B) Postmenopausal women who were taking either estrogens alone (E; n = 38) or estrogens combined with a progestin (E + P; n = 23) made significantly fewer working memory errors on the SPWM than control women who were not on hormone replacement therapy (Con, n = 35) (Duff and Hampson, 2000).

with conjugated equine estrogens versus placebo in a double-blind cross-over trial. Unfortunately, the cognitive task did not have the scope to detect any estrogen-related changes in accuracy.

As a whole, this body of work has shown that estrogen's effects on spatial cognition are not unidirectional. On some tests of spatial memory, even though positional information about objects is involved (defining the task as spatial), effects of estrogens seem to be *positive*. The direction depends on the latent information processing requirements of a task, not necessarily on its surface features.

SEX DIFFERENCES IN NAVIGATIONAL STRATEGIES AND EFFICIENCY

Mental rotation may be a basic adaptation to promote effective navigation or way-finding by allowing us, for example, to recognize objects and scenes from different vantage points. A correlation exists between the accuracy of performance on mental rotation tests and the accuracy of way-finding in natural settings (e.g., Silverman et al., 2000; Saucier et al., 2002) or in virtual environments (Moffat et al., 1998; Astur et al., 2004; Driscoll et al., 2005). Navigation on the human scale is hard to study in a controlled laboratory setting, but recent studies have been able to simulate movement in large-scale space using computer technology. For example, people can be studied while they learn a complex route through a computer-generated virtual environment.

Advanced computer techniques have greatly facilitated the study of navigation-related spatial abilities. Sex differences have been observed in spatial learning: males are quicker than females to learn the layout of a novel virtual environment (Moffat et al., 1998) and show more rapid place learning (Astur et al., 1998). Male and female rats have been shown to use different classes of visual cues to navigate in the radial arm maze (Williams et al., 1990). In humans, too, females exhibit a greater reliance than males on landmark cues (as opposed to the geometry of the environment) to assist in way-finding (e.g., Choi & Silverman, 1996; Sandstrom et al., 1998).

Virtual environments can be combined with fMRI or PET imaging to study the patterns of brain activation evoked during navigation, providing new insights into the network of neural structures that underlies spatial processing. Grön et al. (2000) found different patterns of brain activation in men and women while they navigated a complex, three-dimensional, virtual maze. Whether the sex differences in brain activity reflect the processing of different classes of visual cues in males and females has not been determined.

A remarkable finding from animal studies is the suggestion that male and female reliance on different visual cues may be caused by differential exposure to androgens during early brain development (Williams et al., 1990). If male rats were castrated neonatally or if female rats were treated with estradiol, then as adults they showed a sex reversal relative to same-sex control rats in their preferences for different types of cues when tested in the radial arm maze. This suggests that hormones organize the developing brain to change the salience of, or the responsiveness to, different sorts of visual cues pertinent to navigation. No counterpart to this finding has been demonstrated in humans. But several human studies have raised the possibility of regulation by *adult* hormones. For example, Driscoll et al. (2005) found the concentration of testosterone was correlated with a measure of competence in a virtual maze in men, but not in women. However, Bell and Saucier (2004) found that men with higher testosterone were *less* accurate than men with low testosterone on measures of path integration and piloting in a natural setting.

ORGANIZATIONAL EFFECTS OF STEROIDS

The past 15 years have seen increasing evidence that circulating estradiol concentrations can modulate spatial cognition. The effects fit the classic definition of activational effects in that the behavioral effects seem to be reversible and tied to the presence of active hormone in the bloodstream. Changes over the menstrual cycle are a clear example of reversibility and short-term action. One important question is whether the effects are sufficient to fully explain the sex differences that are observed on many spatial tasks. Unfortunately many of the studies were designed to study endocrine regulation of visuospatial functions, not sex differences. Therefore, men have not always been included. There have been several reports where no significant sex differences were found on spatial tasks when men were explicitly compared with women tested at menses, when ovarian hormones are lowest (e.g., McCormick & Teillon, 2001; Chabanne et al., 2004).

However, we still lack a clear answer to the question of whether there is a residual sex difference once the ovarian cycle is controlled.

A related issue is whether organizational effects of steroids act during early development on the brain systems that control spatial processes. Fetal androgens produced by the developing testes could modify spatial systems in the male brain, for example. Several studies of girls with congenital adrenal hyperplasia (CAH), a condition characterized by excess production of androgens by the fetal adrenal glands, have shown that females with CAH outperformed control females, who were not exposed to excess androgens, on tests of spatial visualization (Resnick et al., 1986; Hampson et al., 1998).

In another study, where androgen levels were measured from specimens of amniotic fluid taken during mid-gestation, the proficiency of healthy normally developing girls on a test of mental rotation was positively correlated with the concentration of testosterone in their amniotic fluid, when they were behaviorally tested at age 7 (Grimshaw et al., 1995). These studies suggest an organizational influence of early androgen exposure. But the data in support of this possibility are not as consistent or as compelling as one would like (c.f., Helleday et al., 1994; Hines et al., 2003).

Several studies have found paradoxical *decreases* in performance on spatial tests in males exposed to higher levels of androgens prenatally (Hampson et al., 1998; Hines et al., 2003; Berenbaum et al., 2006), which is a less tidy fit with the organizational hypothesis. Furthermore, in girls with CAH, childhood and adolescent behaviors, hobbies, and activities are masculinized in several respects (Berenbaum, 1999), leaving open the possibility that differences in spatial aptitude could arise from male-typed gender experiences, not from direct organizational effects of androgens in brain areas that subserve spatial processes. Such considerations make the question of organizational effects a complicated issue.

It is also possible, in theory, that androgens could have an on-line regulatory influence on spatial systems in the adult male brain, parallel to estradiol in females. In men, the average testosterone concentration differs considerably from one person to the next, so that the range considered "normal" is fairly wide. Several menstrual cycle studies have suggested that testosterone is not inert, in that women's scores on visualization tasks were positively correlated with circulating testosterone, but negatively correlated with circulating estradiol concentrations (e.g., Hausmann et al., 2000). It is conceivable, then, that testosterone could exert activational effects in the male brain.

In some studies of healthy young volunteers, individual differences in the level of circulating testosterone have been found to correlate with scores on spatial tasks. Testosterone concentrations predicted visualization scores in young men and women (Moffat & Hampson, 1996; Neave et al., 1999; Silverman et al., 1999) and in elderly men (Moffat et al., 2002). Administering androgens to female-to-male transsexuals has been reported to improve their spatial abilities (Van Goozen et al., 1995; Slabbekoorn et al., 1999; but c.f., Haraldsen et al., 2005), though it is unclear whether or not this represents an activational effect.

In older men experiencing age-related decline in testosterone, treatment with testosterone has been reported to improve spatial cognition and, potentially, some aspects of memory (Janowsky et al., 1994; Cherrier et al., 2001). Likewise, androgen deprivation, a treatment used to slow tumor growth in men with prostate cancer, was said in a recent report to impair performance on a mental rotation test (Cherrier et al., 2003). A dose of testosterone administered orally temporarily improved performance on a mental rotation test in young women (Aleman et al., 2004) relative to placebo, but in men, a single injection of testosterone enanthate did not produce a discernible effect on a spatial rotation task (Wolf et al., 2000).

While some studies therefore do suggest a regulatory influence of testosterone on spatial functioning, the evidence is too scant to be conclusive and there are plenty of inconsistent findings.

BRAIN IMAGING

Studying the mechanisms at the molecular level that underlie effects on cognition is not possible in humans in vivo. What can be done is brain imaging, in order to identify brain areas that are functionally more or less active during different endocrine conditions. One example is the Shaywitz study discussed earlier (Shaywitz et al., 1999), where women underwent fMRI to study the effects of conjugated equine estrogens on brain activation patterns during a memory task. Studies like this are infrequent. This is partly because the view that short-term changes in hormones can perceptibly alter cognition is still new and novel. It also reflects the practicalities and technical difficulties of putting such studies into effect.

One of the first to try to visualize brain-related changes that might underlie the MC effect on mental rotation was Dietrich et al. (2001). Testing the same group of women two times, at menses and during the preovulatory rise in estradiol, visible changes in activation were identified during a mental rotation task. Discrete activation in Brodmann's area 7, the superior parietal cortex, was found in men or in women who were tested at menses, whereas high estradiol was associated with large increases in the numbers of activated voxels and extension into area 39/37 of Brodmann.

AN EVOLUTIONARY HYPOTHESIS

Sex differences in spatial perception and visualization have been recognized for decades. Sex differences in spatial behaviors, especially in spatial navigation, are also found in many other species, in the wild and in animals raised in captivity where experiential variables can be controlled. Differences in other species suggest an evolved origin, as does the modulation of the sex differences by reproductive hormones. It is not out of the question that sex differences in humans could arise through acquired experience, though to the extent that hormonal control is displayed, this seems less likely. An important concept is that different spatial competencies are dissociable entities that, in addition to having separate neurological substrates, may derive from different selection pressures in the ancestral environment. Contemporary evolutionary theories recognize this specificity. For example, the female advantage in remembering the relative positions of static objects within a complex visual scene composed of many different objects has been hypothesized to be linked to foraging pressures (Silverman & Eals, 1992).

Because it is so prominent in many species, special attention has been devoted to the sex difference in navigation. Evolutionary theories propose that differential space use on the part of males and females of a given species, related to the sexual division of labor or to the roles of the two sexes in reproduction, drives the emergence of a sex difference in navigation-related skills. To understand the sex difference, we must identify the source of the selection pressure.

Gaulin and FitzGerald (1986), for example, drew attention to the importance of mating systems as one variable that can influence ranging patterns, and hence spatial abilities. They hypothesized that sex differences in abilities related to navigation will evolve under mating systems that select for sexually dimorphic ranging patterns. Spatial abilities will be enhanced in the sex that does the most ranging. To test their hypothesis, Gaulin and FitzGerald (1986) studied two species of voles ("tundra mice") of the genus *Microtus*, whose phylogenetic history is similar but whose mating systems differed dramatically. In laboratory maze tests, a sex difference in spatial capabilities was present in meadow voles (*M. pennsylvanicus*), a polygynous species where males but not females compete for mates by ranging widely during the breeding season, but not in pine voles (*M. pinetorum*), a closely related species of vole that forms monogamous pair bonds and where both sexes maintain small home ranges that do not differ in size (Gaulin & FitzGerald, 1986). This supports the view that the sex difference in navigational prowess is an adaptation that arises through sexual selection driven by the need for males to travel over greater distances in search of mates.

The theory predicts a reversal of the sex difference in species where females not males are the more widely ranging sex. This occurs in some seahorses and pipefishes (*Syngnathidae*), for instance. As yet, no one has figured out how to test navigational abilities in these species. In humans, various theories have been put forth to explain why some (but not all) spatial functions are amplified in men, relative to women. None of these theories is terribly satisfactory (for a review and critique see Sherry & Hampson, 1997).

In particular, the theories assume a static male advantage, not one that waxes and wanes depending upon women's reproductive status. This sort of dynamic endocrine regulation was not anticipated. One way that the studies reviewed in this chapter have changed our concept of sex differences is by forcing us to turn the tables and ask how dynamic endocrine regulation by ovarian steroids in women might be adaptive. A key fact is that ranging over long distances, though adaptive in many respects, is energetically costly. In contrast to males, where the benefits might outweigh the costs, ranging is *dis*advantageous for reproductive females. Energy balance is critical in female reproduction: a certain percentage of body fat is needed to maintain menstrual cyclicity and ovulatory competence, or even moreso to sustain a viable pregnancy and provide the estimated 16 kg of stored reserves needed for optimal lactation (Frisch & McArthur, 1974). Ranging over long distances jeopardizes optimal reproductive potential and the health of offspring by, among other things, directly competing for precious caloric resources.

High estradiol might serve as a signal for actual or imminent reproductive investment on the part of women, which triggers a set of motivational and behavioral changes that optimize the potential for reproductive success. Down-regulation of the probability of activities (such as long distance ranging) that could pose a threat to successful outcomes might be part of the adaptations that come into play. If down-regulation of navigation-related spatial abilities does occur to reduce the probability of competing energy expenditure, it would be especially important during the highest estrogen conditions of pregnancy. However, estradiol is high during a good part of the menstrual cycle and here, too, energy balance is a nontrivial consideration. In non-pregnant conditions, maintaining threshold body fat is essential to sustain ovulatory competence. About half the cycle is characterized by high estrogen, notably the luteal phase, where there is already an increase in the basal metabolic rate caused by the thermogenic actions of progesterone (Chapter 4). Reduced ranging during critical parts of the menstrual cycle could promote reproductive success, also, through a variety of short-term mechanisms such as optimal availability for mating during fertile periods (near ovulation), or preservation of the implanted embryo (luteal phase).

For a fuller description of Fertility and Parental Care Theory see Sherry and Hampson (1997) and Hampson (2000).

CONCLUSION

The sex difference field today is a vibrant area of research in many areas of medicine and the behavioral sciences. Cognitive sex differences, once considered scientific curiosities only, are still being discovered. Far from being on the fringes of scientific endeavor, many of the sex differences are providing exciting new insights into the brain, into evolutionary theory, and into the functional architecture of the human mind.

This chapter illustrates that spatial abilities have been a fruitful area of study. We don't know if other cognitive sex differences arise the same way, but this body of work can serve as a model for future investigations in other cognitive domains. It must be kept in mind that not all cognitive differences are necessarily

alike. There might well be differences that are exclusively due to the culture-specific environment or upbringing of males and females, i.e., that are learned. This is most likely for differences that have no counterpart in other species, e.g., mathematics.

The evidence presented in this chapter does not rule out some role for experiential variables, but it does suggest that the influence of learning is smaller than anticipated, at least for many spatial sex differences. Researchers often speak as though biology and environment work in an either-or fashion. It is worthwhile to consider the complexities of how the two classes of mechanisms can interact. Experiential factors could, in principle, amplify (or diminish) differences between the sexes, even differences laid down by the endocrine system.

Interactions with the environment are especially important when interpreting the organizational effects of sex steroids. One challenge for future studies will be to clarify whether, for spatial abilities, there is any organizational effect of exposure to sex steroids during early brain development—and if so, to sort out whether the effects are mediated via *direct* actions of hormones on neural systems subserving spatial processes, or are mediated *indirectly* by changing the likelihood that the two sexes will seek out or acquire significant experience with critical activities that form the experiential predecessors of adult spatial abilities.

References

Akar Y, Zulauf M, Yucel I, Akar ME, Erdem U, Trak B. (2005). Menstrual cycle-dependent differences between right and left visual hemifields in perimetry. *Curr Eye Res*, 30:723–727.

Aleman A, Bronk E, Kessels RPC, Koppeschaar HPF, van Honk J. (2004). A single administration of testosterone improves visuospatial ability in young women. *Psychoneuroendocrinology*, 29:612–617.

Astur RS, Ortiz ML, Sutherland RJ. (1998). A characterization of performance by men and women in a virtual Morris water task: A large and reliable sex difference. *Behav Brain Res*, 93:185–190.

Astur RS, Tropp J, Sava S, Constable RT, Markus EJ. (2004). Sex differences and correlations in a virtual Morris water task, a virtual radial arm maze, and mental rotation. *Behav Brain Res*, 151:103–115.

Bell S, Saucier D. (2004). Relationship among environmental pointing accuracy, mental rotation, sex, and hormones. *Environ Behav*, 36:251–265.

Berenbaum SA. (1999). Effects of early androgens on sex-typed activities and interests in adolescents with congenital adrenal hyperplasia. *Horm Behav*, 35:102–110.

Berenbaum SA, Fesi B, Bryk K. (2006). Early androgen effects on spatial and mechanical abilities: Evidence from congenital adrenal hyperplasia. Society for Behavioral Neuroendocrinology Annual Meeting. Pittsburgh, PA.

Breedlove SM, Hampson E. (2002). Sexual differentiation of the brain and behavior. In Becker JB, Breedlove SM, Crews D, McCarthy MM, (Eds.), *Behavioral endocrinology* (pp.75–114). Cambridge, MA: MIT Press.

Chabanne V, Péruch P, Thinus-Blanc C. (2004). Sex differences and women's hormonal cycle effects on spatial performance in a virtual environment navigation task. *Curr Psychol Cogn*, 22:351–375.

Cherrier MM, Asthana S, Plymate S, Baker L, Matsumoto AM, Peskind, E, et al. (2001). Testosterone supplementation improves spatial and verbal memory in healthy older men. *Neurology*, 57:80–88.

Cherrier MM, Rose AL, Higano C. (2003). The effects of combined androgen blockade on cognitive function during the first cycle of intermittent androgen suppression in patients with prostate cancer. *J Urol*, 170:1808–1811.

Choi J, Silverman I. (1996). Sexual dimorphism in spatial behaviors: Applications to route learning. *Evol Cogn*, 2:165–171.

Cohen J. (1988). Statistical power analysis for the behavioral sciences (2nd ed). Hillsdale, NJ: Lawrence Erlbaum.

Cowan RL, Frederick BB, Rainey M, Levin JM, Maas LC, Bang J, et al. (2000). Sex differences in response to red and blue light in human primary visual cortex: A BOLD fMRI study. *Psychiatry Res: Neuroimaging*, 100:129–138.

Dietrich T, Krings T, Neulen J, Willmes K, Erberich S, Thron A, Sturm W. (2001). Effects of blood estrogen level on cortical activation patterns during cognitive activation as measured by functional MRI. *NeuroImage*, 13:425–432.

Driscoll I, Hamilton DA, Yeo RA, Brooks WM, Sutherland RJ. (2005). Virtual navigation in humans: The impact of age, sex, and hormones on place learning. *Horm Behav*, 47:326–335.

Duff SJ, Hampson E. (2000). A beneficial effect of estrogen on working memory in postmenopausal women taking hormone replacement therapy. *Horm Behav*, 38:262–276.

Duff SJ, Hampson E. (2001). A sex difference on a novel spatial working memory task in humans. *Brain Cogn*, 47:470–493.

Epting LK, Overman WH. (1998). Sex-sensitive tasks in men and women: A search for performance fluctuations across the menstrual cycle. *Behav Neurosci*, 112:1304–1317.

Frisch RE, McArthur JW. (1974). Menstrual cycles: Fatness as a determinant of minimum weight for height necessary for their maintenance or onset. *Science*, 185:949–951.

Gaulin SJC, FitzGerald RW. (1986). Sex differences in spatial ability: An evolutionary hypothesis and test. *Am Nat*, 127:74–88.

Grimshaw GM, Sitarenios G, Finegan JK. (1995). Mental rotation at 7 years: Relations with prenatal testosterone levels and spatial play experiences. *Brain Cogn*, 29:85–100.

Grön G, Wunderlich AP, Spitzer M, Tomczak R, Riepe MW. (2000). Brain activation during human navigation: Gender-different neural networks as substrate of performance. *Nature Neurosci*, 3:404–408.

Hampson E. (1990a). Estrogen-related variations in human spatial and articulatory-motor skills. *Psychoneuroendocrinology*, 15:97–111.

Hampson E. (1990b). Influence of gonadal hormones on cognitive function in women. *Clin Neuropharmacol*, 13(Suppl 2):522–523.

Hampson E. (2000). Sexual differentiation of spatial functions in humans. In Matsumoto A (Ed.), *Sexual differentiation of the brain* (pp. 279–300). London: CRC Press.

Hampson E, Kimura D. (1988). Reciprocal effects of hormonal fluctuations on human motor and perceptual-spatial skills. *Behav Neurosci*, 102:456–459.

Hampson E, Moffat SD (2004) The psychobiology of gender: Cognitive effects of reproductive hormones in the adult nervous system. In Eagly AH, Beall AE, Sternberg RJ (Eds.), *The psychology of gender* (pp. 38–64). New York: Guilford Press.

Hampson E, Rovet JF, Altmann D. (1998). Spatial reasoning in children with congenital adrenal hyperplasia due to 21-hydroxylase deficiency. *Dev Neuropsychol*, 14:299–320.

Haraldsen IR, Egeland T, Haug E, Finset A, Opjordsmoen S. (2005). Cross-sex hormone treatment does not change sex-sensitive cognitive performance in gender identity disorder patients. *Psychiatry Res*, 137:161–174.

Hausmann M, Slabbekoorn D, Van Goozen, SHM, Cohen-Kettenis, PT, Güntürkün O. (2000). Sex hormones affect spatial abilities during the menstrual cycle. *Behav Neurosci*, 114:1245–1250.

Helleday J, Bartfai A, Ritzén EM, Forman M. (1994). General intelligence and cognitive profile in women with congenital adrenal hyperplasia (CAH). *Psychoneuroendocrinology*, 19:343–356.

Hines M, Fane BA, Pasterski VL, Mathews GA, Conway GS, Brook C. (2003). Spatial abilities following prenatal androgen abnormality: Targeting and mental rotations performance in individuals with congenital adrenal hyperplasia. *Psychoneuroendocrinology*, 28:1010–1026.

Hogervorst E, Williams J, Budge M, Riedel W, Jolles J. (2000). The nature of the effect of female gonadal hormone replacement therapy on cognitive function in post-menopausal women: A meta-analysis. *Neuroscience*, 101:485–512.

James TW, Kimura D. (1997). Sex differences in remembering the locations of objects in an array: Location-shifts versus location-exchanges. *Evolution and Human Behavior*, 18:155–163.

Janowsky JS, Oviatt SK, Orwoll ES. (1994). Testosterone influences spatial cognition in older men. *Behav Neurosci*, 108:325–332.

Keenan PA, Ezzat WH, Ginsburg K, Moore GJ. (2001). Prefrontal cortex as the site of estrogen's effect on cognition. *Psychoneuroendocrinology*, 26:577–590.

Krug R, Born J, Rasch B. (2006). A three-day estrogen treatment improves prefrontal cortex-dependent cognitive function in postmenopausal women. *Psychoneuroendocrinology*, 31:965–975.

LeBlanc ES, Janowsky J, Chan BKS, Nelson HD. (2001). Hormone replacement therapy and cognition: Systematic review and meta-analysis. *JAMA*, 285:1489–1499.

Maki PM, Rich JB, Rosenbaum RS. (2002). Implicit memory varies across the menstrual cycle: Estrogen effects in young women. *Neuropsychologia*, 40:518–529.

Matarazzo JD. (1972). *Wechsler's measurement and appraisal of adult intelligence* (5th ed). Baltimore, MD: Williams & Wilkins.

Maccoby EE, Jacklin CN. (1974). *The psychology of sex differences*. Stanford, CA: Stanford University Press.

McCarthy G, Blamire AM, Puce A, Nobre AC, Bloch G, Hyder F, et al. (1994). Functional magnetic resonance imaging of human prefrontal cortex activation during a spatial working memory task. *Proc Natl Acad Sci USA*, 91:8690–8694.

McCormick CM, Teillon SM. (2001). Menstrual cycle variation in spatial ability: Relation to salivary cortisol levels. *Horm Behav*, 39:29–38.

McCourt ME, Mark VW, Radonovich KJ, Willison SK, Freeman P. (1997). The effects of gender, menstrual phase and practice on the perceived location of the midsagittal plane. *Neuropsychologia*, 35:717–724.

McEwen BS, Alves SE. (1999). Estrogen actions in the central nervous system. *Endocr Rev*, 20:279–307.

Moffat SD, Hampson E. (1996). A curvilinear relationship between testosterone and spatial cognition in humans: Possible influence of hand preference. *Psychoneuroendocrinology*, 21:323–337.

Moffat SD, Hampson E, Hatzipantelis M. (1998). Navigation in a "virtual" maze: Sex differences and correlation with psychometric measures of spatial ability in humans. *Evol Hum Behav*, 19:73–87.

Moffat SD, Zonderman AB, Metter EJ, Blackman MR, Harman SM, Resnick SM. (2002). Longitudinal assessment of serum free testosterone concentration predicts memory performance and cognitive status in elderly men. *J Clin Endocrinol Metab*, 87:5001–5007.

Moody MS. (1997). Changes in scores on the mental rotations test during the menstrual cycle. *Perc Mot Skills*, 84:955–961.

Neave N, Menaged M, Weightman DR. (1999). Sex differences in cognition: The role of testosterone and sexual orientation. *Brain Cogn*, 41:245–262.

Nichols EL. (1885). On the sensitiveness of the eye to colors of a low degree of saturation. *Am J Sci*, 30:37–41.

Oinonen KA. (2003). The effects of hormones on symmetry detection and perceptions of facial attractiveness. PhD dissertation. Lakehead University, Thunder Bay, ON.

Owen AM, Downes JJ, Sahakian BJ, Polkey CE, Robbins TW. (1990). Planning and spatial working memory following frontal lobe lesions in man. *Neuropsychologia*, 28:1021–1034.

Passingham RE. (1985). Memory of monkeys *(Macaca mulatta)* with lesions in prefrontal cortex. *Behav Neurosci*, 99:3–21.

Penton-Voak IS, Perrett DI, Castles DL, Kobayashi T, Burt DM, Murray LK, Minamisawa R. (1999), Menstrual cycle alters face preference. *Nature*. 399: 741–742.

Petrides M, Alivisatos B, Meyer E, Evans AC. (1993). Functional activation of the human frontal cortex during the performance of verbal working memory tasks. *Proc Natl Acad Sci USA*, 90:878–882.

Phillips K, Silverman I. (1997). Differences in the relationship of menstrual cycle phase to spatial performance on two- and three-dimensional tasks. *Horm Behav*, 32:167–175.

Phillips SM, Sherwin BB. (1992). Effects of estrogen on memory function in surgically menopausal women. *Psychoneuroendocrinology*, 17:485–495.

Postma A, Winkel J, Tuiten A, van Honk J. (1999). Sex differences and menstrual cycle effects in human spatial memory. *Psychoneuroendocrinology*, 24:175–192.

Rapp PR, Morrison JH, Roberts JA. (2003). Cyclic estrogen replacement improves cognitive function in aged ovariectomized rhesus monkeys. *J Neurosci*, 23:5708–5714.

Resnick SM, Berenbaum SA, Gottesman II, Bouchard Jr. TJ. (1986). Early hormonal influences on cognitive functioning in congenital adrenal hyperplasia. *Dev Psychol*, 22:191–198.

Resnick SM, Maki PM, Golski S, Kraut MA, Zonderman AB. (1998). Effects of estrogen replacement therapy on PET cerebral blood flow and neuropsychological performance. *Horm Behav*, 34:171–182.

Rosenberg L, Park S. (2002). Verbal and spatial functions across the menstrual cycle in healthy young women. *Psychoneuroendocrinology*, 27:835–841.

Sandstrom NJ, Kaufman J, Huettel SA. (1998). Males and females use different distal cues in a virtual environment navigation task. *Brain Res Cogn Brain Res*, 6:351–360.

Saucier DM, Green SM, Leason J, MacFadden A, Bell S, & Elias LJ. (2002). Are sex differences in navigation caused by sexually dimorphic strategies or by differences in the ability to use the strategies? *Behav Neurosci*, 116:403–410.

Saucier DM, Kimura D. (1998). Intrapersonal motor but not extrapersonal targeting skill is enhanced during the midluteal phase of the menstrual cycle. *Dev Neuropsychol*, 14:385–398.

Shaywitz SE, Shaywitz BA, Pugh KR, Fulbright RK, Skudlarski P, Mencl WE, et al. (1999). Effect of estrogen on brain activation patterns in postmenopausal women during working memory tasks. *JAMA*, 281:1197–1202.

Shepard RN, Metzler J. (1971). Mental rotation of three-dimensional objects. *Science*, 171:701–703.

Sherry DF, Hampson E. (1997). Evolution and the hormonal control of sexually-dimorphic spatial abilities in humans. *Trends Cogn Sci*, 1:50–56.

Sherwin BB. (1988). Estrogen and/or androgen replacement therapy and cognitive functioning in surgically menopausal women. *Psychoneuroendocrinology*, 13: 345–357.

Silverman I, Choi J, Mackewn A, Fisher M, Moro J, Olshansky E. (2000). Evolved mechanisms underlying wayfinding: Further studies on the hunter-gatherer theory of spatial sex differences. *Evol Hum Behav*, 21:201–213.

Silverman I, Eals M. (1992). Sex differences in spatial abilities: Evolutionary theory and data. In Barkow JH, Cosmides L, Tooby J, (Eds.), *The adapted mind: Evolutionary psychology and the generation of culture* (pp. 533–549). New York: Oxford University Press.

Silverman I, Kastuk D, Choi J, Phillips K. (1999). Testosterone levels and spatial ability in men. *Psychoneuroendocrinology*, 24:813–822.

Silverman I, Phillips K. (1993). Effects of estrogen changes during the menstrual cycle on spatial performance. *Ethol Sociobiol*, 14:257–270.

Slabbekoorn D, van Goozen SHM, Megens J, Gooren LJG, Cohen-Kettenis PT. (1999). Activating effects of cross-sex hormones on cognitive functioning: A study of short-term and long-term hormone effects in transsexuals. *Psychoneuroendocrinology*, 24:423–447.

van Goozen SHM, Cohen-Kettenis PT, Gooren LJG, Frijda NH, Van de Poll NE. (1995). Gender differences in behaviour: Activating effects of cross-sex hormones. *Psychoneuroendocrinology*, 20:343–363.

Voyer D, Voyer S, Bryden MP. (1995). Magnitude of sex differences in spatial abilities: A meta-analysis and consideration of critical variables. *Psychol Bull*, 117:250–270.

Williams CL, Barnett AM, Meck WH. (1990). Organizational effects of early gonadal secretions on sexual differentiation in spatial memory. *Behav Neurosci*, 104:84–97.

Wolf OT, Preut R, Hellhammer DH, Kudielka BM, Schürmeyer TH, Kirschbaum C. (2000). Testosterone and cognition in elderly men: A single testosterone injection blocks the practice effect in verbal fluency, but has no effect on spatial or verbal memory. *Biol Psychiatry*, 47:650–654.

Woolley CS, McEwen BS. (1992). Estradiol mediates fluctuation in hippocampal synapse density during the estrous cycle in the adult rat. *J Neurosci*, 12: 2549–2554.

Part III

Sex Differences in the Neurobiology of Disease

Chapter 17

Sex Differences in Infectious and Autoimmune Diseases

Sabra L. Klein

SEX DIFFERENCES IN DEATH RATES

Men typically die earlier than women, resulting in a significantly longer life expectancy for women (Kinsella & Velkoff, 2001). In Europe and North America, women outlive men by approximately 7 years; in developing countries, the gap between the sexes is smaller and in some cases reversed because of cultural factors (e.g., social status) (Kinsella & Velkoff, 2001). The prevailing hypothesis for why life-span is shorter for males than females is that males are more likely to engage in "risk-taking" behaviors (e.g., aggressive or violent acts) and to be exposed to occupational hazards (Zuk, 1990; Owens, 2002). Alternatively, males may be more susceptible to infectious diseases than females (Zuk & McKean, 1996; Klein, 2000, 2004). In species for which life-span is shorter for males than females, males exhibit higher rates of parasitism than females (Moore & Wilson, 2002).

SEX DIFFERENCES IN DISEASE SUSCEPTIBILITY

Among human and non-human animals, the prevalence (i.e., the proportion of individuals infected) and intensity (i.e., severity) of infectious diseases is higher in males than females (Zuk & McKean, 1996; Klein, 2000; Roberts et al., 2001). Males and females differ in the likelihood of exposure as well as susceptibility to pathogens. Males are more likely to engage in behaviors, such as aggression, dispersal, and grouping, that increase the likelihood of contact with parasites (Zuk & McKean, 1996; Klein, 2000). Males also often are larger than conspecific females, which may make males more obvious targets for parasitism (Moore & Wilson, 2002).

Despite differences in the likelihood of exposure, several studies illustrate that immunological differences exist between the sexes that may underlie increased infection rates in males. Females typically have higher immune responses than males (Zuk & McKean, 1996; Klein, 2000). Elevated immunity among females creates a double-edge sword, it which it is beneficial against infectious diseases, but is detrimental in terms of increased development of autoimmune diseases (Wizemann, 2001). Several field and laboratory studies link sex differences in immune function with circulating steroid hormones (Zuk & McKean, 1996; Klein, 2000; Roberts et al., 2001). Heightened susceptibility to infection is one of the leading causes of increased death rates among men as compared with women in several countries worldwide and this sex difference typically becomes apparent after puberty (Fig. 17.1) (Klein, 2000; Owens, 2002).

Accumulating evidence illustrates that males and females differ in their susceptibility to diseases. The primary goals of this chapter are to: (a) illustrate that sex differences are prevalent in response to both infectious and autoimmune diseases and are pronounced among humans as well as non-human animals; (b) propose that sex differences in infectious and autoimmune diseases are due to immunological differences between the sexes; and (c) review the possible hormonal and genetic mechanisms that may mediate sex differences in response to infectious and autoimmune diseases.

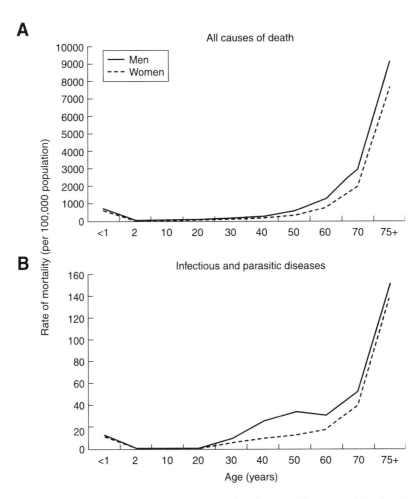

Figure 17.1. Sex differences in rates of mortality from (A) all causes of death and (B) infectious and parasitic infections in the United States for the year 2000 (WHOSIS, 2005). Age-related increases in death rates are apparent for both men and women; death rates, however, are significantly higher for men than women, with this dimorphism becoming most pronounced after puberty.

SEX DIFFERENCES
IN INFECTIOUS DISEASES

Viruses

Males and females differ in their susceptibility to a variety of viral pathogens. Because females typically mount higher immune responses than males, susceptibility to viral infections often is reduced among females. Immune responses to viruses can vary with changes in hormone concentrations caused by natural fluctuations over the menstrual or estrous cycle, contraception use, and pregnancy (Brabin, 2002). Although behavioral factors can influence exposure to viruses, several studies illustrate that physiological differences between males and females cause dimorphic responses to infection.

Sex differences are observed in response to a variety of viral agents that are transmitted sexually. Human immunodeficiency virus (HIV) replication exhibits a sexually dimorphic pattern. The amount of circulating HIV RNA in plasma is one marker of progression to acquired immunodeficiency syndrome (AIDS). HIV RNA levels are consistently lower in women than men (Farzadegan et al., 1998; Sterling et al., 2001; Napravnik et al., 2002). A meta-analysis of published studies revealed that women have approximately 41% less HIV RNA in circulation than do men, despite the fact that CD4+ T cell counts and progression to AIDS are similar between the sexes (Napravnik et al., 2002).

In women, HIV RNA levels are often below the cutoff value for initiation of antiretroviral therapy (Sterling et al., 2001). Because viral load is a factor used in the current guidelines for initiation of antiretroviral therapy, questions have been raised as to whether sex differences in HIV RNA levels may result in delayed treatment of women with HIV (Sterling et al., 2001). This observation is especially disconcerting because the number of people living with HIV/AIDS is expanding faster for women than for men worldwide, with the most noticeable gap occurring in regions experiencing an AIDS epidemic, such as sub-Saharan Africa (Quinn & Overbaugh, 2005).

Whether sex steroids affect HIV replication has not been reported. HIV infection causes hypogonadism (i.e., reduced androgen concentrations) in men, which is associated with wasting syndrome, loss of bone mass, and depression (Grinspoon, 2005). Treatment of patients with anabolic steroids improves muscle mass, bone density, and quality of life in both men and women (Grinspoon, 2005); the immunological consequence of androgen treatment, however, has not been reported.

In parallel with reduced androgen concentrations, estrone and estradiol concentrations increase with the progression of HIV (Christeff et al., 1996; Teichmann et al., 2003). Consequently, estradiol augments transcription of HIV in vitro and this effect can be reversed by exposure to the estrogen receptor (ER) antagonist ICI 182,780 suggesting that the effects of estradiol on HIV are mediated by ERα (Katagiri et al., 2006).

Herpes simplex virus-type 2 (HSV-2) is the causative agent of genital herpes infections and infection of the female reproductive tract is influenced by ovarian sex hormones, including estradiol and progesterone. Consequently, the prevalence of HSV-2 typically is higher in women than men (Wald, 2004). In female mice, susceptibility to HSV-2 varies with stage of the estrous cycle (Gallichan & Rosenthal, 1996). High concentrations of progesterone are associated with reduced survival, increased viral titers in the vagina, vaginal pathology, inflammation, infiltration of leukocytes (e.g., neutrophils), and the expression of chemokines (e.g., CCL5, CXCL2, and CXCL10) and chemokine receptors (e.g., CCR7) in vaginal tissue (Gillgrass et al., 2005). Conversely, administration of estradiol increases survival and reduces signs of inflammation and vaginal pathology during primary HSV-2 infection (Gillgrass et al., 2005). Responses to vaccines against HSV-2 exhibit a sexually dimorphic pattern, in which the vaccine provides protection against the development of symptoms associated with genital herpes in women, but not in men (Stephenson, 2000). Mortality rates following exposure to HSV-type 1 (HSV-1) also are sexually dimorphic, in which male mice exhibit more severe pathology following corneal infection and are more likely to die from infection than are females; treatment of female mice with dihydrotestosterone (DHT) prior to infection significantly increases morbidity and mortality (Han et al., 2001).

Myocarditis or inflammation of the heart can be caused by exposure to viral agents, including group B coxsackieviruses. Mortality rates following inoculation of BALB/c mice with coxsackievirus B-3 are elevated in male (60%) compared with female (25%) mice (Huber & Pfaeffle, 1994). Inoculation of male and female mice with varying doses of coxsackievirus B-3 consistently results in more severe myocarditis in males than females at all doses examined (Lyden et al., 1987).

At low doses of coxsackievirus B-3, severe disease ensues in males, but little or no inflammation is seen in females. Whether the myocardial injury is caused by the virus damaging heart cells or host inflammatory responses is debated. Males, however, develop considerably higher inflammatory responses, including local production of IL-1β, TNF, and IFNγ, than females (Huber & Pfaeffle, 1994; Huber, 2005). In contrast, females develop more robust IL-4 responses during infection than do males (Huber & Pfaeffle, 1994).

Injection of female mice with anti-IL-4 antibody during coxsackievirus B-3 infection significantly increases rates of mortality. Further, adoptive transfer of lymphocytes from infected females into infected male mice increases survival and reduces inflammation of the heart (Huber & Pfaeffle, 1994). Injection of female mice with high doses of testosterone increases, whereas injection of male mice with high doses of estradiol decreases, inflammatory responses (e.g., IFNγ production) and coxsackievirus B-3 virus titers in the heart (Lyden et al., 1987; Huber et al., 1999).

Reported human hantavirus infections in the Americas and Europe, as well as field observations of several rodent-virus systems indicate that more males than females are infected with hantaviruses (Childs et al., 1994; Weigler et al., 1996; White et al., 1996; Mills et al., 1997; Williams et al., 1997; Glass et al., 1998; Mills et al., 1998; Bernshtein et al., 1999). Sex differences in hantavirus infection only become apparent after puberty, suggesting that sex steroid hormones may underlie the dimorphism in infection (Childs et al., 1988; Mills et al., 1997). Sex steroids can modulate sex differences in infection through effects on the immune system or on the expression of behaviors (e.g. aggression) that increase the likelihood of being exposed to hantaviruses (Zuk & McKean, 1996; Root et al., 1999; Klein, 2000, 2004).

Laboratory studies of Norway rats inoculated with Seoul virus (i.e., the hantavirus that naturally infects Norway rats) reveal that when given the same challenge, male and female rats are equally likely to become infected (Klein et al., 2000). After inoculation, however, males shed Seoul virus longer and via more routes (i.e., a combination of saliva, urine, and feces) and have more viral RNA copies present in target organs, such as the lungs, than females (Fig. 17.2) (Klein et al., 2000, 2001; Klein et al., 2002b).

Additionally, the expression of key transcriptional factors (e.g., eIF-2α, NF-κB, IRF-1, NF-IL-6, and STAT6) and genes that encode for antiviral (e.g., IFNγR and Mx proteins), T cell (e.g., CD3 and TCR), and Ig superfamily (e.g., IgM, IgG, and MHC class I and II) proteins is higher in females than males (Klein et al., 2004). Thus, females may be more efficient at transcribing genes that encode for immune responses against Seoul virus infection and that reduce virus replication and viral protein synthesis.

Mx proteins are induced by type I interferons and possess important antiviral properties. Human MxA and rodent Mx2, in particular, confer resistance against hantaviruses, including Seoul virus, Puumala virus, Hantaan virus, and Andes virus, in vitro (Temonen et al., 1995; Jin et al., 2001; Khaiboullina et al., 2005). The suppressed expression of Mx2 in male rats following Seoul virus infection may contribute to increased virus shedding and virus replication in lung tissue (Fig. 17.2) (Klein et al., 2000, 2001; Klein et al., 2002a; Klein et al., 2004).

Although males are more susceptible than females to many viral agents, measles is one virus that causes significantly higher mortality in females than males. Incidence of measles infection is highest among infants and young children. A meta-analysis of deaths caused by exposure to measles from 1950–1989 revealed that female-biased mortality is apparent among infants (<1–4 years), children (5–14 years), and adults (15–44 years) worldwide (Garenne, 1994). The observed sex difference in response to measles virus implies that males and females may respond differently to attenuated viral vaccines.

The standard measles vaccine is a low titer viral vaccine that is offered to infants at 9 months of age. One problem with the standard measles vaccine is that it does not protect infants against infection during the period between when maternal antibody begins to decline and immunization occurs (i.e., from 4–9 months of age). Thus, administration of a high titer measles vaccine to infants <9 months of age was initiated by the World Health Organization in the late 1980s in regions of West Africa. In response to a high titer measles vaccine, mortality rates were consistently higher for girls than boys, which lead to termination of the vaccine trials (Knudsen et al., 1996). Whether girls and boys differed in their immunological responses to the vaccine has not been reported.

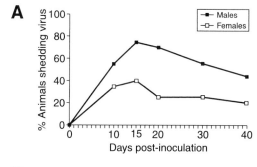

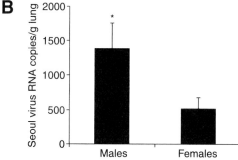

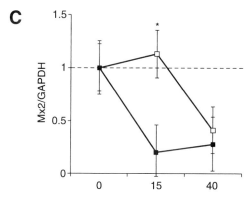

Bacteria

Responses to and colonization of bacterial infections differ between the sexes. For example, rates of infection are higher in male mice infected with *Corynebacterium kutscheri* and in men infected with *Staphylococcus aureus* as compared to females (Komukai et al., 1999; Laupland et al., 2003). Conversely, female mice are more susceptible than males to several bacterial infections, including *Listeria monocytogenes*, *Pseudomonas aeruginosa*, and *Salmonella typhimurium* (Pung et al., 1985; Kita et al., 1989; Guilbault et al., 2002). In response to typhoid infection, excessively high estradiol concentrations reduce survival and increase bacterial growth in female mice (Kita et al., 1989).

Women are more susceptible to sexually transmitted bacterial infections and develop more severe symptoms of disease following infection than do men (Wong et al., 2004). A Canadian retrospective analysis of reported cases of sexually-transmitted bacterial infections from 1991–2000 revealed that while rates of chlamydia infection were higher in women than men, rates of gonorrhea and syphilis were consistently higher in men than women (Wong et al., 2004).

Several factors likely contribute to sex differences in rates of sexually transmitted diseases, including likelihood of engaging in risk-taking sexual behaviors, clinical diagnosis, prevention, and treatment. For gonorrhea, women are much more likely to be asymptomatic than are men suggesting that cases of gonorrhea may be underdiagnosed in women (Judson, 1990). Susceptibility to chlamydia and gonorrhea change during the menstrual cycle and in response to contraceptive use (Sonnex, 1998; Brabin, 2002).

Estrogens and progestins affect bacterial urogenital infections by influencing immune responses and cervical mucus production, which provides an important physical barrier to infection (Sonnex, 1998). Susceptibility of female mice to gonorrhea is increased during proestrous and is associated with estradiol, but not progesterone, concentrations (Braude

Figure 17.2. During Seoul virus infection, male rats are more likely to shed Seoul virus in saliva, have more viral copies in target organs, and have suppressed antiviral responses than are females. (A) Proportion of male and female rats shedding Seoul virus in saliva 0–40 days post-inoculation (p.i.); (B) Number of viral RNA copies in lung tissue collected from infected male and female rats 40 days p.i.; and (C) Gene expression levels for rat Mx2, which is known to have antiviral properties against hantaviruses, in lung tissue collected from male and female rats 0, 15, or 40 days p.i. Gene expression data from infected animals were normalized to the expression levels from same-sex uninfected control animals (i.e., Day 0 p.i.; baseline). Adapted with permission from Klein SL, et al. (2002b). Neonatal sex steroids affect responses to Seoul virus infection in male but not female

Norway rats. *Brain Behav Immun*, 16:736–746, and Klein SL, et al (2004). Differential expression of immunoregulatory genes in male and female Norway rats following infection with Seoul virus. *J Med Virol*, 74:180–190.

et al., 1978; Taylor-Robinson et al., 1990). In vitro data suggest that estrogens facilitate chlamydia attachment and infectivity of vaginal epithelial cells though interactions with ERβ (Guseva et al., 2005).

Tuberculosis is caused by the bacterium *Mycobacterium tuberculosis* and is one of the leading causes of death from infectious diseases worldwide. Sex differences in deaths from pulmonary tuberculosis have been reported in the United States since the late 1800s (Putnam, 1927). Currently, in the United States, tuberculosis can be treated successfully through a combination of antibiotics; thus, deaths from tuberculosis in the United States are low. Based on US hospital admissions data in 2000, disproportionately more men were hospitalized with tuberculosis than were women; of those patients who were hospitalized with tuberculosis, however, mortality rates were similar between the sexes (Hansel et al., 2004).

In less economically, well-developed countries, such as Mexico, India, and Syria, sex significantly influences tuberculosis outcome, in which men are more likely to die from tuberculosis than are women (Bashour & Mamaree, 2003; Balasubramanian et al., 2004; Jimenez-Corona et al., 2006). Although women often are less likely than men to have access to adequate health care in these countries, men are more likely to default from antibiotic treatment and to be retreated for tuberculosis infection than are women (Bashour and Mamaree, 2003; Balasubramanian et al., 2004; Jimenez-Corona et al., 2006).

Even when socioeconomic and cultural barriers to health care are controlled in multivariate regression analyses, men are still more likely to experience a negative health outcome from tuberculosis infection than are women (Bashour & Mamaree, 2003) suggesting that biological differences between the sexes may be involved. In mice infected with M. *marinum*, males are more likely to die from infection and exhibit higher bacterial loads in the lungs and spleen than females (Yamamoto et al., 1991). Castration of males reduces, whereas administration of testosterone increases, susceptibility to M. *marinum* infection in mice (Yamamoto et al., 1991).

Bacillus anthracis is transmitted through aerosolized spores and is of notable interest as a potential bioterrorism agent. Statistical models developed from an outbreak of anthrax in Russia reveal that anthrax spores remain in the lungs of men for a longer duration than in women (Brookmeyer et al., 2005). Inoculation of male and female rabbits with an FDA-licensed anthrax vaccine followed by a challenge with aerosolized anthrax spores results in higher antibody responses in females than males (Little et al., 2006). Survival following infection, however, does not differ between the sexes (Little et al., 2006).

Among US soldiers, reaction to the anthrax vaccine, including development of nodules and injection site erythema, are consistently more pronounced among women then men (Hoffman et al., 2003). Women also report more severe symptoms of malaise (e.g., fatigue) following vaccination than do men (Wolfe et al., 2002; Hoffman et al., 2003). Whether hormones modify responses to anthrax vaccination has not been documented. In vitro, anthrax bacterial toxins repress glucocorticoid receptor, progesterone receptor, and ERα activation in plasmid transfection systems (Webster et al., 2003). Because signaling by these steroid hormone receptors can be anti-inflammatory, reduced signaling may contribute to increased susceptibility to the lethal (i.e., inflammatory) effects of anthrax.

Parasites

Field studies as well as epidemiological studies illustrate that rates of parasitism often are higher in males than females (Klein, 2004). The prevalence and intensity of infection with *Leishmania*, *Plasmodium*, *Entamoeba*, *Necator*, and *Schistosoma* parasites, for example, is higher among men than women (Goble and Konopka, 1973; Jones et al., 1987; Landgraf et al., 1994; Marguerite et al., 1999; Acuna-Soto et al., 2000; Behnke et al., 2000; Degu et al., 2002). Studies of rodents in a controlled laboratory setting reveal that these sex differences may be mediated by endocrine-immune interactions.

One genus of protozoan parasites that causes a pronounced sexual dimorphism in vertebrate hosts is *Plasmodium*. Men and women differ in disease manifestations following infection; men are more likely to develop lymphomas, whereas women are more likely to develop anemia, after infection (Morrow et al., 1976; Brabin et al., 1989; Brabin, 1990).

In general, most studies of malaria in human populations do not distinguish between the responses of males and females and, thus, the prevalence of sex differences may be underreported (Allotey & Gyapong, 2005). A few studies do, however, clearly illustrate that men are more susceptible than women. In a recent prospective study of imported malaria cases in

France, men reported more severe symptoms of malaria infection (e.g., chills, fever, and low platelet counts) than did women (Casalino et al., 2002). Several studies indicate that men tend to have higher parasitemia than women (Molineaux & Gramiccia, 1979; Landgraf et al., 1994; Wildling et al., 1995). Among Ghanaian school children, although the prevalence of *P. falciparum* infection does not differ between the sexes, parasite density is significantly higher for boys than girls around puberty (i.e., from ages 8–16) suggesting that circulating sex steroids may influence this outcome (Landgraf et al., 1994).

Studies of rodent malarias illustrate that mortality rates are higher in males compared with females and may involve endocrine and immunological differences between the sexes (Wunderlich et al., 1991; Benten et al., 1992; Benten et al., 1993; Benten et al., 1997; Zhang et al., 2000; Cernetich et al., 2006). Castration of males reduces, whereas exogenous administration of testosterone increases, mortality following infection with *P. chabaudi* or *P. berghei* in mice (Kamis & Ibrahim, 1989; Wunderlich et al., 1991). In addition to increased mortality rates, male mice recover from *P. chabaudi*-induced weight loss, anemia, and hypothermia slower than females (Sanni et al., 2002; Cernetich et al., 2006).

Recent data from our laboratory further illustrate that gonadally-intact male mice have reduced IFNγ-associated gene expression and IFNγ production during peak parasitemia and produce less antibody during the recovery phase of infection than females (Cernetich et al., 2006). Gonadectomy of female mice significantly reduces these responses suggesting that sex steroid hormones, in particular estrogens, may modulate immune responses to infection. The immunomodulatory effects of testosterone also may underlie increased susceptibility to *Plasmodium* infections in males compared with females. Exposure of adult female mice to testosterone reduces antibody production, decreases major histocompatibility complex (MHC) class II cells in the spleen, and increases CD8+ T cells in the spleen (Benten et al., 1997).

Epidemiological studies of *Leishmania* infections reveal that adult men are more frequently infected than women and that sex differences in behavior (e.g., via occupational exposure) as well host immune responses to infection are involved (Lynch et al., 1982; Jones et al., 1987; Weigle et al., 1993). Sex differences in response to *Leishmania* infection are reported in prepubertal children, in which boys are more likely to

develop visceral leishmaniasis than girls suggesting that if sex steroids are involved, organizational effects on the immune system early in life may be involved (Shiddo et al., 1995).

Experimental studies of *Leishmania* infection in mice also reveal that males are more susceptible to infection than females. Castration of males reduces, whereas administration of testosterone to females increases, susceptibility to *L. major* (Mock & Nacy, 1988). Males also are more susceptible than females to infection with *L. mexicana* and this sex difference appears to be mediated by the effects of estrogens on the synthesis of IFNγ and production of Th1 responses (Fig. 17.3) (Satoskar & Alexander, 1995; Satoskar et al., 1998; Roberts et al., 2001).

Among children and adults, the intensity and prevalence of *Schistosoma* infection in endemic areas is higher in males than females (Marguerite et al., 1999; Degu et al., 2002). Sex differences in the prevalence of infection may be attributed to differences in the amount of time spent in water and, hence, exposure to snails (i.e., the intermediate host) or differences in skin lipids that may influence the ability of *Schistosoma* parasites to penetrate skin and cause infection (Shiff et al., 1972).

Increased parasite burden in males, however, may contribute to elevated pro-inflammatory (e.g., TNF), Th1 (e.g., IFNγ), Th2 (e.g., IgE), and antibody responses in males compared with females (Webster et al., 1997; Abebe et al., 2001; Remoue et al., 2001; Naus et al., 2003). Elevated pro-inflammatory responses against *S. mansoni* are correlated with development of diseases, including hepatosplenomegaly (Mwatha et al., 1998). In contrast, regulatory T-cell responses, including the synthesis of IL-10 and TGFβ, that down-regulate Th1 responses, are higher in females than males (Remoue et al., 2001). IgA production, which provides immunity against reinfection with *Schistosoma* parasites, also is higher in females than males (Remoue et al., 2001). Whether sex steroid hormones mediate sex differences in responses to *Schistosoma* parasites in humans is unclear; estrogens and progestins, however, are hypothesized to regulate elevated IL-10, TGFβ, and IgA production in females (Remoue et al., 2001).

Although males are more susceptible than females to many parasitic infections, males are not more susceptible to all parasites. One of the most well studied parasites for which females are more susceptible than males is *Toxoplasma gondii*. In mouse models, females

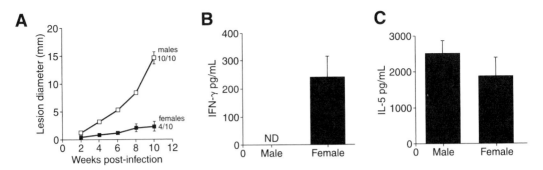

Figure 17.3. Male DBA/2 mice develop larger lesions and produce less IFNγ than females during *Leishmania mexicana* infection. (A). Mean + SE *L. mexicana* lesion diameter on the rumps of male and female mice during the course of *L. mexicana* infection. Numbers represent the proportion of animals with non-healing lesions at week 10 post-inoculation. Mean + SE IFNγ (B) and IL-5 (C) production by white blood cells isolated from the inguinal lymph nodes of male and female mice 10 weeks after inoculation with *L. mexicana* and stimulated in vitro with *L. mexicana*-soluble antigen (20µg/ml). Adapted with permission from Satoskar A, Al-Quassi HH, Alexander J. (1998). Sex-determined resistance against Leishmania mexicana is associated with the preferential induction of a Th1-like response and IFN-gamma production by female but not male DBA/2 mice. *Immunol Cell Biol*, 76:159–166.

develop more severe brain inflammation and are more likely to die following infection than males (Walker et al., 1997). Ovariectomy of female mice reduces, whereas administration of estradiol exacerbates, the development of tissue cysts caused by *T. gondii* infection (Pung & Luster, 1986; Liesenfeld et al., 2001). Male mice produce higher concentrations of TNF, IL-12, and IFNγ than females early during infection (Roberts et al., 1995; Walker et al., 1997). Human studies of sex differences in *T. gondii* infection are scarce because most "healthy" adults are asymptomatic. Among immunocompromised individuals, however, *T. gondii*-induced encephalitis is more prevalent among women than men (Phillips et al., 1994).

Taenia crassiceps is an intestinal cestode for which rodents serve as an intermediate host. Studies of mice reveal that females develop more cysticerci than males (Larralde et al., 1995). Estrogens favor, whereas androgens inhibit, *T. crassiceps* growth and development (Terrazas et al., 1994; Morales-Montor et al., 2002). Males develop higher Th1 responses, including elevated IFNγ synthesis, whereas females exhibit heightened IL-10 production, during the early phase of infection (Terrazas et al., 1998). Because Th1 responses inhibit parasite growth, this is hypothesized to be the mechanism mediating reduced susceptibility to infection in males (Terrazas et al., 1998).

SEX DIFFERENCES IN AUTOIMMUNE DISEASES

Autoimmune diseases are characterized by immunological destruction of host tissues and cells, and occur disproportionately more often in women than men. Approximately 80% of all cases of autoimmunity in the US are women (Jacobson et al., 1997). Sex differences in the incidence of autoimmunity are most pronounced for Sjogren's syndrome, systemic lupus erythematosus (SLE), thyroid disease (Hashimoto's thyroiditis and Graves' disease), scleroderma, and myasthenia gravis in which significantly more women are afflicted with these diseases than are men (Fig. 17.4) (Whitacre, 2001). Animal models have been used to characterize the immunological and endocrinological causes of sex differences in autoimmune diseases.

Current hypotheses about the causes of sex differences in the prevalence and intensity of autoimmune diseases involve the known effects of sex steroids on immune function. Autoimmune disease activity changes dramatically during pregnancy. For autoimmune diseases, including rheumatoid arthritis (RA) and multiple sclerosis (MS), that are caused by elevated cell-mediated immune responses (e.g., excessive production of inflammatory responses) against joint antigens and central nervous system proteins, respectively, symptoms typically decline during the

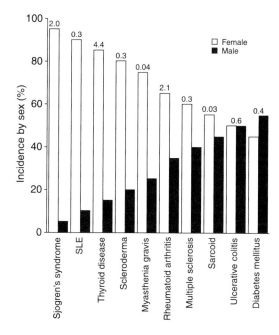

Figure 17.4. The distribution of major autoimmune diseases in men and women. The numbers above each bar refer to the total number of disease cases (x 1,000,000) in the USA. Adapted with permission from Whitacre CC. (2001). Sex differences in autoimmune disease. *Nat Immunol,* 2:777–780.

third trimester of pregnancy when estrogen and progesterone concentrations are high (Klein et al., 1997; Confavreux et al., 1998). Conversely, as concentrations of estrogen and progesterone decline during the post-partum period, symptoms of RA and MS worsen.

For autoimmune diseases caused by antibody production against self-antigens, such as SLE, symptoms are worse during pregnancy, possibly because the hormonal milieu during pregnancy promotes Th2-mediated immunity (Whitacre, 2001). Recent evidence suggests that the contrasting effects of estrogens on autoimmune diseases (i.e., high concentrations relieve symptoms of RA and MS, but exacerbate symptoms of SLE) may be related to the differential expression of ERα and ERβ in secondary lymphoid tissues (Shim et al., 2006).

Animal models have established the causal effects of hormones on sexually dimorphic autoimmune responses. For example, SLE is characterized by the development of antibodies against nucleic acids and immune complex glomerulonephritis. In mouse mod-

els of SLE, females begin developing anti-DNA antibodies and glomerulonephritis sooner than males. Castration of males increases and treatment of females with testosterone decreases morbidity and mortality (Roubinian et al., 1978). Additionally, elevated concentrations of estrogens result in increased auto-antibody titers, more severe renal disease, and earlier death following induction of SLE in mice (Roubinian et al., 1978). Treatment of SLE-susceptible mice with 17β-estradiol rescues autoreactive B cells that normally would be deleted during development via negative selection (Grimaldi et al., 2006). Administration of tamoxifen (i.e., an ER antagonist) reduces disease severity in SLE-prone mice, possibly by suppressing autoreactive B cell maturation (Peeva et al., 2005).

Insulin-dependent diabetes mellitus (IDDM) is an autoimmune condition characterized by cell-mediated immune responses directed against pancreatic β cells. Nonobease diabetic (NOD) mice spontaneously develop autoimmune type 1 diabetes. As in humans, the incidence and severity of type 1 diabetes is higher in female than male NOD mice. The role of sex steroids in mediating the development of IDDM is illustrated by the observation that castration of males increases, whereas ovariectomy of females decreases, the incidence of diabetes (Fitzpatrick et al., 1991; Hawkins et al., 1993).

Further, administration of testosterone to females inhibits the development of diabetes in NOD mice (Hawkins et al., 1993). At a molecular level, estrogens increase, whereas androgens decrease, production of IL-12-induced IFNγ through regulation of the signal transduction factor, STAT4 (Bao et al., 2002). Similar observations have been made using mouse models of myasthenia gravis (Delpy et al., 2005). Thus, estrogens polarize CD4+ T cell responses and disrupt the Th1/Th2 balance to promote development of autoimmune conditions caused by excessively high cell-mediated immune responses.

One of the most well characterized animal models of autoimmune disease is experimental autoimmune encephalomyelitis (EAE). EAE is induced in susceptible mouse strains by immunization with myelin proteins and the subsequent inflammatory demyelination that occurs mimics the pathogenesis seen in MS patients. Similar to MS, females are more susceptible to developing EAE than males. The pathogenesis associated with EAE is caused by excessive activation of inflammatory CD4+ T cells and elevated secretion of cytokines, including IFNγ, which may be mediated by estrogens. Adoptive transfer of autoreactive T cells from females to males leads to increased EAE disease severity in male recipients (Bebo et al., 1998a). EAE disease severity is linked to the sex of the donor T cells suggesting that intrinsic differences (possibly hormonal) during the induction of the initial immune response are a critical determinant of outcome (Bebo et al., 1998a).

The effects of estrogens on EAE severity are biphasic; administration of high doses of estradiol or estriol (an estrogen produced by the placenta during pregnancy) suppresses cell-mediated immune responses and relieves symptoms of EAE, whereas ovariectomy or administration of low doses of estrogens stimulates autoreactive CD4+ T cells and exacerbates EAE pathogenesis (Jansson et al., 1994; Kim et al., 1999; c.f. Bebo et al., 2001). The effects of estrogens on EAE pathogenesis are mediated by ER activity. Administration of the ER antagonist ICI 182,780 increases symptoms of disease, whereas treatment of female mice with the ERα agonist propylpyrazole triol, prior to induction of EAE, reduces disease severity (Elloso et al., 2005). In contrast, treatment of female mice with an ERβ agonist (WAY-202041) prior to induction of EAE has no effect on the development of disease (Elloso et al., 2005).

Although considerable attention has been paid to the role of estrogens in mediating EAE pathogenesis, several studies illustrate that androgens protect males from the development of severe EAE in susceptible strains of mice. Castration of males exacerbates, whereas administration of testosterone or the non-aromatizable androgen DHT reduces, EAE disease severity in male mice (Fig. 17.5) (Bebo et al., 1998b; Palaszynski et al., 2004).

Hypogonadism (i.e., reduced production of testosterone) is a common feature of male MS patients and mice with EAE, which appears to be related to the effects inflammatory cytokines on production of testosterone by Leydig cells (Foster et al., 2003). Thus, administration of testosterone supplements to MS patients may have novel therapeutic applications (Palaszynski et al., 2004).

IMMUNOLOGICAL DIFFERENCES BETWEEN THE SEXES

Sex differences in immune function are well established in vertebrates (Schuurs and Verheul, 1990;

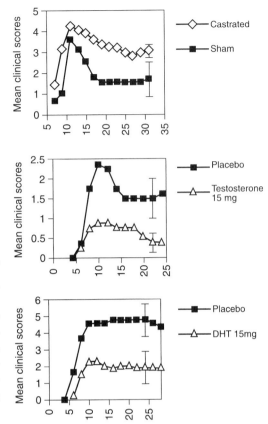

Figure 17.5. Experimental autoimmune encephalomyelitis (EAE) was induced in SJL mice by injection with myelin basic protein. Mean clinical scores based on degree of limb paralysis were assessed daily. Castration significantly increased (A), whereas treatment with testosterone (B) or 5α-dihydrotestosterone (DHT; C) reduced, mean clinical scores for EAE. Adapted with permission from Palaszynski KM, Loo KK, Ashouri JF, Liu HB, Voskuhl RR. (2004). Androgens are protective in experimental autoimmune encephalomyelitis: implications for multiple sclerosis. *J Neuroimmunol*, 146:144–152.

Klein, 2000; Roberts et al., 2001). Males generally exhibit lower immune responses than females (Schuurs & Verheul, 1990; Klein, 2000; Roberts et al., 2001). In particular, innate responses, antibody-mediated responses, and cellular responses typically are higher in females than males. Immunological differences between the sexes may explain why males and females differ in their responses to pathogens and in the development of autoimmune diseases.

Innate Immunity

Innate immunity represents the first-line of defense against pathogens. Because these responses do not require prior exposure or sensitization, they can be initiated immediately following exposure to a novel agent. Males and females differ in their innate immune responses suggesting that some sex differences may be germline encoded. Studies of both humans and rodents illustrate that inflammatory immune responses are generally higher in females than males and may explain why women are more likely to develop inflammatory autoimmune diseases, such as RA and SLE, than men (Da Silva, 1995). Female mice also exhibit stronger delayed-type hypersensitivity reactions to *Schistosoma mansoni* than males (Boissier et al., 2003). Following antigenic stimulation, males produce higher concentrations of the inflammatory mediator, bradykinin, than females and this response is mediated by sex steroid hormones (Green et al., 1999).

The number and activity of cells associated with innate immunity differ between the sexes. Phagocytic cells, including macrophages and neutrophils, can kill pathogens by generating reactive oxygen metabolites and nitric oxide, as well as by secreting enzymes. Among humans and lizards, the phagocytic activity of neutrophils and macrophages is higher in females than males (Mondal & Rai, 1999; Spitzer, 1999). Following parasitic or antigenic stimulation, the production and release of prostaglandin E_2, thromboxane B_2, and nitric oxide is reportedly higher in females than males (Du et al., 1984; Barna et al., 1996; Spitzer, 1999). Other studies, however, demonstrate that plasma concentrations of several pro-inflammatory cytokines, including IL-6 and TNF, are higher in males following trauma (Diodato et al., 2001).

Natural killer (NK) cells also represent a critical first-line of defense against parasites. Women with regular menstrual cycles as well as women tested during the luteal phase of their menstrual cycle have lower NK cell activity than men (Souza et al., 2001; Yovel et al., 2001). Studies of mice illustrate that estradiol can reduce both the number and activity of NK cells (Hanna & Schneider, 1983). Antigen presenting cells (APC) from females are more efficient at presenting peptides than are APC from males (Weinstein et al., 1984). Following infection of the central nervous system, the expression of MHC class II on astrocytes, endothelial cells, and microglia is enhanced in female compared with male mice (Barna et al., 1996).

Although these data illustrate that innate immunity differs between the sexes, whether the sexes differ in their reliance on innate immunity to overcome infection has not been well documented and represents an important area for future research. Immunodeficient mouse models may be utilized to differentiate the roles of innate and acquired immunity in mediating sex differences in response to infection. In response to *P. chabaudi*, WT male mice are more susceptible to infection (i.e., develop higher parasitemia and die faster) than their female counterparts. Deletion of T cells (TCRβδ-/- mice), B cells (μMT mice), or both lymphocyte populations (RAG1 mice) does not abolish the sex differences in morbidity and mortality following *P. chabaudi* inoculation, suggesting that the dimorphism is mediated by innate and not acquired immune responses against infection (Cernetich et al., 2006). In contrast, deletion of IFNγ (IFNγ-/- mice) reduces the sex difference in mortality from *P. chabaudi* and is more detrimental to females than males suggesting that IFNγ may play an important role in mediating sex differences in response to malaria (Fig. 17.6) (Cernetich et al., 2006).

Acquired Immunity

Humoral immune responses (i.e., antibody production by B-cells) are typically elevated in females as compared to males (Falter et al., 1991; Gomez et al., 1993). In mice infected with the parasite *Giardia muris*, females have lower infection rates and higher antibody production than males suggesting a functional advantage for elevated humoral immunity in females (Daniels & Belosevic, 1994).

Cell-mediated immune responses also differ between males and females. T cells, in particular CD4+ helper T cells (Th cells), are functionally and phenotypically heterogeneous and can be differentiated based on the cytokines they release. Reliance on subsets of Th cells (i.e., Th1 or Th2 cells) to overcome infection differs between males and females with females reportedly exhibiting higher Th2 responses (i.e., higher IL-4, IL-5, IL-6, and IL-10 production) than males (Bijlsma et al., 1999; Roberts et al., 2001). There are reports of females having higher Th1 responses (i.e., higher concentrations of IFNγ) than males (Araneo et al., 1991; Barrat et al., 1997). Female rodents also have higher mitogen-stimulated lymphocyte proliferation, faster wound healing, and increased immunological intolerance to foreign

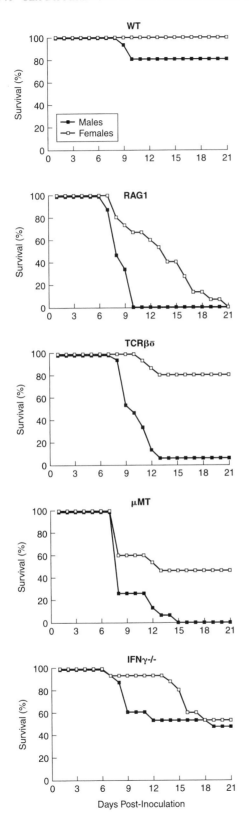

substances than males (Graff et al., 1969; Krzych et al., 1981; Blankenhorn et al., 2003).

Sex differences in Th cell responses may mediate sex differences in response to infection. After experimental inoculation with coxsackievirus, male mice primarily generate Th1 phenotypic responses (i.e., elevated IFNγ, IL-2, IgG2a) and females exhibit predominantly Th2 phenotypic responses (i.e., high IL-4, IL-5, IgG1) (Huber & Pfaeffle, 1994).

Female DBA/2 mice are more resistant to cutaneous *Leishmania mexicana* infection than males (Alexander, 1988). In this case, females produce higher IFNγ responses against *L. mexicana* and ovariectomy of female mice suppresses IFNγ synthesis (Alexander, 1988). Similarly, in humans, women generate a more robust delayed-type hypersensitivity response (i.e., Th1-related), whereas men have higher IgE concentrations (i.e., Th2-related) following infected with *L. mexicana* (Lynch et al., 1982). Female mice are more susceptible to *T. gondii* infection and tend to have lower IL-12 and IFNγ responses than males (Walker et al., 1997). Conversely, females produce higher concentrations of IL-10, which could antagonize IFNγ responses against *T. gondii* (Roberts et al., 1995). Taken together, these data illustrate that sex differences in cytokine responses to infection play a critical role in determining susceptibility to pathogens.

SEX STEROID-IMMUNE INTERACTIONS

The prevailing hypothesis for immunological differences between the sexes is that sex hormones, in

Figure 17.6. Cumulative survival in male and female WT, RAG1, TCRβδ-/-, μMT, and IFNγ-/- mice following ip inoculation with 10^6 *P. chabaudi* AS-infected red blood cells. Deletion of T cells (TCRβδ-/-), B cells (μMT), or both lymphocyte populations (RAG1) is detrimental to both males and females as compared with WT mice, but does not abolish the sexual dimorphism in mortality. In contrast, elimination of IFNγ (IFNγ-/-) significantly reduces the sex difference in mortality and is more detrimental to females than males when compared with their WT counterparts. Adapted with permission from Cernetich A, et al. (2006). Involvement of gonadal steroids and gamma interferon in sex differences in response to blood-stage malaria infection. *Infect Immun*, 74:3190–3203.

particular, testosterone, 17β-estradiol, and progesterone, influence the immune system. The localization of sex hormone receptors in immune cells, including lymphocytes, macrophages, granulocytes, and mast cells, illustrates that there are direct connections between the endocrine and immune systems and that endocrine factors can directly modulate the expression of target genes in immune cells.

Androgens

Sex differences in infectious and autoimmune diseases are mediated, in part, by the effects of androgens, including DHT and testosterone, on the immune system (Olsen & Kovacs, 1996; Roberts et al., 2001; Palaszynski et al., 2004). Androgen receptors have been identified in various lymphoid tissues, including the thymus, bone marrow, and spleen of rodents, as well as in primary cultures of macrophages (Cutolo et al., 1996; Roberts et al., 2001; Wunderlich et al., 2002). Exposure to testosterone in vivo reduces NK cell activity in mice (Hou & Zheng, 1988).

Similarly, stimulation of murine macrophages with testosterone in vitro reduces the synthesis of pro-inflammatory products, including TNF and nitric oxide synthase (D'Agostino et al., 1999). In contrast, testosterone increases synthesis of anti-inflammatory cytokines, such as IL-10 (D'Agostino et al., 1999).

The immunosuppressive effects of testosterone may reflect the inhibitory effects of androgen receptor signaling mechanisms on transcriptional factors (e.g., NF-κB) that mediate the production of pro-inflammatory cytokines (McKay & Cidlowski, 1999). Alternatively, androgens may suppress immune responses by increasing the expression and translation of stress proteins (e.g., heat shock proteins) and apoptosis factors (Hofmann-Lehmann et al., 1998; Vegeto et al., 1999; Jones et al., 2000).

The actions of testosterone contribute to age-related thymic involution that occurs at puberty. Consequently, either surgical or chemical (i.e., via exposure to luteinizing hormone-releasing hormone analogues) castration of young or aged male mice causes profound regeneration of the thymus and can increase T cell numbers and function (Sutherland et al., 2005).

Gonadectomized male mice show greater resistance to several pathogens, including *Leishmania major*, *Plasmodium berghei*, and *P. chabaudi*, but are more susceptible to autoimmune diseases, such as EAE, as compared with gonadally-intact male mice

(Mock & Nacy, 1988; Kamis & Ibrahim, 1989; Wunderlich et al., 1991; Benten et al., 1992; Benten et al., 1993; Benten et al., 1997; Bebo et al., 1998b; Zhang et al., 2000; Palaszynski et al., 2004).

In response to *Angiostrongylus malaysiensis* infection, gonadectomized male rats have reduced numbers of worms, increased numbers of circulating leukocytes, and heavier thymic mass than gonadectomized males injected with testosterone propionate (Kamis et al., 1992). Infection of Indian soft-furred rats with the parasite *Nippostrongylus brasiliensis* results in higher worm burden in gonadally-intact males as compared with females or castrated male rats (Tiuria et al., 1994). Gonadally-intact male reindeer show higher incidence of warble fly (*Hypoderma tarandi*) infestation than both females and castrated male reindeer (Folstad et al., 1989). Although androgens can modify responses to infectious and autoimmune diseases, the mechanisms mediating this effect can be unclear. For example, the effects of testosterone on *P. chabaudi* infection are not mediated by traditional ligand-receptor interactions because pharmacologically blocking either intracellular androgen or estrogen receptors in adulthood has no effect on infection (Benten et al., 1992; Benten et al., 1993). Thus, sex differences in *P. chabaudi* infection cannot solely be explained by the direct actions of testosterone in adulthood suggesting that other mechanisms are involved.

Estrogens

Estrogens modulate immune function in females and appear to contribute to resistance against infectious diseases and susceptibility to autoimmune diseases. Estrogens affect both innate and acquired immune function. Estrogen receptors are expressed in various lymphoid tissue cells as well as in circulating lymphocytes and macrophages (Danel et al., 1983; Cutolo et al., 1996; Roberts et al., 2001). Exposure of human NK cells to 17β-estradiol in vitro enhances NK cytotoxicity (Sorachi et al., 1993). 17β-estradiol also facilitates differentiation of bone marrow precursor cells into functional dendritic cells (DCs) (Paharkova-Vatchkova et al., 2004). Specifically, in vitro exposure to physiological concentrations of E_2 increased the expression of surface receptors, including MHCII, CD80, and CD86, as well as antigen presentation by DCs. Further, the effects of 17β-estradiol on DC differentiation is mediated by the estrogen receptor because blocking the ER with either ICI 182,780 or tamoxifen or utilizing bone marrow precursor cells from ERα−/−mice inhibits DC differentiation (Fig. 17.7) (Paharkova-Vatchkova et al., 2004).

In vitro exposure to 17β-estradiol also increases synthesis of chemokines, including CXCL8 and CCL2, by immature DCs (Bengtsson et al., 2004). Treatment of ovariectomized mice with 17β-estradiol enhances the synthesis of chemokine receptors, CCR1-CCR5, on CD4+ T cells (Mo et al. 2005). Estrogens stimulate synthesis of pro-inflammatory cytokines, including IL-1, IL-6, and TNF (Miller & Hunt, 1996). Estrogens can enhance both cell-mediated and humoral immune responses; there are, however, reports of estrogens suppressing some cell-mediated immune responses (Luster et al., 1984). Estrogens can augment expansion of CD4+CD25+ T-cells in mice (Fig. 17.8) (Polanczyk et al., 2004). The expression of several genes associated with activated CD4+CD25+ T cells (McHugh et al., 2002), including Tnfrsf4, Ltb, CCL3, and Gadd45γ, is

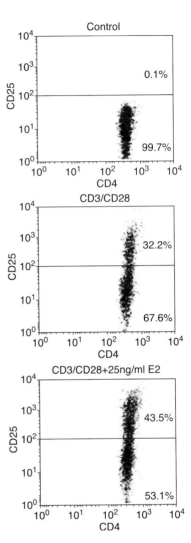

Figure 17.8. In vitro exposure to estradiol augments expansion of CD4+ CD25+ T cells in mice. Flow cytometric analysis of CD4+CD25+ cells isolated from the spleens of C57BL/6 mice and treated in vitro for 24 h with vehicle (control), T cell stimulants (CD3/CD28), or T cell stimulants plus 17β-estradiol (CD3/CD28 + 25ng/ml E₂). Adapted with permission from Polanczyk MJ, et al. (2004). Cutting edge: estrogen drives expansion of the CD4+CD25+ regulatory T cell compartment. *J Immunol*, 173:2227–2230.

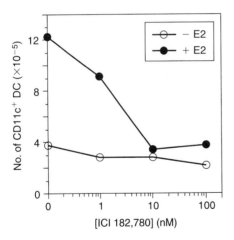

Figure 17.7. Incubation of bone marrow-derived dendritic cells (DCs) with 1nM 17β-estradiol (+E₂) significantly increases DC differentiation relative to DCs exposed to vehicle alone (−E₂). E₂-stimulated DC differentiation is inhibited, in a dose dependent manner, by incubation with the ER antagonist ICI 182,780. Adapted with permission from Paharkova-Vatchkova V, Maldonado R, Kovats S. (2004). Estrogen preferentially promotes the differentiation of CD11c+ CD11b (intermediate) dendritic cells from bone marrow precursors. *J Immunol*, 172:1426–1436.

higher among intact females than intact males and is reduced by gonadectomy of female mice (Cernetich et al., 2006). The cellular and molecular mechanisms mediating estrogenic effects on immune function have not been fully elucidated. The effects of estrogens on transcriptional factors, such as NF-κB, are cell-specific in which estrogens either enhance or inhibit NF-κB signaling pathways depending on the cell type (Kono et al., 2000; Evans et al., 2001). Estrogens also may enhance immune function in females by protecting immune cells against apoptosis (Hofmann-Lehmann et al., 1998; Vegeto et al., 1999).

Progestins

Progestins, primarily progesterone, play a critical role in reproduction, including the maintenance of pregnancy in mammals, and immune function. Progesterone can have both stimulatory and suppressive effects on the immune system, but is typically regarded as immunosuppressive. Progesterone receptors have been identified in epithelial cells, mast cells, granulocytes (e.g., eosinophils), macrophages, and lymphocytes (Miller & Hunt, 1996; Piccinni et al., 2000; Roberts et al., 2001). Progesterone can bind to glucocorticoid receptors, which are more abundant in the immune system than progesterone receptors, and may represent an alternative mechanism for progesterone-induced changes in immune function (Miller & Hunt, 1996).

Progesterone suppresses innate immune responses, including macrophage and NK cell activity as well as NF-κB signal transduction (Furukawa et al., 1984; Toder et al., 1984; Baley & Schacter, 1985; Miller & Hunt, 1996; Savita & Rai, 1998; McKay & Cidlowski, 1999). Progesterone can inhibit nitrite and nitric oxide production as well as TNF mRNA and production by murine macrophages (Miller et al., 1996; Miller & Hunt, 1998; Savita & Rai, 1998). Elevated concentrations of progesterone during pregnancy inhibit the development of Th1 immune responses that can lead to fetal rejection and promote production of Th2 immune responses, including IL-4 and IL-5 production (Piccinni et al., 1995; Piccinni et al., 2000). Thus, progesterone is considered to be an anti-inflammatory hormone.

Progesterone also suppresses antibody production, which may be caused by progesterone inhibiting CD8+ T-cell responses that in turn suppress antibody production by B-cells (Lu et al., 2002). Although the immunomodulatory properties of progesterone are well characterized in both mice and humans, the effects on responses to infectious and autoimmune diseases have not been adequately examined.

GENETIC FACTORS INFLUENCE SEX DIFFERENCES IN DISEASE SUSCEPTIBILITY

Disease Susceptibility Genes

Several studies illustrate that host genes play a critical role in mediating susceptibility and resistance to pathogens as well as autoimmune diseases. Resistance to *P. chabaudi* is polygenic and several loci have been identified that influence susceptibility to infection (termed *Char 1–4*, for *Cha*baudi resistance). Linkage analyses have mapped these loci to chromosomes 9, 8, 17, and 3, respectively. Crosses between resistant and susceptible strains, which result in recombinant inbred strains, reveal that the effects of *Char2* and *Char4* on resistance to infection are more pronounced among females than males (Fortin et al., 2001; Fortin et al., 2002). Thus, genetic resistance to *P. chabaudi* is sex dependent, although the role of sex steroids has not been reported.

Genetic resistance to *L. mexicana* has been mapped to a single locus, *Scl-2* that is located on chromosome 4 and that mediates a 'no lesion growth' phenotype (Roberts et al., 1990). Studies of backcross and F2 recombinant inbred strains of mice (from parental C57BL/6 and DBA/2 mice) reveal that the effect of *Scl-2* on resistance to *L. mexicana* is more pronounced among female than male mice (Roberts et al., 1990). The genes that encode for Janus tyrosine kinases (JAK)-1 and -2 have been mapped into the same region on chromosome 4 which suggests that *Scl-2* may play a role in cytokine-mediated pathways that differ between the sexes (Blackwell, 1996).

Like *P. chabaudi* and *L. mexicana*, susceptibility to mousepox has been mapped to disease-related loci on autosomal chromosomes. Using recombinant inbred strains of mice, 4 loci have been identified, *Rmp1–4* (resistance to mousepox loci), that confer resistance to mousepox. The effects of loci *Rmp2* (on chromosome 2) and *Rmp4* (on chromosome 1) on resistance to infection differ between the sexes, in which these loci confer greater resistance in female than male congenic mice.

If congenic mice are neonatally gonadectomized at 4–7 days of age and infected with mousepox as adults, then the sex difference in resistance is abolished; gonadectomized males and females are equally susceptible to mousepox (Brownstein & Gras, 1995). Neonatal ovariectomy increases female susceptibility to mousepox; whereas, castration of neonatal males has little effect on susceptibility to infection (i.e., castrated males are as susceptible as intact males) (Brownstein & Gras, 1995). Thus, estrogens may enhance as opposed to androgens suppressing genetic resistance to mousepox. These data also indicate that early hormonal manipulation may have profound effects on the expression of disease resistance genes in adulthood.

There is a strong associating between development of autoimmune diseases and MHC genes. Comparisons across inbred mouse strains, based on the expression of sex differences in development of EAE, reveal that H-2s and H-2d haplotypes are associated with female-biased susceptibility to EAE (Yu & Whitacre, 2004).

In addition to genes of the MHC that encode for class I and II proteins, genes found in the MHC class III region, that encode for complement proteins, also appear to be involved in the sex-specific pathogenesis of autoimmune diseases, such as SLE (Yu & Whitacre, 2004). Using recombinant inbred strains of mice several non-MHC loci have been identified that modulate sex-specific susceptibility to autoimmune diseases. Several genetic loci (eae4, eae11, eae12, eae13, eae17, and eae18) that are associated with the development of EAE in mice show sex-specific patterns of expression (Yu & Whitacre, 2004). Similarly, in NOD mice that spontaneously develop symptoms of IDDM, susceptibility loci on chromosome 1 are differentially expressed between the sexes (Boulard et al., 2002). These IDDM-related loci are located on several autosomal chromosomes and are positioned near immunologically-relevant loci (Yu & Whitacre, 2004).

Sex Chromosomes

Although many sexually dimorphic phenotypes are attributed to sex steroids, not all sex differences in physiology are mediated by circulating sex steroid hormones (Arnold, 1997). Sex determination in mammals is mediated by the Sry gene on the Y chromosome which causes the formation of testes that produce and release testosterone. In the presence of both the Sry gene and testosterone, male-typic development ensues (Canning & Lovell-Badge, 2002). In the absence of the Y chromosome and, hence, the Sry gene, ovaries develop (Canning & Lovell-Badge, 2002).

Early hypotheses about the role of host genes in resistance to disease initially speculated that female resistance and male susceptibility to infectious diseases were related to genes on sex chromosomes (Lenz, 1931; Purtilo & Sullivan, 1979). Because there are genes on the X chromosome that regulate immune function and because male mammals are heterogametic, deleterious recessive alleles are more likely to be expressed in males than females. Moreover, even small differences in the effects of alleles are more likely to be evident in males than in females because the phenotype of females results from the average effect of two alleles (Burgoyne et al., 2001). Although sex differences in physiology may be caused by direct effects of sex steroids, an alternative hypothesis is that genes on the X chromosome, the Y chromosome, or both alter the expression of sexually dimorphic phenotypes (via direct, non-hormonal mechanisms).

Whether sex chromosomal genes modulate sex differences in the development of the immune system and susceptibility to disease has recently been considered. To address whether sex differences in susceptibility to autoimmune disease are independent of sex steroids, mice with the Sry gene either deleted (XY⁻Sry) or translocated to an autosomal region (XXSry) were utilized to separate gonadal sex (i.e., the presence of ovaries or testes) from sex chromosome complement (i.e., XX or XY). Use of these mice has provided insight into the causes of sex differences in endocrine and central nervous system development (De Vries et al., 2002). EAE was induced in mice by immunization with myelin basic protein and subsequent immune responses were examined (Palaszynski et al., 2005). The presence of testosterone significantly reduced the production of MBP-specific immune responses. In the absence of gonadal steroids (i.e., following gonadectomy), the presence of the Y chromosome (in XY⁻ female and XY⁻Sry male mice) stimulated autoimmune responses suggesting that sex chromosome complement and sex steroids may have opposing effects on the immune system (Palaszynski et al., 2005).

CONCLUSIONS

The sexes differ in their responses to infectious and autoimmune diseases. The intensity and prevalence of infectious diseases typically are higher in males than females; conversely, the prevalence and severity of autoimmune diseases are greater in females than males. Endocrine-immune interactions play a fundamental role mediating responses to diseases. Because sex steroid concentrations differ dramatically between the sexes, to date, most studies have focused on characterizing the role of sex steroids as mediators of sex differences in immune function. Future studies must continue to examine whether other steroid and peptide hormones contribute to sex differences in disease susceptibility. For example, new evidence suggests that prolactin may be an important regulator of sex differences in response to autoimmune diseases (Grimaldi et al., 2005). Future studies also must continue to establish whether natural hormonal fluctuations associated with puberty, pregnancy, and menstruation affect immune responses to infectious and autoimmune diseases.

The immune systems of males and females differ. There is growing evidence that innate immunity differs substantially between males and females and may regulate differences in the initial responses to pathogens. Pattern recognition receptors, such as toll-like receptors (TLR) in vertebrates, as well as DCs and NK cells are intimately involved in mediating host innate responses to infection and serve as a bridge between innate and acquired immunity. Whether the sexes differ in these innate immunity responses and the extent to which hormones modify these cells and their responses requires additional investigation. Most studies characterizing sex differences in immune responses to infection focus on acquired immune responses, with particular attention paid to the Th1/Th2 dichotomy. Although this approach has yielded valuable information about the causes of sex differences in disease susceptibility, future studies should continue to consider how dimorphic innate and regulatory responses contribute to sex differences in infectious and autoimmune diseases.

The functional significance of sex differences in immune responses to infectious and autoimmune diseases must be considered. This chapter raises the possibility that if males and females differ in their immunological responses to pathogens, they may differ in their responses to treatments as well. Sex differences in the absorption, metabolism, and overall effectiveness of drug treatments are documented (Wizemann, 2001).

The extent to which males and females differ in the immunogenicity of vaccines has not been well characterized and may influence the effectiveness of disease treatments. Studies of both humans and mice reveal that the sexes differ in their responses to vaccines and commonly used vaccine antigens. For example, protection by vaccines developed against *P. chabaudi* is greater for females than males and elevated testosterone concentrations reduces the efficacy of vaccines against *P. chabaudi* in mice (Wunderlich et al., 1993).

Although the prevalence and intensity of *Schistosoma* worms is higher in men than women, men develop higher antibody responses against the worms and surface antigens (e.g., Sh28GST) than women (Remoue et al., 2001; Naus et al., 2003). Consequently, testosterone binds to the *Schistosoma* glutathione S-transferase (GST) protein with high affinity and may modulate host responses to the parasite and to vaccines developed against *Schistosoma* surface antigens (Remoue et al., 2002). The extent to which endocrine-immune interactions affect the immunogenicity of vaccines should be considered. In relation to autoimmunity, whether endocrine treatments have novel therapeutic applications should be explored further. Taken together, the data presented in this chapter illustrate that the occurrence and pathogenesis of autoimmune and infectious diseases differs between males and females, which may be regulated by interactions between the endocrine and immune systems.

Acknowledgments

I thank the students and collaborators who contributed substantially to the data presented from my laboratory, including Brian Bird, Amy Cernetich, Judith Easterbrook, Gregory Glass, Michele Hannah, Ella Hinson, Nirbhay Kumar, Mark Siracusa, and Alan Scott. Support for the data from my laboratory was provided by NIH R01 AI 054995 and a grant from the Johns Hopkins Malaria Research Institute.

References

Abebe F, Gaarder PI, Petros B, Gundersen SG. (2001). Age- and sex-related differences in antibody responses against *Schistosoma mansoni* soluble egg antigen in a cohort of school children in Ethiopia. *Apmis*, 109: 816–824.

Acuna-Soto R, Maguire JH, Wirth DF. (2000). Gender distribution in asymptomatic and invasive amebiasis. *Am J Gastroenterol*, 95:1277–1283.

Alexander J. (1988). Sex differences and cross-immunity in DBA/2 mice infected with L. mexicana and L. major. *Parasitology*, 96 (Pt 2):297–302.

Allotey P, Gyapong M. (2005). *The gender agenda in the control of tropical diseases: a review of current evidence*. Geneva: World Health Organization Special Programme for Research (pp. 1–38).

Araneo BA, Dowell T, Diegel M, Daynes RA. (1991). Dihydrotestosterone exerts a depressive influence on the production of interleukin-4 (IL-4), IL-5, and gamma-interferon, but not IL-2 by activated murine T cells. *Blood*, 78:688–699.

Arnold AP. (1997). Sexual differentiation of the zebra finch song system: positive evidence, negative evidence, null hypotheses, and a paradigm shift. *J Neurobiol*, 33:572–584.

Balasubramanian R, Garg R, Santha T, Gopi PG, Subramani R, Chandrasekaran V, et al. (2004). Gender disparities in tuberculosis: report from a rural DOTS programme in south India. *Int J Tuberc Lung Dis*, 8:323–332.

Baley JE, Schacter BZ. (1985). Mechanisms of diminished natural killer cell activity in pregnant women and neonates. *J Immunol*, 134:3042–3048.

Bao M, Yang Y, Jun HS, Yoon JW. (2002). Molecular mechanisms for gender differences in susceptibility to T cell-mediated autoimmune diabetes in non-obese diabetic mice. *J Immunol*, 168:5369–5375.

Barna M, Komatsu T, Bi Z, Reiss CS. (1996). Sex differences in susceptibility to viral infection of the central nervous system. *J Neuroimmunol*, 67:31–39.

Barrat F, Lesourd B, Boulouis HJ, Thibault D, Vincent-Naulleau S, Gjata B, et al. (1997). Sex and parity modulate cytokine production during murine ageing. *Clin Exp Immunol*, 109:562–568.

Bashour H, Mamaree F. (2003). Gender differences and tuberculosis in the Syrian Arab Republic: patients' attitudes, compliance and outcomes. *East Mediterr Health J*, 9:757–768.

Bebo BF, Jr., Schuster JC, Vandenbark AA, Offner H. (1998a). Gender differences in experimental autoimmune encephalomyelitis develop during the induction of the immune response to encephalitogenic peptides. *J Neurosci Res*, 52:420–426.

Bebo BF, Jr., Zelinka-Vincent E, Adamus G, Amundson D, Vandenbark AA, Offner H. (1998b). Gonadal hormones influence the immune response to PLP 139–151 and the clinical course of relapsing experimental autoimmune encephalomyelitis. *J Neuroimmunol*, 84:122–130.

Bebo BF, Jr., Fyfe-Johnson A, Adlard K, Beam AG, Vandenbark AA, Offner H. (2001). Low-dose estrogen therapy ameliorates experimental autoimmune encephalomyelitis in two different inbred mouse strains. *J Immunol*, 166:2080–2089.

Behnke JM, De Clercq D, Sacko M, Gilbert FS, Ouattara DB, Vercruysse J. (2000). The epidemiology of human hookworm infections in the southern region of Mali. *Trop Med Int Health*, 5:343–354.

Bengtsson AK, Ryan EJ, Giordano D, Magaletti DM, Clark EA. (2004). 17beta-estradiol (E2) modulates cytokine and chemokine expression in human monocyte-derived dendritic cells. *Blood*, 104: 1404–1410.

Benten WP, Wunderlich F, Mossmann H. (1992). Testosterone-induced suppression of self-healing *Plasmodium chabaudi* malaria: an effect not mediated by androgen receptors? *J Endocrinol*, 135:407–413.

Benten WP, Wunderlich F, Herrmann R, Kuhn-Velten WN. (1993). Testosterone-induced compared with oestradiol-induced immunosuppression against *Plasmodium chabaudi* malaria. *J Endocrinol*, 139: 487–494.

Benten WP, Ulrich P, Kuhn-Velten WN, Vohr HW, Wunderlich F. (1997). Testosterone-induced susceptibility to *Plasmodium chabaudi* malaria: persistence after withdrawal of testosterone. *J Endocrinol*, 153:275–281.

Bernshtein AD, Apekina NS, Mikhailova TV, Myasnikov YA, Khlyap LA, Korotkov YS, Gavrilovskaya IN. (1999). Dynamics of Puumala hantavirus infection in naturally infected bank voles (*Clethrinomys glareolus*). *Arch Virol*, 144:2415–2428.

Bijlsma JW, Cutolo M, Masi AT, Chikanza IC. (1999). The neuroendocrine immune basis of rheumatic diseases. *Immunol Today*, 20:298–301.

Blackwell JM. (1996). Genetic susceptibility to leishmanial infections: studies in mice and man. *Parasitology*, 112(Suppl):S67–S74.

Blankenhorn EP, Troutman S, Clark LD, Zhang XM, Chen P, Heber-Katz E. (2003). Sexually dimorphic genes regulate healing and regeneration in MRL mice. *Mamm Genome*, 14:250–260.

Boissier J, Chlichlia K, Digon Y, Ruppel A, Mone H. (2003). Preliminary study on sex-related inflammatory reactions in mice infected with *Schistosoma mansoni*. *Parasitol Res*, 91:144–150.

Boulard O, Fluteau G, Eloy L, Damotte D, Bedossa P, Garchon HJ. (2002). Genetic analysis of autoimmune sialadenitis in nonobese diabetic mice: a major susceptibility region on chromosome 1. *J Immunol*, 168:4192–4201.

Brabin BJ. (1990). An analysis of malaria parasite rates in infants: 40 years after MacDonald. *Bureau of Hygiene and Tropical Diseases*, 87:R1–R21.

Brabin BJ, Brabin L, Crane G, Forsyth KP, Alpers MP, van der Kaay HJ. (1989). Two populations of women with high and low spleen rates living in the same area of Madang, Papua New Guinea, demonstrate different immune responses to malaria. *Trans R Soc Trop Med Hyg*, 83:577–583.

Brabin L. (2002). Interactions of the female hormonal environment, susceptibility to viral infections, and disease progression. *AIDS Patient Care STDS*, 16: 211–221.

Braude AI, Corbeil LB, Levine S, Ito J, McCutchan JA. (1978). Possible influence of cyclical menstrual changes on resistance tot he gonococcus. In Brooks GF (Ed.), *Immunobiology of Neisseria gonorrhoeae* (pp. 328–337). Washington, DC: American Society of Microbiology.

Brookmeyer R, Johnson E, Barry S. (2005). Modelling the incubation period of anthrax. *Stat Med*, 24:531–542.

Brownstein DG, Gras L. (1995). Chromosome mapping of Rmp-4, a gonad-dependent gene encoding host resistance to mousepox. *J Virol*, 69:6958–6964.

Burgoyne PS, Lovell-Badge R, Rattigan A. (2001). Evidence that the testis determination pathway interacts with a non-dosage compensated, X-linked gene. *Int J Dev Biol*, 45:509–512.

Canning CA, Lovell-Badge R. (2002). Sry and sex determination: how lazy can it be? *Trends Genet*, 18:111–113.

Casalino E, Le Bras J, Chaussin F, Fichelle A, Bouvet E. (2002). Predictive factors of malaria in travelers to areas where malaria is endemic. *Arch Intern Med*, 162:1625–1630.

Cernetich A, Garver LS, Jedlicka AE, Klein PW, Kumar N, Scott AL, Klein SL. (2006). Involvement of gonadal steroids and gamma interferon in sex differences in response to blood-stage malaria infection. *Infect Immun*, 74:3190–3203.

Childs JE, Glass GE, Korch GW, LeDuc JW. (1988). The ecology and epizootiology of hantaviral infections in small mammal communities of Baltimore: A review and synthesis. *Bulletin of the Society of Vector Biology*, 13:113–122.

Childs JE, Ksiazek TG, Spiropoulou CF, Krebs JW, Morzunov S, Maupin GO, et al. (1994). Serologic and genetic identification of *Peromyscus maniculatus* as the primary rodent reservoir for a new hantavirus in the southwestern United States. *J Infect Dis*, 169:1271–1280.

Christeff N, Lortholary O, Casassus P, Thobie N, Veyssier P, Torri O, et al. (1996). Relationship between sex steroid hormone levels and CD4 lymphocytes in HIV infected men. *Exp Clin Endocrinol Diabetes*, 104:130–136.

Confavreux C, Hutchinson M, Hours MM, Cortinovis-Tourniaire P, Moreau T. (1998). Rate of pregnancy-related relapse in multiple sclerosis. Pregnancy in Multiple Sclerosis Group. *N Engl J Med*, 339:285–291.

Cutolo M, Accardo S, Villaggio B, Barone A, Sulli A, Coviello DA, et al. (1996). Androgen and estrogen receptors are present in primary cultures of human synovial macrophages. *J Clin Endocrinol Metab*, 81: 820–827.

D'Agostino P, Milano S, Barbera C, Di Bella G, La Rosa M, Ferlazzo V, et al. (1999). Sex hormones modulate inflammatory mediators produced by macrophages. *Ann N Y Acad Sci*, 876:426–429.

Da Silva JA. (1995). Sex hormones, glucocorticoids and autoimmunity: facts and hypotheses. *Ann Rheum Dis*, 54:6–16.

Danel L, Souweine G, Monier JC, Saez S. (1983). Specific estrogen binding sites in human lymphoid cells and thymic cells. *J Steroid Biochem*, 18:559–563.

Daniels CW, Belosevic M. (1994). Serum antibody responses by male and female C57Bl/6 mice infected with *Giardia muris*. *Clin Exp Immunol*, 97:424–429.

De Vries GJ, Rissman EF, Simerly RB, Yang LY, Scordalakes EM, Auger CJ, et al. (2002). A model system for study of sex chromosome effects on sexually dimorphic neural and behavioral traits. *J Neurosci*, 22:9005–9014.

Degu G, Mengistu G, Jones J. (2002). Some factors affecting prevalence of and immune responses to *Schistosoma mansoni* in schoolchildren in Gorgora, northwest Ethiopia. *Ethiop Med J*, 40:345–352.

Delpy L, Douin-Echinard V, Garidou L, Bruand C, Saoudi A, Guery JC. (2005). Estrogen enhances susceptibility to experimental autoimmune myasthenia gravis by promoting type 1-polarized immune responses. *J Immunol*, 175:5050–5057.

Diodato MD, Knoferl MW, Schwacha MG, Bland KI, Chaudry IH. (2001). Gender differences in the inflammatory response and survival following haemorrhage and subsequent sepsis. *Cytokine*, 14:162–169.

Du JT, Vennos E, Ramey E, Ramwell PW. (1984). Sex differences in arachidonate cyclo-oxygenase products in elicited rat peritoneal macrophages. *Biochim Biophys Acta*, 794:256–260.

Elloso MM, Phiel K, Henderson RA, Harris HA, Adelman SJ. (2005). Suppression of experimental autoimmune encephalomyelitis using estrogen receptor-selective ligands. *J Endocrinol*, 185:243–252.

Evans MJ, Eckert A, Lai K, Adelman SJ, Harnish DC. (2001). Reciprocal antagonism between estrogen receptor and NF-kappaB activity in vivo. *Circ Res*, 89:823–830.

Falter H, Persinger MA, Reid K. (1991). Sex differences in primary humoral responses of albino rats to human serum albumin. *Immunol Lett*, 28:143–145.

Farzadegan H, Hoover DR, Astemborski J, Lyles CM, Margolick JB, Markham RB, et al. (1998). Sex differences in HIV-1 viral load and progression to AIDS. *Lancet*, 352:1510–1514.

Fitzpatrick F, Lepault F, Homo-Delarche F, Bach JF, Dardenne M. (1991). Influence of castration, alone or combined with thymectomy, on the development of diabetes in the nonobese diabetic mouse. *Endocrinology*, 129:1382–1390.

Folstad I, Nilssen AC, Halvorsen O, Andersen J. (1989). Why do male reindeer (*Rangifer t. tarandus*) have higher abundance of second and third instar larvae of *Hypoderma tarandi* than females? *Oikos*, 55:87–92.

Fortin A, Stevenson MM, Gros P. (2002). Complex genetic control of susceptibility to malaria in mice. *Genes Immun*, 3:177–186.

Fortin A, Cardon LR, Tam M, Skamene E, Stevenson MM, Gros P. (2001). Identification of a new malaria susceptibility locus (Char4) in recombinant congenic strains of mice. *Proc Natl Acad Sci U S A*, 98:10793–10798.

Foster SC, Daniels C, Bourdette DN, Bebo BF, Jr. (2003). Dysregulation of the hypothalamic-pituitary-gonadal axis in experimental autoimmune encephalomyelitis and multiple sclerosis. *J Neuroimmunol*, 140:78–87.

Furukawa K, Itoh K, Okamura K, Kumagai K, Suzuki M. (1984). Changes in NK cell activity during the estrous cycle and pregnancy in mice. *J Reprod Immunol*, 6:353–363.

Gallichan WS, Rosenthal KL. (1996). Effects of the estrous cycle on local humoral immune responses and protection of intranasally immunized female mice against herpes simplex virus type 2 infection in the genital tract. *Virology*, 224:487–497.

Garenne M. (1994). Sex differences in measles mortality: a world review. *Int J Epidemiol*, 23:632–642.

Gillgrass AE, Fernandez SA, Rosenthal KL, Kaushic C. (2005). Estradiol regulates susceptibility following primary exposure to genital herpes simplex virus type 2, while progesterone induces inflammation. *J Virol*, 79:3107–3116.

Glass GE, Livingstone W, Mills JN, Hlady WG, Fine JB, Biggler W, et al. (1998). Black Creek Canal Virus infection in *Sigmodon hispidus* in southern Florida. *Am J Trop Med Hyg*, 59:699–703.

Goble FC, Konopka EA. (1973). Sex as a factor in infectious disease. *Transactions of the New York Academy of Sciences*, 35:325–346.

Gomez E, Ortiz V, Saint-Martin B, Boeck L, Diaz-Sanchez V, Bourges H. (1993). Hormonal regulation of the secretory IgA (sIgA) system: estradiol- and progesterone-induced changes in sIgA in parotid saliva along the menstrual cycle. *Am J Reprod Immunol*, 29:219–223.

Graff RJ, Lappe MA, Snell GD. (1969). The influence of the gonads and adrenal glands on the immune response to skin grafts. *Transplantation*, 7:105–111.

Green PG, Dahlqvist SR, Isenberg WM, Strausbaugh HJ, Miao FJ, Levine JD. (1999). Sex steroid regulation of the inflammatory response: sympathoadrenal dependence in the female rat. *J Neurosci*, 19:4082–4089.

Grimaldi CM, Jeganathan V, Diamond B. (2006). Hormonal regulation of B cell development: 17beta-estradiol impairs negative selection of high-affinity DNA-reactive B cells at more than one developmental checkpoint. *J Immunol*, 176:2703–2710.

Grimaldi CM, Hill L, Xu X, Peeva E, Diamond B. (2005). Hormonal modulation of B cell development and repertoire selection. *Mol Immunol*, 42:811–820.

Grinspoon S. (2005). Androgen deficiency and HIV infection. *Clin Infect Dis*, 41:1804–1805.

Guilbault C, Stotland P, Lachance C, Tam M, Keller A, Thompson-Snipes L, Cowley E, et al. (2002). Influence of gender and interleukin-10 deficiency on the inflammatory response during lung infection with *Pseudomonas aeruginosa* in mice. *Immunology*, 107:297–305.

Guseva NV, Dessus-Babus SC, Whittimore JD, Moore CG, Wyrick PB. (2005). Characterization of estrogen-responsive epithelial cell lines and their infectivity by genital *Chlamydia trachomatis*. *Microbes Infect*, 7:1469–1481.

Han X, Lundberg P, Tanamachi B, Openshaw H, Longmate J, Cantin E. (2001). Gender influences herpes simplex virus type 1 infection in normal and gamma interferon-mutant mice. *J Virol*, 75:3048–3052.

Hanna N, Schneider M. (1983). Enhancement of tumor metastasis and suppression of natural killer cell activity by beta-estradiol treatment. *J Immunol*, 130:974–980.

Hansel NN, Merriman B, Haponik EF, Diette GB. (2004). Hospitalizations for tuberculosis in the United States in 2000: predictors of in-hospital mortality. *Chest*, 126:1079–1086.

Hawkins T, Gala RR, Dunbar JC. (1993). The effect of neonatal sex hormone manipulation on the incidence of diabetes in nonobese diabetic mice. *Proc Soc Exp Biol Med*, 202:201–205.

Hoffman K, Costello C, Menich M, Grabenstein JD, Engler RJ. (2003). Using a structured medical note for determining the safety profile of anthrax vaccine for US soldiers in Korea. *Vaccine*, 21:4399–4409.

Hofmann-Lehmann R, Holznagel E, Lutz H. (1998). Female cats have lower rates of apoptosis in peripheral blood lymphocytes than male cats: correlation with estradiol-17beta, but not with progesterone blood levels. *Vet Immunol Immunopathol*, 65:151–160.

Hou J, Zheng WF. (1988). Effect of sex hormones on NK and ADCC activity of mice. *Int J Immunopharmacol*, 10:15–22.

Huber SA. (2005). Increased susceptibility of male BALB/c mice to coxsackievirus B3-induced myocarditis: role for CD1d. *Med Microbiol Immunol*, (Berl) 194:121–127.

Huber SA, Pfaeffle B. (1994). Differential Th1 and Th2 cell responses in male and female BALB/c mice infected with coxsackievirus group B type 3. *J Virol*, 68:5126–5132.

Huber SA, Kupperman J, Newell MK. (1999). Hormonal regulation of CD4(+) T-cell responses in coxsackievirus B3-induced myocarditis in mice. *J Virol*, 73:4689–4695.

Jacobson DL, Gange SJ, Rose NR, Graham NM. (1997). Epidemiology and estimated population burden of selected autoimmune diseases in the United States. *Clin Immunol Immunopathol*, 84:223–243.

Jansson L, Olsson T, Holmdahl R. (1994). Estrogen induces a potent suppression of experimental autoimmune encephalomyelitis and collagen-induced arthritis in mice. *J Neuroimmunol*, 53:203–207.

Jimenez-Corona ME, Garcia-Garcia L, Deriemer K, Ferreyra-Reyes L, Bobadilla-Del-Valle M, et al. (2006). Gender differentials of pulmonary tuberculosis transmission and reactivation in an endemic area. *Thorax*, 61:348–353.

Jin HK, Yoshimatsu K, Takada A, Ogino M, Asano A, Arikawa J, Watanabe T. (2001). Mouse Mx2 protein inhibits hantavirus but not influenza virus replication. *Arch Virol*, 146:41–49.

Jones KJ, Alexander TD, Brown TJ, Tanzer L. (2000). Gonadal steroid enhancement of facial nerve regeneration: role of heat shock protein 70. *J Neurocytol*, 29:341–349.

Jones TC, Johnson WD, Jr., Barretto AC, Lago E, Badaro R, Cerf B, et al. (1987). Epidemiology of American cutaneous leishmaniasis due to *Leishmania braziliensis braziliensis*. *J Infect Dis*, 156:73–83.

Judson FN. (1990). Gonorrhea. *Med Clin North Am*, 74:1353–1366.

Kamis AB, Ibrahim JB. (1989). Effects of testosterone on blood leukocytes in *Plasmodium berghei*-infected mice. *Parasitol Res*, 75:611–613.

Kamis AB, Ahmad RA, Badrul-Munir MZ. (1992). Worm burden and leukocyte response in *Angiostrongylus malaysiensis*-infected rats: the influence of testosterone. *Parasitol Res*, 78:388–391.

Katagiri D, Hayashi H, Victoriano AF, Okamoto T, Onozaki K. (2006). Estrogen stimulates transcription of human immunodeficiency virus type 1 (HIV-1). *Int Immunopharmacol*, 6:170–181.

Khaiboullina SF, Rizvanov AA, Deyde VM, St Jeor SC. (2005). Andes virus stimulates interferon-inducible MxA protein expression in endothelial cells. *J Med Virol*, 75:267–275.

Kim S, Liva SM, Dalal MA, Verity MA, Voskuhl RR. (1999). Estriol ameliorates autoimmune demyelinating disease: implications for multiple sclerosis. *Neurology*, 52:1230–1238.

Kinsella K, Velkoff VA. (2001). An Aging World: 2001. In: (Bureau USC, ed): U.S. Government Printing Office.

Kita E, Yagyu Y, Nishikawa F, Hamuro A, Oku D, Emoto M, Katsui N, Kashiba S. (1989). Alterations of host resistance to mouse typhoid infection by sex hormones. *J Leukoc Biol*, 46:538–546.

Klein SL. (2000). The effects of hormones on sex differences in infection: from genes to behavior. *Neurosci Biobehav Rev*, 24:627–638.

Klein SL. (2004). Hormonal and immunological mechanisms mediating sex differences in parasite infection. *Parasite Immunol*, 26:247–264.

Klein SL, Bird BH, Glass GE. (2000). Sex differences in Seoul virus infection are not related to adult sex steroid concentrations in Norway rats. *J Virol*, 74:8213–8217.

Klein SL, Bird BH, Glass GE. (2001). Sex differences in immune responses and viral shedding following Seoul virus infection in Norway rats. *Am J Trop Med Hyg*, 65:57–63.

Klein SL, Hairston JE, Devries AC, Nelson RJ. (1997). Social environment and steroid hormones affect species and sex differences in immune function among voles. *Horm Behav*, 32:30–39.

Klein SL, Wisniewski AB, Marson AL, Glass GE, Gearhart JP. (2002a). Early exposure to genistein exerts long-lasting effects on the endocrine and immune systems in rats. *Mol Med*, 8:742–749.

Klein SL, Marson AL, Scott AL, Ketner G, Glass GE. (2002b). Neonatal sex steroids affect responses to Seoul virus infection in male but not female Norway rats. *Brain Behav Immun*, 16:736–746.

Klein SL, Cernetich A, Hilmer S, Hoffman EP, Scott AL, Glass GE. (2004). Differential expression of immunoregulatory genes in male and female Norway rats following infection with Seoul virus. *J Med Virol*, 74:180–190.

Knudsen KM, Aaby P, Whittle H, Rowe M, Samb B, Simondon F, Sterne J, Fine P. (1996). Child mortality following standard, medium or high titre measles immunization in West Africa. *Int J Epidemiol*, 25:665–673.

Komukai Y, Amao H, Goto N, Kusajima Y, Sawada T, Saito M, Takahashi KW. (1999). Sex differences in susceptibility of ICR mice to oral infection with *Corynebacterium kutscheri*. *Exp Anim*, 48:37–42.

Kono H, Wheeler MD, Rusyn I, Lin M, Seabra V, Rivera CA, et al. (2000). Gender differences in early alcohol-induced liver injury: role of CD14, NF-kappaB, and TNF-alpha. *Am J Physiol Gastrointest Liver Physiol*, 278:G652–661.

Krzych U, Strausser HR, Bressler JP, Goldstein AL. (1981). Effects of sex hormones on some T and B cell functions as evidenced by differential immune expression between male and female mice and cyclic pattern of immune responsiveness during the estrous cycle. *Prog Clin Biol Res*, 70:145–150.

Landgraf B, Kollaritsch H, Wiedermann G, Wernsdorfer WH. (1994). Parasite density of *Plasmodium falciparum* malaria in Ghanaian schoolchildren: evidence for influence of sex hormones? *Trans R Soc Trop Med Hyg*, 88:73–74.

Larralde C, Morales J, Terrazas I, Govezensky T, Romano MC. (1995). Sex hormone changes induced by the parasite lead to feminization of the male host in murine *Taenia crassiceps* cysticercosis. *J Steroid Biochem Mol Biol*, 52:575–580.

Laupland KB, Church DL, Mucenski M, Sutherland LR, Davies HD. (2003). Population-based study of the epidemiology of and the risk factors for invasive *Staphylococcus aureus* infections. *J Infect Dis*, 187:1452–1459.

Lenz F (1931). *Morbidic hereditary factors*. New York: Macmillan Press.

Liesenfeld O, Nguyen TA, Pharke C, Suzuki Y. (2001). Importance of gender and sex hormones in regulation of susceptibility of the small intestine to peroral infection with *Toxoplasma gondii* tissue cysts. *J Parasitol*, 87:1491–1493.

Little SF, Ivins BE, Webster WM, Fellows PF, Pitt ML, Norris SL, Andrews GP. (2006). Duration of protection of rabbits after vaccination with *Bacillus anthracis* recombinant protective antigen vaccine. *Vaccine*, 24:2530–2536.

Lu FX, Abel K, Ma Z, Rourke T, Lu D, Torten J, McChesney M, Miller CJ. (2002). The strength of B cell immunity in female rhesus macaques is controlled by CD8+ T cells under the influence of ovarian steroid hormones. *Clin Exp Immunol*, 128:10–20.

Luster MI, Hayes HT, Korach K, Tucker AN, Dean JH, Greenlee WF, Boorman GA. (1984). Estrogen immunosuppression is regulated through estrogenic responses in the thymus. *J Immunol*, 133:110–116.

Lyden DC, Olszewski J, Feran M, Job LP, Huber SA. (1987). Coxsackievirus B-3-induced myocarditis. Effect of sex steroids on viremia and infectivity of cardiocytes. *Am J Pathol*, 126:432–438.

Lynch NR, Yarzabal L, Verde O, Avila JL, Monzon H, Convit J. (1982). Delayed-type hypersensitivity and immunoglobulin E in American cutaneous leishmaniasis. *Infect Immun*, 38:877–881.

Marguerite M, Gallissot MC, Diagne M, Moreau C, Diakkhate MM, Roberts M, et al. (1999). Cellular immune responses of a Senegalese community recently exposed to *Schistosoma mansoni*: correlations of infection level with age and inflammatory cytokine production by soluble egg antigen-specific cells. *Trop Med Int Health*, 4:530–543.

McHugh RS, Whitters MJ, Piccirillo CA, Young DA, Shevach EM, Collins M, et al. (2002). CD4(+) CD25(+) immunoregulatory T cells: gene expression analysis reveals a functional role for the glucocorticoid-induced TNF receptor. *Immunity*, 16:311–323.

McKay LI, Cidlowski JA. (1999). Molecular control of immune/inflammatory responses: interactions between nuclear factor-kappa B and steroid receptor-signaling pathways. *Endocr Rev*, 20:435–459.

Miller L, Hunt JS. (1996). Sex steroid hormones and macrophage function. *Life Sci*, 59:1–14.

Miller L, Hunt JS (1998). Regulation of TNF-alpha production in activated mouse macrophages by progesterone. *J Immunol*, 160:5098–5104.

Miller L, Alley EW, Murphy WJ, Russell SW, Hunt JS. (1996). Progesterone inhibits inducible nitric oxide synthase gene expression and nitric oxide production in murine macrophages. *J Leukoc Biol*, 59:442–450.

Mills JN, Ksiazek TG, Ellis BA, Rollin PE, Nichol ST, Yates TL, et al. (1997). Patterns of association with host and habitat: antibody reactive with Sin Nombre virus in small mammals in the major biotic communities of the southwestern United States. *Am J Trop Med Hyg*, 56:273–284.

Mills JN, Johnson JM, Ksiazek TG, Ellis BA, Rollin PE, Yates TL, et al. (1998). A survey of hantavirus antibody in small-mammal populations in selected United States National Parks. *Am J Trop Med Hyg*, 58:525–532.

Mock BA, Nacy CA. (1988). Hormonal modulation of sex differences in resistance to *Leishmania major* systemic infections. *Infect Immun*, 56:3316–3319.

Molineaux L, Gramiccia G. (1979). The Garki project: research on the epidemiology and control of malaria in the Sudan Savannah of West Africa. In. Geneva: World Health Organization.

Mondal S, Rai U. (1999). Sexual dimorphism in phagocytic activity of wall lizard's splenic macrophages and its control by sex steroids. *Gen Comp Endocrinol*, 116:291–298.

Moore SL, Wilson K. (2002). Parasites as a viability cost of sexual selection in natural populations of mammals. *Science*, 297:2015–2018.

Morales-Montor J, Baig S, Hallal-Calleros C, Damian RT. (2002). *Taenia crassiceps*: androgen reconstitution of the host leads to protection during cysticercosis. *Exp Parasitol*, 100:209–216.

Morrow RH, Kisuule A, Pike MC, Smith PG. (1976). Burkitt's lymphoma in the Mengo districts of Uganda: epidemiologic features and their relationship to malaria. *J Natl Cancer Inst*, 56:479–483.

Mwatha JK, Kimani G, Kamau T, Mbugua GG, Ouma JH, Mumo J, et al. (1998). High levels of TNF, soluble TNF receptors, soluble ICAM-1, and IFN-gamma, but low levels of IL-5, are associated with hepatosplenic disease in human schistosomiasis mansoni. *J Immunol*, 160:1992–1999.

Napravnik S, Poole C, Thomas JC, Eron JJ, Jr. (2002). Gender difference in HIV RNA levels: a meta-analysis of published studies. *J Acquir Immune Defic Syndr*, 31:11–19.

Naus CW, Booth M, Jones FM, Kemijumbi J, Vennervald BJ, Kariuki CH, Ouma JH, et al. (2003). The relationship between age, sex, egg-count and specific antibody responses against *Schistosoma mansoni* antigens in a Ugandan fishing community. *Trop Med Int Health*, 8:561–568.

Olsen NJ, Kovacs WJ. (1996). Gonadal steroids and immunity. *Endocr Rev*, 17:369–384.

Owens IP. (2002). Ecology and evolution. Sex differences in mortality rate. *Science*, 297:2008–2009.

Paharkova-Vatchkova V, Maldonado R, Kovats S. (2004). Estrogen preferentially promotes the differentiation of CD11c+ CD11b(intermediate) dendritic cells from bone marrow precursors. *J Immunol*, 172:1426–1436.

Palaszynski KM, Loo KK, Ashouri JF, Liu HB, Voskuhl RR. (2004). Androgens are protective in experimental autoimmune encephalomyelitis: implications for multiple sclerosis. *J Neuroimmunol*, 146:144–152.

Palaszynski KM, Smith DL, Kamrava S, Burgoyne PS, Arnold AP, Voskuhl RR. (2005). A yin-yang effect between sex chromosome complement and sex hormones on the immune response. *Endocrinology*, 146:3280–3285.

Peeva E, Venkatesh J, Diamond B. (2005). Tamoxifen blocks estrogen-induced B cell maturation but not survival. *J Immunol*, 175:1415–1423.

Phillips AN, Antunes F, Stergious G, Ranki A, Jensen GF, Bentwich Z, et al. (1994). A sex comparison of rates of new AIDS-defining disease and death in 2554 AIDS cases. AIDS in Europe Study Group. *AIDS*, 8:831–835.

Piccinni MP, Scaletti C, Maggi E, Romagnani S. (2000). Role of hormone-controlled Th1- and Th2-type cytokines in successful pregnancy. *J Neuroimmunol*, 109:30–33.

Piccinni MP, Giudizi MG, Biagiotti R, Beloni L, Giannarini L, Sampognaro S, et al. (1995) Progesterone favors the development of human T helper cells producing Th2-type cytokines and promotes both IL-4 production and membrane CD30 expression in established Th1 cell clones. *J Immunol*, 155:128–133.

Polanczyk MJ, Carson BD, Subramanian S, Afentoulis M, Vandenbark AA, Ziegler SF, Offner H. (2004). Cutting edge: estrogen drives expansion of the CD4+CD25+ regulatory T cell compartment. *J Immunol*, 173:2227–2230.

Pung OJ, Luster MI. (1986). *Toxoplasma gondii*: decreased resistance to infection in mice due to estrogen. *Exp Parasitol*, 61:48–56.

Pung OJ, Tucker AN, Vore SJ, Luster MI. (1985). Influence of estrogen on host resistance: increased susceptibility of mice to *Listeria monocytogenes* correlates with depressed production of interleukin 2. *Infect Immun*, 50:91–96.

Purtilo DT, Sullivan JL. (1979). Immunological bases for superior survival of females. *Am J Dis Child*, 133:1251–1253.

Putnam P. (1927). Sex differences in pulmonary tuberculosis deaths. *The American Journal of Hygiene*, 7:663–705.

Quinn TC, Overbaugh J. (2005). HIV/AIDS in women: an expanding epidemic. *Science*, 308:1582–1583.

Remoue F, Mani JC, Pugniere M, Schacht AM, Capron A, Riveau G. (2002). Functional specific binding of testosterone to *Schistosoma haematobium* 28-kilodalton glutathione S-transferase. *Infect Immun*, 70:601–605.

Remoue F, To Van D, Schacht AM, Picquet M, Garraud O, Vercruysse J, et al. (2001). Gender-dependent specific immune response during chronic human *Schistosomiasis haematobia*. *Clin Exp Immunol*, 124:62–68.

Roberts CW, Cruickshank SM, Alexander J. (1995). Sex-determined resistance to *Toxoplasma gondii* is associated with temporal differences in cytokine production. *Infect Immun*, 63:2549–2555.

Roberts CW, Walker W, Alexander J. (2001). Sex-associated hormones and immunity to protozoan parasites. *Clin Microbiol Rev*, 14:476–488.

Roberts M, Alexander J, Blackwell JM. (1990). Genetic analysis of *Leishmania mexicana* infection in mice: single gene (Scl-2) controlled predisposition to cutaneous lesion development. *J Immunogenet*, 17:89–100.

Root JJ, Calisher CH, Beaty BJ. (1999). Relationships of deer mouse movement, vegetative structure, and prevalence of infection with Sin Nombre virus. *J Wildl Dis*, 35:311–318.

Roubinian JR, Talal N, Greenspan JS, Goodman JR, Siiteri PK. (1978). Effect of castration and sex hormone treatment on survival, anti-nucleic acid antibodies, and glomerulonephritis in NZB/NZW F1 mice. *J Exp Med*, 147:1568–1583.

Sanni LA, Fonseca LF, Langhorne J. (2002). Mouse models for erythrocytic-stage malaria. *Methods Mol Med*, 72:57–76.

Satoskar A, Alexander J. (1995). Sex-determined susceptibility and differential IFN-gamma and TNF-alpha mRNA expression in DBA/2 mice infected with *Leishmania mexicana*. *Immunology*, 84:1–4.

Satoskar A, Al-Quassi HH, Alexander J. (1998). Sex-determined resistance against *Leishmania mexicana* is associated with the preferential induction of a Th1-like response and IFN-gamma production by female but not male DBA/2 mice. *Immunol Cell Biol*, 76:159–166.

Savita, Rai U. (1998). Sex steroid hormones modulate the activation of murine peritoneal macrophages: receptor mediated modulation. *Comp Biochem Physiol C Pharmacol Toxicol Endocrinol*, 119:199–204.

Schuurs AH, Verheul HA. (1990). Effects of gender and sex steroids on the immune response. *J Steroid Biochem*, 35:157–172.

Shiddo SA, Aden Mohamed A, Akuffo HO, Mohamud KA, Herzi AA, Herzi Mohamed H, et al. (1995). Visceral leishmaniasis in Somalia: prevalence of markers of infection and disease manifestations in a village in an endemic area. *Trans R Soc Trop Med Hyg*, 89:361–365.

Shiff CJ, Cmelik SH, Ley HE, Kriel RL. (1972). The influence of human skin lipids on the cercarial penetration responses of *Schistosoma haematobium* and *Schistosoma mansoni*. *J Parasitol*, 58:476–480.

Shim GJ, Gherman D, Kim HJ, Omoto Y, Iwase H, Bouton D, et al. (2006). Differential expression of oestrogen receptors in human secondary lymphoid tissues. *J Pathol*, 208:408–414.

Sonnex C. (1998). Influence of ovarian hormones on urogenital infection. *Sex Transm Infect*, 74:11–19.

Sorachi K, Kumagai S, Sugita M, Yodoi J, Imura H. (1993). Enhancing effect of 17 beta-estradiol on human NK cell activity. *Immunol Lett*, 36:31–35.

Souza SS, Castro FA, Mendonca HC, Palma PV, Morais FR, Ferriani RA, et al. (2001). Influence of menstrual cycle on NK activity. *J Reprod Immunol*, 50:151–159.

Spitzer JA. (1999). Gender differences in some host defense mechanisms. *Lupus*, 8:380–383.

Stephenson J. (2000). Genital herpes vaccine shows limited promise. *JAMA*, 284:1913–1914.

Sterling TR, Vlahov D, Astemborski J, Hoover DR, Margolick JB, Quinn TC. (2001). Initial plasma HIV-1 RNA levels and progression to AIDS in women and men. *N Engl J Med*, 344:720–725.

Sutherland JS, Goldberg GL, Hammett MV, Uldrich AP, Berzins SP, Heng TS, et al. (2005). Activation of thymic regeneration in mice and humans following androgen blockade. *J Immunol*, 175:2741–2753.

Taylor-Robinson D, Furr PM, Hetherington CM. (1990). *Neisseria gonorrhoeae* colonises the genital tract of oestradiol-treated germ-free female mice. *Microb Pathog*, 9:369–373.

Teichmann J, Schmidt A, Lange U, Stracke H, Discher T, Friese G, et al. (2003). Longitudinal evaluation of serum estradiol and estrone in male patients infected with the human immunodeficiency virus. *Eur J Med* Res, 8:77–80.

Temonen M, Lankinen H, Vapalahti O, Ronni T, Julkunen I, Vaheri A. (1995). Effect of interferon-alpha and cell differentiation on Puumala virus infection in human monocyte/macrophages. *Virology*, 206:8–15.

Terrazas LI, Bojalil R, Govezensky T, Larralde C. (1994). A role for 17-beta-estradiol in immunoendocrine regulation of murine cysticercosis (*Taenia crassiceps*). *J Parasitol*, 80:563–568.

Terrazas LI, Bojalil R, Govezensky T, Larralde C. (1998). Shift from an early protective Th1-type immune response to a late permissive Th2-type response in murine cysticercosis (*Taenia crassiceps*). *J Parasitol*, 84:74–81.

Tiuria R, Horii Y, Tateyama S, Tsuchiya K, Nawa Y. (1994). The Indian soft-furred rat, *Millardia meltada*, a new host for *Nippostrongylus brasiliensis*, showing androgen-dependent sex difference in intestinal mucosal defence. *Int J Parasitol*, 24:1055–1057.

Toder V, Nebel L, Elrad H, Blank M, Durdana A, Gleicher N. (1984). Studies of natural killer cells in pregnancy. II. The immunoregulatory effect of pregnancy substances. *J Clin Lab Immunol*, 14:129–133.

Vegeto E, Pollio G, Pellicciari C, Maggi A. (1999). Estrogen and progesterone induction of survival of monoblastoid cells undergoing TNF-alpha-induced apoptosis. *FASEB J*, 13:793–803.

Wald A. (2004). Herpes simplex virus type 2 transmission: risk factors and virus shedding. *Herpes*, 11(Suppl 3):130A–137A.

Walker W, Roberts CW, Ferguson DJ, Jebbari H, Alexander J. (1997). Innate immunity to *Toxoplasma gondii* is influenced by gender and is associated with differences in interleukin-12 and gamma interferon production. *Infect Immun*, 65:1119–1121.

Webster JI, Tonelli LH, Moayeri M, Simons SS, Jr., Leppla SH, Sternberg EM. (2003). Anthrax lethal factor represses glucocorticoid and progesterone receptor activity. *Proc Natl Acad Sci U S A*, 100:5706–5711.

Webster M, Libranda-Ramirez BD, Aligui GD, Olveda RM, Ouma JH, Kariuki HC, et al. (1997). The influence of sex and age on antibody isotype responses to *Schistosoma mansoni* and *Schistosoma japonicum* in human populations in Kenya and the Philippines. *Parasitology*, 114 (Pt 4):383–393.

Weigle KA, Santrich C, Martinez F, Valderrama L, Saravia NG. (1993). Epidemiology of cutaneous leishmaniasis in Colombia: environmental and behavioral risk factors for infection, clinical manifestations, and pathogenicity. *J Infect Dis*, 168:709–714.

Weigler BJ, Ksiazek TG, Vandenbergh JG, Levin M, Sullivan WT. (1996). Serological evidence for zoonotic hantaviruses in North Carolina rodents. *J Wildl Dis*, 32:354–357.

Weinstein Y, Ran S, Segal S. (1984). Sex-associated differences in the regulation of immune responses controlled by the MHC of the mouse. *J Immunol*, 132:656–661.

Whitacre CC. (2001). Sex differences in autoimmune disease. *Nat Immunol*, 2:777–780.

White DJ, Means RG, Birkhead GS, Bosler EM, Grady LJ, Chatterjee N, et al. (1996). Human and rodent hantavirus infection in New York State: public health significance of an emerging infectious disease. *Arch Intern Med*, 156:722–726.

WHOSIS. (2005). Number and rates of registered deaths. In: www.who.int/whosis.

Wildling E, Winkler S, Kremsner PG, Brandts C, Jenne L, Wernsdorfer WH. (1995). Malaria epidemiology in the province of Moyen Ogoov, Gabon. *Trop Med Parasitol*, 46:77–82.

Williams RJ, Bryan RT, Mills JN, Palma RE, Vera I, De Velasquez F, et al. (1997). An outbreak of hantavirus pulmonary syndrome in western Paraguay. *Am J Trop Med Hyg*, 57:274–282.

Wizemann TM, Pardue, M., (Ed.). (2001). *Exploring the biological contributions to human health: does sex matter?* Washington DC: National Academy Press.

Wolfe J, Proctor SP, Erickson DJ, Hu H. (2002). Risk factors for multisymptom illness in US Army veterans of the Gulf War. *J Occup Environ Med*, 44:271–281.

Wong T, Singh A, Mann J, Hansen L, McMahon S. (2004). Gender differences in bacterial STIs in Canada. *BMC Womens Health*, 4(Suppl 1):S26.

Wunderlich F, Maurin W, Benten WP, Schmitt-Wrede HP. (1993). Testosterone impairs efficacy of protective vaccination against *P. chabaudi* malaria. *Vaccine*, 11:1097–1099.

Wunderlich F, Marinovski P, Benten WP, Schmitt-Wrede HP, Mossmann H. (1991). Testosterone and other gonadal factor(s) restrict the efficacy of genes controlling resistance to *Plasmodium chabaudi* malaria. *Parasite Immunol*, 13:357–367.

Wunderlich F, Benten WP, Lieberherr M, Guo Z, Stamm O, Wrehlke C, et al. (2002). Testosterone signaling in T cells and macrophages. *Steroids*, 67:535–538.

Yamamoto Y, Saito H, Setogawa T, Tomioka H. (1991). Sex differences in host resistance to *Mycobacterium marinum* infection in mice. *Infect Immun*, 59: 4089–4096.

Yovel G, Shakhar K, Ben-Eliyahu S. (2001). The effects of sex, menstrual cycle, and oral contraceptives on the number and activity of natural killer cells. *Gynecol Oncol*, 81:254–262.

Yu CY, Whitacre CC. (2004). Sex, MHC and complement C4 in autoimmune diseases. *Trends Immunol*, 25:694–699.

Zhang Z, Chen L, Saito S, Kanagawa O, Sendo F. (2000). Possible modulation by male sex hormone of Th1/Th2 function in protection against *Plasmodium chabaudi chabaudi* AS infection in mice. *Exp Parasitol*, 96:121–129.

Zuk M. (1990). Reproductive strategies and disease susceptibility: an evolutionary viewpoint. *Parasitol Today*, 6:231–233.

Zuk M, McKean KA. (1996). Sex differences in parasite infections: patterns and processes. *Int J Parasitol*, 26:1009–1023.

Chapter 18

Sex Differences in Neuroimmunology

Steven S. Zalcman

Initially a fledgling field of study with a unique focus, neuroimmunology has become an expansive multi-disciplinary area of research. Accordingly, the term *neuroimmunology* means different things to different people. The present chapter uses as its center the Besedovsky model of neuroimmune interactions: During the course of an orchestrated immune response, immune-derived messengers induce changes in neural activity that in turn modulates the ongoing response (Besedovsky & del Rey, 1996). This model permits an analysis of: (a) the effects of immunogenic substances and immune messengers (notably cytokines) on neurotransmitter and neuroendocrine activity, and behavior; and (b) the immunomodulatory effects of the hypothalamic-pituitary-adrenal (HPA)-axis and sympathetic nervous system (Figure 18.1).

Major historical shifts have resulted from this perspective. For example, the brain is no longer viewed as being completely immune privileged. Thus, the doors have opened for studies examining the ability of pathogens, immune cells, antibody molecules, and cytokines to enter the brain and potently modulate neurotransmitter function, neuroendocrine activity, and behavior (Banks, 2006). Indeed, it has become clear that substances (notably cytokines) produced by cells of the immune system are also produced in the brain where they act as potent neuromodulators in immune-dependent and immune-independent manners (Maier et al., 2001). In parallel, this model has stimulated studies examining central nervous system (CNS) regulation of peripheral immunity.

It has become increasingly clear that gonadal hormones play principal roles in mediating reciprocal interactions between the immune and central nervous systems. The following review will focus on aspects of neuroimmune interactions shown to be sexually dimorphic. This includes interactions between immunogenic substances, cytokines, and neuroendocrine hormones, CNS abnormalities associated with immune activation, the relationship between stress, development and immunity, and behavioral changes associated with immune responding.

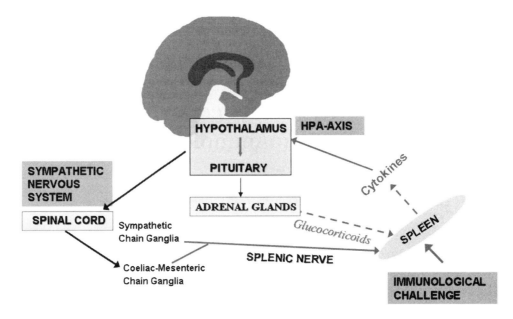

Figure 18.1. Schematic diagram illustrating neuroimmune interactions. Diagram shows bi-directional communication between the brain and immune system during an orchestrated immune response. Following immunological challenge, an immune response is mounted in lymphoid organs (e.g., spleen). Cytokines released during the response induce changes in neural activity, which in turn activate the HPA-axis and sympathetic outflow to lymphoid organs. In the former regard, glucocorticoids released by the adrenal glands serve to modulate (notably suppress) an ongoing immune response. The sympathetic nervous system (e.g., via the splenic nerve, which is formed when the sympathetic chain ganglia and coeliac-mesenteric chain ganglia unite) also mediates neuroimmune interactions. Dotted lines represent humoral factors, including cytokines (which may directly or indirectly influence brain activity) and glucocorticoids.

SEXUAL DIMORPHISM IN THE IMMUNE-NEUROENDOCRINE RELATIONSHIP

A fundamental tenet of neuroimmunology is that a negative feedback loop exists between the brain and immune system that regulates an ongoing orchestrated immune response (Besedovsky & del Rey, 1996). An essential component of this regulatory loop is the HPA axis. Increases in HPA axis activity during an immune response can have immuno-enhancing or -suppressive effects (Guyre et al., 1984; Dhabhar & McEwen, 1999; Silverman et al., 2005). Immune cells bear glucocorticoid receptors, the stimulation of which can up- or down-regulate immune function. With regard to negative feedback loops, relatively high levels of corticosterone or cortisol inhibit immune function. Thus, an important role of HPA activation following immunological challenge is suppression of an ongoing immune response. This serves an adaptive purpose since an unrestrained immune response would be expected to result in autoimmune phenomena (Theophilopoulos, 1995).

The HPA axis interacts with the hypothalamic-pituitary-gonadal (HPG) axis to regulate sex steroid hormone production. Conversely, sex hormones play important roles in regulating HPA activity. Of further importance, a close relationship exists between immune responding, HPA-axis activity and sex steroid hormones. Indeed, the HPA-axis and the HPG-axis play fundamental roles in immune system development and in regulating immune function (Morale et al., 2001). Thus, considerable attention has focused on the relationship between immune responding and neuroendocrine hormones.

The immune–neuroendocrine relationship has been extensively studied using endotoxin/LPS challenge. In this section, I will briefly summarize this model. This will be followed by a discussion of representative findings of sexual dimorphism in neuroendocrine alterations induced by LPS challenge or proinflammatory cytokine administration, and the role of sex steroid hormones in mediating such effects.

The Endotoxin—LPS Model

Endotoxin and LPS are often used synonymously to refer to a structural component of the cell wall of Gram-negative bacteria (e.g., *E. coli*, *Salmonella*). LPS is released when bacteria are lysed, and plays fundamental roles in the pathogenesis of Gram-negative bacterial infections (e.g., it mediates pathogen-host interactions) (Ulevitch et al., 2004; Miller et al., 2005).

When bacteria are lysed, LPS is released into the bloodstream and binds lipid proteins, which in turn, interact with CD14 receptors on monocytes and macrophages. CD14 receptors, via MD2 proteins, interact with toll-like receptor-4 to stimulate macrophages (and endothelial cells) to produce and release proinflammatory cytokines, notably IL-1β, IL-6, IL-8, TNFα, and interferon (IFN)γ. Proinflammatory cytokines stimulate production of prostaglandins and leukotrienes. The end results of these actions include inflammation, fever, as well as neuroendocrine and behavioral alterations. In addition to its peripheral effects, LPS stimulates proinflammatory cytokine activity in brain (Rivest, 2003). Experimentally, LPS can be injected in purified form to induce a spectrum of immunophysiological and behavioral changes that are characteristic of Gram-negative bacterial infections.

LPS-induced Alterations
of Neuroendocrine Activity

LPS potently activates the HPA axis (Turnbull & Rivier, 1995; Dantzer et al., 1999; Beishuizen & Thijs, 2003). There is an increasing amount of evidence indicating that HPA responses to LPS challenge are sexually dimorphic. For example, increases in plasma ACTH and corticosterone levels following exposure to endotoxin are more pronounced in randomly cycling female rats than male rats (Spinedi et al., 1992; da Silva et al., 1993; Rivier, 1994; Watonobe et al., 1996).

LPS-induced corticosterone increases are further augmented in ovariectomized mice and rats (Spinedi et al., 1992; da Silva et al., 1993; Rivier, 1994). HPA responses of ovariectomized females receiving progesterone do not appreciably differ from those of intact females, however (da Silva et al., 1993). The investigators also showed that gonadectomy enhances inflammation-induced corticosterone variations in males, and that this effect is blocked by administration of 5 alpha-dihydrotestosterone. In contrast with the effects of gonadectomy on LPS-induced increases in corticosterone levels, ovariectomy attenuates LPS-induced increases in ACTH in female rats, and ovariectomy with estrogen $(E)_2$ supplementation eliminates these increases in ACTH (Watanobe & Yoneda, 2003). In males, testosterone replacement restores LPS-induced ACTH alterations.

Thus, there is a consensus that LPS-induced increases in HPA axis activity are sexually dimorphic, and mediated by sex steroid hormones. However, whereas LPS-induced increases in corticosterone concentrations are enhanced by gonadectomy, ACTH responses are attenuated by this treatment. It remains to be determined whether these differential effects are due to differences in LPS-induced alterations in ACTH and corticosterone levels, or to organismic variables such as species and strain of animal used across studies (see Watonobe & Yoneda, 2003). In the latter regard, Frederic et al. (1993) underscored the importance of genetic factors by showing that gonadectomy attenuates LPS-induced increases in corticosterone levels in C57Bl/6 mice but not in CBA mice. It is also important to consider that neuroendocrine responses to LPS may vary across developmental periods, and that this occurs in a sexually dimorphic manner. For example, Spinedi et al. (1997) found that whereas juvenile female rats showed a hyporesponsive HPA response to LPS challenge, no effect was observed in males. Of further significance, maximal responses to LPS peaked by postnatal day 30 in males, and by day 45 in females (i.e., after puberty).

Sex differences in these responses also persist beyond puberty: among 15-month-old mice, female HPA responses to LPS exceed male responses (Suescun et al., 1994). It is important to note that sex differences in basal levels of corticosterone and ACTH were also noted at this and other developmental periods. This was attributed to the fact that estradiol enhances and testosterone suppresses HPA function. The fact that the immune and neuroendocrine systems interact during various developmental stages suggests that alterations in one system could have long-lasting consequences on the other system. Thus, altered immunity during critical developmental periods could result in alterations in neuroendocrine activity in adulthood.

In support of this hypothesis, adult rats that were exposed to LPS within 5 days of birth showed increases in circulating ACTH and corticosterone levels as well as potentiated HPA responses following stressor exposure (Shanks et al., 1994, 1995). In the latter regard, it was suggested that the potentiated HPA responses were related to altered negative feedback sensitivity to glucocorticoids. Since there were sex differences in basal levels of CRH in the median eminence and paraventricular nucleus of the hypothalamus, it is possible that different mechanisms mediated this effect in males and females. Of further importance, neonatal gonadectomy (2 days prior to LPS challenge) differentially influenced HPA measures in males and females. Specifically, LPS-induced increases in ACTH and corticosterone levels were attenuated in females. In males, gonadectomy resulted in a potentiation of corticosterone, while ACTH levels were unaffected. Moreover, adult female rats that received LPS during early life also showed increases in testosterone levels, insulin sensitivity, locomotor activity, and glucocorticoid receptor densities in the hypothalamus (Nilsson et al., 2001). The fact that basal levels of hormones are altered by neonatal LPS challenge suggests that organizational changes are engendered by this treatment.

Along the same lines, adult offspring of mothers exposed to LPS during pregnancy show a range of physiological and endocrine abnormalities that vary among males and females. For example, increased basal levels of corticosterone and testosterone were increased in female offspring (Nilsson et al., 2001). Male offspring displayed elevated levels of 17β-estradiol, progesterone leptin, as well as increased body weight and food intake. Males also showed a reduced corticosterone response to stressor exposure coupled with an upregulation of hippocampal glucocorticoid receptor protein. Thus, exposure to LPS during critical developmental periods can result in long-term sexually dimorphic abnormalities in HPA axis activity. More research is needed to explore these effects, particularly in light of disorders associated with in utero or neonatal exposure to infectious agents.

Cytokine-induced Alterations of Neuroendocrine Activity

Proinflammatory cytokines (notably IL-1β, TNFα, and IL-6) released following LPS challenge also stimulate HPA axis activity. Thus, it is thought that they play important roles in mediating subsequent alterations of HPA axis activity (see Dantzer et al., 1999; Rivest, 2003) as well as LPS-induced behavioral changes (see section Sex Differences in Behavioral and Physiological Alterations Associated with Immune Activation, in this chapter). However, these cytokines are not equipotent in stimulating HPA activity: IL-1β induces the most potent effects, followed by TNFα and IL-6 (Besedovsky et al., 1985; Dunn, 1992; Zalcman et al., 1994; see Dunn, 2000).

Considerable attention has focused on IL-1β as a prime mediator of LPS-induced alterations of HPA activity. There are parallels in the abilities of LPS and IL-1β to stimulate HPA axis activity. Of unique importance, IL-1β like LPS, stimulates HPA activity in a sexually dimorphic manner. For example, female HPA responses to an injection of LPS exceed those of males. As well, IL-1β-induced increases in corticosterone concentrations are further augmented by gonadectomy (Spinedi et al., 1992; Lee & Rivier, 1993; Rivier, 1994; but see da Silva et al., 1993).

In light of these findings, it is not surprising that estradiol (E$_2$) replacement attenuates IL-1β-induced stimulation of the HPA-axis (Xiao et al., 2000). It is also important to note that sex differences in HPA responses to IL-1β vary across stages of sexual maturation. For example, plasma ACTH levels are increased by IL-1β administration (0.5 or 2.0 micrograms/kg) in immature (21 to 22-day-old) male and female rats (Rivier, 1994). Females show more pronounced increases in corticosterone levels, but only to the 0.5 dose (possibly owing to ceiling effects at the higher dose). A similar sexual dimorphism is evident in forty- and seventy day-old animals.

TNFα and IL-6 are also thought to play roles in mediating LPS-induced stimulation of the HPA axis. There are few studies examining sex differences in the HPA consequences of these cytokines, however. Nonetheless, Watanobe (2002) showed that ACTH and corticosterone responses to an injection of TNFα, like IL-1β, were higher in females than males. In contrast, no sex differences were associated with IL-6-induced increases in these measures. Silva et al. (2002) similarly found that men and women had similar cortisol responses to an injection of IL-6. Curiously, a sex difference was found with respect to ACTH production, which was higher in men, suggesting that there are sex differences in the sensitivity of the adrenal glands to IL-6 (Silva et al., 2002).

It is also important to note that sex steroid hormones mediate effects of IL-6 on HPA activity. Xiao et al. (2001) showed in ovariectomized female rhesus monkeys that IL-6-induced increases in ACTH levels are further augmented by E_2. In contrast, testosterone attenuated the HPA activating effects of IL-6 (Papadopoulos & Wardlaw, 2000).

Thus, there is limited evidence that the effects of TNFα and IL-6 on HPA axis activity are sexually differentiated. However, this does not preclude a role for these cytokines (along with IL-1β) in mediating the sexually dimorphic effects of LPS on HPA axis activity. As mentioned, IL-1β's effects on HPA-activity are reduced by E_2 replacement (Xiao et al., 2001), whereas IL-6's effects are further augmented by E_2. The fact that E_2 differentially affects IL-1β- and IL-6-induced HPA variations raises the possibility that these cytokines modulate each other's effects through negative feedback loops. This notion is supported but the finding that IL-1β-induced increases in ACTH levels occurred coincident with a suppression of IL-6 (Xiao et al., 2001). Based on these observations, these authors suggested that IL-1β-induced increases in ACTH are related to E_2's inhibitory effects on IL-6 release.

Inasmuch as neuroimmune feedback loops modulate peripheral cytokine activity, it should also be considered that the central response to peripheral proinflammatory cytokines released following LPS plays an important role in mediating subsequent stimulation of the HPA axis. Intriguing support for this hypothesis stems from a study by Watanobe and Yoneda (2003) who showed that altering the sex steroid hormone milieu results in an increase in the number of IL-1β and TNF-α binding sites in mediobasal hypothalamus. The direction of these effects paralleled the LPS-induced ACTH response. Thus, it was suggested that sexually dimorphic HPA responses to LPS are related to the sensitivity of the hypothalamus to peripheral proinflammatory cytokines (i.e., IL-1β and TNF-α) that are released following LPS challenge, and to levels of circulating sex steroids.

To be sure, more research is needed to unravel the role of peripheral and central proinflammatory cytokines in mediating sexually dimorphic effects of LPS on HPA axis activity. Nonetheless, the mentioned studies underscore the need to consider that complex interactions between cytokine-ergic feedback loops and sex steroid hormone regulation of brain cytokine activity play important roles. Studies of adaptive alterations of neuroendocrine activity (and behavior) during the course of an orchestrated immune response and following cytokine challenge have stimulated further work assessing the contribution of immune elements to psychiatric abnormalities (e.g., depression) and immunologically based disorders (e.g., autoimmunity). It should also be emphasized that because cytokine administration influences HPA activity in the absence of an ongoing immune response, their HPA (and other) effects are not uniquely associated with responses to infectious agents.

Neuroendocrine Hormones, Gonadal Steroids and Autoimmunity

As mentioned, glucocorticoids serve to down regulate an ongoing immune response. Thus, blunted HPA activity would be expected to result in enhanced immune activity. This, in turn, would favor the development and expression of autoimmune phenomena (i.e., immune responses directed against the self). As discussed, HPA responses to LPS challenge or proinflammatory cytokine administration are more robust in females than males. It is thought that this augmented response helps to restrain the potentiated immune response in females. It follows, however, that blunted HPA responses would favor enhanced immunity and thus, development and expression of autoimmune phenomena.

The incidence of autoimmune disorders is higher in women than men. Studies have shown that reduced levels of circulating glucocorticoids are evident in individuals with autoimmune disorders (e.g., rheumatoid arthritis, systemic lupus erythematosus; see Chrousos, 1995; Harbuz, 2002; Tonelli et al., 2001). In parallel, blunted HPA responses (including changes in corticosterone, ACTH, and central corticotropin releasing hormone (CRH)) are evident in strains of animals predisposed to developing autoimmune disorders(e.g., Lewis (LEW/N) rats (see Tonelli et al., 2001).

The fact that autoimmune disorders are more prevalent in females implies that gonadal hormones play a role. An intriguing hypothesis by Marques-Deak and colleagues (2005) suggested that developmental alterations in the relative expression of glucocorticoid and estrogen receptors might predispose females to autoimmune disorders. The rationale for this proposal is that before puberty, glucocorticoid receptor expression predominates and favors immunosuppressive effects. However, B cell expression of ERα and ERβ, which is associated with immunoenhancing effects, is increased in post-pubertal females. Thus, it was suggested that a shift from a predominance of pre-pubertal glucocorticoid receptors to post-pubertal estrogen receptors favors an immunoenhancement and thus, an increased vulnerability to auto-immune phenomena (see Marques-Deak et al., 2005).

It should also be considered that interplay between systems that regulate peripheral immunity contributes to the development and expression of autoimmune conditions. The sympathetic nervous system plays a major role in mediating neuroimmune interactions (Williams et al., 1981; Nance et al., 1987; MacNeil et al., 1996; see Sanders & Munson, 1985; Felten et al., 1987; Sanders et al., 2001; Bellinger et al., 2001). It is thus of unique interest that important interactions occur between glucocorticoids, catecholamines, and cytokines, which in turn are thought to influence the development of autoimmune disorders (Sundar et al., 1990; Brown et al., 1991; Zalcman et al., 1994; see Bellinger et al., 1992; Elenkov et al., 2000). The extent to which interactions between gonadal hormones and the sympathetic nervous system contributes to autoimmune phenomena remains to be determined.

SEX DIFFERENCES IN DEVELOPMENT, STRESS, AND INFLAMMATION

It has become increasingly clear that pre- or postnatal exposure to environmental stimuli (notably infectious agents and stressful events) can produce long-lasting changes in immunity. In the present section, I will briefly discuss evidence that such effects, including variations in T cell activity, natural killer (NK) cell activity, and neuroinflammation are sexually differentiated.

Development, Stress, and Immunity

As discussed earlier, pre- or postnatal exposure to bacterial endotoxin results in long-lasting and sexually differentiated alterations in HPA-axis activity. There is evidence that LPS challenge during critical developmental periods also produces long-lasting immuno-logical changes in a sexually dimorphic manner. For example, Hodgson et al. (2002) showed that LPS challenge during the first week post-partum resulted in suppressed NK cell activity and increased tumor metastases in chronically stressed male, but not female Fischer 344 rats.

Other early life events may also produce long-lasting and sexually dimorphic alterations in immune responsivity. Hermes et al. (2005) showed that a complex interaction occurs between development, stressor exposure, gender, and granuloma formation. The authors used carrageenin (seaweed) to produce a granuloma. The inflammatory response is characterized by macrophage and neutrophil activity and the actions of proinflammatory cytokines (notably IL-1 and TNF).

First, the authors showed that long-term social isolation similarly delayed carrageenin-induced granuloma in male and female rats. However, there were sex differences in inflammatory responses to additional exposure to an acute stressor (restraint), with female responses being more robust than male responses. Inasmuch as the end result of this response is tissue healing, these findings have important implications on the effects of long- and short-term stressors on resilience to immunologically based disorders.

The authors suggested that these findings could help explain increases in disease vulnerability and mortality in men with low levels of social integration. Inasmuch as female responses were potentiated compared to male responses, these findings may also have important implications for the increased prevalence of autoimmune disorders in women. Indeed, as the authors point out, autoimmune rats show enhanced inflammatory responses to carrageenin exposure.

The immunological consequences of stressor exposure in adults may also be compromised in a sexually dimorphic manner by other environmental manipulations during critical developmental periods. For example, Giberson and Weinberg (1995) showed that the number of thymic and blood pan T cells and blood CD4+ T cells were reduced in chronically stressed offspring of mothers that received ethanol prenatally. This effect was most pronounced in male offspring. These findings are consistent with those of Redei et al. (1993) who showed that in utero exposure to alcohol induces a long lasting reduction in mitogen-induced T cell proliferation in pre- and peripubertal male offspring but not in female offspring. Of further significance, these effects were inhibited by maternal adrenalectomy.

Together, these studies show that different environmental challenges (bacterial endotoxin, social isolation, and ethanol) during critical pre- or postnatal periods can produce long-lasting and sexually dimorphic changes in vulnerability to stressor-induced alterations of immunity. The extents to which given sex differences are activational in nature or whether they also reflect organizational effects remain to be elucidated. Parenthetically, inasmuch as certain cytokines that mediate the individual's response to endotoxin challenge also act as neurodevelopmental factors (Hornig et al., 2002), it is likely that long-term changes in neural circuitry or neural responses that are produced by pre- or post-natal endotoxin challenge are mediated by those cytokines. The roles of other mediators, including maternal behavior, sex steroid hormones, HPA activity, and genetic factors, among others, remain to be elucidated.

Sex Steroid Hormones and Neuroinflammation

As mentioned, the Besedovsky model of neuroimmune interactions has helped opened the door for studies of immune responses in brain. Accordingly, it has become apparent that the brain is not completely immune privileged. To be sure, protective barriers exist; nonetheless, it is clear that immune responding extends to brain. An increasing amount attention is being focused on neuroinflammation (see Rivest, 2003), particularly across developmental periods (Godbout et al., 2005).

Inasmuch as estrogen is known to be neuroprotective (Czlonkowska et al, 2006), it might be expected that there are sex differences in inflammatory responses in brain. In support of this hypothesis, Soucy et al. (2005) examined the role of sex steroid hormones in brain expression of transcripts of proinflammatory cytokines following LPS challenge. These investigators found that expression was attenuated in ovariectomized mice, and that this effect was reversed by E_2 replacement therapy.

A role for ERα was also suggested since ERα deficient mice did not mount an appropriate response to LPS. This suggests an intriguing way in which estrogens may be neuroprotective, namely by helping to mount effective responses against inflammatory agents. Moreover, in female rats, estrogen has been shown to reduce central (and peripheral) production of proinflammatory cytokines associated with a severe brain insult (Nordell et al., 2003). Inasmuch as this was evident in young but not senescent rats, it was suggested that estrogen treatment might not be indicated in older individuals.

Moreover, it is important to note that there are sex differences in the incidence of multiple sclerosis (MS), which is characterized by neuroinflammation associated with autoreactive T cell responses against myelin basic protein (see Whitacre et al., 1998). Work stemming from an animal model of MS, namely experimental autoimmune encephalomyelitis (EAE), indicates that stressor exposure attenuates clinical manifestations and related pathology of EAE to a greater extent in females than males, possibly due to potentiated HPA responses in females (Griffin et al., 1993; Whitacre et al., 1998). To be sure other factors are involved. For example, clinical manifestations of EAE are reduced by treatment with E2 and T cell receptor peptides (Offner & Vandenbark, 2005).

SEX DIFFERENCES IN BEHAVIORAL AND PHYSIOLOGICAL ALTERATIONS ASSOCIATED WITH IMMUNE ACTIVATION

In 1988, Benjamin Hart suggested that behavioral changes during illness serve an adaptive purpose (Hart, 1988). In subsequent years, seminal work by Dantzer and Kelley and others (see Dantzer et al., 1999; Dantzer, 2001) established that following exposure to certain immunological challenges, a series of adaptive behavioral and physiological changes are induced that help the individual mount an effective immune response. This is consistent with the Besedovsky model in which adaptive alterations of neural function occur following antigenic challenge that serve to regulate the ongoing immune response. Indeed, sickness behaviors are mediated centrally through cytokine-neurotransmitter interactions (see Dantzer et al., 1999). Here, a brief description of the sickness model will be followed by a discussion of sex differences in various symptoms of sickness behavior.

Symptoms of Sickness Behavior

The classic symptoms of sickness behavior include an increased expression of depressive-like behaviors, hypoactivity, social withdrawal, lethargy, anhedonia, as well as anorexia, fever, cognitive difficulties, and altered sleep patterns (Dantzer et al., 1999). These behaviors are intimately linked to the central actions of cytokines released during the host response to an infectious agent.

Indeed, brain cytokines are induced following systemic administration of proinflammatory cytokines, and highly selective cytokine-neurotransmitter interactions occur in brain regions underlying the observed behavioral effects (Laye et al., 1994). The behaviors comprising sickness behavior serve adaptive purposes during an immune response. For example, reduced activity during illness reduces metabolic demands thereby making resources available to the immune system. It also conserves body heat, which helps augment immune function.

Of further importance, reduced activity limits exposure to other pathogens, the response to which would be compromised. Sick animals are also more vulnerable to predators; hence hypoactivity also limits exposure to aggressive encounters. Moreover, a reduction in appetitive behaviors helps deprive an infectious agent of nutrients while social withdrawal limits the spread of an infections agent and exposure to other pathogens. However, abnormal or protracted increases would be expected to result in psychopathological outcomes. In support of this hypothesis, depressive-like episodes develop in patients receiving cytokine therapy, and cytokines have been implicated in the etiology of clinical depression (see Maes et al., 1999).

Sex Differences in Sickness Behavior

Exploration and Locomotion

Hypoactivity and reduced social exploration are characteristic symptoms of sickness behavior (see Dantzer et al., 1999; Dantzer, 2001). There are many studies showing that novelty-induced locomotion and exploration or social exploration (i.e., investigation of a juvenile conspecific) are reduced during infection or following proinflammatory cytokine administration.

Given that there are sex differences in general activity levels, it might be expected that male and female activity levels would also differ during illness. However, with regard to novelty-induced activity, intact males and estrous females show comparable reductions in locomotion and exploration following a single injection of LPS (Avitsur et al., 1997), or a single injection of IL-1β (Avitsur et al., 1995; Yirmiya et al., 1995).

Engeland and colleagues (2003a) also found that locomotion following challenge with LPS or muramyl dipeptide (MDP, a synthetic analog of a component of the cell wall of gram positive bacteria) was similarly reduced in males and females. Thus, a single injection of gram-negative or gram-positive bacteria induces comparable reductions in locomotion and exploratory activity in male and females rats. Nonetheless, these authors found subtle differences in behavioral tolerance to LPS.

Upon repeated exposure to LPS, tolerance develops to the effects of LPS. This serves to limit further development of inflammation. It is this of unique interest that although behavioral tolerance to repeated intermittent injections of LPS were observed in male and female rats, it developed more quickly in females (i.e., after the second injection) (Engeland et al., 2003a).

Of further importance, behavioral tolerance to LPS did not develop in rats receiving LPS during proestrous (Engeland et al., 2006). Tolerance to LPS was similarly not seen in long day female meadow voles coincident with increased circulating levels of progesterone (Engeland et al., 2003b). Moreover, combined LPS and MDP treatment exaggerated measures of horizontal and vertical activity in females but not in males (Engeland et al., 2003). The authors pointed out, however, that since baseline activity measures were lower in males, it is possible that a floor effect may have limited or precluded appreciable sex differences.

Weil et al., (2006) recently suggested that the individual's 'immediate social environment' influences the extent to which activity is altered following LPS challenge. Specifically, these investigators showed in males that LPS-induced reductions in social exploration, which is a classic symptom of sickness behavior (see Dantzer et al., 1999), are more pronounced when males are exposed to a female conspecific than when they are exposed to a male conspecific.

Like LPS, IL-1β induces comparable reductions of activity in males and females (Avitsur et al., 1995; Yirmiya et al., 1995), although its effects on locomotor behavior are less pronounced in females that are not in the estrous phase of the cycle (Avitsur et al., 1995). In the latter regard, a role for progesterone was suggested since its administration to ovariectomized animals potentiated the behavioral response to IL-1β. In males, IL-1β-induced decreases in social exploration are more pronounced in castrated than intact males, suggesting that gonadal hormones influence this behavioral effect (Dantzer et al., 1991).

These investigators further showed that intracerebroventricular administration of arginine vasopressin (AVP) reduces IL-1β's behavioral effects, particularly in castrated males. Administration of a vasopressin receptor antagonist enhances these effects in intact males. Based on these findings, these authors suggested that behavioral consequences of central IL-1β are opposed by AVP and that this occurs in an androgen-dependent manner.

Feeding and Anorexia

It has been well established that LPS, other inflammatory-inducing substances, and proinflammatory cytokines influence feeding and induce anorectic effects. For example, significant reductions in consumption of standard chow and palatable substances are evident following exposure to LPS (see Dantzer et al, 1999; Dunn, 2001), and following peripheral or central injections of pro-inflammatory cytokines involved in the host's response to LPS challenge (notably, IL-1β, IL-6 and TNFα) (see Dantzer et al., 1999; Plata-Salaman, 1999; Merali et al., 2003; Asarian & Langahns, 2005).

Cytokines also play important roles in feeding under physiological conditions (see Plata-Salaman, 2001). Cytokine regulation of feeding can occur at various levels, including the gut and brain. In the latter regard, cytokines are potent modulators of neural activity in brain sites (e.g., hypothalamus) that control feeding (see Dantzer et al., 1999).

There is evidence that LPS-induced anorexia is sexually differentiated. Geary and colleagues (2004) showed that anorexia following LPS challenge was greater in cycling female rats during diestrus or estrus than in males. In response to a higher dose of LPS, females in estrous consumed less food than females during diestrous. This was due to reductions in meal frequency. Furthermore, ovariectomy plus cyclic estradiol treatment resulted in a greater reduction in spontaneous meal frequency than ovariectomy alone.

Parenthetically, in another model of illness anorexia, decreases in food intake in tumor bearing female rats were due to a reduction in meal number (Varma et al., 2001). In male rats, LPS-induced anorectic effects were due to reductions meal number

and meal size (Geary et al., 2004). Lennie (2004) also showed that among females, the severity of anorexia varied with the stage of the estrous cycle, being more pronounced when estradiol levels were at their peak (proestrous/estrous). In parallel, anorexia was potentiated in animals receiving estradiol injections prior to induction of an inflammatory response, and was more severe in rats that were pre-treated with progesterone. This finding is consistent with that of Wurtman and Baum (1980) who showed that cyclic decreases in food intake occur coincident with increases in estradiol levels. IL-1β-induced anorexia is similarly enhanced by estradiol (Butera et al., 2002).

Thus, there is a convergence of findings on the relationship between estradiol, anorexia and inflammation. However, there are disparities in the literature regarding the severity of anorexia in males and females during an inflammatory response. In contrast with Geary et al. (2004), who showed that anorexia was more severe in female rats than in males, Lennie (2004) showed that males ate less than females.

One possible explanation for these differential findings relates to the fact that different substances were used to induce an inflammatory response. Whereas the former study used LPS, the latter used turpentine, which induces a more localized inflammation. It is also possible that differences in the profile of cytokine and hormone activation induced by these challenges (Geisterfer & Gauldie, 1996; Nadeau & Rivest, 1999) contributed to the differential findings. Along these lines, it was suggested that an increase in anti-inflammatory cytokines in female rats in response to turpentine may have limited the severity of weight loss (Lennie, 2004). This suggestion is consistent with the hypothesis that the severity of anorexia during an inflammatory response is related to the ratio of pro- and anti-inflammatory cytokines (Plata-Salaman, 1999).

There are other factors that may explain differential findings across studies, even those utilizing the same substance to induce inflammation. For example, there is a recent report that sex differences in LPS-induced weight loss are subject to seasonal effects. Owen-Ashley et al. (2006) showed that LPS-induced decreases in food and water intake were more pronounced on long days than short days in male birds. In contrast, length of day did not appreciably affect food intake in females. Moreover, there may be sex differences in the mechanisms underlying anorectic effects induced during an inflammatory response, and in baseline differences in circulating levels of cytokines. In one study, it was shown that circulating concentrations of leptin, which is an adipocyte-secreted hormone and putative cytokine that is induced after LPS challenge, were more pronounced in female rats than males (Gayle et al., 2006). Further to the point, Dixon et al. (2004) showed that circulating levels of TNFα, a proinflammatory cytokine linked with leptin, were higher in non-obese girls than obese girls. Finally, the possibility should be considered that the estrous cycle is disrupted during an inflammatory response, thereby confounding interpretation of findings (see Lennie, 2004).

In summary, evidence is beginning to accumulate suggesting that altered food consumption and anorexia during an inflammatory response occurs in a sexually dimorphic manner. However, there are disparities with regard to the direction of effects, possibly owing to differences in species used and methods used to induce inflammation, among other factors. To be sure, we are at an early stage in our understanding of the important relationship between immune activation, sex steroid hormones, and feeding.

Maternal Behaviors

As discussed earlier, Weil et al., (2006) suggested that the effects of LPS on social exploration are influenced by the individual's immediate environment. Effects of LPS on maternal behaviors are also influenced by environmental factors. For example, although nest building is compromised in lactating dams treated with LPS at room temperature, this effect is not observed at relatively low temperatures that could threaten pup survival (Aubert et al., 1997).

Paralleling these findings, in lactating dams aggressive behavior against a male intruder, which serves to protect the pups and thus, increase survival rates, is not altered following LPS challenge (except at a very high dose of LPS) (Weil et al., 2006). It has also been shown in female cats that defensive rage behavior, a form of aggression that is expressed when an animal's kittens are threatened, is potently modulated by IL-1β (see Zalcman and Siegel, 2006). Using a model of aggression elicited by electrical stimulation of the midbrain periaqueductal gray, it was shown that IL-1β in medial hypothalamus (Hassanain et al., 2003, 2005; see also Bhatt and Siegel, 2006) facilitates feline defensive rage behavior. Taken together, these studies show that in contrast with the profile of hypoactivity

associated with LPS challenge or IL-1β administration, forms of maternal aggression that are designed to protect the offspring from threatening stimuli are not compromised by endotoxin challenge, and are facilitated by IL-1β.

Reproductive Behaviors

The relationship between immunological challenge and reproductive behaviors has been studied on various levels. In a series of experiments, Avitsur and Yirmiya, and colleagues studied sexual behavior in rats at various time frames following LPS challenge. Significant inhibition of proceptive behaviors and the lordosis reflex was observed in female rats for up to six hours following LPS challenge (Avitsur et al., 1997). In contrast, male sexual behavior (including mounting, intromission, and ejaculation) was unaffected by LPS challenge, except at the highest doses tested. Paralleling these findings, Klein and Nelson (1999) showed that sexually active female prairie voles spend less time with LPS-treated males than those receiving saline. Meadow voles did not show this effect, suggesting that genetic factors play a role in underlying these effects. Of further importance, while LPS-treated female prairie voles spent more time with familiar males than with unfamiliar ones, male prairie voles displayed no such preferences (Bilbo et al., 1999).

IL-1β is released peripherally and centrally within the time frame during which LPS-induced alterations of sexual behavior occur. Given this fact coupled with the finding that IL-1β inhibits the proestrous LH surge and ovulation (Rivier & Vale, 1990), Avitsur et al. (1999) hypothesized that IL-1β influences sexual activity in a manner similar to LPS. Paralleling findings with LPS, a single peripheral injection of IL-1β inhibited female, but not male sexual behavior (Yirmiya et al., 1995). The relationship between IL-1β and sexual attractivity was also explored. It was found that male rats displayed less sexual behavior toward an IL-1β-treated female than one receiving saline. In contrast, non-treated females spent similar amounts of time with IL-1β-treated males and controls (except males receiving a very high dose of IL-1β). In females, IL-1β inhibited proceptive behavior and the lordosis response (see Avitsur et al., 1999). These effects were antagonized by pretreatment with cyclo-oxygenase inhibitors, suggesting a principal role for prostaglandin synthesis in mediating these behavioral effects of IL-1β.

TNFα is another pro-inflammatory cytokine released following LPS challenge that induces symptoms of sickness behavior. It is thus of unique interest that TNFα induced a dose-dependent suppression of sexual behaviors in estrous females (see Avitsur et al., 1999). In light of the parallel effects of LPS, IL-1β and TNFα on sexual behavior, it was hypothesized that these cytokines mediate such effects of LPS. It was shown that combined antagonism of the IL-1 type I receptor and inhibition of TNF synthesis (by pentoxifylline) was required to inhibit LPS-induced suppression of sexual behavior in females. Pretreatment with an IL-1 receptor antagonist alone did not block LPS-induced effects; pentoxifylline blocked the lordosis reflex but not other sexual behaviors.

In summary, there are sex differences in the effects of LPS challenge or proinflammatory cytokine administration on sexual behavior. Since male sexual behavior is relatively unaltered by immune activation, it was suggested that males tend to hide their health status to attract a mate (see Avitsur & Yirmiya, 1999). In contrast, suppressed female responses during illness may be related to the fact that ovulation is prevented in chronic states of immune activation. Thus, physiological and endocrine mechanisms that mediate this effect may likewise mediate suppression of female sexual activity following LPS challenge or cytokine administration.

Fever

Elevated body temperature during an immune response serves to potentiate immune function and decrease survival of invading pathogens (see Blatteis, 2006). Proinflammatory cytokines and prostaglandin (PGE_2) in the brain underlie the febrile response to LPS. LPS-induced febrile responses are sexually differentiated. For example, Murakimi and Ono (1987) showed that LPS induced greater increases in rectal temperature and thermal response index in male mice compared with females. The authors suggested that sex hormones contributed to the male febrile response since castration attenuated this effect in males but not females. Further to the point, the febrile response of adult females that had received a subcutaneous injection of testosterone propionate on postnatal day 1 was similar to those induced in males. Mouihate and Pittman (2003) further showed in ovariectomized rats that LPS-induced fever was at-

tenuated by estrogen and progesterone replacement compared with ovariectomized controls. This effect occurred coincident with decreases in hypothalamic cyclooxygenase-2 expression and plasma IL-1β concentrations.

Numerous cytokines have been shown to play a role in febrile responses (see Leon, 2002), and there is evidence that some of their effects on fever are sexually dimorphic. Mouihate et al. (1998) underscored the importance of gonadal hormones in the febrile response to IL-1β. These investigators reported that in females, IL-1β-induced fever was higher and of longer duration in proestrus than in diestrus. A prominent role for ovarian hormones was suggested by the finding that in ovariectomized females, IL-1β-induced fever was highest in rats receiving injections of estradiol 17β and progesterone compared with rats that received estradiol 17β alone. There is evidence that the febrile response varies as an interaction between gender, age, and type of immunological challenge. For example, older females show an increased response to LPS-induced fever (Wachulec et al., 1997), but their response to a yeast infection is reduced compared to males (Refinetti et al., 1990).

CONCLUSIONS

The Besedovsky model of neuroimmune interactions has opened the door for integrated analyses of the relationship between the immune and central nervous systems. Many aspects of this relationship are sexually differentiated, including the immune-neuroendocrine relationship and behavioral changes associated with immune responding. Studies examining the relationship between development, stress, gender, and immunity have also revealed that pre- and postnatal exposure to infectious agents, stressful events, and other environmental stimuli may produce long-lasting changes in CNS activity and immune function. Of further importance, certain immunologically based disorders (e.g., autoimmune disorders) show different prevalence rates in males and females. Thus, sex differences should be considered as fundamental mediators of many aspects of neuroimmune interactions. Our understanding of these differences has important basic and clinical implications, and future studies should shed more light on mechanisms underlying these differences.

References

Asarian L, Langhans W. (2005). Current perspectives on behavioural and cellular mechanisms of illness anorexia. *Int Rev Psychiatry*, 17(6):451–459.

Aubert A, Goodall G, Dantzer R, Gheusi G. (1997). Differential effects of lipopolysaccharide on pup retrieving and nest building in lactating mice. *Brain Behav Immun*, 11(2):107–118.

Avitsur R, Donchin O, Barak O, Cohen E, Yirmiya R. (1995). Behavioral effects of interleukin-1 beta: modulation by gender, estrus cycle, and progesterone. *Brain Behav Immun*, 9(3):234–241.

Avitsur R, Pollak Y, Yirmiya R. (1997). Different receptor mechanisms mediate the effects of endotoxin and interleukin-1 on female sexual behavior. *Brain Res*, 773(1–2):149–161.

Avitsur R, Cohen E, Yirmiya R. (1997). Effects of interleukin-1 on sexual attractivity in a model of sickness behavior. *Physiol Behav*, 63(1):25–30.

Avitsur R, Yirmiya R. (1999). The immunobiology of sexual behavior: gender differences in the suppression of sexual activity during illness. *Pharmacol Biochem Behav*, 64(4):787–796.

Banks, WA. (2006). The blood-brain barrier in psychoneuroimmunology. *Neuro Clin* 24(3):413–419.

Beck RD Jr, Wasserfall C, Ha GK, Cushman JD, Huang Z, Atkinson MA, Petitto JM. (2005). Changes in hippocampal IL-15, related cytokines, and neurogenesis in IL-2 deficient mice. *Brain Res*, 1041(2):223–230.

Bellinger DL, Lorton D, Felten SY, Felten DL. (1992). Innervation of lymphoid organs and implications in development, aging, and autoimmunity. *Int J Immunopharmacol*, 14:329–344.

Bellinger DL, Lorton D, Lubahn C, Felten DL. (2001). Innervation of lymphoid organs-associations of nerves with cells of the immune system and their implications in disease. Ader R, Felten DL, Cohen N (Eds.), *Psychoimmunology*, 3rd Ed. (pp. 55–112). San Diego: Academic Press.

Beishuizen A, Thijs LG. (2003). Endotoxin and the hypothalamo-pituitary-adrenal (HPA) axis. *J Endotoxin Res*, 9(1):3–24.

Besedovsky H, del Rey A, Sorkin E, Da Prada M, Burri R, Honegger C. (1983). The immune response evokes changes in brain noradenergic neurons. *Science*, 221:564–565.

Besedovsky HO, del Rey AE, Sorkin E. (1985). Immuneneuroendocrine interactions. *J Immunol*, 135(2 Suppl):750s–754s.

Besedovsky HO, del Rey, A. (1996). Immune-neuroendocrine interactions: facts and hypotheses. *Endoc Rev*, 17:64–102.

Bhatt S, Siegel A. (2006). Potentiating role of interleukin 2 (IL-2) receptors in the midbrain periaqueductal gray (PAG) upon defensive rage behavior in the cat: role of neurokinin NK(1) receptors. *Behav Brain Res*, 28;167(2):251–260.

Bilbo SD, Klein SL, DeVries AC, Nelson RJ. (1999). Lipopolysaccharide facilitates partner preference behaviors in female prairie voles. *Physiol Behav*, 68(1–2):151–156.

Blatteis CM. (2006). Endotoxic fever: new concepts of its regulation suggest new approaches to its management. *Pharmacol Ther*, 111(1):194–223.

Brown R., Li Z., Vriend CY, Nirula, R, Janz L, Falk J, Nance, DM, Dyck, DG, Greenberg AH. (1991). Suppression of splenic macrophage interleukin-1 secretion following intracerebroventricular injection of interleukin-1 beta: evidence for pituitary-adrenal and sympathetic control. *Cell Immunol*, 132:84–93.

Butera PC, Doerflinger AL, Roberto F. (2002). Cyclic estradiol treatment enhances the effects of interleukin-1beta on food intake in female rats. *Brain Behav Immun*, 16(3):275–281.

Chisari AN, Gaillard RC, Giovambattista A, Voirol M-J, Piermaria J, Spinedi E. (2000). Sexual dimorphism in the hypothalamo-pituitary-adrenal (HPA) axis and TNFalpha responses to phospholipase A2-related neurotoxin (from *Crotalus durissus terrificus*) challenge. *J Endocrinol Invest*, 23(7):440–448.

Chrousos GP. (1995). The hypothalamic-pituitary-adrenal axis and immune-mediated inflammation. *N Engl J Med*, 332(20):1351–1362.

Czlonkowska A, Ciesielska A, Gromadzka G, Kurkowska-Jastrzebska I. (2006). Gender differences in neurological disease: role of estrogens and cytokines. *Endocrine*, 29(2):243–256.

Dantzer R, Bluthe RM, Kelley KW. (1991). Androgendependent vasopressinergic neurotransmission attenuates interleukin-1-induced sickness behavior. *Brain Res*, 557(1–2):115–120.

Dantzer R, Aubert, A, Bluthe RM, Gheusi G, Cremona S, Laye S, et al. (1999). Mechanisms of the behavioural effects of cytokines. *Adv Exp Med Biol*, 461:83–105.

Dantzer R. (2001). Cytokine-induced sickness behavior: mechanisms and implications. *Ann N Y Acad Sci*, 917:608–617.

Da Silva JA, Peers SH, Perretti M, Willoughby DA. (1993). Sex steroids affect glucocorticoid response to chronic inflammation and to interleukin-1. *J Endocrinol*, 136:389–397.

Demas GE, Johnson C, Polacek KM. (2004). Social interactions differentially affect reproductive and immune responses of Siberian hamsters. *Physiol Behav*, 83(1):73–79.

Dixon D, Goldberg R, Schneiderman N, Delamater A. (2004). Gender differences in TNF-alpha levels among obese vs nonobese Latino children. *Eur J Clin Nutr*, 58(4):696–699.

Dhabhar FS, McEwen BS. (1999). Enhancing versus suppressive effects of stress hormones on skin immune function. *Proc Natl Acad Sci U S A*, 96(3):1059–1064.

Dunn AJ. (1992). The role of interleukin-1 and tumor necrosis factor alpha in the neurochemical and neuroendocrine responses to endotoxin. *Brain Res Bull*, 29(6):807–812.

Dunn AJ. (2000). Cytokine activation of the HPA axis. *Ann NY Acad Sci*, 917:608–617.

Dunn, AJ. (2001). Effects of cytokines and infection on brain neurochemistry. In: Ader, R., Felten, D.L., Cohen, N. (Eds.), *Psychoneuroimmunology*. San Diego: Academic Press, (pp. 649–666).

Elenkov IJ, Wilder RL, Chrousos GP, Vizi ES. (2000). The sympathetic nerve—an integrative interface between two supersystems: the brain and the immune system. *Pharmacol Rev*, 52(4):595–638.

Engeland CG, Kavaliers M, Ossenkopp KP. (2003a). Sex differences in the effects of muramyl dipeptide and lipopolysaccharide on locomotor activity and the development of behavioral tolerance in rats. *Pharmacol Biochem Behav*, 74:433–447.

Engeland CG, Kavaliers M, Ossenkopp KP. (2003b). The influence of photoperiod and sex on lipopolysaccharide-induced hypoactivity and behavioral tolerance development in meadow voles (*Microtus pennsylvanicus*). *Psychoneuroendocrinology*. 2003 8:970–991.

Engeland CG, Kavaliers M, Ossenkopp KP. (2006). Influence of the estrous cycle on tolerance development to LPS-induced sickness behaviors in rats. *Psychoneuroendocrinology*, 31:510–525.

Felten DL, Felten SY, Bellinger DL, Carlson SL, Ackerman KD, Madden KS, et al. (1987). Noradrenergic sympathetic neural interactions with the immune system: structure and function. *Immunol Rev*, 100:225–260.

Frederic F, Oliver C, Wollman E, Delhaye-Bouchaud N, Mariani J. (1993). IL-1 and LPS induce a sexually dimorphic response of the hypothalamo-pituitary-adrenal axis in several mouse strains. *Eur Cytokine Netw*, 4:321–329.

Giberson PK, Weinberg J. (1995). Effects of prenatal ethanol exposure and stress in adulthood on lymphocyte populations in rats. *Alcohol Clin Exp Res*, (5):1286–1294.

Gaillard RC, Spinedi E. (1998). Sex- and stress-steroids interactions and the immune system: evidence for a neuroendocrine-immunological sexual dimorphism. *Domest Anim Endocrinol*, 15:345–352.

Gayle DA, Desai M, Casillas E, Beloosesky R, Ross MG. (2006). Gender-specific orexigenic and anorexigenic mechanisms in rats. *Life Sci*, 79(16):1531–1536.

Geary N, Asarian L, Sheahan J, Langhans W. (2004). Estradiol-mediated increases in the anorexia induced by intraperitoneal injection of bacterial lipopolysaccharide in female rats. *Physiol Behav*, 82:251–261.

Geisterfer M, Gauldie J. (1996). Regulation of signal transducer, GP130 and the LIF receptor in acute inflammation in vivo. *Cytokine*, 8(4):283–287.

Godbout JP, Chen J, Abraham J, Richwine AF, Berg BM, Kelley KW, Johnson, RW. (2005). Exaggerated neuroinflammation and sickness behavior in aged mice following activation of the peripheral innate immune system. *FASEB J*, 19(10):1329–1331.

Guyre PM, Bodwell JE, Munck A. (1984). Glucocorticoid actions on lymphoid tissue and the immune system: physiologic and therapeutic implications. *Prog Clin Biol Res*, 142:181–194

Hadid R, Spinedi E, Giovambattista A, Chautard T, Gaillard RC. (1996). Decreased hypothalamo-pituitary-adrenal axis response to neuroendocrine challenge under repeated endotoxemia. *Neuroimmunomodulation*, 3(1):62–68.

Harbuz M. (2002). Neuroendocrine function and chronic inflammatory stress. *Exp Physiol*, 87(5):519–525.

Hart BL. (1988). Biological basis of the behavior of sick animals. *Neurosci Biobehav Rev*, 12(2):123–137.

Hassanain M, Zalcman S, Bhatt S, Siegel A. (2003). Interleukin-1 beta in the hypothalamus potentiates feline defensive rage: role of serotonin-2 receptors. *Neuroscience*, 120(1):227–233.

Hassanain M, Bhatt S, Zalcman S, Siegel A. (2005). Potentiating role of interleukin-1beta (IL-1beta) and IL-1beta type 1 receptors in the medial hypothalamus in defensive rage behavior in the cat. *Brain Res*, 1048(1–2):1–11.

Hermes GL, Rosenthal L, Montag A, and McClintock MK. (2005). Social isolation and the inflammatory response: sex differences in the enduring effects of a prior stressor. *Am J Physiol Regul Integr Comp Physiol*, 290: R273–R282.

Hodgson DM, Knott B. (2002). Potentiation of tumor metastasis in adulthood by neonatal endotoxin exposure: sex differences. *Psychoneuroendocrinology*, (7):791–804.

Hornig M, Mervis R, Hoffman K, Lipkin WI. (2002). Infectious and immune factors in neurodevelopmental damage. *Mol Psychiatry*, 7(Suppl 2):S34–S35.

Klein SL, Nelson RJ. (1999). Activation of the immune-endocrine system with lipopolysaccharide reduces affiliative behaviors in voles. *Behav Neurosci*, 113(5):1042–1048.

Laye S, Parnet P, Goujon E, Dantzer R. (1994). Peripheral administration of lipopolysaccharide induces the expression of cytokine transcripts in the brain and pituitary of mice. *Brain Res Mol Brain Res*, 27:157–162.

Lee S, Rivier C. (1993). Effect of exposure to an alcohol diet for 10 days on the ability of interleukin-1 beta to release ACTH and corticosterone in the adult ovariectomized female rat. *Alcohol Clin Exp Res*, 17:1009–1013.

Lennie TA. (2004). Sex differences in severity of inflammation-induced anorexia and weight loss. *Biol Res Nurs*, 5(4):255–264.

Leon LR, White AA, Kluger MJ. (1998). Role of IL-6 and TNF in thermoregulation and survival during sepsis in mice. *Am J Physiol*, 275:R269–277.

Leon LR. (2002). Invited review: cytokine regulation of fever: studies using gene knockout mice. *J Appl Physiol*, 92(6):2648–2655.

MacNeil BJ, Jansen AH, Greenberg AH, Nance DM. (1996). Activation and selectivity of splenic sympathetic nerve electrical activity response to bacterial endotoxin. *Am J Physiol*, 270:R264–R270.

Maes M. (1999). Major depression and activation of the inflammatory response system. *Adv Exp Med Biol*, 461:25–46.

Maier SF Watkins LR Nance DM. (2001). Multiple routes of of action of interleukin-1 on the nervous system. In Ader, R., Cohen, N., Felten, D.L. (Eds.), *Psychoneuroimmunology* (pp. 563–583), San Diego: Academic Press.

Merali Z, Brennan K, Brau P, Anisman H. (2003). Dissociating anorexia and anhedonia elicited by interleukin-1beta: antidepressant and gender effects on responding for "free chow" and "earned" sucrose intake. *Psychopharmacology* (Berl), 165:413–418.

Miller SI, Ernst RK, Bader MW. (2005). LPS, TLR4 and infectious disease diversity. *Nat Rev Microbiol*, 3(1): 36–46.

Morale MC, Gallo F, Tirolo C, Testa N, Caniglia S, Marletta N, et al. (2001). Neuroendocrine-immune (NEI) circuitry from neuron-glial interactions to function: Focus on gender and HPA-HPG interactions on early programming of the NEI system. *Immunol Cell Biol*, 79:400–417.

Mouihate A, Chen X, Pittman QJ. (1998). Interleukin-1beta fever in rats: gender difference and estrous cycle influence. *Am J Physiol*, 275:R1450–R1454

Mouihate A, Pittman QJ. (2003). Neuroimmune response to endogenous and exogenous pyrogens is differently modulated by sex steroids. *Endocrinology*, 144(6): 2454–2460.

Murakami N, Ono T. (1987). Sex-related differences in fever development of rats. *Am J Physiol*, 252(2 Pt 2):R284–R289.

Nadeau S, Rivest S. (1999). Regulation of the gene encoding tumor necrosis factor alpha (TNF-alpha) in the rat brain and pituitary in response in different models of systemic immune challenge. *J Neuropathol Exp Neurol*, 58(1):61–77.

Nance DM, Hopkins, DA, Bieger, D. (1987). Re-investigation of the innervation of the thymus gland in mice and rats. *Brain Behav Immun*, 1(2):134–147.

Nilsson C, Larsson BM, Jennische E, Eriksson E, Bjorntorp P, York DA, Holmang A. (2002). Maternal endotoxemia results in obesity and insulin resistance in adult male offspring. *Endocrinology*, 142(6): 2622–2630.

Nordell VL, Scarborough MM, Buchanan AK, Sohrabji F. (2003). Differential effects of estrogen in the injured forebrain of young adult and reproductive senescent animals. *Neurobiol Aging*, 24(5):733–743.

Offner H, Vandenbark AA. (2005). Congruent effects of estrogen and T-cell receptor peptide therapy on regulatory T cells in EAE and MS. *Int Rev Immunol*, 24(5–6):447–477.

Owen-Ashley NT, Turner M, Hahn TP, Wingfield JC. (2006). Hormonal, behavioral, and thermoregulatory responses to bacterial lipopolysaccharide in captive and free-living white-crowned sparrows (*Zonotrichia leucophrys gambelii*). *Horm Behav*, 49(1):15–29.

Papadopoulos AD, Wardlaw SL. (1999). Endogenous alpha-MSH modulates the hypothalamic-pituitary-adrenal response to the cytokine interleukin-1beta. *J Neuroendocrinol*, 11(4):315–319.

Papadopoulos AD, Wardlaw SL. (2000). Testosterone suppresses the response of the hypothalamic-pituitary-adrenal axis to interleukin-6. *Neuroimmunomodulation*, 8(1):39–44.

Plata-Salaman CR. (2001). Cytokines and feeding. *Int J Obes Relat Metab Disord*, 25(Suppl 5):S48–S52.

Prendergast BJ, Hotchkiss AK, Bilbo SD, Nelson RJ. (2004). Peripubertal immune challenges attenuate reproductive development in male Siberian hamsters (*Phodopus sungorus*). *Biol Reprod*, 70:813–820.

Refinetti R, Ma H, Satinoff E. (1990). Body temperature rhythms, cold tolerance, and fever in young and old rats of both genders. *Exp Gerontol*, 25(6):533–243.

Redei E, Halasz I, Li LF, Prystowsky MB, Aird F. (1993). Maternal adrenalectomy alters the immune and endocrine functions of fetal alcohol-exposed male offspring. *Endocrinology*, 133:452–460.

Rivest S. (2003). Molecular insights on the cerebral innate immune system. *Brain Behav Immun*, 17:13–19.

Rivier C, Vale W. (1990). Cytokines act within the brain to inhibit luteinizing hormone secretion and ovulation in the rat. *Endocrinology*, 127(2):849–856.

Rivier C. (1994). Stimulatory effect of interleukin-1 beta on the hypothalamic-pituitary-adrenal axis of the rat: influence of age, gender and circulating sex steroids. *J Endocrinol*, 140:365–372.

Rivier C. (1999). Gender, sex steroids, corticotropin-releasing factor, nitric oxide, and the HPA response to stress. *Pharmacol Biochem Behav*, 64(4):739–751.

Sanders VM, Munson AE. (1985). Norepinephrine and the antibody response. *Pharmacol Rev*, 37(3):229–248.

Sanders VM, Kasprowicz DJ, Kohm AP, Swanson MA. (2001). Neurotransmitter receptors on lymphocytes and other lymphoid cells. In Ader, R., Felten, DL, Cohen N (Eds.), *Psychoneuroimmunology*, 3rd Ed, (pp. 161–196). San Diego: Academic Press.

Shanks N, McCormick CM, Meaney MJ. (1994). Sex differences in hypothalamic-pituitary-adrenal responding to endotoxin challenge in the neonate: reversal by gonadectomy. *Brain Res Dev Brain Res*, 79:260–266.

Shanks N, Larocque S, Meaney MJ. (1995). Neonatal endotoxin exposure alters the development of the hypothalamic-pituitary-adrenal axis: early illness and later responsivity to stress. *J Neurosci*, 15(1 Pt 1):376–384.

Silva C, Ines LS, Nour D, Straub RH, da Silva JA. (2002). Differential male and female adrenal cortical steroid hormone and cortisol responses to interleukin-6 in humans. *Ann N Y Acad Sci*, 966:68–72.

Silverman MN, Pearce BD, Biron CA, Miller AH. (2005). Immune modulation of the hypothalamic-pituitary-adrenal (HPA) axis during viral infection. *Viral Immunol*, 18(1):41–78.

Soucy G, Boivin G, Labrie F, Rivest S. (2005). Estradiol is required for a proper immune response to bacterial and viral pathogens in the female brain. *J Immunol*, 174(10):6391–6398.

Spinedi E, Suescun MO, Hadid R, Daneva T, Gaillard RC. (1992). Effects of gonadectomy and sex hormone therapy on the endotoxin-stimulated hypothalamo-pituitary-adrenal axis: evidence for a neuroendocrine-immunological sexual dimorphism. *Endocrinology*, 131(5):2430–2436.

Spinedi E, Chisari A, Pralong F, Gaillard RC. (1997). Sexual dimorphism in the mouse hypothalamic-pituitary-adrenal axis function after endotoxin and insulin stresses during development. *Neuroimmunomodulation*, 4:77–83.

Suescun M, Chisari AN, Carino M, Hadid R, Gaillard RC, Spinedi E. (1994). Sex steroid regulation of the hypothalamo-pituitary-adrenal axis activity in middle-aged mice during endotoxic shock. *Neuroimmunomodulation*, 1(5):315–320.

Sundar SK, Cierpial MA, Kilts C, Ritchie JC, Weiss JM. (1990). Brain IL-1-induced immunosuppression occurs through activation of both pituitary-adrenal axis and sympathetic nervous system by corticotropin-releasing factor. *J Neurosci*, 10(11):3701–3706.

Silverman MN, Pearce BD, Biron CA, Miller AH. (2005). Immune modulation of the hypothalamic-pituitary-adrenal (HPA) axis during viral infection. *Viral Immunol*, 18:41–78.

Theofilopoulos AN. (1995). The basis of autoimmunity: Part I. Mechanisms of aberrant self-recognition. *Immunol Today*, 16(2):90–98.

Tonelli L, Webster JI, Rapp KL, Sternberg E. (2001). Neuroendocrine responses regulating susceptibility and resistance to autoimmune/inflammatory disease in inbred rat strains. *Immunol Rev*, 184:203–211.

Turnbull AV, Rivier C. (1995). Regulation of the HPA axis by cytokines. *Brain Behav Immun*, 9(4):253–275.

Ulevitch RJ, Mathison JC, da Silva Correia J. (2004). Innate immune responses during infection. *Vaccine*, 22(Suppl 1):S25–S30.

Varma M, Chai JK, Meguid MM, Yang ZJ. (2001). Gender differences in tumor-induced anorectic feeding pattern in Fischer-344 rats. *Physiol Behav*, 74(1–2):29–35.

Wachulec M, Peloso E, Satinoff E. (1997). Individual differences in response to LPS and psychological stress in aged rats. *Am J Physiol*, 272(4 Pt 2):R1252–R1257.

Watanobe H. (2002). Sexual dimorphism in the pituitary-adrenal response to tumor necrosis factor-alpha, but not to interleukin-6, in the rat. *Brain Res Bull*, 57(2):151–155.

Watanobe H, Yoneda M. (2003). A mechanism underlying the sexually dimorphic ACTH response to lipopolysaccharide in rats: sex steroid modulation of cytokine binding sites in the hypothalamus. *J Physiol*, 547:221–232.

Weil ZM, Bowers SL, Dow ER, Nelson RJ. (2006). Maternal aggression persists following lipopolysaccharide-induced activation of the immune system. *Physiol Behav*, 87(4):694–699.

Whitacre CC, Dowdell K, Griffin AC. (1998). Neuroendocrine influences on experimental autoimmune encephalomyelitis. *Ann N Y Acad Sci*, 840:705–716.

Williams JM, Peterson RG, Shea PA, Schmedtje JF, Bauer DC, Felten DL. (1981). Sympathetic innervation of murine thymus and spleen: evidence for a functional link between the nervous and immune systems. *Brain Res Bull*, 6(1):83–94.

Wurtman JJ, Baum MJ. (1980). Estrogen reduces total food and carbohydrate intake, but not protein intake, in female rats. *Physiol Behav*, 24(5):823–827.

Xiao E, Xia-Zhang L, Ferin M, Wardlaw SL. (2001). Differential effects of estradiol on the adrenocorticotropin responses to interleukin-6 and interleukin-1 in the monkey. *Endocrinology*, 142(7):2736–2741.

Yirmiya R, Avitsur R, Donchin O, Cohen E. (1995). Interleukin-1 inhibits sexual behavior in female but not in male rats. *Brain Behav Immun*, 9(3):220–233.

Zalcman S, Green-Johnson JM, Murray L, Nance, DM, Dyck, DG, Anisman, H, et al. (1994). Cytokine-specific central monoamine alterations induced by interleukin (IL)-1, IL-2 and IL-6. *Brain Res*, 643:40–49.

Zalcman S, Green-Johnson JM, Murray L, Wan W, Nance DM, Greenberg AH. (1994). Interleukin-2-induced enhancement of an antigen-specific IgM plaque-forming cell response is mediated by the sympathetic nervous system. *J Pharmacol Exp Ther*, 271(2):977–982.

Zalcman SS, Siegel A. (2006). The neurobiology of aggression and rage: role of cytokines. *Brain Behav Immun*, 20(6):507–514.

Chapter 19

Sex Differences in Pain

Emeran A. Mayer, Jennifer S. Labus,
and Karen J. Berkley

Pain scientists and clinicians were among the first to respond to challenges in the biomedical research community to include women in clinical trials (NIH Guide1994) and to study sex and gender differences (Berkley, 1992; Ruda, 1993; Institute of Medicine [U.S.] et al., 2001). Reviews of information on sex differences in pain began appearing in the mid-nineties (Unruh, 1996; Fillingim & Maixner, 1996; Berkley, 1997). However, information at that time, while plentiful, was difficult to find, because it had to be obtained primarily by scouring through the methods and results sections of individual articles; few studies addressed the issue directly. These early reviews on pain forecast what would become a consensus for all sex difference research in the late 1990s: i.e., that sex/gender differences, while complex, were potent, and studies of the differences were maturing from a descriptive into a hypothesis-driven field.

Since then, the number of articles describing research specifically directed at some particular aspect of sex differences in pain have steadily increased. Thus,

a PubMed search in June 2006 using the phrases "sex differences in pain" and "gender differences in pain" revealed that in the 19 years between 1972 and 1990 only ~4 papers/year were published; from 1991 through 1995, 21/year were published; from 1996 through 2000, 45/year were published; and finally, from 2000 until mid-2006, ~100 papers/year were published. In addition, a book (Fillingim, 2000), special issues of two journals (Keogh & Arendt-Nielsen, 2004; Berkley et al., 2006), and more reviews have recently appeared (e.g., Aloisi, 2003; Craft, 2003a, 2003b, 2004; Mayer et al., 2004; Arendt-Nielsen et al., 2004; Wiesenfeld-Hallin, 2005; Kuba & Quinones-Jenab, 2005; Aloisi & Bonifazi, 2006; Chang et al. 2006b). Furthermore, chapters in pain textbooks are now regularly written (e.g., Baranowski & Holdcroft, 2005; Holdcroft & Berkley, 2005; Holdcroft, 2006).

Given this plethora of readily-available information, we present here a brief overview of the field, providing citations to appropriate recent papers, and we discuss at greater length some intriguing new directions, in particular those involving brain imaging studies on sex-related pain differences. First, we consider what is known about sex differences in pain in healthy individuals and those with chronic pain conditions, along with the factors that influence the differences. Next, we review what is known about sex differences in the efficacy and usage of different treatments. We then discuss potential mechanisms that contribute to the differences. A special section follows that describes new data emerging from brain imaging studies. Finally, we conclude with an overview of the clinical implications of these findings.

SEX DIFFERENCES IN PAIN IN HEALTHY INDIVIDUALS

Psychophysical Studies—Skin

Almost all reviews conclude that for stimulation of the skin, females have lower thresholds and less tolerance to noxious stimulation than males (Riley III et al., 1999). Of importance, however, is that the *overall* sex differences are not large. Instead, the magnitude (and sometimes the direction) of the differences vary considerably depending on the particular type of stimulus used (Riley III et al., 1999), its temporal characteristics (e.g., repetitive or single; Sarlani & Greenspan 2002; Robinson et al., 2004), its bodily location (Harju, 2002), the subjects' age (Harju, 2002), ethnicity (Kim et al., 2004), gender role (Robinson et al., 2004), level of anxiety (Robinson et al., 2004), family factors (Fillingim et al., 2000), past history (Rollman et al., 2004), and genetic characteristics (Mogil et al., 2003; Kim et al., 2004). Another factor that influences sex differences on skin pain is the stage of the woman's menstrual cycle (Riley III et al., 1999) or hormonal status (e.g., pregnancy), although consensus on this issue is impeded by inconsistencies in nomenclature and hormone assessment across studies (Sherman & LeResche 2006).

Muscle and visceral pain: Less research has been carried out on sex differences in muscle and visceral pain than on skin pain in healthy individuals, in part because the test stimuli are more aversive and invasive. So far, the results overall appear to indicate less of a sex difference in pain evoked by stimulation of muscles and visceral organs than by stimulation of the skin or even a reversal in the sex differences (i.e., women report less pain than men) (Chang et al., 2006a). However, there is no clear consensus yet.

Thus, in studies that examined pain produced by limb exercise, men reported more pain than women (Cook et al., 1998; Poudevigne et al., 2002; Dannecker et al., 2005); and in a more recent study, men reported higher affective ratios (Dannecker et al., 2005). Other studies showed no sex difference. For example, pain thresholds to electrical stimulation of arm or leg muscles do not differ in men and women (Giamberardino et al., 1997), nor does delayed muscle soreness following eccentric shoulder exercise (Nie et al., 2005). In contrast, pain after chewing or biting exercises or glutamate injections into the masseter muscle was greater in women than in men (Plesh et al., 1998; Cairns et al., 2001; Karibe et al., 2003; Ge et al., 2005).

In studies that examined pain produced by visceral stimulation, rectosigmoid distension produces no sex differences unless the stimuli are repeated, in which case women exhibit more pain then men (Mayer et al., 2004). For the esophagus, males report more pain to mechanical and chemical (hydrochloric acid) stimulation and develop more acid-evoked hyperalgesia than females, but females exhibit larger pain referral areas than men (Reddy et al., 2005). It remains to be determined if some of these differences are related to the nature of the pain stimulus used (phasic, tonic, repetitive), to the site of stimulation (pelvic vs. thoracic), subject selection or other parameters. For example, while prolonged stimuli are thought to engage the endogenous opioid system, transient phasic stimuli do not. Thus sex differences in the subjective responses to sustained pain stimuli, may reflect sex differences in the endogenous opioid system.

In summary, contrary to common belief, sex differences in the subjective responses to experimentally pain stimuli, not only cutaneous, but also deep muscular and visceral stimuli, are small, variable and highly stimulus and context dependent.

The perception of pain is a multidimension experience reflecting the integration of many inputs with different underlying mechanisms, including the encoding and ascending transmission of nociceptive input, and the multiple mechanisms of endogenous modulation. The selection of individuals willing to undergo experimental pain studies, and the unique context of an experimental pain testing session (for example the a priori knowledge that the pain will be within an ethically justifiable range, and will not be associated with tissue injury) is likely to affect endogenous pain modulation systems in a unique way.

It is plausible to assume that while some of the components of this experience are sex neutral, others are sex-related. Of the latter group, some may be related to fluctuation of sex steroid levels, whereas others may be due to organizational effects of sex steroids in brain development or due to direct effects of the x or y chromosomes.

In order to advance our understanding of the true prevalence and relevance of such sex-related differences in the experience of pain, it will be necessary to identify those components in the processing of nociceptive information and in the modulation of the pain experience that are sex related, and those that are not. For example, sex differences may play a greater role in the stress-related modulation of pain than sex differences in the ascending transmission of nociceptive afferent input. Functional brain imaging techniques provide a unique way for this deconstruction of the integrated subjective pain experience into such individual components and are likely to play an increasing role in this field (see section on Brain Imaging, below).

Clinical Application of Experimental Pain Assessments

One common and not surprising finding is that experimental pain assessments can be influenced by the existence of clinical pain conditions. For example, temporal summation of pain (i.e., the increase in pain intensity with repetitive noxious stimulation of constant intensity) induced by heat stimulation applied to the skin of a finger is increased in individuals with temporomandibular disorder (Sarlani & Greenspan 2005). Similarly, rectal pain thresholds induced by repetitive sigmoid distension are reduced in patients with irritable bowel syndrome, but not in those with a functional abdominal pain syndrome (Nozu et al., 2006). Furthermore, the presence of dysmenorrhea reduces muscle (but not skin) pain thresholds in women.

Thus, the question arises as to whether the sex differences observed in healthy individuals have any predictive value clinically. For example, it has been suggested that the greater susceptibility of women to the development of temporal summation of muscle pain to repeated injections of glutamate into the trapezius muscle or to heat stimulation of the skin might contribute to the higher female prevalence, respectively, of neck shoulder pain (Ge et al., 2005) and temporomandibular disorder (Sarlani & Greenspan 2005). Similarly, it has also been suggested that the

fact that males are more sensitive to mechanical and chemical stimulation of the esophagus contributes to their prevalence of heartburn or acid reflux, whereas the fact that females exhibit larger pain referral areas of esophageal stimulation contributes to their prevalence of functional chest pain (Reddy et al., 2005).

This important issue also relates to current efforts to use psychophysical methods (e.g., experimental pain responses or quantitative sensory testing [QST]) as an aid for diagnosis, for developing therapeutic strategies, and for assessing therapeutic efficacy. Thus, in a recent review, Edwards et al. (2005) conclude: "Collectively, the findings . . . suggest that experimental pain responses relate to clinical pain report in a variety of samples (i.e., greater pain sensitivity is associated with greater clinical pain), that such responses predict the risk of acute procedural pain, [and] that these responses also correlate with treatment outcome."

With respect to sex differences, however, questions arise as to whether QST indeed reflects clinical pain intensity or predicts therapeutic outcomes. For example, regarding QST and clinical pain intensity, Fillingim et al., (2000) measured experimental thermal pain responses and used questionnaires to assess overall pain symptoms during the previous month in males and females. Whereas experimental thermal and clinical pains were greater in women than in men, thermal pain sensitivity correlated with clinical pain reports only in women.

Similarly, regarding therapeutic outcomes, Walker and Carmody (1998) tested the efficacy of ibuprofen for reducing nociception induced by electrical stimulation of the ear lobe, and found that, despite similar blood levels of ibuprofen, analgesia was less in women than men. In contrast, however, in a clinical pain setting, Averbuch and Katzper (2000) found no sex differences in efficacy of ibuprofen for dental pain.

Regarding visceral pain, controlled pressure distension of colon, stomach or esophagus is commonly used to assess visceral pain sensitivity in various patient populations with common visceral pain conditions. In general, the perceptual sensitivity measures (both in terms of sensory and affective sensitivity) obtained with these techniques shows only moderate correlations with clinical symptom severity, and sex differences in such responses have not been used to predict differences in symptom severity or treatment responses (Azpiroz et al., 2007).

Thus, while the use of QST as a pain assessment tool in the clinic shows great promise, more work needs to be done to understand how it can be used most effectively. Given the issues discussed earlier in the interpretation of sex-related differences in the pain response to experimental stimuli in healthy volunteers, it is not surprising that there is not a better correlation between those studies in healthy subjects and sex differences in clinic patients with chronic pain.

SEX DIFFERENCES IN CHRONIC PAIN CONDITIONS

It has been known for some time that more painful diseases and syndromes, particularly those of autoimmune etiology, show a higher female prevalence. Thus, as detailed and referenced in Box 75.1 of Holdcroft and Berkley (2005), there is a higher female prevalence of many conditions of the head and neck (e.g., migraine, burning mouth, temporomandibular disorder, trigeminal neuralgia), limbs (e.g., carpel tunnel syndrome, piriformis syndrome, Raynaud's disease, complex regional pain syndrome type I [reflex sympathetic dystrophy]), internal organs (e.g., interstitial cystitis, gall bladder disease, proctalgia fugax, irritable bowel syndrome [but not functional esophageal or gastroduodenal disorders; (Chang et al., 2006b)]), and more general conditions (e.g., fibromyalgia, postherpetic neuralgia, multiple sclerosis, rheumatoid arthritis).

In addition, some conditions and syndromes are more likely to co-occur in women than in men (e.g., irritable bowel syndrome, fibromyalgia, interstitial cystitis, migraine; Mayer et al., 1999; Berkley 2005; Heitkemper & Jarrett 2005). In contrast, there is a male prevalence of a much smaller number of conditions: e.g., cluster headache, brachial plexus neuropathy, gout, duodenal ulcer, Pancoast tumor, myralgia parasthetica, and pancreatic disease, and less evidence for co-occurrence of conditions.

In addition to known diseases and syndromes, many "everyday" pains also appear to burden women more than men. Thus, epidemiological studies consistently find that women report more severe pain, more frequent pain, pain of longer duration, and pain in more bodily areas than men (e.g., Dao & LeResche 2000). Part of the reason may be the greater prevalence across the lifespan of painful obstetric and gynecological conditions than of painful male-specific conditions. Thus, common painful conditions such as dysmenorrhea may predispose women to more widespread musculoskeletal pains (Giamberardino et al., 1997; Bajaj et al., 2002) as well as to the coexistence of multiple painful conditions (Berkley 2005).

FACTORS THAT INFLUENCE SEX DIFFERENCES IN PAIN PREVALENCE

Overall, the discussion above indicates that despite the generally small sex differences in experimental pain perception in healthy individuals, the burden of pain is much greater for females than for males. This conclusion is oversimplified, however, because the size of sex differences in pain as well as its direction can be influenced by many factors.

One major factor affecting sex differences in pain prevalence is the apparent greater *willingness* of women in Western cultures to report pain and to seek healthcare (Isacson and Bingefors 2002). This factor may underlie the fact that the female prevalence of a number of diseases is consistently greater in epidemiological studies of clinical compared with community samples, as seen for example in irritable bowel syndrome (Hungin et al., 2003) and temporomandibular disorder (LeResche 2000).

Second, the *signs and symptoms* by which several diseases and syndromes are diagnosed differ in females and males, which can lead to misleading prevalence estimates. This issue has only recently been recognized, and is slowly becoming incorporated into changes in criteria for diagnosing disorders such as irritable bowel syndrome (Longstreth et al., 2006), migraine (Kirchmann 2006), chronic pelvic pain/interstitial cystitis (Hanno 2007) and coronary artery disease (Philpott et al., 2001; Eastwood & Doering 2005).

A third factor is that the prevalence patterns of various pains changes with *age*, some appearing only after puberty, others diminishing, disappearing, or even reversing with increasing age afterwards (LeResche 2000; Macfarlane 2005).

A fourth factor is *reproductive status*. Thus, the severity of pain in number of chronic pain conditions (e.g., migraine: Brandes, 2006) can vary with the menstrual cycle, menopausal status, and pregnancy. Although interpretation of the nature of these variations is confounded by methodological issues (Sherman & LeResche 2006), whatever the fluctuations are, they obviously can influence any assessment of sex differences depending on the reproductive status of the women at the time assessments are made.

A fifth complex of factors can be generally classed as *psychosocial* or *environmental*. There are many of these types of factors, all of which impact assessments of sex differences in pain, either by reducing or increasing the differences or accounting for the these differences. Examples include gender role expectations (Robinson et al., 2004), interpersonal aspects of the experimental environment (Jackson et al., 2005), the individual's coping strategy and state of anxiety (Edwards et al. 2004; Robinson et al., 2004; Emery et al., 2006; Keogh & Eccleston 2006), family role models (Edwards et al., 1985), cultural differences in pain expression (Chang et al., 2006b), socioeconomic factors (Bingefors & Isacson 2004), and past pain history (Robinson & Wise 2004).

A sixth complex of factors that affect or help acount for sex differences are assorted *physiological* characteristics such as the bodily site (Heinberg et al., 2004), taste factors (Lewkowski et al., 2003; Bhattacharjee & Mathur 2005) and blood pressure (Maixner & Humphrey 1993; Bragdon et al., 2002; Lewkowski et al., 2003).

Finally, of considerable importance is that sex differences are primarily seen in many stress-sensitive so called functional pain disorders, and tend to disappear when *pain becomes severe and chronic* (Turk & Okifuji 1999; Edrington et al., 2004; Heinberg et al., 2004).

SEX DIFFERENCES IN EFFICACY AND USE OF TREATMENTS

In addition to sex differences in reported experiences of pain, studies are now beginning to demonstrate sex differences in efficacy and usage of pain treatments. As previously described, there are three categories of therapy used to treat pain: drugs, somatic manipulations, and situational adjustments (Berkley 1997). Sex differences are beginning to be found in each category (Holdcroft & Berkley 2005).

For example, for drugs, kappa opioids appear to be more effective analgesics in females than males (Gear et al., 1999), but only at certain doses (Gear et al., 2003), and possibly only in women with certain genetic characteristics (Mogil et al., 2003). Serotonin agents used to treat irritable bowel also appear to be more effective in women than men, but the conclusions are hindered by the fact that the studies were

likely underpowered for men (Cremonini & Talley 2004). Sex differences in drug efficacy are also associated with sex differences in and the effect of reproductive status on pharmacokinetics (Tanaka, 1999). For example, such a situation appears to be the case for µ-opioid analgesics, where sex differences in the ratio of active metabolites of morphine contribute to the greater efficacy of morphine in females as well as to explain contradictory findings in rodents in whom the greater efficacy of morphine in males may be because some metabolites are not formed (reviewed in Holdcroft & Berkley, 2005).

Another example is acetaminophen, whose pharmacokinetics vary significantly with the menstrual cycle (Gugilla et al., 2002). Sex differences in drug efficacy are also influenced by other factors, such as sex differences in smoking and alcohol consumption (Tanaka, 1999), as well as the greater overall willingness of women to use more over-the-counter analgesic and adjuvant medications, which can increase side effects of prescription drugs and therefore their use (Roe et al., 2002).

Sex differences in the efficacy or usage of somatic therapies (physical interventions) are also beginning to be found. For example, women are more willing to use simple interventions such as relaxation or massage than men (Unruh et al., 1999), whereas exercise and nerve blocks have been found less effective in women than men for improving symptoms (Fronek et al., 2003); and women are at higher risk of adverse events after many surgical procedures (e.g., Myles et al., 1997; Stadler et al., 2003).

Sex differences in the efficacy and use of situational adjustments also exist. Women are more likely to use and to benefit from cognitive therapies (Jensen et al., 1994) and to use lifestyle-changing approaches such as aromatherapy, gardening, support groups and diet alterations (Unruh et al., 1999; Keogh et al., 2005).

MECHANISMS OF SEX DIFFERENCES IN PAIN

There is now a huge, rapidly growing literature accumulating from many areas of research on the many factors that contribute to the sex differences that were summarized above. In addition, it is important to note that, even when observed sex differences themselves appear small, the mechanisms by which the pain is brought about can differ in females and males.

Contributing factors include: genetics, peripheral organ physiology and bodily structure, nervous system structure and physiology, peripheral and central neuroactive agents, sex steroid hormones, interactions between the nervous and immune systems, stress, lifespan events, lifestyle and cultural roles. What is immediately obvious is that no single factor on its own can explain the differences. Although each factor will be discussed individually below, it should be kept in mind that, as illustrated in Figure 19.1, the factors continuingly interact and combine in a myriad of ways as individuals progress through their lifespan. Thus, it will become evident that despite many significant differences between females and males in pain and pain mechanisms, individual differences remain the most important.

Peripheral Organ Physiology and Bodily Structure

It is well known that women relative to men have higher blood pressure, more body fat, and less muscle mass. All of these differences have been shown to contribute to various aspects of sex differences in pain (e.g., Maixner & Humphrey, 1993; Sinaki et al., 2001; Vilming et al., 2001). Very few animal studies have been done, however, to address these factors further (Ramos et al., 2002).

Another obvious physiological difference is the female-specific ovarian cycle, whose influences on pain are pervasive and under intense study in both women (Sherman & LeResche, 2006) and experimental animals (discussed further).

Finally, as discussed, sex differences in reproductive and other pelvic organs likely contributes to sex differences in the co-occurrence of painful clinical conditions. Mechanisms underlying this issue are only just beginning to be studied in animal models (Berkley, 2005; Morrison et al., 2006).

Nervous System Structure and Physiology

The book in which this chapter is published documents numerous ways in which the anatomy and physiology of the nervous system is influenced by the sex of the individual. One could argue that virtually all of these sex differences can influence pain experiences in individuals, because, as discussed above and below, so many aspects of an individual's life influence the pain experience. This conclusion is particularly important for pain that is chronic or intense, because the activity of more regions of the brain is influenced under those circumstances (Coghill et al., 1999, 2003). One aspect of this very rapidly expanding and exciting area of research—brain imaging—will be considered in further detail.

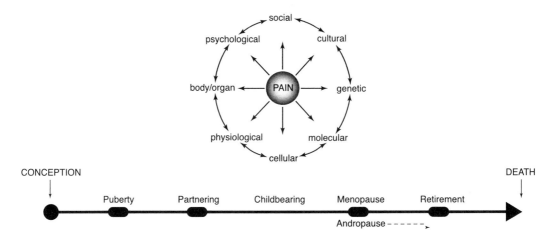

Figure 19.1. Conceptualization of factors that can interact dynamically, evolving and changing as events occur across an individual's lifespan and influencing pain in men and women differently. Adapted with permission from Holdcroft AI and Berkley KJ. (2005). Sex and gender differences in pain. In: McMahon SB, Koltzenberg M. (Eds.) *Wall and Melzack's textbook of pain*, 5th edition. Edinburgh: Elsevier Ltd, Churchill Livingstone.

Peripheral and Central Neurotransmitters/neuromodulators

The expression and functioning of a large number of neuroactive agents and their receptors in peripheral sensory receptors, sensory neurons (spinal and vagal primary afferents), or neurons in the spinal cord and brain have been shown to exhibit a sex difference or to be influenced by reproductive status or hormone manipulations in humans or experimental animals in a manner that influences pain. Some of these agents are listed and referenced in review publications (Berkley et al., 2002; Holdcroft & Berkley, 2005). In addition, receptors for many of these and other agents are co-expressed with estrogen receptors in sex-specific manner that influences nociception (e.g., Vanderhorst et al., 2005) or antinociception (e.g., Murphy et al., 1999; Flores et al., 2003).

Animal research in this area is currently quite vigorous. For example, recent studies have extended investigations of acute opioid-mediated antinociception for somatic stimulation in rodents to opioid-mediated antinociception of persistent and visceral nociception (Ji et al., 2006; Wang et al., 2006) and to NMDA-associated morphine tolerance (Bryant et al., 2006). The former two studies confirmed morphine's greater potency in female rodents, while the third study suggests that the morphine tolerance in females is less sensitive to modifications of the NMDA system than it is in males. What is still not well understood are reasons for the apparent difference between rodents and humans in the direction of morphine-related sex differences (Fillingim, 2004).

One new direction is studies of sex differences in the involvement in nociception of non-opioid agents. Examples of such agents include: cyclooxygenase enzymes (Cox-1 in particular; Chillingworth et al., 2006), acid-sensing ion channels (ASISs; Chanda & Mogil, 2006) and both endocannabinoids in the brain and exogenously-administered cannabinoids (which show sex and ovarian cyclical modifications; Craft, 2005; Bradshaw et al., 2006).

Genetics

Genetic influences on sex differences in pain reveal themselves in at least four ways. First are sex-linked inherited genetic diseases such as male-prevalent hemophilic arthropathy (Tann, 1979) and Fabry's disease (Masson et al., 2004), female-prevalent peroneal muscular atrophy (Fryns & Van den, 1980) and acute intermittent porphyria (Smith et al., 1990). Second are genetic variations in liver enzyme metabolizing systems such as the cytochrome P450 (CYP 2 and 3) families that affect the pharmacological activity of analgesics in a sex-specific manner (Ciccone & Holdcroft, 1999; Anakk et al., 2003; Stamer et al., 2005). Third are sex specific effects on gene expression, such as those associated with the modulation by estradiol of receptors for neuroactive agents involved in nociception and analgesia. Examples include the augmenting influence of estradiol on nerve growth factor, calcitonin gene-related peptide, galanin, enkephalin and substance P (reviewed in Holdcroft & Berkley, 2005).

Fourth are genetic variations that exert their influences on nociceptive sensitivity, endogenous pain modulation, or analgesia in a sex-specific manner, that only very recently have come under study in both humans and animal models. Three examples concern genetic variations in the μ-opioid receptor gene (OPRM1), the melanocortin-1 receptor gene (MC1R), and the CGRP gene. Thus, a single nucleotide polymorphism of the OPRM1 gene is associated with lower thermal nociceptive pain ratings in men and higher pain ratings in women (Fillingim et al., 2005). Non-functional MC1R genes in both mutant mice and humans show increased analgesia to kappa opioid analgesia only in females (Mogil et al., 2003), as well as reduced sensitivity to noxious stimuli and increased analgesia to morphine-6-glucoronide in both sexes (Mogil et al., 2005b). And finally, differences in sensitivity to noxious heat stimulation of the skin that are found among different strains of mice (some of which show sex differences; Mogil et al., 2000) can be accounted for by differential responsiveness of primary afferent thermal nociceptors to heat stimuli (Mogil et al., 2005a).

In a population-based sample, Diatchenko identified 3 haplotypes of the gene encoding COMT which they referred to as low (LPS), average (APS) and high (HPS), and which encompass 96% of the population (Diatchenko et al., 2006). Five variations of these haplotypes were strongly associated with variations in the sensitivity to a battery of experimental pain stimuli. The presence of even a single LPS haplotype diminished the risk of developing temporomandibular joint disorder (TMD), a functional pain syndrome frequently co-occurring with IBS, by as much as 2.3 times. The associations of COMT genotypes with pain sensitivity appears to be stimulus specific: while the val[158]met genotype (present in about 50% of the population) was associated with the rate of temporal summation of heat pain, the COMT *haplotype* exerts a greater influence on resting nociceptive activity to transient pain stimuli: LPS/LPS homozygotes showed the least, APS/APS homozygotes the highest, and APS/LPS heterozygotes showed the greatest pain responsiveness to such transient stimuli.

Although these new results using sophisticated genetic techniques are exciting, it is important to be careful not to attribute all sex differences to genetic factors. Thus, how these recently discovered genetic variations interact with sex differences in environmental and lifespan factors presents a major challenge, which is only just beginning to be addressed experimentally. For example, Chesler and colleagues (2002) have found that large sources of variance in rat nociceptive reflexes (tail flick) include the experimenter who is testing the rats and other aspects of the rat's social environment such as the order in which rats in a group of rats are studied.

Sex Steroid Hormones

Three recent articles provide excellent reviews of the extensive literature concerning the influence of sex steroid hormones on pain in humans and experimental animals (Aloisi 2003; Craft et al., 2004; Aloisi & Bonifazi, 2006). In short, the influence of these hormones—estrogens, progesterone, and testosterone and their metabolites—is pervasive, affecting not only virtually all central and peripheral nervous system function (as discussed in this book), as well as the expression of neuroactive agents and metabolism of pharmaceutical agents as described briefly above, but also the immune system (e.g., female prevalence of painful autoimmune diseases (Ackerman 2006); influence of testosterone or estradiol on inflammation (Flake et al., 2006)) and the hypothalamic-pituitary-adrenal (HPA) axis (e.g., Kudielka & Kirschbaum, 2005).

This pervasiveness means that actions of the hormones are complex. Furthermore, conclusions are confounded by several circumstances, such as the means by which hormonal influences are studied (Becker et al., 2005). It is not well understood, for example how results from studies in which hormonal manipulations were exogenous (e.g., ovariectomy, hormone replacement) versus endogenous (e.g., puberty, ovarian cyclicity, reproductive senescence) can be reconciled. Thus, the significance of the location of exogenous delivery (e.g., systemic, local, spinal cord, brain, etc.; Ji et al., 2006), the duration and timing of delivery, which hormones are delivered and in what combination, all remain uncertain. Although it is tempting to generalize about the effects of individual hormones (e.g., that estradiol increases and testosterone reduces pain and analgesia), such generalizations are risky, and exceptions abound (Stoffel et al., 2003; Aloisi & Bonifazi, 2006).

Neuroimmune System Interactions

It is difficult to underestimate the importance for improving our understanding of pain and the impact of sex differences on pain. It is a rapidly emerging area of research that concerns the profound regulatory interactions between the nervous and immune systems. It is encouraging therefore that one relevant area—the involvement of neuron-glia interactions in the spinal cord in chronic pain—has recently become a major focus of research (Banks & Watkins, 2006; Watkins et al., 2007).

Not only do nervous and immune system interactions influence the effects of acute injury, but they also affect the occurrence and symptomatology of painful diseases via systemic, regional and local routes that involve a complex interplay between the central nervous system, the HPA axis and the sympathetic and parasympathetic nervous systems (Marques-Deak et al., 2005; Rittner et al., 2005; Watkins & Maier, 2005; Wieseler-Frank et al., 2005; Zhang & Oppenheim, 2005; Hains & Waxman, 2006; Sternberg 2006; Frank et al., 2007). How sex differences manifest themselves in the context of this interaction or influence this interaction is not yet understood, but the effects are likely to be far-reaching because all components of interacting systems can be influenced not only by sex steroid hormones as mentioned above, but also by sex-specific environmental factors (e.g., stress, next section).

Stress

Sex differences in the mechanisms and consequences of stress have been reported in virtually every realm of biomedical inquiry, with considerable relevance to sex differences in pain (Mayer, 2000; Holdcroft & Berkley, 2005). In fact, some of the sex differences in the prevalence and clinical presentation of patients with common, stress-sensitive functional pain disorders, including IBS, pelvic pain/IC and fibromyalgia may be due to sex differences in stress-induced pain modulation. New approaches and hypotheses are emerging from research in this area. For example, a review of results from animal research prompted Kajantie and Phillips (2006) to hypothesize that sex differences in response to acute stressors are a result of "the need to protect the fetus from the adverse effects of maternal stress responses, in particular excess glucocorticoid exposure."

Another hypothesis regarding sex-related differences in the stress response which is also related to protection of the offspring was proposed by Taylor (2002). The author proposed that female-specific modulatory systems involving oxytocin and female sex hormones have evolved, the activation of which can result in a "tend and befriend" response, characterized by affiliative behavior. The hypothesis further suggests that such a system has evolved since it is more adaptive in terms of survival of offspring to attenuate or inhibit the fight and flight response in the mother caring for the young. The consequences of these different stress response systems for sex differences in the pain sensitivity result from the fact that while the fight and flight response includes powerful stress-induced analgesia systems, the tend and befriend response may be associated with greater cutaneous and possibly visceral sensitivity.

Lifespan Events, Lifestyle, Sociocultural Aspects

Although sex differences in pain expression are already observable in neonates (Guinsburg et al., 2000; Fuller 2002), females and males continue to have different experiences throughout their lifespan that can affect pain. These experiences are both universally associated with stages of development and individually unique (Fig. 19.1). They are either sex-specific (e.g., hormonal changes) or more likely to occur in one sex than the other due to sex differences in lifestyle (e.g., smoking, violent behaviors, dangerous occupations, coping behaviors; (Rollman et al., 2004; Keogh & Eccleston, 2006), social roles (e.g., Robinson et al., 2001), and cultural expectations (e.g., Hobara, 2005). Although research on how lifespan psychosocial factors influence pain abounds (e.g., Gallagher, 2004; Fillingim, 2005; Halpert & Drossman, 2005; Mayer,

2007), studies directed specifically on sex/gender influences are only just beginning to appear (Holdcroft & Berkley, 2005; Chang et al., 2006b).

One currently active translational research area concerns the influence of events very early in life on pain in adulthood. Anand and colleagues (2006) have recently published a review and a consensus statement on this topic. The review summarizes many epidemiological and experimental findings in humans and other animals that vividly demonstrate the profound effects of various noxious events during the neonatal period on adult pain and other behaviors. The review/consensus also calls for more consistent and active use worldwide of deliberate procedures to minimize injury and stress during the neonatal period.

In addition to the influence of physically noxious early life-events on adult pain, aversive psychosocial life events, in particular those related to the quality of the early life environment and the availability of the primary care giver can have a profound effect on the vulnerability for chronic pain conditions in the adult (Mayer and Collins 2002). Importantly and not surprisingly, the adult consequences of neonatal noxious events are not uniform (Anand 2000). In many cases, repetitive injury delivered to nearly any part of the body (i.e., both visceral and somatic) or other stressors (e.g., maternal separation) in the neonate leads to *increased* pain and other abnormally enhanced behaviors in adulthood (e.g., Al-Chaer et al., 2000; Fitzgerald & Beggs, 2001; Coutinho et al., 2002). In other situations, however, neonatal injury and stress leads to widespread hypoalgesia or dampened behavioral responses to noxious events (Anand, 2000; Ren et al., 2004; Wang et al., 2004), or to very little change (Anand & Birch, 2002; Howard et al., 2005).

Sex differences in these effects are just beginning to be studied, mostly in experimental animals. For example, Sternberg and Ridgway (2003), studying rats, found that three types of early stress—prenatal, postnatal, or both pre- and postnatal-influenced nociceptive thresholds, morphine analgesia, and stress-induced analgesia in adult females and males in different ways. Similarly, Kalinichev and colleagues (2001) reported that maternal separation in the early post-natal period alters sensitivity to chronic morphine administration in a sex-dependent manner. Other studies in which hormonal manipulations were made at different developmental periods found that adult sex differences in morphine analgesia and stress-induced analgesia could be attributed to the hormonal environment in the neonatal period (Sternberg et al., 1995; Krzanowska et al., 2002).

BRAIN IMAGING STUDIES

Less than a decade of research has focused on differences in brain activity underlying the subjective pain experience in women and men. This newly emerging field, using various neuroimaging methodologies including PET, fMRI, MEG, and radioligand studies has examined sex differences in somatic and visceral pain studies, both in healthy subject and in patient populations. Due to the novelty and growing impact of this new field in pain research on a better understanding of the neurobiological basis of sex differences, the following section provides greater detail in the discussion of published studies. Key features of all published studies are summarized in Table 19.1.

Neuroimaging Studies of Sex-related Differences in Somatic Pain

In the first published neuroimaging study to examine sex differences in the brain's response to pain, Paulson and colleagues (1998) demonstrated that a noxious 50°C heat (as compared to nonxious heat [40°C] delivered to the left forearm using $H_2^{15}0$ PET) was associated with increased rCBF activity in healthy adult women (n = 10) compared to men (n = 10) when administered in the anterior insula, thalamus, and in bilateral prefrontal cortex (BA 9/46) (Paulson et al., 1998). However, because women retrospectively reported the fixed painful stimulus as more intense than men, interpretation of the results were limited since greater brain responses in women could be attributable to either differences in pain sensitivity or alterations in brain mechanisms.

Improving upon the experimental paradigm of Paulson et al., (1998), Derbyshire and colleagues (Derbyshire et al., 2002) equalized the subjective experience of the pain stimuli. Specifically, the intensity level of the stimulus was individually adjusted to maintain fixed levels of self-reported pain ratings throughout the study. Specifically, a laser stimulus was used to deliver non-painful, mild and moderate thermal pain heat to the back of the right hand of 10 women and 11 men, and brain response was measure using $H_2^{15}0$ PET.

The statistical analysis examined what brain regions were most positively correlated with retrospective subjective pain intensity ratings of non-painful, mild and moderate thermal pain. Of particular note, the authors chose not to examine whether any regions were significantly negatively correlated with self-report ratings, an equally important question.

Results of this study indicated that anterior and posterior insula, bilateral parietal (BA 40), left primary and secondary sensory, and prefrontal (BA 46) cortices were more positively correlated in men as compared to women. Additionally, in women as compared to men the rCBF response of the perigenual cingulate (pACC; BA 24/25) showed greater positive correlations with ratings but this difference was due to the lack of a positive relationship between this area and ratings in men.

The authors speculated that their findings might be related to differential activation of brain circuits associated with the affective response to pain. An alternative explanation for the observed greater pACC response in women and the greater insula response in men could be the fact that women engage more affective circuits, while men engage primarily sensory circuits in response to the noxious stimulus.

Most recently, Moulton and colleagues (2006) have demonstrated sex differences in central pain response in 28 healthy adults (17 females). Brain response to nonpainful (40° C), and painful (~46°C) thermal stimuli applied to the left foot was measure using fMRI. Stimulus intensity levels were determined on an individual basis successfully maintaining equality in the subjective experience of the pain.

Blood oxygenation level-dependent (BOLD) signal amplitude was found to be greater in men for primary somatosensory cortex, mid-anterior cingulate, and dorsolateral prefrontal cortex. However, using a novel statistical approach the authors demonstrated that these differences were the result of greater negative BOLD signal change or deactivations in women in most areas. In other words, in women there was a greater spatial extent of deactivations in left primary somatosensory, dorsolateral prefrontal and right anterior insula. These areas are also consistent with Derbyshire et al. (1998) and support the notion that men show greater engagement of sensory circuits, and possibly different coping mechanisms (dorsolateral PFC) in response to the noxious somatic stimulus.

Of note, Becerra et al. (1998) examined differences in the brain's response to pain between 10 men

Table 19.1. Brain Imaging Studies on Sex-differences in Pain[*]

Reference	Type of Imaging	Condition of Subjects	Stimulus	Comments	Results	Possible sex Differences
Somatic pain studies						
Paulson et al., 1998	$H_2^{15}O$-PET	Healthy women (n = 10) and men (n = 10)	Phasic noxious thermal heat delivered to left hand with thermode	Women had higher retrospective pain ratings Fixed stimulus intensity	Women had greater activation in contralateral thalamus, insula and prefrontal cortex	Activation in some areas greater for women (but women have higher pain ratings)
Derbyshire et al., 2002	$H_2^{15}O$- PET	Healthy women (n = 11) and men (n = 10)	Phasic noxious thermal heat delivered to right hand by laser	Retrospective pain ratings equal for women and men Individually adjusted stimulus intensities	Left anterior/posterior insula, prefrontal, S1, S2 and parietal cortices were more positively associated with retrospective pain ratings in men; In women positive correlation was observed in perigenual ACC	Greater positive correlation in several areas in men, with the exception of perigenual ACC, which was greater in women
Moulton et al., 2006	fMRI	Healthy women (n = 17) and men (n = 11)	Phasic noxious thermal stimuli delivered to dorsum of the left foot via thermode	Real-time pain ratings equal between women and men Individually adjusted stimulus intensities	Greater BOLD signal *amplitude* for men in S1, mid-ACC, and dorsolateral PFC, largely attributable to a greater proportion of voxels in these regions demonstrating significant negative BOLD signal changes in women vs. men.	Women in comparison to men demonstrated a greater proportion of deactivations in S1, mid-ACC, and anterior insula
Visceral pain studies						
Berman et al., 2000	$H_2^{15}O$- PET	Two samples of 30 male and female IBS patients - sample 1, n = 13 (7 women) -sample 2, n = 17 (6 women)	Phasic aversive visceral stimulus (rectal distension)	Retrospective ratings of non-painful distensions equal Fixed stimulus intensities	Overall activation patterns greater in men than in women; the insula was activated bilaterally only in men	Activation greater in men, especially in insula

(continued)

Table 19.1. (continued)

Reference	Type of Imaging	Condition of Subjects	Stimulus	Comments	Results	Possible sex Differences
Naliboff et al., 2003	$H_2^{15}O$- PET	Male (n = 19) and female (n = 23) patients with IBS	Phasic aversive visceral stimulus (moderate rectal distension or anticipation of rectal distension)	Retrospective ratings of non-painful distensions equal Fixed stimulus intensities	For both stimulation and expectation of the visceral stimulus, women showed greater activation in ventromedial PFC, right rostral ACC, and left amygdala; men showed greater activation in right dorsolateral PFC, insula, and dorsal pons	In patients with IBS, men show greater activation in some areas, women showed greater activation in other areas
Hobson et al., 2005	MEG and CEP	Healthy men and women -sample 1, n = 16 (8 women) -sample 2, n = 11 (5 women)	Phasic esophageal electrical stimuli	Retrospective pain ratings equivalent between women and men Individually adjusted stimulus intensities	For women and men, neural activity in parallel within the S1 and S2 cortex and posterior insula followed by activity in the anterior insula and mid-ACC and then posterior and perigenual ACC	No sex differences were observed in the observed temporal patterns
Berman et al., 2006	fMRI	Healthy men (n = 5) and women (n = 6)	Rectal distension	Pain ratings equivalent between women and men Fixed stimulus intensity	Women demonstrated greater proportion of deactivated voxels during uncomfortable rectal distension in the amygdala, ventral striatum, thalamus, and dorsal brainstem where as men showed more activations in the insula.	Greater deactivations of brain areas in women
mu-opiod receptor Studies						
Zubieta et al., 1999	PET: μ-opioid receptor binding with [11C]carfentanil, a selective μ-opioid receptor agonist	Two groups of healthy men and women of different ages; Sample 1, n = 36 (12 women) scans were studied retrospectively Sample 2, n = 30 (18 women), scans were studied prospectively	No stimulation	-	μ-opioid binding potential increased with age in some parts of neocortex and putamen; higher μ-opioid binding in women was observed in several cortical and subcortical areas; the sex differences changed with age. In particular, μ-opioid binding diminished in postmenopausal women to levels below those in men in the ...	There was generally higher μ-opioid binding potential (receptor density) in women than in men, but the differences diminished and sometimes reversed with age as the women became postmenopausal

382

| Zubieta et al., 2002 | PET: μ-opioid receptor binding with [^{11}C]carfentanil, a selective μ-opioid receptor agonist | Healthy men (n = 14) and women (n = 14), with cycling women in the early follicular phase of their cycle (low, slowly rising levels of estradiol) | Tonic somatic pain stimulus (Injection of hypertonic versus normal saline into masseter muscle) | Real-time ratings of pain between groups equal Individually adjusted stimulus intensities | During muscle pain, men had larger magnitudes of μ-opioid receptor activation than those in women in anterior thalamus, ventral basal ganglia, and amygdala; however, women showed reductions of μ-opioid receptor activation in nucleus accumbens | During pain, there was generally higher μ-opioid receptor activation in men, with women showing reduced activation in an area that has been shown in animals to produce hyperalgesia when its opioid receptors are blocked |
| Smith et al., 2006 | fMRI & PET:μ-opioid receptor binding with ^{11}C | Healthy men (n = 8) and women (n = 8), with women in follicular phase of cycle and additional scanning of healthy women after 7–9 day treatment with transdermal estradiol patch (high estradiol phase, not replicating natural physiological state) | Tonic somatic pain stimulus (Injection of hyper-tonic vs. isotonic saline into masseter muscles) | Pain ratings equivalent between groups

Individually adjusted stimulus intensities | Similar to men, during a high estradiol, low progesterone state as compared to a low estradiol, low progesterone state, sustained pain induced greater endogenous opioid transmission in brain regions involved in supraspinal modulation of pain (thalamus, hypothalamus, nucleus accumbens, and amygdala) | Sex differences observed in μ-opioid receptor concentrations and in the release of endogenous opioids appear to be influenced by circulating levels of estradiol in women |

(continued)

Table 19.1. (*continued*)

Reference	Type of Imaging	Condition of Subjects	Stimulus	Comments	Results	Possible sex Differences
Serotonin Synthesis Studies						
Nakai et al., 2003	PET: serotonin synthesis, with tracer (α-[^{11}C]methyl-L-tryptophan)	Male (n = 6) and female (n = 6) non-constipation predominant IBS patients and 12 age-matched healthy controls (6 women)	No stimulation	-	Serotonin synthesis greater in female IBS patients in right medial temporal gyrus when compared with healthy female controls; no differences in male IBS patients compared with healthy male controls	When comparing healthy subjects with patients with IBS, only women showed differences, i.e., women with IBS had higher levels in one cortical area compared with healthy women; the authors argue that the sex differences were unrelated to plasma total or free tryptophan concentrations in the groups
Nakai et al., 2005	PET: Serotonin synthesis With α-[^{11}C]methyl-L-tryptophan	Men (n = 6) and women (n = 5) with non-constipation predominant IBS	Aversive visceral stimulus (rectal distension)	Pain ratings equivalent between groups Individually adjusted stimulus intensities	Serotonin synthesis greater in posterior cingulate in men and infragenual cingulate in women; differences in the basal ganglia and fusiform gyrus were also noted	Men and women demonstrated differences in serotonin synthesis; authors argue sex differences were unrelated to plasma total or free tryptophan levels

and 10 women in their mid-follicular and mid-luteal phase of the menstrual cycle. Preliminary results indicated that activation patterns were the same for men and for women in midfollicular phase, but greater activation of ACC, insula, and frontal cortex was observed in men when compared with women in mid-luteal phase (Becerra et al., 1998). This effort represents the earliest documented attempt to determine the effects of hormonal status in women on sex differences in pain.

Neuroimaging Studies of Sex-differences in Visceral Pain

Berman et al. reported the first study of brain responses in two samples of a total of 30 IBS patients (13 females; 6 with constipation-predominant bowel habit) with $H_2^{15}O$-PET in response to rectal distension (Berman et al., 2000). Specifically, in the first sample of 13 patients (7 females) after insertion of a rectal balloon, rCBF activity was measured during a resting baseline, noxious visceral stimulation (45 and 60 mmHg) and expectation. Brain responses in the second sample (11 males) were also taken during a resting baseline, noxious visceral stimulation (45 mmHg), and expectation. In this second sample, an additional sigmoid balloon was inserted before rCBF activity was measured, but the sigmoid balloon was never inflated.

During the expectation condition, after having received a 45-mmHg rectal balloon inflation patients were told they would "receive an even larger inflation than they had previously received" but this inflation was never given. Although stimulus intensities were fixed (e.g., 45 and 60 mmHg), subjective stimulus ratings were equal in men and women. Overall, regional brain activations were stronger in males. Also, in males, but not females, rectal distension was associated with activation of regions within the "central pain matrix" (including anterior insula and dACC). Insula activation correlated most strongly with the objective intensity of the stimulus (rectal pressure), whereas dACC activation correlated most strongly with the subjective discomfort rating of the stimulus. Greater insula activation was similar to that found by Derbyshire using a somatic pain stimulus (Derbyshire et al., 2002). The authors interpreted their findings in IBS patients as possibly being related to the greater sympathetic nervous system responses to rectal distension seen in male patients (Tillisch et al., 2005).

Naliboff et al. studied brain responses in 42 (23 females) non-constipated IBS patients to a visceral (rectal) stimulus of moderate intensity and during expectation using $H_2^{15}O$-PET (Naliboff et al., 2003). Specifically, rCBF activity was measured before and after sigmoid balloon stimulation during a resting baseline, 45-mmHg rectal balloon inflation, and an anticipation condition. In response to the visceral stimulus, both male and female patients showed activation of the expected pain regions (dACC, anterior insula) in addition to prefrontal and brainstem regions. Female patients showed greater activation in limbic (amygdala) and paralimbic regions (ventromedial PFC, infra-genual cingulate cortex and dACC), whereas male patients showed greater activation of the midposterior insula, dorsolateral PFC and dorsal pons. Similar sex-related differences were observed during the expectation condition. This study replicated the finding from the earlier study showing greater activation by male patients of the insular cortex and the dorsolateral PFC. The findings also suggested that female patients in response to a pelvic aversive stimulus show greater responses of limbic and paralimbic regions, while male patients show greater activation of regions belonging to a corticolimbic pain inhibition system.

In a more recent study, Berman et al. (2006) studied brain responses in 13 healthy adults (6 women) during 15 seconds of cued rectal distension at two pressures: 25 mmHg (uncomfortable), and 45 mmHg (mild pain), as well as during an expectation condition (no distension). The 45-mmHg pressure significantly activated the insula and dACC in both sexes. However, when the number of activated voxels, number of deactivated voxels, and ratio of deactivated voxels to total voxels affected were assessed via random effects mixed-model analyses combining subject data at the region level, greater insula activation in men compared to women was seen during the expectation condition and during the 25-mmHg distension. In contrast, greater *deactivations* in women were seen in the amygdala (25-mmHg distension) and midcingulate (45-mmHg distension). Women had a significantly higher proportion of deactivated voxels than men in all four subcortical structures during the 25-mmHg distension. These results are surprisingly consistent with the greater proportion of regional deactivations in women found by Moulton et al. (2006) using a somatic pain stimulus.

Hobson et al. (2005) have conducted a novel study examining sex differences in the temporal dynamics of the brain's response to noxious visceral stimulation in regions commonly activated by noxious stimuli. Specifically, scalp recorded electrical cortical evoked potential (CEP) and magnetoencephalography (MEG) were used to examine the temporal dynamics of the brain's response to noxious electrical esophageal stimuli in healthy adults (8 women). MEG, which is better at localizing cortical activity than EEG, has a poorer spatial resolution than PET and fMRI, but an improved temporal resolution on the scale of milliseconds (Liu et al., 2006).

Results indicated that for women and men, neural activity following noxious stimulation occurs first within the primary (S1) and secondary (S2) somatosensory cortex and posterior insula, followed by activity in the anterior insula and midcingulate cortex and finally in the posterior and perigenual cingulate. Interestingly, and in contrast to the observed sex differences of the brain to pelvic visceral stimuli using fMRI and PET, no sex differences were observed in the observed temporal patterns of the brain regions associated with esophageal stimulation.

As pointed out earlier, lack of an appropriate control condition makes it problematic to ascribe a pain-specific function to the reported regions. However, the findings provide the first evidence regarding lack of sex differences in the temporal dynamics operating within neural networks. This evidence supports the notion that instead of differences in the time scale, directionality, and specificity (location, destination) of information transfer between the brain regions within a network, observed sex differences in central responses to noxious stimulation (or during the pain experience or in brain activation patterns during the pain experience) are likely related to the differential engagement of the regions with a network as indexed by neural activity (e.g., differences in response to incoming signal, difference in efferent signal magnitude).

Applying network analyses, Labus et al. (2006) examined sex-differences in the effective connectivity of functional neural networks in IBS. Specifically, 46 IBS patients (24 females) received $H_2^{15}O$ PET scans during resting baseline, rectal distension and expectation conditions. Using sophisticated multivariate statistical techniques including partial least squares and structural equation modeling, significant sex-differences were observed in well-characterized amygdala modulatory circuitry during anticipation, including amygdala efferents to the pons, midbrain,

and infragenual ACC and afferent input to the amygdala from the supragenual ACC.

The authors concluded that during expectation of rectal discomfort, male patients show normal feedback inhibition within a network circuit involving infra- and supra-genual ACC, and amygdala resulting in a suppression of limbic activity. In contrast, female patients show strong connectivity between amygdala and infragenual ACC, but not in feedback inhibition, resulting in stronger infragenual ACC activation. These results are consistent with a greater responsiveness in female patients of a circuit regulating amygdala reactivity to emotionally salient stimuli. It is of interest that in contrast to the patients, such a sex difference in amygdala responsiveness was not observed in healthy control subjects (unpublished observations).

Of relevance to this conclusion are two other studies. Kern and colleagues examined sex differences in non-painful and subliminal visceral stimuli. First, Kern et al. (2001) studied brain responses in 28 healthy control subjects (15 women) to non-painful rectal distension using fMRI (Kern et al., 2001). Subjects received individualized distension intensities that were either below (subliminal) or just above the perception threshold. In both sexes, increasing stimulus intensity was associated with increases in brain activation. Volume of cortical activity during distension was significantly greater in women at all distension levels. Men showed localized clusters of fMRI activity primarily in the sensory motor cortex and parieto-occipital regions, whereas women also showed activity in the insular cortex, dACC and PFC regions.

Using a high-resolution functional magnetic resonance imaging sequence optimized for the cingulate cortex, Lawal et al. (2005) examined sex-differences in response to visceral stimulation and to external anal and sphincter contraction (EASC) in healthy controls. Specifically, activity in the cingulate gyrus (anterior and posterior cingulate was measured during rectal distensions below (subliminal), at (liminal) and above (supraliminal) perceptual threshold, and during an EASC protocol. Results indicated that volume of cortical activity during liminal and supraliminal distension was greater in females than males. In women, the volume of cortical activity was significantly greater in the ACC compared to the PCC. This difference was not observed in men.

In both sexes, increasing stimulus intensity was associated with increases in brain activation. Additionally, increasing stimulus intensity was associated with increased cortical activity in women only. Sex differences were not observed during EASC. Together, these findings are consistent with the greater involvement of affective circuits during visceral stress in women.

Neurochemical Pathway Studies

Opioid System

Jon-Kar Zubieta and colleagues have examined the μ-opioid receptor system as a potential candidate underlying sex differences in the regulation of the somatic pain experience (Zubieta et al., 1999; Smith et al., 2006). First, sex differences in μ-opiod receptor binding were examined using [^{11}C]carfentinil and PET in a total of 66 subjects (30 females) (Zubieta et al., 1999). No pain stimuli were delivered and the only condition was a resting baseline. Higher μ-opioid receptor availability/ binding was observed in healthy women compared to men in the amygdala, pons, thalamus, caudate nucleus, cerebellum and anterior cingulate, prefrontal cortex, temporal, and parietal cortices. Generally, there was higher μ-opioid binding in women than in men, but the differences diminished and sometimes reversed with age as the women became postmenopausal. Specifically, women showed a higher binding potential than men during the reproductive years and less binding post-menopause in the amygdala, thalamus, and pons.

Next, sex differences in μ-opioid receptor binding were examined using [^{11}C]carfentinil and PET in 28 subjects (14 females) during tonic pain and saline control periods (Zubieta et al., 2002). During the painful condition a steady state of deep somatic pain was maintained at an average intensity of 50 on a 101-point visual analogue scale by continuous infusion of hypertonic saline into the masseter muscle while isotonic saline was infused in a similar manner during the control condition. Overall, results indicate that men have greater activation of the μ-opioid system in the anterior thalamus, hypothalamus ventral basal ganglia, and amygdala than women who demonstrate less activation in nucleus accumbens in response to sustained pain (Zubieta et al., 2002, 2003), suggesting that sex differences in endogenous opioid receptor activation during painful stimulation might contribute to sex differences in pain.

Zubieta and collegues have extended the findings of the above study by examining the effects of hormonal status in women on the μ-opioid system (Smith et al., 2006). Using the same experimental paradigm, sex differences in μ-opioid receptor binding were examined in healthy men and women controlling for circulating levels of estradiol in women. Women were studied during low and high-estrogen states and high estradiol states were induced via long term (7–9 days) of transdermal micronized estradiol (0.4 mg/day) patches. Similar to men, during a high estradiol, low progesterone state as compared to a low estradiol, low progesterone state, sustained pain induced greater endogenous opioid transmission in brain regions involved in supraspinal modulation of pain (thalamus, hypothalamus, nucleus accumbens, and amygdala). This study provides the first evidence that sex differences observed in μ-opioid receptor concentrations and in the release of endogenous opioids appear to be influenced by circulating levels of estradiol in women.

Serotonin System

Nakai and colleagues have examined how the serotonin receptor system might contribute to sex differences in visceral pain in patients with IBS and healthy controls (Nakai et al., 2003, 2005). Female IBS patients demonstrated greater serotonin synthesis in the right medial temporal gyrus in comparison to female controls, where as male IBS patients did not show differences from healthy male controls. In a second study examining female versus male IBS patients, serotonin synthesis was greater in the posterior cingulate and areas of the basal ganglia in men as compared to women who show greater serotonin synthesis in the infragenual cingulate, fusiform gyrus, and areas of the fusiform gyrus. Results suggest that sex differences in serotonin synthesis during rectal distension might contribute to sex differences in visceral pain.

Summary and Perspectives for Future Brain Imaging Studies

Not surprisingly, given the infancy of the neuroimaging field, the published somatic and visceral pain studies with PET and fMRI examining sex-differences in brain responses to noxious stimuli represent a wide range of neuroimaging techniques, experimental paradigms, and statistical analyses. This makes it difficult to interpret and generalize the results, as well as aggregating studies (as we have attempted in Table 19.1).

Nevertheless, this review provides a starting point for generating future hypotheses regarding sex-differences in pain, illustrating the strengths of current experimental paradigms and statistical analyses and emphasizing the improvements necessary to move this field forward. Future studies will need to establish group differences in brain activation to standardized stimuli between healthy males and females, and between female and male patients groups (e.g., IBS, chronic lower back pain, fibromyalgia) while accounting for hormonal status.

The fMRI studies reviewed above employed a variety of analytic techniques and dependent variables (change in BOLD response and rCBF activity correlations, time series). A careful choice of statistical analysis technique (univariate vs multivariate, activation versus correlation, looking at both activations and de-activation) is important as indicated by the work of Moulton (2006) and Berman (2006). However, activation analyses are unable to reveal how cognitive processes interact or how brain regions interact with one another in the context of larger neural networks. Therefore network analyses such as effective connectivity modeling are a valuable complementary analysis technique.

CLINICAL IMPLICATIONS

The information reviewed above has considerable implications for the evaluation, diagnosis and therapy of male and female patients with acute and chronic pain, despite the fact that our understanding of the precise neurobiological mechanisms underlying the reported sex-related differences in prevalence, clinical presentation and treatment responses is still in its infancy. For example, different strategies in the initial history taking, which include taking into account the greater prevalence in female pain patients of comorbid conditions (other pain conditions as well as disorders of mood and affect) and the greater willingness of women to report physical symptoms of pain and distress, may yield valuable information for diagnosis and treatment planning.

The consideration of the importance of stress in chronic pain conditions, and sex differences in the prevalence of relevant stressors, such as sexual abuse and early life trauma, can have important implications for diagnosis and treatment strategies. Similarly, individualized dosing of pharmacologic interventions

(including opioids, and certain IBS drugs) may reduce side effects and increase effectiveness. The greater openness of women to "holistic" treatment approaches, including combinations of cognitive behavioral and drug therapies is important in optimizing treatment outcomes. Finally, as new pharmacologic treatments are being evaluated in clinical trials, it is important that studies are powered sufficiently to allow for separate analyses in female and male patients.

SUMMARY

During the past decade, tremendous progress has been made in the basic and clinical understanding of sex and gender differences in various aspects of pain, including pain sensitivity in healthy individuals, in the clinical presentation of pathological pain states, in the responsiveness of various acute and chronic pain conditions to therapy, and in sex differences in the pathophysiology of chronic pain. This progress is reflected in an increasing number of preclinical and clinical publications on the epidemiology, on treatment responses, and on the neurobiological mechanisms underlying sex differences in healthy individuals and chronic pain patients.

These new insights are beginning to have direct translational implications for the diagnosis and treatment of common chronic pain syndromes. A new investigative strategy is proposed to further improve the understanding of sex differences in chronic pain conditions. The deconstruction of the multidimensional subjective experience of pain into several interacting components, ranging from the encoding of nociceptive information in peripheral organs, transmission via ascending pathways to the brain, endogenous modulation (both inhibitory and facilitatory) of the nociceptive transmission and the subjective experience by multiple neural and neuroendocrine and hormonal systems may make it possible to investigate which of these subsystems contributes to the observed sex differences in healthy subjects and in patients with chronic pain syndromes.

CONCLUSIONS

The literature reviewed in this chapter demonstrates that significant progress has been made in addressing possible sex-related differences in pain sensitivity, in the prevalence of many common, chronic pain conditions and in the neurobiology underlying such behavioral differences. However, significant gaps in our knowledge still prevent us from tying these observations together with the emerging results from brain imaging studies and from a growing animal literature on sex differences in pain. In particular, the apparent discrepancy between relatively small, and sometimes contradictory sex-related differences observed in experimental pain studies in healthy control subjects and the robust differences seen in the prevalence of many chronic pain disorders requires further study. It is proposed that similar to the emerging efforts in relating different subjective and biological components of the multidimensional pain experience to different genetic polymorphisms (Diatchenko et al., 2006), a strategy of deconstructing the pain experience into components which are sex-specific and those which are sex-neutral may be helpful.

To continue the comparison with emerging genetic approaches to chronic human pain, studies to examine sex-gene and sex-gene-environment interactions may further improve our understanding of the precise role of sex and gender factors in chronic pain syndromes. Such an approach may also make it possible to identify specific neurobiological mechanisms, such as brain networks or central receptor systems which are truly sex related (and influenced by organizational or activational sex steroid actions) from those that are sex neutral.

References

Ackerman LS. (2006). Sex hormones and the genesis of autoimmunity. *Arch Dermatol*, 142:371–376.

Al-Chaer ED, Kawasaki M, Pasricha PJ. (2000). A new model of chronic visceral hypersensitivity in adult rats induced by colon irritation during postnatal development. *Gastroenterology*, 119:1276–1285.

Aloisi AM. (2003). Gonadal hormones and sex differences in pain reactivity. *Clin J Pain*, 19:168–174.

Aloisi AM, Bonifazi M. (2006). Sex hormones, central nervous system and pain. *Horm Behav*, 50:1–7.

Anakk S, Ku CY, Vore M, Strobel HW. (2003). Insights into gender bias: rat cytochrome P450 3A9. *J Pharmacol Exp Ther*, 305:703–709.

Anand KJ. (2000). Pain, plasticity, and premature birth: a prescription for permanent suffering? *Nat Med*, 6: 971–973.

Anand KJ, Aranda JV, Berde CB, Buckman S, Capparelli EV, Carlo W, et al. (2006). Summary proceedings from the neonatal pain-control group. *Pediatrics*, 117:S9–S22.

Anand P, Birch R. (2002). Restoration of sensory function and lack of long-term chronic pain syndromes after brachial plexus injury in human neonates. *Brain*, 125:113–122.

Arendt-Nielsen L, Bajaj P, Drewes AM. (2004). Visceral pain: gender differences in response to experimental and clinical pain. *Eur J Pain*, 8:465–472.

Averbuch M, Katzper M. (2000). A search for sex differences in response to analgesia. *Arch Intern Med*, 160:3424–3428.

Azpiroz F, Bouin M, Camilleri M, Mayer EA, Poitras P, Spiller RC. (2007). Mechanisms of hypersensitivity in IBS and functional disorders. *Neurogastroenterol Motil*, 19:62–88.

Bajaj P, Bajaj P, Madsen H, Arendt-Nielsen L. (2002). A comparison of modality-specific somatosensory changes during menstruation in dysmenorrheic and nondysmenorrheic women. *Clin J Pain*, 18:180–190.

Banks WA, Watkins LR. (2006). Mediation of chronic pain: not by neurons alone. *Pain*, 124:1–2.

Baranowski A, Holdcroft A (2005) Gender and pain. In Holdcroft A, Jaggar SI, (Eds.), *Core Topics in Pain* (pp. 195–200). Cambridge: Cambridge University Press.

Becerra L, Comite A, Breiter H, Gonzalez RG, Borsook D. (1998). Differential CNS activation following a noxious thermal stimulus in men and women: An fMRI study. *Soc Neurosci Abstr*, 24:1136.

Becker JB, Arnold AP, Berkley KJ, Blaustein JD, Eckel LA, Hampson E, et al. (2005). Strategies and methods for research on sex differences in brain and behavior. *Endocrinology*, 146:1650–1673.

Berkley KJ. (1992). Vive la difference! *Trends Neurosci*, 15:331–332.

Berkley KJ. (1997). On the dorsal columns: translating basic research hypotheses to the clinic. *Pain*, 70: 103–107.

Berkley KJ. (2005). A life of pelvic pain. *Physiol Behav*, 86:272–280.

Berkley KJ, Hoffman GE, Murphy AZ, Holdcroft A (2002) Pain: Sex/gender differences. In Pfaff DW, Arnold AP, Etgen AM, Fahrbach SE, Rubin R, (Eds.), *Hormones, Brain and Behavior* (pp. 409–442). New York: Academic Press.

Berkley KJ, Zalcman SS, Simon VR. (2006). Sex and gender differences in pain and inflammation: a rapidly maturing field. *Am J Physiol Regul Integr Comp Physiol*, 291:R241–R244.

Berman S, Munakata J, Naliboff B, Chang L, Mandelkern M, Silverman DH, et al. (2000). Gender differences in regional brain response to visceral pressure in IBS patients. *Eur J Pain*, 4:157–172.

Berman SM, Naliboff BD, Suyenobu B, Labus JS, Stains J, Bueller JA, et al. (2006). Sex differences in regional brain response to aversive pelvic visceral stimuli. *Am J Physiol Regul Integr Comp Physiol*, 291:R268–R276.

Bhattacharjee M, Mathur R. (2005). Antinociceptive effect of sucrose ingestion in the human. *Indian J Physiol Pharmacol*, 49:383–394.

Bingefors K, Isacson D. (2004). Epidemiology, co-morbidity, and impact on health-related quality of life of self-reported headache and musculoskeletal pain—a gender perspective. *Eur J Pain*, 8:435–450.

Bradshaw HB, Rimmerman N, Krey JF, Walker JM. (2006). Sex and hormonal cycle differences in rat brain levels of pain-related cannabimimetic lipid mediators. *Am J Physiol Regul Integr Comp Physiol*, 291:R349–R358.

Bragdon EE, Light KC, Costello NL, Sigurdsson A, Bunting S, Bhalang K, Maixner W. (2002). Group differences in pain modulation: pain-free women compared to pain-free men and to women with TMD. *Pain*, 96:227–237.

Brandes JL. (2006). The influence of estrogen on migraine: a systematic review. *JAMA*, 295:1824–1830.

Bryant CD, Eitan S, Sinchak K, Fanselow MS, Evans CJ. (2006). NMDA receptor antagonism disrupts the development of morphine analgesic tolerance in male, but not female C57BL/6J mice. *Am J Physiol Regul Integr Comp Physiol*, 291:R315–R326.

Cairns BE, Hu JW, Arendt-Nielsen L, Sessle BJ, Svensson P. (2001). Sex-related differences in human pain and rat afferent discharge evoked by injection of glutamate into the masseter muscle. *J Neurophysiol*, 86:782–791.

Chanda ML, Mogil JS. (2006). Sex differences in the effects of amiloride on formalin test nociception in mice. *Am J Physiol Regul Integr Comp Physiol*, 291:R335–R342.

Chang L, Naliboff BD, Labus JS, Schmulson M, Lee OY, Olivas TI, Stains J, Mayer EA. (2006a). Effect of sex on perception of rectosigmoid stimuli in irritable bowel syndrome. *Am J Physiol Regul Integr Comp Physiol*, 291:R277–R284.

Chang L, Toner BB, Fukudo S, Guthrie E, Locke GR, Norton NJ, Sperber AD. (2006b). Gender, age, society, culture, and the patient's perspective in the functional gastrointestinal disorders. *Gastroenterology*, 130:1435–1446.

Chesler EJ, Wilson SG, Lariviere WR, Rodriguez-Zas SL, Mogil JS. (2002). Identification and ranking of genetic and laboratory environment factors influencing a behavioral trait, thermal nociception, via computational analysis of a large data archive. *Neurosci Biobehav Rev*, 26:907–923.

Chillingworth NL, Morham SG, Donaldson LF. (2006). Sex differences in inflammation and inflammatory pain in cyclooxygenase-deficient mice. *Am J Physiol Regul Integr Comp Physiol*, 291:R327–R334.

Ciccone GK, Holdcroft A. (1999). Drugs and sex differences: a review of drugs relating to anaesthesia. *Br J Anaesth*, 82:255–265.

Coghill RC, McHaffie JG, Yen YF. (2003). Neural correlates of interindividual differences in the subjective experience of pain. *Proc Natl Acad Sci U S A*, 100:8538–8542.

Coghill RC, Sang CN, Maisog JM, Iadarola MJ. (1999). Pain intensity processing within the human brain: a bilateral, distributed mechanism. *J Neurophysiol*, 82:1934–1943.

Cook DB, O'Connor PJ, Oliver SE, Lee Y. (1998). Sex differences in naturally occurring leg muscle pain and exertion during maximal cycle ergometry. *Int J Neurosci*, 95:183–202.

Coutinho SV, Plotsky PM, Sablad M, Miller JC, Zhou H, Bayati AI, et al. (2002). Neonatal maternal separation alters stress-induced responses to viscerosomatic nociceptive stimuli in rat. *Am J Physiol Gastrointest Liver Physiol*, 282:G307–G316.

Craft RM. (2003a). Sex differences in drug- and non-drug-induced analgesia. *Life Sci*, 72:2675–2688.

Craft RM. (2003b). Sex differences in opioid analgesia: "from mouse to man." *Clin J Pain*, 19:175–186.

Craft RM. (2005). Sex differences in behavioral effects of cannabinoids. *Life Sci*, 77:2471–2478.

Craft RM, Mogil JS, Aloisi AM. (2004). Sex differences in pain and analgesia: the role of gonadal hormones. *Eur J Pain*, 8:397–411.

Cremonini F, Talley NJ. (2004). Diagnostic and therapeutic strategies in the irritable bowel syndrome. *Minerva Med*, 95:427–441.

Dannecker EA, Hausenblas HA, Kaminski TW, Robinson ME. (2005). Sex differences in delayed onset muscle pain. *Clin J Pain*, 21:120–126.

Dao TT, LeResche L. (2000). Gender differences in pain. *J Orofac Pain*, 14:169–184.

Derbyshire SW, Nichols TE, Firestone L, Townsend DW, Jones AK. (2002). Gender differences in patterns of cerebral activation during equal experience of painful laser stimulation. *J Pain*, 3:401–411.

Derbyshire SWG, Jones AKP, Townsend D, Gyulai F, Smith GS, Firestone L. (1998). Gender differences in the central response to pain controlled for stimulus intensity. *Soc Neurosci Abstr*, 24:528.

Diatchenko L, Anderson AD, Slade GD, Fillingim RB, Shabalina SA, Higgins TJ, et al. (2006). Three major haplotypes of the beta2 adrenergic receptor define psychological profile, blood pressure, and the risk for development of a common musculoskeletal pain disorder. *Am J Med Genet B Neuropsychiatr Genet*, 141:449–462.

Eastwood JA, Doering LV. (2005). Gender differences in coronary artery disease. *J Cardiovasc Nurs*, 20:340–351.

Edrington JM, Paul S, Dodd M, West C, Facione N, Tripathy D, et al. (2004). No evidence for sex differences in the severity and treatment of cancer pain. *J Pain Symptom Manage*, 28:225–232.

Edwards PW, Zeichner A, Kuczmierczyk AR, Boczkowski J. (1985). Familial pain models: the relationship between family history of pain and current pain experience. *Pain*, 21:379–384.

Edwards RR, Haythornthwaite JA, Sullivan MJ, Fillingim RB. (2004). Catastrophizing as a mediator of sex differences in pain: differential effects for daily pain versus laboratory-induced pain. *Pain*, 111:335–341.

Edwards RR, Sarlani E, Wesselmann U, Fillingim RB. (2005). Quantitative assessment of experimental pain perception: multiple domains of clinical relevance. *Pain*, 114:315–319.

Emery CF, Keefe FJ, France CR, Affleck G, Waters S, Fondow MD, et al. (2006). Effects of a brief coping skills training intervention on nociceptive flexion reflex threshold in patients having osteoarthritic knee pain: a preliminary laboratory study of sex differences. *J Pain Symptom Manage*, 31:262–269.

Fillingim RB. (2000). Sex, gender and pain. Seattle: IASP Press.

Fillingim RB. (2004). Sex differences in opioid analgesia: clinical and experimental findings. *Eur J Pain*, 8:413–425.

Fillingim RB. (2005). Individual differences in pain responses. *Curr Rheumatol Rep*, 7:342–347.

Fillingim RB, Edwards RR, Powell T. (2000). Sex-dependent effects of reported familial pain history on recent pain complaints and experimental pain responses. *Pain*, 86:87–94.

Fillingim RB, Kaplan L, Staud R, Ness TJ, Glover TL, Campbell CM, et al. (2005). The A118G single nucleotide polymorphism of the mu-opioid receptor gene (OPRM1) is associated with pressure pain sensitivity in humans. *J Pain*, 6:159–167.

Fillingim RB, Maixner W. (1996). The influence of resting blood pressure and gender on pain responses. *Psychosom Med*, 58:326–332.

Fitzgerald M, Beggs S. (2001). The neurobiology of pain: developmental aspects. *Neuroscientist*, 7:246–257.

Flake NM, Hermanstyne TO, Gold MS. (2006). Testosterone and estrogen have opposing actions on inflammation-induced plasma extravasation in the rat temporomandibular joint. *Am J Physiol Regul Integr Comp Physiol*, 291:R343–R348.

Flores CA, Shughrue P, Petersen SL, Mokha SS. (2003). Sex-related differences in the distribution of opioid receptor-like 1 receptor mRNA and colocalization with estrogen receptor mRNA in neurons of the spinal trigeminal nucleus caudalis in the rat. *Neuroscience*, 118:769–778.

Frank MG, Baratta MV, Sprunger DB, Watkins LR, Maier SF. (2007). Microglia serve as a neuroimmune substrate for stress-induced potentiation of CNS pro-inflammatory cytokine responses. *Brain Behav Immun*, 21:47–59.

Fronek KS, Schmelz M, Kruger S, Hohenberger W, Schick CH. (2003). Effects of gender and level of surgical sympathetic block on vasoconstrictor function. *Clin Auton Res*, 13:I74–I78.

Fryns JP, Van den BH. (1980). Sex-linked recessive inheritance in Charcot-Marie-Tooth disease with partial clinical manifestations in female carriers. *Hum Genet*, 55:413–415.

Fuller BF. (2002). Infant gender differences regarding acute established pain. *Clin Nurs Res*, 11:190–203.

Gallagher RM. (2004). Biopsychosocial pain medicine and mind-brain-body science. *Phys Med Rehabil Clin N Am*, 15:855–882.

Ge HY, Madeleine P, Arendt-Nielsen L. (2005). Gender differences in pain modulation evoked by repeated injections of glutamate into the human trapezius muscle. *Pain*, 113:134–140.

Gear RW, Gordon NC, Miaskowski C, Paul SM, Heller PH, Levine JD. (2003). Sexual dimorphism in very low dose nalbuphine postoperative analgesia. *Neurosci Lett*, 339:1–4.

Gear RW, Miaskowski C, Gordon NC, Paul SM, Heller PH, Levine JD. (1999). The kappa opioid nalbuphine produces gender- and dose-dependent analgesia and antianalgesia in patients with postoperative pain. *Pain*, 83:339–345.

Giamberardino MA, Berkley KJ, Iezzi S, de Bigontina P, Vecchiet L. (1997). Pain threshold variations in somatic wall tissues as a function of menstrual cycle, segmental site and tissue depth in non-dysmenorrheic women, dysmenorrheic women and men. *Pain*, 71:187–197.

Gugilla SR, Boinpally RR, Bolla SM, Devaraj R. (2002). Influence of menstrual cycle on the pharmacokinetics of paracetamol through salivary compartment in healthy subjects. *Ther Drug Monit*, 24:497–501.

Guinsburg R, de Araujo PC, Branco de Almeida MF, de C, X, Cassia BR, Tonelotto J, Kopelman BI. (2000). Differences in pain expression between male and female newborn infants. *Pain*, 85:127–133.

Hains BC, Waxman SG. (2006). Activated microglia contribute to the maintenance of chronic pain after spinal cord injury. *J Neurosci*, 26:4308–4317.

Halpert A, Drossman D. (2005). Biopsychosocial issues in irritable bowel syndrome. *J Clin Gastroenterol*, 39:665–669.

Hanno PM. (2007). Painful bladder syndrome/interstitial cystitis and related disorders. In Wein AJ, Kavoussi LR, Novick AC, Partin AW, Peters CA, (Eds.), *Campbell-Walsh urology*, Philadelphia, PA: W.B. Saunders Co.

Harju EL. (2002). Cold and warmth perception mapped for age, gender, and body area. *Somatosens Mot Res*, 19:61–75.

Heinberg LJ, Fisher BJ, Wesselmann U, Reed J, Haythornthwaite JA. (2004). Psychological factors in pelvic/urogenital pain: the influence of site of pain versus sex. *Pain*, 108:88–94.

Heitkemper M, Jarrett M. (2005). Overlapping conditions in women with irritable bowel syndrome. *Urol Nurs*, 25:25–30.

Hobara M. (2005). Beliefs about appropriate pain behavior: cross-cultural and sex differences between Japanese and Euro-Americans. *Eur J Pain*, 9:389–393.

Hobson AR, Furlong PL, Worthen SF, Hillebrand A, Barnes GR, Singh KD, Aziz Q. (2005). Real-time imaging of human cortical activity evoked by painful esophageal stimulation. *Gastroenterology*, 128:610–619.

Holdcroft A. (2006). Gender differences in clinical pain management. In Mao J (Ed.), *Translational pain research, comparing preclinical studies and clinical pain management* (pp. 277–294). Hauppauge, NY, Nova Science Publishers, Inc.

Holdcroft AI, Berkley KJ. (2005). Sex and gender differences in pain. In McMahon SB, Koltzenburg M (Eds.), *Wall and Melzack's textbook of pain* (pp. 1181–1197). Edinburgh: Churchill Livingstone.

Howard RF, Walker SM, Mota PM, Fitzgerald M. (2005). The ontogeny of neuropathic pain: postnatal onset of mechanical allodynia in rat spared nerve injury (SNI) and chronic constriction injury (CCI) models. *Pain*, 115:382–389.

Hungin AP, Whorwell PJ, Tack J, Mearin F. (2003). The prevalence, patterns and impact of irritable bowel syndrome: An international survey of 40,000 subjects. *Aliment Pharmacol Ther*, 17:643–650.

Institute of Medicine (U.S.), Wizemann TM, Pardue ML (2001) *Exploring the biological contributions to human health: does sex matter?* Washington, DC: National Academies Press.

Isacson D, Bingefors K. (2002). Epidemiology of analgesic use: a gender perspective. *Eur J Anaesthesiol*, Suppl 26:5–15.

Jackson T, Iezzi T, Chen H, Ebnet S, Eglitis K. (2005). Gender, interpersonal transactions, and the perception of pain: an experimental analysis. *J Pain*, 6:228–236.

Jensen I, Nygren A, Gamberale F, Goldie I, Westerholm P. (1994). Coping with long-term musculoskeletal pain and its consequences: is gender a factor? *Pain*, 57:167–172.

Ji Y, Murphy AZ, Traub RJ. (2006). Sex differences in morphine-induced analgesia of visceral pain are supraspinally and peripherally mediated. *Am J Physiol Regul Integr Comp Physiol*, 291:R307–R314.

Kajantie E, Phillips DI. (2006). The effects of sex and hormonal status on the physiological response to acute psychosocial stress. *Psychoneuroendocrinology*, 31:151–178.

Kalinichev M, Easterling KW, Holtzman SG. (2001). Early neonatal experience of Long-Evans rats results in long-lasting changes in morphine tolerance and dependence. *Psychopharmacology* (Berl), 157:305–312.

Karibe H, Goddard G, Gear RW. (2003). Sex differences in masticatory muscle pain after chewing. *J Dent Res*, 82:112–116.

Keogh E, Arendt-Nielsen L. (2004). Sex differences in pain. *Eur J Pain*, 8:395–396.

Keogh E, Bond FW, Hanmer R, Tilston J. (2005). Comparing acceptance- and control-based coping instructions on the cold-pressor pain experiences of healthy men and women. *Eur J Pain*, 9:591–598.

Keogh E, Eccleston C. (2006). Sex differences in adolescent chronic pain and pain-related coping. *Pain*, 123:275–284.

Kern MK, Jaradeh S, Arndorfer RC, Jesmanowicz J, Hyde J, Shaker R. (2001). Gender differences in cortical representation of rectal distension in healthy humans. *Am J Physiol Gastrointest Liver Physiol*, 281: G1512–G1523.

Kim H, Neubert JK, San Miguel A, Xu K, Krishnaraju RK, Iadarola MJ, et al. (2004). Genetic influence on variability in human acute experimental pain sensitivity associated with gender, ethnicity and psychological temperament. *Pain*, 109:488–496.

Kirchmann M. (2006). Migraine with aura: new understanding from clinical epidemiologic studies. *Curr Opin Neurol*, 19:286–293.

Krzanowska EK, Ogawa S, Pfaff DW, Bodnar RJ. (2002). Reversal of sex differences in morphine analgesia elicited from the ventrolateral periaqueductal gray in rats by neonatal hormone manipulations. *Brain Res*, 929:1–9.

Kuba T, Quinones-Jenab V. (2005). The role of female gonadal hormones in behavioral sex differences in persistent and chronic pain: clinical versus preclinical studies. *Brain Res Bull*, 66:179–188.

Kudielka BM, Kirschbaum C. (2005). Sex differences in HPA axis responses to stress: a review. *Biol Psychol*, 69:113–132.

Labus J, Mayer EA, Berman S, Suyenobu B, Chang L, Naliboff BD. (2006). Sex-specific differences in a brain network functioning during anticipation of rectal discomfort in irritable bowel syndrome patients (IBS). *Gastroenterology*, 130:A-93.

Lawal A, Kern M, Sanjeevi A, Hofmann C, Shaker R. (2005). Cingulate cortex: a closer look at its gut-related functional topography. *Am J Physiol Gastrointest Liver Physiol*, 289:G722–G730.

LeResche L. (2000). Epidemiologic perspectives on sex differences in pain. In Fillingim RB, (Ed.), *Sex, gender, and pain* (pp. 233–249). Seattle: IASP Press.

Lewkowski MD, Ditto B, Roussos M, Young SN. (2003). Sweet taste and blood pressure-related analgesia. *Pain*, 106:181–186.

Liu Z, Ding L, He B. (2006). Integration of EEG/MEG with MRI and fMRI. *IEEE Eng Med Biol Mag*, 25:46–53.

Longstreth GF, Thompson WG, Chey WD, Houghton LA, Mearin F, Spiller RC. (2006). Functional bowel disorders. *Gastroenterology*, 130:1480–1491.

Macfarlane GJ. (2005). Looking back: developments in our understanding of the occurrence, aetiology and prognosis of chronic pain 1954–2004. *Rheumatology*, (Oxford) 44 Suppl 4:iv23–iv26.

Maixner W, Humphrey C. (1993). Gender differences in pain and cardiovascular responses to forearm ischemia. *Clin J Pain*, 9:16–25.

Marques-Deak A, Cizza G, Sternberg E. (2005). Brain-immune interactions and disease susceptibility. *Mol Psychiatry*, 10:239–250.

Masson C, Cisse I, Simon V, Insalaco P, Audran M. (2004). Fabry disease: a review. *Joint Bone Spine*, 71:381–383.

Mayer EA. (2000). The neurobiology of stress and gastrointestinal disease. *Gut*, 47:861–869.

Mayer EA. (2007). Somatic manifestations of traumatic stress. In Kirmayer L, Barad M, Lemelson R (Eds.), *Inscribing trauma: cultural, psychological, and biological perspectives on terror and its aftermath*, Cambridge: Cambridge University Press.

Mayer EA, Berman S, Chang L, Naliboff BD. (2004). Sex-based differences in gastrointestinal pain. *Eur J Pain*, 8:451–463.

Mayer EA, Collins SM. (2002). Evolving pathophysiologic models of functional gastrointestinal disorders. *Gastroenterology*, 122:2032–2048.

Mayer EA, Naliboff B, Lee OY, Munakata J, Chang L. (1999). Review article: gender-related differences in functional gastrointestinal disorders. *Aliment Pharmacol Ther*, 13:65–69.

Mogil JS, Chesler EJ, Wilson SG, Juraska JM, Sternberg WF. (2000) Sex differences in thermal nociception and morphine antinociception in rodents depend on genotype. *Neurosci Biobehav Rev*, 24:375–389.

Mogil JS, Miermeister F, Seifert F, Strasburg K, Zimmermann K, Reinold H, et al. (2005a). Variable sensitivity to noxious heat is mediated by differential expression of the CGRP gene. *Proc Natl Acad Sci U S A*, 102:12938–12943.

Mogil JS, Ritchie J, Smith SB, Strasburg K, Kaplan L, Wallace MR, et al. (2005b). Melanocortin-1 receptor gene variants affect pain and mu-opioid analgesia in mice and humans. *J Med Genet*, 42:583–587.

Mogil JS, Wilson SG, Chesler EJ, Rankin AL, Nemmani KV, Lariviere WR, et al. (2003). The melanocortin-1 receptor gene mediates female-specific mechanisms of analgesia in mice and humans. *Proc Natl Acad Sci USA*, 100:4867–4872.

Morrison TC, Dmitrieva N, Winnard KP, Berkley KJ. (2006). Opposing viscerovisceral effects of surgically induced endometriosis and a control abdominal surgery on the rat bladder. *Fertil Steril*, 86:1067–1073.

Moulton EA, Keaser ML, Gullapalli RP, Maitra R, Greenspan JD. (2006). Sex differences in the cerebral BOLD signal response to painful heat stimuli. *Am J Physiol Regul Integr Comp Physiol*, 291:R257–R267.

Murphy AZ, Shupnik MA, Hoffman GE. (1999). Androgen and estrogen (alpha) receptor distribution in the periaqueductal gray of the male rat. *Horm Behav*, 36:98–108.

Myles PS, Hunt JO, Moloney JT. (1997). Postoperative 'minor' complications: comparison between men and women. *Anaesthesia*, 52:300–306.

Nakai A, Diksic M, Kumakura Y, D'souza D, Kersey K. (2005). The effects of the 5-HT3 antagonist, alosetron, on brain serotonin synthesis in patients with irritable bowel syndrome. *Neurogastroenterol Motil*, 17:212–221.

Nakai A, Kumakura Y, Boivin M, Rosa P, Diksic M, D'souza D, Kersey K. (2003). Sex differences of brain serotonin synthesis in patients with irritable bowel syndrome using alpha-[11C]methyl-L-tryptophan, positron emission tomography and statistical parametric mapping. *Can J Gastroenterol*, 17:191–196.

Naliboff BD, Berman S, Chang L, Derbyshire SWG, Suyenobu B, Vogt BA, et al. (2003). Sex-related differences in IBS patients: central processing of visceral stimuli. *Gastroenterology*, 124:1738–1747.

Nie H, Kawczynski A, Madeleine P, Arendt-Nielsen L. (2005). Delayed onset muscle soreness in neck/shoulder muscles. *Eur J Pain*, 9:653–660.

NIH (1994) NIH Guide.

Nozu T, Kudaira M, Kitamori S, Uehara A. (2006). Repetitive rectal painful distention induces rectal hypersensitivity in patients with irritable bowel syndrome. *J Gastroenterol*, 41:217–222.

Paulson PE, Minoshima S, Morrow TJ, Casey KL. (1998). Gender differences in pain perception and patterns of cerebral activation during noxious heat stimulation in humans. *Pain*, 76:223–229.

Philpott S, Boynton PM, Feder G, Hemingway H. (2001). Gender differences in descriptions of angina symptoms and health problems immediately prior to angiography: the ACRE study. Appropriateness of Coronary Revascularisation study. *Soc Sci Med*, 52: 1565–1575.

Plesh O, Curtis DA, Hall LJ, Miller A. (1998). Gender difference in jaw pain induced by clenching. *J Oral Rehabil*, 25:258–263.

Poudevigne MS, O'Connor PJ, Pasley JD. (2002). Lack of both sex differences and influence of resting blood pressure on muscle pain intensity. *Clin J Pain*, 18: 386–393.

Ramos A, Kangerski AL, Basso PF, Silva Santos JE, Assreuy J, Vendruscolo LF, et al. (2002). Evaluation of Lewis and SHR rat strains as a genetic model for the study of anxiety and pain. *Behav Brain Res*, 129:113–123.

Reddy H, Arendt-Nielsen L, Staahl C, Pedersen J, Funch-Jensen P, Gregersen H, Drewes AM. (2005). Gender differences in pain and biomechanical responses after acid sensitization of the human esophagus. *Dig Dis Sci*, 50:2050–2058.

Ren K, Anseloni V, Zou SP, Wade EB, Novikova SI, Ennis M, et al. (2004). Characterization of basal and re-inflammation-associated long-term alteration in pain responsivity following short-lasting neonatal local inflammatory insult. *Pain*, 110:588–596.

Riley III JL, Robinson ME, Wise EA, Price DD. (1999). A meta-analytic review of pain perception across the menstrual cycle. *Pain*, 81:225–235.

Rittner HL, Machelska H, Stein C. (2005). Leukocytes in the regulation of pain and analgesia. *J Leukoc Biol*, 78:1215–1222.

Robinson ME, Riley JL, III, Myers CD, Papas RK, Wise EA, Waxenberg LB, Fillingim RB. (2001). Gender role expectations of pain: relationship to sex differences in pain. *J Pain*, 2:251–257.

Robinson ME, Wise EA. (2004). Prior pain experience: influence on the observation of experimental pain in men and women. *J Pain*, 5:264–269.

Robinson ME, Wise EA, Gagnon C, Fillingim RB, Price DD. (2004). Influences of gender role and anxiety on sex differences in temporal summation of pain. *J Pain*, 5:77–82.

Roe CM, McNamara AM, Motheral BR. (2002). Gender- and age-related prescription drug use patterns. *Ann Pharmacother*, 36:30–39.

Rollman GB, Abdel-Shaheed J, Gillespie JM, Jones KS. (2004). Does past pain influence current pain: biological and psychosocial models of sex differences. *Eur J Pain*, 8:427–433.

Ruda MA. (1993). Gender and pain. *Pain*, 53:1–2.

Sarlani E, Greenspan JD. (2002). Gender differences in temporal summation of mechanically evoked pain. *Pain*, 97:163–169.

Sarlani E, Greenspan JD. (2005). Why look in the brain for answers to temporomandibular disorder pain? *Cells Tissues Organs*, 180:69–75.

Sherman JJ, LeResche L. (2006). Does experimental pain response vary across the menstrual cycle? A methodological review. *Am J Physiol Regul Integr Comp Physiol*, 291:R245–R256.

Sinaki M, Nwaogwugwu NC, Phillips BE, Mokri MP. (2001). Effect of gender, age, and anthropometry on axial and appendicular muscle strength. *Am J Phys Med Rehabil*, 80:330–338.

Smith AG, Francis JE, Green JA, Greig JB, Wolf CR, Manson MM. (1990). Sex-linked hepatic uroporphyria and the induction of cytochromes P450IA in rats caused by hexachlorobenzene and polyhalogenated biphenyls. *Biochem Pharmacol*, 40:2059–2068.

Smith YR, Stohler CS, Nichols TE, Bueller JA, Koeppe RA, Zubieta JK. (2006). Pronociceptive and antinociceptive effects of estradiol through endogenous opioid neurotransmission in women. *J Neurosci*, 26:5777–5785.

Stadler M, Bardiau F, Seidel L, Albert A, Boogaerts JG. (2003). Difference in risk factors for postoperative nausea and vomiting. *Anesthesiology*, 98:46–52.

Stamer UM, Bayerer B, Stuber F. (2005). Genetics and variability in opioid response. *Eur J Pain*, 9:101–104.

Sternberg EM. (2006). Neural regulation of innate immunity: a coordinated nonspecific host response to pathogens. *Nat Rev Immunol*, 6:318–328.

Sternberg WF, Mogil JS, Kest B, Page GG, Leong Y, Yam V, Liebeskind JC. (1995). Neonatal testosterone exposure influences neurochemistry of non-opioid swim stress-induced analgesia in adult mice. *Pain*, 63:321–326.

Sternberg WF, Ridgway CG. (2003). Effects of gestational stress and neonatal handling on pain, analgesia, and stress behavior of adult mice. *Physiol Behav*, 78:375–383.

Stoffel EC, Ulibarri CM, Craft RM. (2003). Gonadal steroid hormone modulation of nociception, morphine antinociception and reproductive indices in male and female rats. *Pain*, 103:285–302.

Tanaka E. (1999). Gender-related differences in pharmacokinetics and their clinical significance. *J Clin Pharm Ther*, 24:339–346.

Tann G. (1979). Recent advances in hemophilia. *Southeast Asian J Trop Med Public Health*, 10:218–228.

Taylor SE. (2002). *The tending instinct: how nurturing is essential for who we are and how we live*. New York, NY: Times Books.

Tillisch K, Labus JS, Naliboff BD, Bolus R, Shetzline M, Mayer EA, Chang L. (2005). Characterization of the alternating bowel habit subtype in patients with irritable bowel syndrome. *Am J Gastroenterol*, 100: 896–904.

Turk DC, Okifuji A. (1999). Does sex make a difference in the prescription of treatments and the adaptation to chronic pain by cancer and non-cancer patients? *Pain*, 82:139–148.

Unruh AM. (1996). Gender variations in clinical pain experience. *Pain*, 65:123–167.

Unruh AM, Ritchie J, Merskey H. (1999). Does gender affect appraisal of pain and pain coping strategies? *Clin J Pain*, 15:31–40.

Vanderhorst VG, Gustafsson JA, Ulfhake B. (2005). Estrogen receptor-alpha and -beta immunoreactive neurons in the brainstem and spinal cord of male and female mice: relationships to monoaminergic, cholinergic, and spinal projection systems. *J Comp Neurol*, 488:152–179.

Vilming ST, Kloster R, Sandvik L. (2001). The importance of sex, age, needle size, height and body mass index in post-lumbar puncture headache. *Cephalalgia*, 21:738–743.

Walker JS, Carmody JJ. (1998). Experimental pain in healthy human subjects: gender differences in nociception and in response to ibuprofen. *Anesth Analg*, 86:1257–1262.

Wang G, Ji Y, Lidow MS, Traub RJ. (2004). Neonatal hind paw injury alters processing of visceral and somatic nociceptive stimuli in the adult rat. *J Pain*, 5:440–449.

Wang X, Traub RJ, Murphy AZ. (2006). Persistent pain model reveals sex difference in morphine potency. *Am J Physiol Regul Integr Comp Physiol*, 291:R300–R306.

Watkins LR, Hutchinson MR, Ledeboer A, Wieseler-Frank J, Milligan ED, Maier SF. (2007). Glia as the "bad guys": Implications for improving clinical pain control and the clinical utility of opioids. *Brain Behav Immun*, 21:131–146.

Watkins LR, Maier SF. (2005). Immune regulation of central nervous system functions: from sickness responses to pathological pain. *J Intern Med*, 257: 139–155.

Wieseler-Frank J, Maier SF, Watkins LR. (2005). Immune-to-brain communication dynamically modulates pain: physiological and pathological consequences. *Brain Behav Immun*, 19:104–111.

Wiesenfeld-Hallin Z. (2005). Sex differences in pain perception. *Gend Med*, 2:137–145.

Zhang N, Oppenheim JJ. (2005). Crosstalk between chemokines and neuronal receptors bridges immune and nervous systems. *J Leukoc Biol*, 78:1210–1214.

Zubieta JK, Dannals RF, Frost JJ. (1999). Gender and age influences on human brain mu-opioid receptor binding measured by PET. *Am J Psychiatry*, 156:842–848.

Zubieta JK, Ketter TA, Bueller JA, Xu Y, Kilbourn MR, Young EA, Koeppe RA. (2003). Regulation of human affective responses by anterior cingulate and limbic mu-opioid neurotransmission. *Arch Gen Psychiatry*, 60:1145–1153.

Zubieta JK, Smith YR, Bueller JA, Xu Y, Kilbourn MR, Jewett DM, et al. (2002). mu-opioid receptor-mediated antinociceptive responses differ in men and women. *J Neurosci*, 22:5100–5107.

Chapter 20

Sex Differences in Anxiety Disorders

Margaret Altemus and Laura Epstein

Anxiety disorders are common in both men and in women, but women suffer with disproportionately higher rates of illness. Thirty-one percent of women versus 19% of men will experience an anxiety disorder during their lifetime (Kessler et al., 1994). Anxiety disorders are often chronic conditions that create a substantial level of disability. All anxiety disorders are characterized by symptoms of anxiety, but there are distinct characteristics of each disorder. The Diagnostic and Statistical Manual of Mental Disorders (DSM-IV) (American Psychiatric Association, 1994) describes panic disorder, agoraphobia, generalized anxiety disorder, obsessive-compulsive disorder, posttraumatic stress disorder, and specific phobias including social phobia and situational phobia.

CLINICAL FEATURES OF ANXIETY DISORDERS

Panic disorder is diagnosed when an individual has recurrent panic attacks and associated avoidance be-

haviors. Panic attacks are discrete, paroxysmal periods of intense anxiety. The symptoms of a panic attack may be somatic or cognitive and typically last between 10 to 30 minutes.

Patients may describe a fear that they are "going crazy" or that they are experiencing a life-threatening illness (eg., heart attack) and will die. Symptoms of panic attacks include palpitations, shortness of breath, choking, nausea, dizziness, numbness or tingling, hot flashes, and fear of dying or losing control. It is important to realize that although panic attacks are the primary symptom in panic disorder, panic attacks are also commonly associated with other anxiety disorders and can occur episodically in individuals who do not meet criteria for any anxiety disorder.

Panic disorder is diagnosed when there is no clear stimulus for the initial panic attacks and patients are apprehensive about recurrence of panic attacks. The prevalence of panic disorder in a recent large epidemiological study, the National Comorbidity Survey, was 5% in women versus 2% in men (Kessler et al., 1994). The sex difference in prevalence of panic disorder is apparent as early as age 6 (Lewinsohn et al., 1998). Women are more likely to experience palpitations, shortness of breath, nausea, and feeling smothered during attacks whereas men are more likely to experience sweating and stomach pain (Sheikh et al., 2002; Chambliss & Mason, 1986). Women are also 3 times more likely to relapse after resolution of panic disorder (Yonkers et al., 2003).

Agoraphobia, the most disabling consequence of panic disorder, is fear of having a panic attack or the fear of confined spaces leading to restriction of independent activities or activities outside the home. Research indicates that agoraphobia may be more severe in women than men, causing a greater degree of impairment in quality of life (Starcevic et al., 1998; Turgeon et al., 1998). Lifetime prevalence rates of agoraphobia in the Virginia Adult Twin Study and National Comorbidity Survey were 3%–4% of men and 7%–9% of women (Kessler et al., 1994; Hettema et al., 2005).

Generalized anxiety disorder is uncontrollable worrying about multiple problems. The worry is about realistic issues, but the degree of worry is excessive. Additional symptoms can include muscle tension, fatigue, insomnia, restlessness, poor concentration, and irritability. Generalized anxiety disorder symptoms are more continuous and do not occur in the brief explosive bursts characteristic of panic disorder. The lifetime prevalence in the National Comorbidity study was 4% in men and 7% in women (Kessler et al., 1994). To date, no significant sex differences in clinical course of generalized anxiety disorder have been found (Yonkers et al., 2000).

Obsessive-compulsive disorder (OCD) is different from generalized anxiety disorder in that worries in OCD are more idiosyncratic and unrealistic. Patients with OCD often perform ritualistic compulsions in order to relieve obsessions about contamination, harm, and symmetry. Common compulsions are checking, cleaning, and counting. To meet diagnostic criteria, the obsessions and compulsions must take up more than one hour per day and significantly impair social or occupational functioning.

In adulthood, OCD is 1.5 times more prevalent in women than in men (Karno et al., 1988; Weissman et al., 1994; Bogetto et al., 1999; Lochner et al., 2004). OCD is a chronic disorder and chronicity has not been shown to differ by gender. However, symptoms differ among sexes: women have a higher prevalence of intrusive aggressive thoughts, cleaning and checking for harm compulsions and lower prevalence of the symmetry/ordering symptoms than do men (Mataix-Cols et al., 2002). Men have more comorbid tic disorders than women (Holzer et al., 1994; Zohar et al., 1997). Women are more likely to have an onset of OCD after the age of 20 (Karno et al., 1988; Weissman et al., 1994), particularly in association with pregnancy (Neziroglu et al., 1992).

Exposure to trauma such as accidents or sexual or physical violence can cause post-traumatic stress disorder (PTSD). PTSD is characterized by the re-experiencing of a traumatic event through dreams or flashbacks along with hyperarousal, hypervigilance, and avoidance of thoughts or experiences related to the event. Although men are more likely to experience trauma in general population samples (Breslau et al., 1991; Stein et al., 1997), women may experience trauma earlier in life as a result of sexual assault (Kilpatrick et al., 1992). Kessler et al. (1992) estimated that the lifetime prevalence of PTSD is 10% in women and 5% in men (Kessler et al., 1995). Even when controlling for type of traumatic event, women are more likely than men to develop PTSD (Breslau et al., 1991; Gianconia et al., 1995).

A phobia is an excessive fear of a particular object or situation. In the Virginia Adult Twin Study, animal phobia had a lifetime prevalence of 5% in men and 11% in women; situational phobia (flying, elevators, bridges) had a lifetime prevalence of 9% in men and 12% in women (Hettema et al., 2005). In a separate study, social phobia had a lifetime prevalence of 11% in men and 16% in women (Kessler et al., 1994). Like generalized anxiety disorder, the clinical course of phobias has not been shown to differ significantly between men and women (Bourdon et al., 1988; Yonkers et al., 2001a).

DETERMINANTS OF SEX DIFFERENCES

There is very strong evidence from family studies that genetic factors play a role in all anxiety disorders. At this point, however, few candidate gene studies have been replicated. One mechanism through which genetic factors may contribute to the sex difference in anxiety disorders is through differential prevalence of potential vulnerability alleles.

One study revealed a higher frequency of the 5HT2C receptor Ser23 allele in females as compared to males (Fehr et al., 2000) and four other studies found a nonsignificant increased frequency of the allele in females (Ebstein et al., 1997; Oruc et al., 1997; Gutierrez et al., 1999; Samochowiec et al., 1999). 5HT2C agonists have anxiogenic effects in healthy volunteers and exacerbate symptoms of OCD and panic in individuals with those disorders (Wood, 2003).

It is also possible that sex-specific hormonal milieu and other sex-specific biological factors differentially affect expression or the downstream effects of vulnerability genes for anxiety in men versus women. One study of the catechol-o-methyltransferase (COMT) gene found that there was association between low activity allele and OCD in females only (Alsobrook et al., 2002). However, two other studies found the opposite—that the low activity gene was associated with OCD in males only (Karayiorgou et al., 1997; Karayiorgou et al., 1999).

There is little evidence that genetic or environmental factors play a greater role in the etiology of anxiety disorders in women versus men. Although one study found that familial environmental factors played a greater role in women with social phobia (Kendler et al., 2002), there was no evidence of sex differences in the relative contribution of genetic and environmental risk factors for other phobias (Kendler et al., 2002), obsessive-compulsive disorder (Hudziak et al., 2004), generalized anxiety disorder (Hettema et al., 2005; Mackintosh et al., 2006), or panic (Hettema et al., 2005).

Examination of sex differences in brain structure and function provide an opportunity to consider processes downstream of genetic and environmental factors which also may shed light to sex differences in anxiety disorder prevalence and clinical course. There is emerging evidence that differences between the sexes include brain anatomy, neurochemistry, and patterns of activation and response to environmental stimuli.

Sex differences in brain structure and function are primarily determined during development under the influence of circulating gonadal steroids, but may also arise in part from other sex chromosome effects (Arnold et al., 2003; see also chapter 2) as well as sex-specific environmental factors. Gender differences in the physiology and pathophysiology of other body systems also have been identified which may impact the etiology and course of anxiety disorders (Institute of Medicine, 2001). Sex differences in immune responses and autonomic regulation may be particularly important in this regard.

Anxiety disorders and the stress response are tightly linked. There is a large body of evidence that biological aspects of gender modulate the effects of acute and chronic stress on hormonal stress responses (see chapter 6), neural systems (Shors et al., 2001), and behavior (Wood & Shors, 1998; Luine, 2002; Jackson et al., 2005). Multiple studies have shown that patients with anxiety disorders have hyperactivated stress systems including corticotropin-releasing hormone (CRH), vasopressin, and norepinephrine (Charney et al., 1987; Altemus et al., 1992; Baker et al., 1999). The same systems have also been shown to be hyperactivated in animal models of anxiety disorders (Coplan et al., 1996; Heim et al., 1997).

There is evidence that blood pressure and pulse are more reactive to stress in women compared to men (Kario et al., 2001), and that women are more sensitive to the effects of catecholamines on emotional memory consolidation (Cahill, 2003). Rumination, or perseverative focus on emotional reactions, is a feature of anxiety and more common in women and girls (Nolen-Hoeksema & Girgus, 1994; Nolen-Hoeksema et al., 1999; Garneski et al., 2002). In addition, given the same amount of anxiogenic stimulation by CO_2 inhalation, women and men had similar physiological responses, but women experienced more subjective fear and panic symptoms (Kelly et al., 2006). Together, these characteristics may increase stress sensitivity and suggest another potential biological pathway to disproportionate generation of anxiety disorders in women.

Finally, it is likely that gender-specific economic, cultural, and psychosocial experiences may contribute to sex differences in anxiety, independent of innate biological differences. For example, women experience more sleep disruption associated with child care and also are more likely to diet. Food restriction is known to alter brain serotonergic function (Attenburrow et al., 2003), which may increase risk of anxiety in women who diet. During childhood, girls tend to be reinforced for empathy and less assertiveness, while boys tend to be reinforced for more assertive, active, and independent behavior—differences which also may influence propensity to develop anxiety disorders (Chambliss Mason, 1986).

Studies of depression suggest that there are likely to be sex differences in the relative influence of specific environmental factors. In one study, men were more sensitive to depressogenic effects of separation and work problems while women were more sensitive to the depressogenic effects of problems such as getting along with individuals in their proximal network (Kendler et al., 2001).

HORMONAL INFLUENCE ON ANXIETY DISORDERS: EVIDENCE FROM PREGNANCY AND LACTATION

Naturalistic studies of anxiety during pregnancy, lactation, and the menstrual cycle are sparse, but provide evidence that shifts in reproductive hormones may change the course of anxiety disorders.

Pregnancy may be associated with reduction in panic symptoms, and then worsening of symptoms postpartum(Cowley & Roy-Byrne, 1989; Sholomskas et al., 1993; Klein et al., 1995). These observations are consistent with evidence that progesterone and progesterone metabolites enhance $GABA_A$ receptor sensitivity, and that panic disorder is particularly sensitive to benzodiazepine treatment. Vulnerability to experimentally-induced panic is reduced in the luteal phase of the menstrual cycle, when progesterone levels are highest (Perna et al., 1995).

Another change during pregnancy is that both catecholamine and HPA axis stress response systems are suppressed (Barron et al., 1986; Schulte et al., 1990; Matthews & Rodin, 1992). These stress response systems are also suppressed during lactation (Altemus et al., 1995; Heinrichs et al., 2001; Mezzacappa et al., 2003). These and several other brain neurochemical systems known to modulate anxiety and fear, including oxytocin and prolactin appear to be altered in parallel during pregnancy and lactation (Altemus et al., 2004).

Rapid weaning or lack of breastfeeding postpartum may precipitate more rapid decreases in these anxiolytic hormones, destabilizing stress responses and exacerbating anxiety symptoms. Behavioral studies have demonstrated suppression of multiple fear behaviors and stress-induced gene responses in lactating rats and mice (Hansen & Ferreira, 1986; Abbud et al., 1993; Toufexis et al., 1999) and decreased anxiety and depression in breast-feeding compared to bottle-feeding mothers (Lane et al., 1997; Yonkers et al., 2001b; Mezzacappa & Katkin, 2002).

Until relatively recently, women spent much of their adult lives either pregnant or lactating. To balance these protective processes, women may have evolved a higher underlying "set-point" of stress reactivity and anxiety, which is dampened by reproductive hormones. Now that women are spending many years of their adult lives not pregnant or lactating, their underlying higher "set-point" may be unmasked, thus making women more reactive to stress and more susceptible to anxiety disorders.

In contrast to panic, women seem to experience an exacerbation of OCD symptoms premenstrually (Dillon & Brooks, 1992), as well as during pregnancy (Neziroglu et al., 1992; Williams & Koran, 1997; Altemus, 2001), suggesting exacerbation of OCD by gonadal steroids. In addition, suppression and blockade of gonadal steroids appears to ameliorate symptoms of OCD (Casas et al., 1986; Chouinard et al., 1996).

Because pregnancy, lactation, and the menstrual cycle each are associated with changes in multiple hormones, it is not possible to link changes in anxiety symptoms in these studies to any particular hormone. Although there have been no studies of the effects of estrogen treatment on anxiety disorders in humans, a few clinical studies suggest that estrogen can blunt anxiety. Preliminary reports indicate that subclinical anxiety symptoms are reduced in menopausal women treated with estrogen and estrogen receptor agonists (Ditkoff et al., 1991; Baksu et al., 2005; Gulseren et al., 2005); and anxiety symptoms are reduced in depressed, menopausal women treated with estrogen (Soares et al., 2001). Estrogen also seems to blunt autonomic responses to stress in postmenopausal women (Lindheim et al., 1992).

ANTITHYROID ANTIBODIES AND ANXIETY

Presence of antithyroid antibodies is another potentially important risk factor for increased anxiety in women because presence of these antibodies is associated with a high risk for hyperthyroidism postpartum, which in turn can induce panic attacks and generalized anxiety symptoms. Antithyroid antibodies are present in 14% of women of reproductive age (Lazarus et al., 1996). Although not usually clinically significant, antithyroid antibodies are strongly associated with autoimmune thyroiditis postpartum, conferring an 11-fold increased risk of thyroiditis. By 6 months postpartum, 15%–42% of women with antithyroid antibodies meet laboratory criteria for hyperthyroidism (Sakaihara et al., 2000).

CONCLUSION

Ongoing effort will be needed to sort out whether particular sex differences in the prevalence, phenomenology, and course of anxiety disorders arise from biological determinants, environmental determinants or interactions between biology and the environment. The fact that women have much greater and more frequent fluxes in reproductive hormones over a lifespan may enhance the potential for dysregulation of a wide variety of brain neurochemical systems. Sex differences in anxiety disorders and hormonal modulation of anxiety disorders are likely to provide an important window into the pathophysiology of these illnesses. Better understanding of the pathophysiology of anxiety disorders should enhance diagnosis and treatment for both women and men.

References

Abbud R, Hoffman GE, Smith MS. (1993). Cortical refractoriness to N-methyl-D,L-aspartic acid (NMDA) stimulation in the lactating rat: recovery after pup removal and blockade of progesterone receptors. *Brain Research*, 604:16–23.

Alsobrook J, Zohar A, Leboyer M, Chabane N, Ebstein R, Pauls D. (2002). Association between the COMT locus and obsessive-compulsive disorder in females but not males. *Am J Med Genet*, 114:116–120.

Altemus M. (2001). Obsessive-compulsive disorder during pregnancy and postpartum. In Yonkers K, Little B (Eds.), *Management of psychiatric disorders in pregnancy* (pp. 149–163). London: Arnold.

Altemus M, Deuster P, Galliven E, Carter S, Gold P. (1995). Suppression of hypothalamic-pituitary-adrenal axis responses to stress in lactating women. *J Clin Endo Metab*, 80:2954–2959.

Altemus M, Fong J, Yang R, Damast S, Luine V, Ferguson D. (2004). Changes in cerebrospinal fluid neurochemistry during pregnancy. *Bio Psychiatry*, 56:386–392.

Altemus M, Pigott T, Kalogeras KT, Demitrack M, Dubbert B, Murphy DL, Gold PW. (1992). Abnormalities in the regulation of vasopressin and corticotropin releasing factor secretion in obsessive-compulsive disorder. *Arch Gen Psychiatry*, 49:9–20.

American Psychiatric Association. (1994). *Diagnostic and Statistical Manual of Mental Disorders*. 4th Edition. Washington, DC: American Psychiatric Association.

Arnold A, Rissman E, DeVries G. (2003). Two perspectives on the origin of sex differences in the brain. *Ann NY Acad Sci*, 1007:176–188.

Attenburrow M, Williams C, Odontiadis J, Powell J, Van de Ouderaa F, Williams M, Cowen P. (2003). The effect of a nutritional source of tryptophan on dieting-induced changes in brain 5-HT function. *Psychological Medicine*, 33:1381–1386.

Baker D, West S, Nicholson W, Ekhator N, Kasckow J, Hill K, et al. (1999). Serial CSF corticotropin-relesing hormone levels and adrenocortical activity in combat veterans with posttraumatic stress disorder. *Am J Psychiatry*, 156:585–588.

Baksu A, Ayas B, Citak S, Kalan A, Basku B, Goker N. (2005). Eficacy of tibolone and transdermal estrogen therapy on psychological symptoms of menopause. *Int J Genaecol & Obst*, 91:58–62.

Barron WM, Mujais SK, Zinaman M, Bravo EL, Lindheimer MD. (1986). Plasma catecholamine responses to physiologic stimuli in normal human pregnancy. *Am J Obstet Gynecol*, 154:80–84.

Bogetto F, Venturello S, Albert U, Maina G, Ravizza L. (1999). Gender-related clinical differences in obsessive-compulsive disorder. *Eur J Psychiatry*, 14:434–441.

Bourdon K, Boyd J, Rae D, Burns J, Thompson J, Locke B. (1988). Gender differences in phobias: results of the ECA community survey. *J Anxiety Disorders*, 2:227–241.

Breslau N, Davis G, Andreski P, Peterson E. (1991). Traumatic events and post-traumatic stress disorder in an urban population of young adults. *Arch Gen Psychiatry*, 48:216–222.

Cahill L. (2003). Sex-related influences on the neurobiology of emotionally influenced memory. *Ann NY Acad Sci*, 985:163–173.

Casas M, Alvarez E, Duro P, Garcia-Ribera C, Udina C, Velat A, et al. (1986). Antiandrogenic treatment of obsessive-compulsive neurosis. *Acta Psychiatr Scand*, 73:221–222.

Chambliss D, Mason J. (1986). Sex, sex-role stereotyping and agoraphobia. *Behav Res Ther*, 24:231–235.

Charney D, Woods S, Goodman W, Heninger G. (1987). Neurobiological mechanisms of panic anxiety: biochemical and behavioral correlates of yohimbine-induced panic attacks. *Am J Psychiatry*, 144:1030–1036.

Chouinard G, Belanger M, Beauclair L, Sultan S, Pearson-Murphy B. (1996). Potentiation of fluoxetine by aminoglutethimide, an adrenal steroid suppressant, in obsessive-compulsive disorder resistant to SSRIs: a case report. *Prog Neuro-psychopharmacology Biol Psychiatry*, 20:1067–1079.

Coplan J, Andrews M, Rosenblum L, Owens M, Friedman S, Gorman J, Nemeroff C. (1996). Persistent elevations of cerebrospinal fluid concentrations of corticotropin-releasing factor in adult nonhuman primates exposed to early-life stressors: implications for the pathophysiology of mood and anxiety disorders. *Proc of the Nat Acad of Sci USA*, 93:1619–1623.

Cowley DS, Roy-Byrne PP. (1989). Panic disorder during pregnancy. *J Psychosom Obstet Gyn*, 10:193–210.

Dillon K, Brooks D. (1992). Unusual cleaning behavior in the luteal phase. *Psychological Reports*, 70:35–39.

Ditkoff EC, Crary WG, Cristo M, Lobo RA. (1991). Estrogen improves psychological function in asymptomatic postmenopausal women. *Obstet Gynecol*, 78:991–995.

Ebstein R, Segman R, Benjamin J, Osher Y, Nemanov L, Belmaker R. (1997). 5-HT2C (HTR2C) serotonin receptor gene polymorphism associated with the human personality trait of reward dependence: interaction with dopamine D4 receptor (D4DR) and dopamine D3 receptor (D3DR) polymorphisms. *Am J Med Genet*, 74:65–72.

Fehr C, Szegedi A, Anghelescu I, Klawe C, Hiemke C, Dahemn N. (2000). Sex differences in allelic frequencies of the 5-HT2C Cys23Ser polymorphism in psychiatric patients and health volunteers: Findings from an association study. *Psychiatric Genetics*, 10: 59–66.

Garnefski N, Teerds J, Kraaij V, Legerstee J, Van den Kommer T. (2004). Cognitive emotion regulation strategies and depressive symptoms: differences between males and females. *Pers Individ Dif*, 36:267–276.

Gianconia R, Reinherz H, Siverman A, Pakiz B, Frost A, Cohen E. (1995). Traumas and posttraumatic stress disorder in a community population of older adolescents. *J Acad Child Adolesc Psychiatry*, 34:1369–1380.

Gulseren L, Kalafat D, Mandaci H, Gulseren S, Camli L. (2005). Effects of tibolone on the qulaity of life, anxiety-depression levels and cognitive functions in natural menopause: an observational follow-up study. *Aust N Z J Obstet Gynaecol*, 45:71–73.

Gutierrez B, Fananas L, Arranz M, Valles V, Guillamat R, van Os J, Collier D. (1999). Allelic association analysis of the 5-HT2C receptor gene in bipolar affective disorder. *Neurosci Lett*, 212:65–67.

Hansen S, Ferreira A. (1986). Food intake, aggression and fear behavior in the mother rat: control by neural systems concerned with milk ejection and maternal behavior. *Behav Neurosci*, 100:410–415.

Heim C, Owens M, Plotsky O, Nemeroff C. (1997). Persistent changes in corticotropin-releasing factor systems due to ealy life stress: relationship to the pathophysiology of major depression and post-traumatic stress disorder. *Psychopharmocology Bulletin*, 33: 185–192.

Heinrichs M, Meinlschmidt G, Neumann I, Wagner S, Kirschbaum C, Ehlert U, Helhammer D. (2001). Effects of suckling on hypothalamic-pituitary-adrenal axis responses to psychosocial stress in postpartum lactating women. *J Clin Endo Metab*, 86:4798–4804.

Hettema J, Prescott C, Myers J, Neale M, Kendler K. (2005). The structure of genetic and environmental risk factors for anxiety disorders in men and women. *Arch Gen Psychiatry*, 62:182–189.

Holzer J, Goodman W, McDougle C, Baer L, Boyarsky B, Leckman J, Price L. (1994). Obsessive compulsive disorder with and without a chronic tic disorder: a comparison of symptoms in 70 patients. *Br J of Psychiatry*, 164:469–473.

Hudziak J, van Beijsterveldt C, Althoff R, Stanger C, Rettew D, Nelson E, et al. (2004). Genetic and environmental contributions to the child behavior checklist obsessive-compulsive scale. A cross-cultural twin study. *Arch Gen Psychiatry*, 61(6):608–16.

Institute of Medicine. (2001). *Exploring the Biological Contributions to Human Health: Does Sex Matter?* Washington, D.C.: National Academy Press.

Jackson E, Payne J, Nadel L, Jacobs W. (2005). Stress differentially modulates fear conditioning in healthy men and women. *Biol Psychiatry*, 59:516–522.

Karayiorgou M, Altemus M, Galke B, Goldman D, Murphy D, Ott G, Gogos J. (1997). Genotype determining low catechol-O-methyltransferase activity as a risk factor for obsessive-compulsive disorder. *Proc Natl Acad of Sci*, 94(9):4572–4575.

Karayiorgou M, Sobin C, Blundell M, Galke B, Malinova L, Goldberg O, Ott J, Gogos J. (1999). Family-based association studies support a sexually dimorphic effect of COMT and MAOA on genetic susceptibility to obsessive-compulsive disorder. *Biol Psychiatry*, 45(9):1178–89.

Kario K, Schwartz J, Davidson K, Pickering T. (2001). Gender differences in associations of diurnal blood pressure variation. *Hypertension*, 38:997–1002.

Karno M, Golding J, Sorenson S, Burnam M. (1988). The epidemiology of obsessive-compulsive disorder in five US communities. *Arch Gen Psychiatry*, 45:1094–1099.

Kelly M, Forsyth J, Karekla M. (2006). Sex differences in response to a panicogenic challenge procedure: An experimental evaluation of panic vulnerabllity in a non-clinical sample. *Behav Res Ther*, 44:1421–1430.

Kendler K, Thornton L, Prescott C. (2001). Gender differences in the rates of exposure to stressful life events and sensitivity to their depressogenic effects. *Am J Psychiatry*, 158:587–593.

Kendler K, Jacobson K, Myers J, Prescott C. (2002). Sex differences in genetic and environmental risk factors for irrational fears and phobias. *Psychological Medicine*, 32:209–217.

Kessler R, Sonnega A, Bromet E, Hughes M, Nelson C. (1995). Post-traumatic stress disorder in the National Comorbidiy Survey. *Arch Gen Psychiatry*, 52:1048–1060.

Kessler R, McGonagle K, Zhao S, Nelson C, Hughes M, Eshleman S, et al. (1994). Lifetime and 12 month prevalences of DSM-III-R psychiatric disorders in the US. Results from the national comorbidity survey. *Arch Gen Psychiatry*, 51:8–19.

Kilpatrick D, Edmunds C, Seymour A. (1992). *Rape in America: A report to the nation*. In. Charleston, SC: Crime Victims Research and Treatment Center.

Klein D, Skrobala A, Garfinkel R. (1995). Preliminary look at the effects of pregnancy on the course of panic disorder. *Anxiety*, 1:227–232.

Lane A, Keville R, Morris M, Kinsella A, Turner M, Barry S. (1997). Post-natal depression and elation among mothers and their partners: prevalence and predictors. *Br J Psychiatry*, 171:550–555.

Lazarus J, Hall R, Othman S, Parkes A, Richards C, McCulloch B, Harris B. (1996). The clinical spectrum of postpartum thyroid disease. *QJM*, 89:429–435.

Lewinsohn P, Lewinsohn M, Gotlib I, Seeley J, Allen N. (1998). Gender differences in anxiety disorders and anxiety symptoms in adolescents. *J Abnormal Psychiatry*, 107:109–117.

Lindheim SR, Legro RS, Bernstein L, Stanczyk FZ, Vijod MA, Presser SC, et al. (1992). Behavioral stress responses in premenopausal and postmenopausal women and the effects of estrogen. *Am J Obstet Gyn*, 167:1831–1836.

Lochner C, Hemmings S, Kinnear C, Moolman-Smook J, Corfield V, Knowles J, et al. (2004). Gender in obsessive-compulsive disorder: Clinical and genetic findings. *Eur J Neuropsychopharmacology*, 14:437–445.

Luine V. (2002). Sex differences in chronic stress effects on memory in rats. *Stress*, 5:205–216.

Mackintosh M, Gatz M, Wetherell J, Pedersen N. (2006). A twin study of lifetime generalized anxiety disorder (GAD) in older adults: genetic and environmental influences shared by neuroticism and GAD. *Twin Research and Human Genetics* 9:30–37.

Mataix-Cols D, Rauch S, Baer L, Eisen J, Shera D, Goodman W, et al. (2002). Symptom stability in adult obsessive-compulsive disorder: data from a naturalistic two-year follow-up study. *Am J Psychiatry*, 159:263–268.

Matthews KA, Rodin J. (1992). Pregnancy alters blood pressure responses to psychological and physical challenge. *Psychophysiology*, 29:232–240.

Mezzacappa E, Yu A, Myers M. (2003). Lactation and weaning effects on physiological and behavioral responses to stressors. *Physiol Behav*, 78:1–9.

Mezzacappa ES, Katkin ES. (2002). Breast-feeding is associated with reductions in perceived stress and negative mood in mothers. *Health Psychol*, 21:187–193.

Neziroglu F, Anemone R, Yaryura-Tobias J. (1992). Onset of obsessive-compulsive disorder in pregnancy. *Am J Psychiatry*, 149:947–950.

Nolen-Hoeksema S, Girgus J. (1994). The emerence of gender differences in depression during adolescence. *Psychol Bull*, 115:424–443.

Nolen-Hoeksema S, Larson J, Grayson C. (1999). Explaining the gender difference in depressive symptoms. *J Pers Soc Psychol*, 77:1061–1072.

Oruc L, Verheyen G, Furac I, Jakovljevic M, Ivezic S, Raeymaekers P, et al. (1997). Association alalysis of the 5-HT2C receptor and 5-HAT transporter genes in bipolar disorder. *Am J Med Genet*, 74:504–506.

Perna G, Brambilla F, Arancio C, Bellodi L. (1995). Menstrual cycle-related sensitivity to 35% CO2 in panic patients. *Biol Psychiatry*, 37:528–532.

Sakaihara M, Yamada H, Kato E, Ebina Y, Shimada S, Kobashi G, et al. (2000). Postpartum thyroid dysfunction in women with normal thyroid function during pregnancy. *Clin Endocrinol*, 53:487–492.

Samochowiec J, Smolka M, Winterer G, Rommelspacher H, Schmidt L, Sander T. (1999). Association analysis between a Cys23Ser substitution polymorphism of the human 5-HT2C receptor gene and neuronal hyperexcitability. *Am J Med Genet*, 88(2):126–30.

Schulte HM, Weisner D, Allolio B. (1990). The corticotropin releasing hormone test in late pregnancy: lack of adrenocorticotropin and cortiol response. *Clin Endocrinol*, 33:99–106.

Sheikh J, Leskin G, Klein D. (2002). Gender differences in panic disorder: findings from the National Comorbidity Survey. *Am J Psychiatry*, 159:55–58.

Sholomskas D, Wickamaratne P, Dogolo L, O'Brien D, Leaf P, Woods S. (1993). Postpartum onset of panic disorder: a coincidental event? *J Clin Psychiatry*, 54:476–480.

Shors T, Chua C, Falduto J. (2001). Sex differences and opposite effects of stresss on dendritic spine density in the male versus female hippocampus. *J Neuroscience*, 21:6292–6297.

Soares C, Almeida O, Joffe H, Cohen L. (2001). Efficacy of estradiol for the treatment of depressive disorder in perimenopausal women. *Arch Gen Psychiatry*, 58:529–534.

Starcevic V, Djordjevic A, Latas M, Bogojevic G. (1998). Characteristics of agoraphobia in women and men with panic disorder and agoraphobia. *Depression and Anxiety*, 8:8–13.

Stein M, Walker J, Hazen A, Forde D. (1997). Full and partial posttraumatic stress disorder: findings from a community survey. *Am J Psychiatry*, 154:1114–1119.

Toufexis DJ, Rochford J, Walker CD. (1999). Lactation-induced reduction in rats' acoustic startle is associated with changes in noradrenergic neruotransmission. *Behav Neurosci*, 113:176–184.

Turgeon L, Marchand A, Dupuis G. (1998). Clinical features in panic disorder with agoraphobia. *J Anxiety Disord*, 12:539–553.

Weissman M, Bland R, Canino G, Greenwald S, Hwu H, Lee C, et al. (1994) The cross national epidemiology of obsessive compulsive disorder. The Cross National Collaborative Group. *J Clin Psychiatry*, 55:5–10.

Williams K, Koran L. (1997). Obsessive-compulsive disorder in pregnancy, the puerperium and the premenstrum. *J Clin Psychiatry*, 58:330–334.

Wood GE, Shors TJ. (1998). Stress facilitates classical conditioning in males, but impairs classical conditioning in female through activational effects of ovarian hormones. *Proc Natl Acad Sci USA*, 95:4066–4071.

Wood M. (2003). Therapeutic potential of 5-HT2C receptor antagonists in the treatment of anxiety disorders. *Current Drug Targets—CNS & Neurological Disorders* 2:383–387.

Yonkers K, Dyck I, Keller M. (2001a). An eight-year longitudinal comparison of clinical course and characteristics of social phobia among men and women. *Psychiatric Services*, 52:637–643.

Yonkers K, Dyck I, Warshaw M, Keller M. (2000). Factors predicting the clinical course of generalized anxiety disorders. *Br J of Psychiatry*, 176:544–549.

Yonkers K, Bruce S, Dyck I, Keller M. (2003). Chronicity, relapse and illness—course of panic disorder, social phobia and generalized anxiety disorer: Findings in men and women from 8 years follow-up. *Depression and Anxiety*, 17:173–179.

Yonkers K, Ramin SM, Rush AJ, Navarrete CA, Carmod T, March D, et al. (2001b). Onset and persistence of postpartum depression in an inner-city maternal health clinic system. *Am J Psychiatry*, 158:1856–1863.

Zohar A, Pauls D, Ratzoni G, Apter A, Dycian A, Binder M, et al. (1997). Obsessive-compulsive disorder with and without tics in an epidemiological sample of adolescents. *Am J Psychiatry*, 154:274–276.

Chapter 21

Hormones and Mood

Meir Steiner and Elizabeth A. Young

The lifetime prevalence of depressive disorders in women is approximately twice that of men (Kessler et al, 2003). This higher incidence of depression in women is primarily seen from puberty on and is less marked in the years after menopause (Weissman & Olfson, 1995) with the exception of an additional perimenopausal blip (Kessler et al., 1993; Freeman et al, 2004; Schmidt et al, 2004; Schmidt, 2005). The underlying causality of gender difference in mood-related disorders is not clear at this time. Since mood disorders occur in both men and women it is assumed that a unified basis for the development of these diseases exists.

The principal constituent of this unified theory is believed to be related to genetic predisposition. Multiple environmental stressful events cause biochemical changes in a host of neuroendocrine systems and neuroanatomical areas. The genetic predisposition, which is multi-factorial, determines how stressful life events are interpreted and predicts the response, which can lead to the development of mood disorders. The higher prevalence of mood disorders in women could be related to an increased genetic predisposition, an increased vulnerability/exposure to stressful life events, modulation of the neuroendocrine system by fluctuating gonadal hormones, or a combination of any or all of these factors (Noble, 2005).

We have previously proposed a biological susceptibility hypothesis to account for gender differences in the prevalence of mood disorders based on the idea that there is a disturbance in the interaction between the HPG axis and other neuromodulators in women (Steiner & Dunn, 1996; Dunn & Steiner, 2000). According to this hypothesis, the neuroendocrine rhythmicity related to female reproduction is vulnerable to change and is sensitive to psychosocial, environmental and physiological factors. Thus, premenstrual dysphoric disorder (PMDD), depression with post-partum onset (PPD), and mood disorders associated with the perimenopause or with menopause, may all be related to hormone-modulated changes in neurotransmitter function.

Control of mood and behavior involves many different neurotransmitter systems, including glutamate, GABA, acetylcholine (ACh), serotonin (5-HT), dopamine (DA), noradrenaline (NA) and neuropeptides. Given the observation that prevalence and symptomatology of mood disorders is often different between males and females, it is presumed that gonadal steroid hormones are somehow involved. For example, declining levels of estrogen in women have been associated with postnatal depression and postmenopausal depression, and the cyclical variations of estrogens and progesterone are probably the trigger of premenstrual complaints in women with premenstrual syndrome (Fink et al., 1996). The interaction between neurotransmitters and steroid hormones is extremely complex and delicately balanced. Each system appears to have a modulatory function on the other, and changes in one system may have dramatic effect on the other systems.

Gonadal steroid receptors vary in abundance across different regions of the brain. Estrogen receptors are found in the amygdala, hippocampus, basal forebrain, cortex, cerebellum, locus coeruleus, midbrain raphe nuclei, the pre-optic area, and the ventromedial and arcuate areas of the hypothalamus, as well as the pituitary gland (Stomati et al., 1998; McEwen, 1988; Herbison et al., 1995).

Activation of cholinergic, dopaminergic or adrenergic neurotransmitter systems can alter concentrations of cytosolic hypothalamic estrogen receptors. Muscarinic agonists and antagonists can increase estrogen-binding sites in the female rat hypothalamus (Lauber & Whalen, 1988). Estrogen, progesterone, and glucocorticoid receptors can also be activated by insulin-like growth factor 1 (IGF-1), epidermal growth factor (EGF), transforming growth factor alpha (TGF-alpha), cyclic AMP, protein kinase activators and by various neurotransmitters (Culig et al., 1995). Thus activation of neurotransmitter systems can have a direct modulatory effect on binding of gonadal hormones in the central nervous system (CNS).

Conversely, steroid hormones such as estrogen can modulate neuronal transmission by a variety of mechanisms. They may affect the synthesis and/or release of neurotransmitters, as well as the expression of receptors, membrane plasticity, and permeability. It has been suggested that steroid hormone receptors function as general transcription factors to achieve integration of neural information in the CNS (Mani et al., 1997).

Steroids are believed to act primarily by classical genomic mechanisms through intracellular receptors to modulate transcription and protein synthesis. This mechanism involves the binding of the steroid to a cytoplasmic or nuclear receptor. The hormone-receptor complex then binds to DNA to trigger RNA dependent protein synthesis. The response time for this mechanism is on the order of several minutes, hours or days. Recently however, it has been shown that steroids can also produce rapid effects on electrical excitability and synaptic function through direct membrane mechanisms, such as ligand-gated ion-channels, G-proteins, and neurotransmitter transporters (Wong et al., 1996).

These short-term (seconds to minutes) effects of steroids may occur through binding to the cell membrane, binding to membrane receptors, modulation of ion-channels, by direct activation of second messenger systems, (Moss et al., 1997) or by activation of receptors by factors such as cytokines and dopamine (Brann et al., 1995). Topical application of estrogen or progesterone to nervous tissue has been shown to result in a rapid change in membrane potential and sex steroids can affect membrane fluidity thereby modifying ion transport or receptor function (Maggi & Perez, 1985).

Gender differences also exist in brain activity, which may have an important implication in the development of mood disorders. Several studies have shown greater functional connectivity between the amygdala and subgenual prefrontal cortex in women (Kilpatrick et al., 2006). Considering that the subgenual prefrontal cortex has been associated with depression, the greater incidence of depressed mood in females may be attributed to this cause (Drevets et al., 1998; Hirayasu et al., 1999; Botteron et al., 2002).

The role and potential relevance of estrogen and other sex steroids to psychiatric disorders is the focus of current scientific attention. Estrogen has been described as a 5-HT, NA and ACh agonist; it also modulates DA_2 receptors. The implications to the reproductive life cycle of women will be briefly reviewed. Specifically, the impact of hormonal fluctuations during menarche, premenstrually, during pregnancy and postpartum, and perimenopausally will be discussed.

MENARCHE AND MOOD DISORDERS IN ADOLESCENCE

Epidemiological studies consistently show that beginning at menarche, mood disorders are at least twice more common in women than in men. Why these gender differences exist and why they start at puberty is perhaps one of the most intriguing and least understood phenomenon in clinical psychiatry (Lewinsohn et al., 1998).

Prior to adolescence, the rates of depression are similar in girls and boys, or are slightly higher in boys (Twenge & Nolen-Hoeksma, 2002). Wiith the onset of puberty, the gender proportion of depression dramatically shifts to a 2:1 female to male ratio (Kessler & Walters, 1998; Lewinsohn et al., 1998). In the U.S. general population, the lifetime prevalence of major depression (MD) in adolescents and young adults (15–24 years of age) has been reported as 20.6% for females and 10.5% for males (Kessler & Walters, 1998). Lifetime rates of MD in early- as well as late-maturing females, were even higher (30% vs. 22% and 34% vs. 22%, respectively) when compared to "on-time" girls.

There is conflicting opinion regarding the age at which gender differences in rates of MD emerge: researchers are divided between the 12 to 14 and the 15 to 19 year age brackets (Cohen et al., 1993; Hankin et al., 1998; Lewinsohn et al., 1998). The transition from childhood to adolescence is clearly associated with susceptibility to depressive symptoms in females and is illustrated through the following findings: girls' depression scores generally decrease from 9 to 11 years of age, but increase from 12 to 17 years of age; conversely, boys' depression scores decrease overall from 9 to 17 years of age (Angold et al., 2002). Moreover, adolescent girls have a tendency to display higher levels of depressive symptoms, lower levels of self-esteem, and higher cortisol and dihydroepiandrosterone (DHEA) levels than boys (Goodyer et al., 2000; Angold, 2003).

An integrative theory of depression in adolescents has been introduced (Lewinsohn et al., 1998), although a persuasive explanation of the sharp rise in the prevalence of depression in females after menarche has yet to be elucidated.

The onset of puberty is heralded by a growth spurt, which begins with rapid growth in height and weight typically between 7.5 and 11.5 years of age. Following this initial burst, physical growth continues at a slow pace for several years. The first sign of sexual maturation in girls is breast budding at about 10.5 years, followed by growth of pubic hair which begins at about 11.5 years, growth of the uterus and vagina, and the enlargement of the labia and clitoris. Menstruation begins after these changes occur. Finally, axillary

hair appears, hips broaden, and fat deposits increase. On average, these changes take four to five years; however, considerable variation exists in the sequence and tempo of these events.

In North America and Europe, the age of menarche has declined about 4 months per decade since 1850; in North America, menarche now occurs around 12.5 years of age on average (Tanner, 1968). This dramatic decline in the age at which girls reach puberty is one of the strongest examples of environmental factors that affect hormonal responses. The search to isolate the particular environmental factors involved in this acceleration, however, has been only marginally helpful. It has been suggested that urbanization has a major role in this change as well as improvements in general health, nutrition, and other sociocultural factors. However, other environmental factors also seem to be implicated in the timing of menarche.

Girls who are blind with some perception of light reach menarche earlier than normally-sighted girls, and totally blind girls with no light perception reach puberty even earlier (Zacharias & Wurtman, 1964). In comparison, girls with major depressive disorder have also been shown as having lower exposure to light (and lower circadian amplitude) versus healthy controls (Armitage et al., 2004). This may correlate with the fact that girls who experience the onset of menarche at an earlier age have elevated risk for depression. Moreover, fewer girls start to menstruate during spring and summer time as compared to during seasons of reduced amounts of daylight (fall and winter) (Bojlen & Bentzon, 1974).

The relationship between psychosocial development and physical maturation has been widely examined. Girls undergoing pubertal change are thought to experience greater distress and to be more vulnerable to stress than pre- or postpubertal girls (Caspi & Moffitt, 1991). Two parameters of pubertal change in particular have received much attention: *pubertal status* and *pubertal timing*. *Pubertal status* is defined as the current level of physical development of an adolescent relative to the overall process of pubertal change (a biological factor), usually denoted by a series of stages from prepubertal (Stage I) to adult (Stage V) according to Tanner (Tanner, 1962). *Pubertal timing*, on the other hand, is defined as the maturation of an adolescent relative to her peers (a psychosocial factor).

There appears to be a relatively sharp demarcated period in mid-puberty when girls become more vulnerable to depression than boys. In a recent report on 1073 U.S. children 9 to 13 years of age, the depression rates in girls rose significantly in mid-puberty, i.e., with the transition to Tanner Stage III. In contrast, the prevalence of depression in boys *declines* from Tanner Stage II (Angold et al., 1998). Further, it has been determined that in girls, *pubertal status* (versus the age at puberty per se) better predicted the emergence of the sex ratio in depression rates. Thus, the onset of menarche may signal an increased, but latent biological vulnerability to mood dysregulation in women (Nolen-Hoeksema & Girgus, 1994).

Moreover, a follow-up study indicated that risk for depression was actually correlated with elevated levels of testosterone and estrogen rather than changes in body morphology (Angold et al., 1999). Although hormones affect rates of physical development during puberty, it is important to note that Tanner Stage III may only be the physical manifestation of the underlying hormonal cause.

Although changes in affect, mood, and behavior are considered to be related to cyclic hormonal changes, studies of female adolescents and premenstrual syndrome (PMS) are inconclusive. One study reports no relationship between menstrual cycle phase and negative affect (Golub & Harrington, 1981) whereas others show that PMS is associated with other distress factors in this age group (Raja et al., 1992; Freeman et al., 1993; Derman et al., 2004). Notwithstanding, relationships between changes in pubertal hormones and negative affect in female adolescents have been observed. For example, investigators have found that negative affect was significantly related to a rapid increase in estradiol levels (Warren & Brooks-Gunn, 1989). Negative affect in healthy girls was also associated with higher levels of testosterone and cortisol, and lower levels of sulphated DHEA (Susman et al., 1991).

There is both indirect and limited direct evidence of the involvement of the serotonergic system in the etiology of depressive disorders in child and adolescent depression. In a comparative study of psychiatric inpatients and normal controls (aged 7–17 years), levels of whole-blood 5-HT (which may correlate with CNS serotonin) were lowest in patients with mood disorders (Hughes et al., 1996). There is some indication of the responsiveness of children and adolescents with MD to serotonergic but not noradrenergic agents; researchers have hypothesized that, in childhood, the serotonergic systems may mature at an earlier rate than the noradrenergic systems (Ryan & Varma, 1998).

Gonadal hormones affect the production of 5-HT receptors at the transcriptional level, and the altered distribution or function of 5-HT receptor subtypes brought on by changes in the hormonal milieu at menarche may increase vulnerability to mood disorders.

A study in female cynomolgus monkey with depressive behaviors supports the notion that mood disorders are associated with alterations in 5-HT receptors (Shively et al., 2006). Decreased 5-HT$_{1A}$ binding potential was found in the raphe, amygdala, hippocampus, and anterior cingulate cortex of depressed monkeys versus non-depressed controls. Furthermore, greater periods of depression were associated with lower levels of 5-HT$_{1A}$ binding potential. Although the factors associated with decreased binding potential are unknown, these studies support the hypothesis that decreases in 5-HT receptor availability or receptor affinity are related to etiology of depression.

Furthermore, the heritability of depression has also been demonstrated in several studies (Beardslee et al., 1998; Rice at al., 2002; Sullivan et al., 2000). Recently, research on 5-HT related genes suggest that certain individuals may be genetically predisposed to the development of depression (Caspi et al., 2003; Kauffman et al., 2004; Grabe et al., 2005; Kendler et al., 2005). A functional polymorphism in the promoter region of the 5-HT transporter gene (5HTTL PR) is associated with lower activity and elevated risk of depression as a result of negative life events. Moreover, adults whom were either heterozygous or homozygous for this variant allele had a higher rate of depression versus those who did not possess a copy of this mutant, even though all subjects were exposed to the same levels of stress. These results were replicated in a subsequent study on adolescent girls 12 to 17 years of age; however, these findings were not observed in adolescent boys (Eley et al., 2004).

Nevertheless, it is still unclear how the dramatic changes in the hormonal milieu associated with menarche and a host of psychosocial stressors combine to produce depressive symptoms. One possible unifying hypothesis suggests that disruption of biological rhythms, such as disturbed sleep patterns (Armitage et al., 2001) or irregular menstrual cycles, together with psychosocial losses causing the disruption of social rhythms (also known as "social zeitgebers") could trigger the onset of a major depressive episode in vulnerable individuals (Ehlers et al., 1988).

Another complementary theory emphasizes the neurobiology of stress and the dysregulation of affect during female biological transitions such as menarche—a transition which may be associated with changes in the reactivity of the stress system (Dorn & Chrousos, 1997). However, despite the observation that adolescent girls are exposed to more stressors after the age of 13, only 20%–50% of girls who experience severe, negative life events actually become clinically depressed. These data suggest other significant contributors to the onset of depression (Lewinsohn et al., 1994; Ge et al., 2001, Hankin et al., 2004).

The newly fluctuating levels of gonadal hormones as well as gonadotropins, which mark the onset of menarche and the establishment of menstrual cycles, introduce a major change in the hormonal milieu to which all bodily systems have to adjust. This is the period of time during which the hypothalamic-pituitary-adrenal (HPA) axis has to mature and be sensitized to a variety of new feedback mechanisms. This is also the time period during which the HPA axis may be more vulnerable to external psychosocial stressors, to sleep deprivation, and to the influences of nicotine, alcohol and other drugs. Enhanced HPA axis vulnerability may result in a higher incidence of stress hormone dysregulation and mood instability.

Taken together, it is suggested that pubertal and other hormonal changes should be monitored prospectively along with individual, genetic, constitutional, and psychological characteristics in our efforts to predict the development of negative affect during puberty (Steiner et al., 2000).

PREMENSTRUAL DYSPHORIA

The recent inclusion of research diagnostic criteria for PMDD in the DSM-IV recognizes the fact that some women in their reproductive years have extremely distressing emotional and behavioral symptoms premenstrually (APA, 1994a). Through the use of these criteria, PMDD can be differentiated from *premenstrual syndrome* (PMS) which has milder physical symptoms, i.e. breast tenderness, bloating, headache and minor mood changes (WHO, 1996a). PMDD can also be differentiated from *premenstrual magnification* (concurrent diagnoses of PMS or PMDD *and* a major psychiatric or an unstable medical condition) and from *premenstrual exacerbation* of a current psychiatric disorder or medical condition (Steiner & Wilkins, 1996).

Epidemiological surveys have estimated that as many as 75% of women with regular menstrual cycles experience some symptoms of premenstrual syndrome (Johnson, 1987). PMDD, on the other hand, is much less common. It affects only 3% to 8% of women in this group (Johnson et al., 1988; Ramcharan et al., 1992; Angst et al. 2001), but it is more severe and exerts a much greater psychological toll. These women report premenstrual symptoms that seriously interfere with their lifestyle and relationships (Freeman et al., 1985; O'Brien et al., 1995) as well as with their work productivity (Dean & Borenstein, 2004). An additional group of women who marginally miss the PMDD/DSM-IV criteria, but who suffer from moderate to severe PMS has recently been identified (Wittchen et al., 2002; Steiner et al, 2003).

The etiology of PMS and PMDD is still largely unknown. That PMS and PMDD are biological phenomena (as opposed to psychological or psychosocial events) is primarily underscored by recent, convincing evidence of the heritability of premenstrual symptoms (Kendler et al., 1998) and the elimination of premenstrual complaints with suppression of ovarian activity (Schmidt et al., 1998) or surgical menopause (Casson et al., 1990). The current consensus seems to be that normal ovarian function rather than simple hormone imbalance is the cyclic trigger for biochemical events within the central nervous system and other target tissues that unleash premenstrual symptoms in vulnerable women (Roca et al.,1996). This viewpoint is attractive in that it encourages investigation of the neuroendocrine-modulated central neurotransmitters and the role of the hypothalamic-pituitary-gonadal axis in PMDD. Notwithstanding, a surge of recent research has encompassed other etiological influences including female biological rhythms (sleep, body temperature), and psycho-social factors.

The role of the female sex hormones in premenstrual symptomatology has been considered of central importance, yet in women with PMDD, the ovarian axis is apparently functioning normally with normal hormone (estrogen and progesterone) levels (Schmidt et al., 1998). Recently, attention has shifted from a focus on estrogen and progesterone to the role of androgens in premenstrual dysphoria.

Early investigations of androgens have suggested that women with PMS or PMDD have elevated levels of serum testosterone in the luteal phase compared with controls (although still within the normal range), which may contribute primarily to the symptom of irritability (Eriksson et al., 1992; Ho et al., 2001). This hypothesis of increased androgenicity is backed both by animal and human studies of androgen enhancement of irritability and/or aggression.

Androgens promote sexual drive in both males and females, and also, have been tentatively linked with mood (e.g. depression, and premenstrual irritability) and impulsive behavior (e.g. compulsions, and binge eating). Enhanced serotonin availability (e.g., with the use of SSRIs), on the other hand, is associated with reduction in irritability, depression, impulsive behavior, and reduced libido. An inverse relationship between serotonin and androgens, and their effects on human behavior has been proposed; the behavioral effects of androgens may be therefore partly mediated by a reduction in serotonin activity (Eriksson et al., 2000).

Reduction of premenstrual dysphoria with androgen antagonists in women with PMS who showed higher mean levels of total testosterone in the late luteal phase also lends support to the idea of increased androgenicity (Rowe & Sasse, 1986; Burnet et al., 1991). Others, however, have not observed differences in plasma testosterone in comparisons of women with or without PMS (Dougherty et al., 1997), and one study has reported significantly *lower* total and free plasma testosterone levels in a sample of 10 women with PMS (Bloch et al., 1998). Further comparative studies of women with PMS and PMDD are therefore required.

There is increasing attention to the metabolite of progesterone, allopregnanolone in the manifestation of premenstrual symptoms. Treatment studies have suggested that progesterone and progestagens may actually provoke, rather than ameliorate, the cyclical symptom changes of PMDD (Hammarback et al., 1985). Allopregnanolone, on the other hand, is thought to modulate gamma aminobutyric acid (GABA) receptor functioning and produce an anxiolytic effect (Rapkin et al., 1997).

Quantitative differences in progesterone and allopregnanolone levels between PMS subjects and controls have been examined. The findings to date in women are contradictory (Rapkin et al., 1997; Schmidt et al., 1994; Wang et al., 1996; Bicikova et al., 1998; Monteleone et al., 2000), although a recent study in an animal model is more promising. In a progesterone-withdrawal paradigm, designed to mimic PMS and postpartum depression in female rats, Smith and colleagues have found that decreased levels of allo-

pregnanolone lead to increased production of the α4 subunit of the GABA$_A$ receptor. This in turn changes the sensitivity of the GABA$_A$ receptor to endogenous ligands, resulting in symptoms associated with PMS (Smith et al., 1998).

An alternative strategy to measuring various hormone plasma levels in an attempt to discern the etiology of PMDD has been to search for endocrine abnormalities that have been repeatedly associated with other forms of mood changes. The main advantage of this approach is its potential to help further our understanding of PMDD as well as its relation to other psychiatric disorders. The current literature suggests that thyroid dysfunction, which can produce depressive symptoms, may be found in a small group of women with premenstrual symptoms but that PMDD should not be viewed as a masked form of hypothyroidism (Schmidt et al., 1993; Korzekwa et al., 1996).

Of the neurotransmitters studied to date, increasing evidence suggests that 5-HT may be important in the pathogenesis of PMDD (Rapkin, 1992; Steiner et al., 1997). PMDD shares many features of other mood and anxiety disorders linked to serotonergic dysfunction. In addition, reduction in brain 5-HT neurotransmission is thought to lead to poor impulse control, depressed mood, irritability, and increased carbohydrate craving—all mood and behavioral symptoms associated with PMDD.

The serotonergic system has a reciprocal relationship with gonadal hormones. Brain serotonergic activity is influenced by estrogen, progesterone and testosterone (Bethea et al., 1998; Fink et al., 1999). In the hypothalamus, estrogen induces a diurnal fluctuation in 5-HT (Cohen and Wise, 1988), whereas progesterone increases the turnover rate of 5-HT (Ladisich, 1977).

More recently, several studies concluded that 5-HT *function* may also be altered in women with PMDD. Some studies used models of serotonin function (such as whole blood 5-HT levels, platelet uptake of 5-HT, and platelet tritiated imipramine binding) and found altered 5-HT function during all phases of the menstrual cycle (Ashby et al., 1988; Rapkin, 1992; Steege et al., 1992).

Other studies that used challenge tests (with L-tryptophan, fenfluramine, buspirone, m-chlorophenylpiperazine) suggested abnormal serotonin function in symptomatic women but differed in their findings as to whether the response to 5-HT is blunted or heightened (Bancroft et al., 1991; Bancroft & Cook 1995; FitzGerald et al., 1997; Su et al., 1997; Steiner et al., 1999).

Acute tryptophan depletion (suppressing brain 5-HT synthesis) was significantly associated with exacerbation of premenstrual symptoms, in particular irritability (Menkes et al., 1994). Treatment with pyridoxine (vitamin B6) may alleviate symptoms by serving as a cofactor for tryptophan hydoxylase and, hence, increasing the synthesis of serotonin (Eriksson & Humble, 1990). Additional evidence suggesting the involvement (although not necessarily etiologic) of the serotonergic system has emerged from treatment studies: drugs facilitating serotonergic transmission, such as selective serotonin reuptake inhibitors (SSRIs), are very effective in reducing premenstrual symptoms (Pearlstein, 2002; Steiner et al., 2006). These studies imply, at least in part, a possible change in 5-HT receptor sensitivity in women with premenstrual dysphoria (Steiner & Born, 2000).

The current consensus is that women with premenstrual dysphoria may be behaviorally or biochemically sub- or supersensitive to biological challenges of the serotonergic system. It is not yet clear whether these women present with a trait or state marker (alternatively, both conditions could be possible) of premenstrual syndromes.

The close reciprocal relationship between the serotonergic system and gonadal hormones identifies the former as a plausible target for interventions. In support of this hypothesis, the SSRIs are more effective treatment option than lifestyle adjustment and stress management, or more extreme interventions that eliminate ovulation altogether (e.g. ovarian suppression, using long-term treatment with GnRH agonists, which is not only associated with the untoward effects of introducing early menopause but may also increase depressive symptoms (Warnock et al, 1998).

Results from several randomized placebo-controlled trials in women with PMDD, with predominantly psychological symptoms of irritability, tension, dysphoria, and lability of mood, have clearly demonstrated that the SSRIs have excellent efficacy and minimal side effects. More recently, several studies indicate that intermittent (premenstrually only) treatment with SSRIs is equally effective in these women and, thus, may offer an attractive treatment option for a disorder that is itself intermittent (Steiner et al., 2006).

POSTPARTUM DEPRESSION

The specific link and the uniqueness of psychiatric disorders precipitated or triggered by pregnancy or childbirth have recently been acknowledged by the American Psychiatric Association (APA, 1994b). Based primarily on the work of the Task Force on the DSM-IV (Purnine & Frank, 1996), the manual now has a course-specific designation "postpartum onset," that can be applied to both psychotic and non-psychotic postpartum mental disorders. Thus, major depressive disorders, bipolar disorders (manic and depressed), schizoaffective disorders, and psychotic disorders (not otherwise specified) will have the qualifier "with postpartum onset."

Postpartum blues is considered the most mild of the postpartum mood disturbances; its prevalence has been reported to be 26%–85%, depending on the diagnostic criteria used (Stein et al., 1981). The symptoms of this syndrome typically begin within the first week following childbirth, peak on the fifth day and resolve by the twelfth day postpartum. Symptoms include dysphoria, mood lability, crying, anxiety, insomnia, poor appetite, and irritability. The mood disturbance characterizing postpartum "blues" is considered transient and insufficient in and of itself to cause serious impairment of a woman's functioning (O'Hara et al., 1991). In some women, however, the disturbance may persist beyond the initial postpartum period, leading to more serious PPD (Cox et al., 1993; Josefsson et al, 2001).

Epidemiologic studies of the nature, prevalence and course of an episode of major PPD have found that between 10%–15% of women exhibit depressive symptoms in the first weeks following delivery (Carothers & Murray, 1990; Pop et al., 1993), and that the great majority of these depressive episodes resolve spontaneously within three to six months (Cox et al., 1993; Cooper & Murray, 1995). The symptom profile of PPD resembles that of a major depressive episode experienced at other times in life, but it is unique in its timing and in that it always involves at least the mother-baby dyad and in most cases an entire family unit.

Postpartum psychosis is much more rare and severe than either depression or the so-called postpartum "blues." It has a prevalence of approximately 1 in 500–1000 births, and a rapid onset within the first few days to 2 weeks postpartum (Brockington et al., 1982). Postpartum psychosis, believed to be in most cases an episodic presentation of a manic-depressive illness, severely impairs the affected woman's ability to function. In the most extreme cases, the risks of suicide or infanticide are high (Millis & Kornblith, 1992), requiring admission to a psychiatric hospital (Kendell et al., 1987).

Pregnancy and childbirth have an enormous combined psychological, physiologic, and endocrine effect on a woman's body and mind. Since the changes in mood coincide with these profound changes in hormones and other humoral agents related to pregnancy and childbirth, a causal link has been supposed probable (Steiner, 1998).

In the animal kingdom, maternal behavior is mediated by hormonal and neurochemical changes associated with reproduction (Rosenblatt et al., 1988). In animals, it has been suggested that the various neuromodulators be divided into groups that define their proposed role in maternal response: primers—most important during late pregnancy (e.g. steroid hormones and prolactin); triggers—released during parturition (e.g. oxytocin); and modifiers—specifically, of oxytocin release (e.g. beta-endorphins, other neurotransmitters) (Keverne & Kendrick, 1994). There is, of course, a considerable scope for interactions between these changes and varying repertoires of maternal behavior across different species (Fleming & Corter, 1988) and the relevance to human behavior is as yet unclear.

The peak in mood disturbance during the blues at around the fifth day postpartum coincides with extreme hormonal fluctuations that are a natural consequence of parturition. These hormones act within the central nervous system at a variety of limbic sites known to be involved in emotional responses, arousal and reinforcement. Only a handful of studies attempted to measure these changes, especially in gonadal hormones and prolactin. To date, the results do not seem to correlate strongly with changes in mood and are mostly disappointing and inconsistent. For example, a rapid fall in progesterone showed a weak but significant relationship to the development of "the blues" in one study (Harris et al., 1994) but not in another (Heidrich et al., 1994).

Similarly, increased plasma cortisol levels correlated with "the blues" and with PPD in one study (Okano & Nomura, 1992), but not in others (Smith et al., 1990; O'Hara et al., 1991). Preliminary results suggest that natural killer-cell activity is lower in postpartum dysphorics and that this decrease is related

to higher levels of cortisol (Pedersen et al., 1993). In contrast, negative or false-positive results with the dexamethasone suppression test do not correlate with mood changes indicating that the HPA axis is physiologically 'hyperactive' postpartum ('ceiling effect') and measurements along this axis as an indicator for depression in this population are probably invalid (Steiner et al.,1986; Smith et al., 1990; O'Hara et al., 1991).

The HPA, rather than the HPG axis may in fact play a unique role in human maternal behavior. Euthymic new mothers with positive maternal attitudes and high levels of cortisol postpartum exhibit the highest level of postpartum maternal approach behavior (Fleming et al., 1987). None of the other hormones measured (estradiol, progesterone, testosterone and thyroid indices) were correlated with any of the maternal behaviors measured (Fleming et al., 1987; 1995). These results suggest that cortisol does not induce maternal behavior directly but it probably facilitates maternal attitudes, which may then be expressed as emotions and/or behavior.

Thyroid dysfunction is implicated in mood disorders and it is suggested that transient thyroid dysfunction following childbirth is associated with PPD (Pedersen, 1999). In some women, pregnancy and the postpartum period are associated with pathological changes in thyroid function. A review of the literature in this area clearly indicates the possibility that a subgroup of women with PPD have a basis for the depressed mood in thyroid disorder. More specifically, in some women depressive symptoms are associated with positive thyroid antibody status during the postpartum period (Harris et al., 1992). It is believed that 1% of all postpartum women will show a mood disorder associated with transient thyroid dysfunction and treatment of the thyroid condition must be part of the management.

The direct and/or indirect effect of the rate of the postpartum withdrawal of some of the other major hormones and neuromodulators involved is intriguing. It is suggested that women who experience a more rapid beta-endorphin withdrawal are more prone to mood changes (Smith et al., 1990). A sharp fall in circulating estrogen concentrations after delivery has been associated with acute onset of postpartum psychosis (Wieck et al., 1991). These changes are believed to trigger a cascade of changes in central and peripheral monoamine systems. Very preliminary data suggest an increased sensitivity of dopamine receptors in acute postpartum psychosis (Wieck et al., 1991) and an abnormality in alpha$_2$-adrenoceptor sensitivity associated with "the blues" (Best et al., 1988). Changes in serotonergic receptor sensitivities are documented in PPD (Hannah et al., 1992), but not in women with "the blues" (Katona et al., 1985).

More recently it has been hypothesized that PPD may be caused by transient-hypothalamic corticotropin-releasing hormone (CRH) supression (Magiakou et al., 1996). The HPA axis is progressively hyperactive throughout pregnancy, with increasing levels of circulating CRH (of placental origin) and decreasing levels of CRH-binding protein. Both these phenomena, together with pregnancy-associated increases in estradiol, particularly during the third trimester (also stimulating the HPA axis), may contribute to the elevated levels of CRH, ACTH and cortisol (Cizza et al., 1997). After parturition the source of placental CRH is removed, and together with the postpartum estrogen withdrawal which is further prolonged by breastfeeding (Kim et al., 2000) may lead to a prolonged state of HPA axis hypoactivity. Indeed, it has been demonstrated that a subgroup of women with PPD, the suppression of the HPA axis was more severe and lasted longer than that of women who had no postpartum mood instability (Magiakou et al., 1996).

Corticotropin-releasing hormone is associated with the neurobiology of stress and depression (Chrousos & Gold, 1992). Postpartum depression also appears within the context of central CRH dysregulation. With the additional established evidence of direct estrogenic regulation of the CRH gene expression (Vamvakopoulos & Chrousos, 1993), it is not surprising that estrogen is proposed as a treatment for PPD (Sichel et al., 1995; Gregoire et al., 1996; Ahokas et al., 2001). In the only double-blind, placebo-controlled study published to date, a 3-month course of 200 µg/day of 17ß-estradiol significantly improved the clinical symptoms of severely depressed women postpartum (Gregoire et al., 1996). Unfortunately further research on the role of estrogen therapy for PPD has not yet emerged. Similarly, progesterone has been widely used for the treatment of postnatal depression but without controlled trials (O'Brien & Pitt 1994).

The reciprocal relationship between the serotonergic system and gonadal hormones has not as yet been studied during pregnancy or in postpartum women. However, preliminary results from studies in postpartum rats indicate that 5-HT receptor changes in the limbic area are negatively correlated with progesterone levels (Glaser et al., 1990). It is argued that postpartum withdrawal of gonadal hormones may cause changes along the serotonergic cascade that can lead to a mood disorder in vulnerable or genetically predisposed women. It should therefore be possible to treat the disturbance by "adjusting" the levels of the hormone (the trigger) (Henderson et al., 1991) or by reversing the sensitivity (predisposition).

Results from some preliminary studies on preventative interventions with lithium prophylaxis (Stewart et al., 1991; Cohen et al., 1995) and with SSRIs (Stowe et al., 1995; Appleby et al., 1997) are very encouraging. Since mood disorders associated with childbearing have different times of onset in different women and are heterogenous in their presentation, concomitant measurements of the temporal changes in gonadal hormones and the biochemical changes in the monoamine system are crucial.

Further evidence of a biological component of postpartum mood disorders comes from family and family-history studies. In our own study of women with postpartum mood disturbances and their first-degree relatives we found that at least one family member met criteria for a past or present psychiatric disorder in 71% of the cases for which the information was available. Positive histories for MD and alcoholism were found in 48% and 30% of these families respectively (Steiner & Tam, 1999). Further analysis of these data revealed an interesting gender distribution of psychiatric disorders in the first-degree relatives of the postpartum women. A female:male ratio greater than 2:1 was found in relatives with a past or present diagnosis of MD, in the case of alcoholism, a male:female ratio of 4:1 was evident. This lifetime prevalence of mood-related disorders in the first-degree relatives of women presenting with postpartum mood disorders is much higher than in the population at large and may indicate potential genetic or familial components of the disorders.

Despite the fact that most animals share the same physiological events at parturition, the differences in behavioral response between humans (as well as other primates) and non-primate mammals are remarkable. The differences between primates and non-primates are mainly in the organization of social structures, the complex influences of the family unit, and the constant exposure of all members of a group to the young. Therefore, it is easy to assume that, in humans, even thinking about children may be sufficient to stimulate maternal responsiveness. The psychosocial literature to date has advanced several psychological and social stress factors as potential etiologic theories of primary non-psychotic PPD. These factors include lack of social support, negative life events, occupational instability, lack of prior experience with children, unplanned pregnancy and antenatal "pessimism," dissatisfaction with the marital relationship (or being unmarried), and a poor relationship between the affected woman and her own mother (Paykel et al., 1980; Murray et al., 1995).

As previously mentioned, postpartum mood disorders affect not only the mother but also quite possibly the infant. Hence, changes in maternal mood and behavior associated with the postpartum period may render lasting effects on neonatal development. Indeed, the quantity, quality, and regularity of interactions between mother and infant may affect an infant's temperament and subsequently its levels of arousal, attention and reactions to environmental stimuli (Susman et al., 2001). In addition, animal models demonstrate that early-life experiences can permanently alter not only an infant's hormonal response to stress (Anisman et al., 1998), but also the regulation of brain neurochemistry (Polan & Hoffer, 1999). Moreover, behavioral problems are consistently found in children whose mothers were affected by a postpartum mood disorder (Goodman & Gotlib, 1999; Breznitz & Friedman, 1988; Hart et al., 1998; Hay et al., 2003; Murray, 1992; Sohr-Preston & Scaramella, 2006).

In summarizing these studies, no unifying conclusion can be reached, and it is impossible at this stage to translate any of these results into predictive, diagnostic, therapeutic, prognostic or preventative applications. It seems more likely that intrinsic abnormal reactions to some of the hormonal changes, rather than the changes themselves, are responsible for the disorder. If the psychobiological factors (or their interactions) responsible for the emotional disorders associated with childbearing could be shown, our understanding of the etiology not only of PPD but also of a wider range of psychiatric disorders might be enhanced.

PERIMENOPAUSE, MENOPAUSE AND BEYOND

The transition into menopause is a major hormonal event and is associated in many women with both physical and psychosocial symptoms. The term perimenopause describes the period immediately before the menopause—from the time when the hormonal and clinical features of approaching menopause commence till the end of the first year after menopause (WHO, 1996b).

The physiologic hallmark of the transition into menopause is gradual estrogen depletion. In the 1960s and '70s "depletion" was equated with "deficiency" and menopause, representing a state of estrogen deficiency, was therefore considered a medical disorder warranting treatment. A famous quote from that era highlights this approach: "It sometimes seems as if the only thing worse than being subjected to the raging hormonal influences of the female cycle is to have those influences subside" (Parlee, 1976). The notion of universal hormone replacement for *all* menopausal women was so rampant that the WHO convened a special session and eventually came out with a consensus statement to counter the above which read: "Menopause is part the normal aging process which in itself does not require therapeutic intervention. The health status of women during this period is not recognized as being a simple endocrine-deficiency state which could or should be corrected by attempting to create for each woman a premenopausal normal environment" (WHO, 1981).

Changes most commonly associated with estrogen depletion (and/or unpredictable fluctuations) include vasomotor symptoms such as hot flushes and night sweats (Guthrie et al., 1996; Freedman, 2000), urogenital dryness/atrophy causing dyspareunia as well as an increased risk over time of osteoporosis and cardiovascular disease (Mitchell & Woods, 1996). The relationship between the perimenopause/menopause and mood disorders is less well understood. The majority of postmenopausal women do not experience prominent symptoms of depression (epidemiologic data), but a higher than expected prevalence of depressive-like symptoms has been observed in peri-and postmenopausal women attending gynaecologic clinics (clinic-based surveys) (Avis & McKinlay, 1991; Schmidt & Rubinow, 1991).

It is unclear whether there is decline in new onset episodes of major depression in females of this age group as suggested by the Epidemiological Catchment Area study, a finding not supported by data from the National Comorbidity Survey. The role of sociocultural factors and demographic differences have been the focus of much study but the results are controversial (Anderson et al., 1987; Hay et al., 1994).

Some cross-cultural differences are nevertheless noteworthy: Japanese women experience very few physical or emotional symptoms associated with menopause. It is proposed that these findings are indicative not only of cultural and demographic differences but also reflect the influence of biological, genetic and nutritional/dietary factors (Lock, 1994; Nagata et al., 1998).

The most prevalent mood symptoms during the perimenopausal include irritability, tearfullness, anxiety, depressed/labile mood, lack of motivation/energy, poor concentration and interrupted sleep. These symptoms have been linked to predictable fluctuations in estradiol, especially abrupt withdrawal from very high erratic levels, rather than to times when levels are slowly and gradually declining (Prior, 1998).

Several lines of evidence point to the link between estrogen depletion/deficiency and mood disorders in vulnerable or predisposed women. Estrogen has direct effects on the CNS in areas which are not strictly relevant to reproduction. For example, estrogen regulates synaptogenesis, has a general trophic effect on cholinergic neurons and stimulates a significant increase in 5-HT_{2A} binding sites in areas that are involved in regulating both mood and cognition. Therefore, it is not surprising that estrogen improves psychological functioning and well-being in non-depressed postmenopausal women (Ditkoff et al., 1991; Palinkas & Barret-Connor, 1992) or that estrogen replacement therapy (ERT) has a positive effect on mood states (Zweifel & O'Brien, 1997).

The ability of estrogen to act as a 5HT agonist/modulator is of particular significance. Estrogens not only increases the number of 5HT_{2A} receptor binding sites, but also increases 5HT synthesis, uptake and 3H-imipramine binding. Estrogens also decrease 5HT_1 receptor binding sites and 5HT transporter mRNA and increases the prolactin response to 5HT agonists—all in line with antidepressant-like action (Biegon & McEwen., 1982; Halbreich et al., 1995; Fink et al., 1996; Pecins-Thompson et al., 1998). The clinical relevance of these effects to the pathophysiology of women-specific mood and anxiety disorders remains to be determined.

The strongest evidence to date for the ability of estrogens to improve mood and cognitive functioning comes from studies in young surgically menopausal women treated with ERT (Sherwin, 1988; Sherwin & Suranyi-Cadotte, 1990). It is encouraging to note that several very preliminary studies seem to indicate the beneficial effects of combining estrogen replacement therapy (ERT) with SSRIs in the treatment of postmenopausal depressed women (Schneider et al., 1997). Preliminary evidence also indicates the efficacy of transdermal 17ß-estradiol alone in the treatment of perimenopasual women with major and minor depression (Schmidt et al., 2000; Soares et al., 2001).

Estrogens specifically maintain verbal memory in women and may prevent or forestall the deterioration in short- and long-term memory that occurs with age (Sherwin., 1999a). There is also evidence that estrogen may have a role in the prevention and treatment of Alzheimer's disease (AD). Theoretically estrogen could be a good anti-Alzheimer's treatment (Garcia-Segura et al., 2001). Estrogen has the properties of an antioxidant, can modify inflammatory response, increases growth of ACh neurons, can affect amyloid precursor protein cleavage, inhibits ApoE levels, increases glucose utilization and increase cerebral blood flow, but stimulates glucocorticoid secretion.

Unfortunately the clinical data to date are somewhat mixed: the estimated risk of AD decreases significantly in women who have been on long-term ERT (Paganini-Hill & Henderson, 1994; Kawas et al., 1997); but others have reported only 50% reduction in incidence (Waring et al., 1999), with some benefit in early onset AD only and some protection against further deterioration (Costa et al., 1999) whereas others have seen no beneficial effect at all (Mulnard et al., 2000).

The use of ERT continues to be controversial with the risk of breast and endometrial cancer in long-term users still looming. At the same time, the search for the perfect Selective Estrogen Receptor Modulator (SERM) is ongoing. The "ideal" SERM would have negative receptor activity on breast and endometrial cells and positive receptor activity on bone, cardiovascular and brain. So far, there is evidence that raloxifene is effective in preventing osteoporosis and has protective cardiovascular properties and also seems to reduce the risk for breast cancer (Delmas et al., 1997; Cauley et al., 2001), but its effect on cognitive function in humans has not been established. There is some indication that it may lower the risk of decline in attention and memory (Yaffe et al., 2001) and in animals there is some indication that raloxifene plus estradiol induces neurite outgrowth to a greater extent than raloxifene or estradiol alone (Nilsen et al., 1998).

Progesterone, which in the past has been promoted by some as an antidepressant, can by itself not only cause depression but seems also to reverse the estrogen induced receptor expression. Progestogens also have potent anaesthetic properties and dampen brain excitability; they also increase the concentration of monoamine oxidase, the enzyme that catabolizes 5HT in the brain, whereas estrogen decreases the enzyme, thereby increasing the concentration of 5HT (Luine et al., 1975; Sherwin, 1999b).

Testosterone is also an extremely important psychoactive compound and its relevance to women's well-being is just beginning to be recognized (Tuiten et al., 2000). While we are awaiting results of the ongoing long-term prospective studies with ERT and SERM, it is important to recognize that depressive symptoms are a significant risk factor for mortality in older women (Whooley & Browner, 1998). Whether depressive symptoms are a marker for or a cause of—life-threatening conditions remain to be determined. Nevertheless, treatment for depression may not only enhance the quality of life, but may also reduce mortality in this population.

REPRODUCTIVE HORMONE ABNORMALITIES IN MAJOR DEPRESSION

While the focus of this chapter is on mood during times of estrogen changes, such as puberty and postpartum, we thought it useful to add some information on reproductive hormones in women with depression that occurs outside of puberty, postpartum, and menopausal contexts. Stress is strongly linked to the onset of depression; and overactivity of the main stress hormone axis as manifested by an increase in cortisol secretion is a well-established phenomenon in depression (Sachar et al., 1973; Carroll et al., 1976). Later studies have continued to validate this hypercortisolemia in depression (Rubin et al., 1987; Halbreich et al., 1985; Pfohl et al., 1985; Carroll et al, 2007). Our own studies (Young et al., 2001) also found increased cortisol in women with major depression compared to age and menstrual cycle day matched control women. Furthermore, we have consistently found greater HPA axis dysregulation in depressed women than depressed men (Young, 1995; Young & Ribiero, 2006).

Stress is known to inhibit the reproductive axis, with the report of Christian (1971) demonstrating infertility secondary to high population density

often cited as a seminal report. Shortly after the isolation and sequencing of CRH, studies by Rivier and Vale (1984) demonstrated that CRH inhibited LH secretion in rats. Later studies cannulating the hypophyseal portal system in rats demonstrated that CRH inhibited GnRH secretion (Petraglia et al, 1987).

Studies in non-human primates by the group of Michel Ferin also demonstrated inhibition of LH secretion by injection of CRH (Olster & Ferin, 1987). Anatomical studies demonstrate that CRH neurons synapse with GnRH neurons (MacLusky et al., 1988). Studies in primates by the Knobil laboratory (Williams et al, 1990) recording multi-unit activity from the arcuate nucleus (i.e. the GnRH pulse generator) demonstrated that CRH administration induced inhibition of the rhythmic firing of the arcuate nucleus accompanying LH secretory pulses, as well as abolishing LH pulses. Studies with a CRH antagonist, alpha-helical CRF_{9-41}, demonstrated the antagonist's ability to reverse stress induced LH suppression in rats, confirming a central CRH based mechanism by which stress inhibits LH secretion (Rivier et al, 1986).

Glucocorticoids also exert inhibitory effects on GnRH secretion or LH responsiveness to GnRH, including direct effects of cortisol on the gonadotrope (Sutter & Schwartz, 1985). Radovic et al. (1988) have demonstrated a glucocorticoid responsive element (GRE) on the GnRH gene, providing the potential for glucocorticoids to modulate GnRH gene expression. Our recent studies in ewes have found: clear inhibition of LH secretory amplitude by stress; blockade of the effects of stress or endotoxin by metyrapone inhibition of cortisol synthesis; and, infusion of stress levels of cortisol can produce inhibition of LH pulse amplitude which is blocked by RU486, a glucocorticoid receptor antagonist (Breen et al., 2004; Debus et al., 2002). Diminished LH response to GnRH following long term prednisolone treatment is found in women (Sakakura et al., 1975). Patients with Cushing's disease, where cortisol is increased but central CRH is likely to be low because of gluccorticoid feedback on PVN CRH, show inhibition of LH secretion.

In depression, a number of studies have been conducted examining either basal levels of reproductive hormones or response to GnRH. Almost all of the studies included patients of both sexes and did not analyze the data separately by sex, menstrual phase, or menopausal status. Using a high dose of GnRH (250 µg), Winokur and co-workers reported a normal

LH and FSH response to GnRH in a group of male and female depressed patients that included both pre- and postmenopausal women (Winokur et al., 1982).

Measurements of LH concentration in a single blood sample revealed lower basal LH concentrations in depressed than control postmenopausal women. The sample size was not large enough to analyze the baseline data or response to GnRH stimulation data separately for men and pre- versus postmenopausal women. However, unless GnRH secretion is markedly reduced, an abnormal response to GnRH would not be expected, since altered GnRH secretion is a central, not peripheral, phenomenon. Brambilla et al. (1990) used a lower dose of GnRH (150 μg) to examine LH response to GnRH in 15 premenopausal and 32 postmenopausal depressed women. They noted a decreased LH response to GnRH in both groups of depressed patients.

Measurement of serum LH in 4 samples drawn over the course of one hour again demonstrated lower baseline LH concentrations in postmenopausal depressed women than in their matched controls. It is possible that increased secretion of LH following removal of the negative feedback of gonadal steroids in postmenopausal women unmasks a defect in LH secretion that is not as easily observed in women with intact estrogen and progesterone feedback. Studies by Unden et al. (1988), again examining depressed patients of both sexes which were not analyzed separately, observed no change in baseline or GnRH stimulated LH and FSH secretion. However, given the major differences in LH pulse amplitude and mean LH levels between follicular and luteal phase it would be extremely difficult to observe a difference in basal LH secretion between MDD and control women without strict control of menstrual cycle phase.

Only recently have studies began to focus on the pulsatile rhythm of LH secretion in MDD women. Thus far there have been only four published studies examining pulsatile LH secretion in depressed women, two by Meller et al. (2001, 1997), one by us (Young et al., 2000) and a fourth looking at both the data from Young et al. and Meller et al. with spectral analysis (Grambsch et al., 2004).

The data from the Meller et al. studies showed altered power in slower LH frequencies in the follicular phase. Our data revealed significantly lower estradiol in the follicular phase in a small sample of depressed women (Young et al, 2000). Since our publication, a large scale epidemiological study by Harlow et al.

(2003) has found earlier menopause accompanied by lower estradiol in perimenopausal depressed women. Thus three recent studies have found evidence of reproductive axis abnormalities in depressed women. One study of the reproductive axis in men with major depression (Schweiger et al., 1999) also revealed decreased testosterone and a trend for slower LH pulses, suggesting that abnormalities in the reproductive axis are also found in men. As discussed earlier these changes in estrogen (or testosterone) levels likely impact central serotonergic function.

CONCLUSION

The complex integration of the neurotransmitter and steroid hormone systems implies that circulating steroid hormones from peripheral endocrine glands can directly regulate brain function and modulate behavior. Regulation occurs through a variety of mechanisms including, for example, direct interaction with or up-regulation of specific receptors on neuronal cells. Thus, the hormonal milieu surrounding a neuronal cell will, in part, determine the response of that cell to various stimuli.

Adrenal and gonadal steroids regulate the transcription of most of the major neurotransmitter system. Steroid hormones also have direct effects on neuronal cell function by non-genomic mechanisms influencing the sensitivity and responsiveness of the neurons.

Levels of estrogen and progesterone vary significantly across the female lifespan. At puberty there is an increase in estrogen and initiation of cyclic and diurnal variation in estrogen production. The sudden appearance of higher levels of estrogen in puberty alters the sensitivity of the neurotransmitter systems. Behaviors such as moodiness, irritability and conflicts with parents around this time may in part reflect this increased sensitivity. The constant flux of estrogen and progesterone levels continues throughout the reproductive years.

The neurotransmitter systems are thus constantly being attenuated or amplified. PMS and PMDD may be the result of an altered activity (or sensitivity) of certain neurotransmitter systems. Pregnancy and delivery produce dramatic changes in estrogen and progesterone levels as well as significant changes in the HPA axis, possibly increasing vulnerability to depression. Finally, at menopause, estrogen levels decline while pituitary LH and FSH levels increase.

The loss of modulating effects of estrogen and progesterone may underlie the development of perimenopausal mood disorders in vulnerable women.

Since these hormonal changes occur in all women, it seems safe to speculate that the development of mood disorders requires more than just fluctuating levels of hormones, but also a genetic predisposition. These genetic as yet unidentified "defects" probably relate to subtle alterations in number and function of various receptors and enzymes and to subtle structural and anatomical differences in the CNS. These differences caused by genetic polymorphism, combined with the flux in the hormonal milieu determine how the system reacts to multiple environmental stresses and predicts the development of mood disorders. Further research into this complex system is needed to be able to identify specific "genetic markers" which might help us better understand how the balance between estrogen, progesterone, testosterone, and other steroid hormones affect neurotransmitter function.

References

Ahokas A, Kaukoranta J, Wahlbeck K, Aito M. (2001). Estrogen deficiency in postpartum depression: successful treatment with sublingual physiologic 17ß-estradiol: a preliminary study. *J Clin Psychiatry*, 62: 332–336.

American Psychiatric Association. (1994a). *DSM-IV: Diagnostic and Statistical Manual of Mental Disorders*, 4th edition, (pp. 717–718), Washington, DC: American Psychiatric Association.

American Psychiatric Association. (1994b). *DSM-IV: Diagnostic and Statistical Manual of Mental Disorders*, 4th edition, (pp. 386–387), Washington, DC: American Psychiatric Association.

Anderson E, Hamburger S, Liu JH, Rebar RW. (1987). Characteristics of menopausal women seeking assistance. *Am J Obstet Gynecol* 156:428–433.

Angold A, Costello EJ, Worthman CM. (1998). Puberty and depression: the roles of age, pubertal status and pubertal timing. *Psychol Med*, 28:51–61.

Angold A, Costello EJ, Erkanli A, Worthman CM. (1999). Pubertal changes in hormone levels and depression in girls. *Psychol Med*, 29:1043–1053.

Angold A, Erkanli A, Silberg J, Eaves L, Costello EJ. (2002). Depression scale scores in 8–17 year-olds: effects of age and gender. *J Child Psychol Psychiatry*, 43:1052–1063.

Angold A. (2003). Adolescent depression, cortisol and DHEA. *Psychol Med*, 33:573–581.

Angst J, Sellaro R, Merikangas KR, Endicott J. (2001). The epidemiology of perimenstrual psychological symptoms. *Acta Psychiatr Scand*, 104:110–116.

Anisman H, Zaharia MD, Meaney MJ, Merali Z. (1998). Do early-life events permanently alter behavioral and hormonal responses to stressors? *Int J Dev Neurosci*, 16:149–164.

Appleby L, Warner R, Whitton A, Faragher B. (1997). A controlled study of fluoxetine and cognitive-behavioral counselling in the treatment of postnatal depression. *BMJ*, 314:932–936.

Armitage R, Emslie GJ, Hoffmann RF, Rintelmann J, Rush JA. (2001). Delta sleep EEG in depressed adolescent females and healthy controls. *J Affect Disord* 63:139–148.

Armitage R, Hoffmann R, Emslie G, Rintelman J, Moore J, Lewis K. (2004). Rest-activity cycles in childhood and adolescent depression. *J Am Acad Child Adolesc Psychiatry*, 43:761–769.

Ashby CR Jr, Carr LA, Cook CL, Steptoe MM, Franks DD. (1988). Alteration of platelet serotonergic mechanisms and monoamine oxidase activity in premenstrual syndrome. *Biol Psychiatry*, 24:225–233.

Avis NE, McKinlay SM. (1991). A longitudinal analysis of women's attitudes toward the menopause: results from the Massachusetts Women's Health Study. *Maturitas*, 13, 65–79.

Bancroft J, Cook A. (1995). The neuroendocrine response to d-fenfluramine in women with premenstrual depression. *J Affect Disord*, 36:57–64.

Bancroft J, Cook A, Davidson D, Bennie J, Goodwin G. (1991). Blunting of neuroendocrine responses to infusion of L-tryptophan in women with premenstrual mood change. *Psychol Med*, 21:305–312.

Beardslee WR, Versage EM, Gladstone TRG. (1998). Children of affectively ill parents: a review of the past 10 years. *J Am Acad Child Adolesc Psychiatry*, 37:1134–1141.

Best NR, Wiley M, Stump K, Elliott JM, Cowen PJ. (1988). Binding of tritiated yohimbine to platelets in women with maternity blues. *Psychol Med*, 18:837–842.

Bethea CL, Pecins-Thompson M, Schutzer WE, Gundlah C, Lu ZN. (1998). Ovarian steroids and serotonin neural function. *Mol Neurobiol*, 18:87–123.

Bicikova M, Dibbelt L, Hill M, Hampl R, Starka L. (1998). Allopregnanolone in women with premenstrual syndrome. *Horm Metab Res*, 30:227–230.

Biegon A, McEwen BS. (1982). Modulation by estradiol of serotonin receptors in brain. *J Neurosci*, 2:199–205.

Bloch M, Schmidt PJ, Su TP, Tobin MB, Rubinow DR. (1998). Pituitary-adrenal hormones and testosterone across the menstrual cycle in women with premenstrual syndrome and controls. *Biol Psychiatry*, 43: 897–903.

Bojlen K, Bentzon MW. (1974). Seasonal variation in the occurrence of menarche. *Dan Med Bull*, 21: 161–68.

Botteron KN, Raichle ME, Drevets WC, Heath AC, Todd RD. (2002). Volumetric reduction in left subgenual prefrontal cortex in early onset of depression. *Biol Psychiatry*, 51:342–344.

Brambilla F, Maggioni M, Ferrari E, Scarone S, Catalano M. (1990). Tonic and dynamic gonadotropin secretion in depressive and normothymic phases of affective disorders. *Psychiatry Res*, 32:229–339.

Brann DW, Hendry LB, Mahesh VB. (1995). Emerging diversities in the mechanism of action of steroid hormones. *J Steroid Biochem Mol Biol*, 52:113–133.

Breen KM, Stackpole CA, Clarke IJ, Pytiak AV, Tilbrook AJ, Wagenmaker ER. et al. (2004). Does the type II glucocorticoid receptor mediate cortisol-induced suppression in pituitary responsiveness to gonadotropin-releasing hormone? *Endocrinology*, 145:2739–2746.

Breznitz Z, Friedman SL. (1988). Toddlers' concentration: Does maternal depression make a difference? *J Child Psychol Psychiatry*, 29:267–279.

Brockington IF, Winokur G, Dean C. (1982). Puerperal psychosis. In Brockington IF, Kumar R. (Eds.), *Motherhood and mental illness* (pp. 37–69). London: Academic Press.

Burnet RB, Radden HS, Easterbrook EG, McKinnon RA. (1991). Premenstrual syndrome and spironolactone. *Aust N Z J Obstet Gynaecol*, 31:366–368.

Carroll BJ, Curtis GC, Mendels J. (1976). Neuroendocrine regulation in depression I. Limbic system-adrenocortical dysfunction. *Arch Gen Psychiatry*, 33:1039–1044.

Carroll BJ, Cassidy F, Naftolowitz D, Tatham NE, Wilson WH, Iranmanesh A, et al. (2007). Pathophysiology of hypercortisolism in depression. *Acta Psychiatr Scand*, Suppl(433):90–103.

Carothers AD, Murray L. (1990). Estimating psychiatric morbidity by logistic regression: application to postnatal depression in a community sample. *Psychol Med*, 20:695–702.

Caspi A, Moffitt TE. (1991). Individual differences are accentuated during periods of social change: the sample case of girls at puberty. *J Pers Soc Psychol*, 61:57–68.

Caspi A, Sugden K, Moffitt TE, Taylor A, Craig IW, Harrington H, et al. (2003). Influence of life stress on depression: moderation by a polymorphism in the 5-HTT gene. *Science*, 301:386–389.

Casson P, Hahn PM, Van Vugt DA, Reid RL. (1990). Lasting response to ovariectomy in severe intractable premenstrual syndrome. *Am J Obstet Gynecol*, 162:99–105.

Cauley JA, Norton L, Lippman ME, Eckert S, Krueger KA, Purdie DW, et al. (2001). Continued breast cancer risk reduction in postmenopausal women treated with raloxifene: 4-year results form the MORE trial. Multiple outcomes of raloxifene evaluation. *Breast Cancer Res Treat*, 65:125–134.

Christian JJ. (1971). Population density and reproductive efficiency. *Biology of Reproduction*, 4:248–294.

Chrousos GP, Gold PW (1992). The concepts of stress and stress system disorders: overview of physical and behavioral homeostasis. *JAMA*, 267:1244–1252.

Cizza G, Gold PW, Chrousos GP. (1997). High dose transdermal estrogen, corticotropin-releasing hormone, and postnatal depression. *J Clin Endocrinol Metab*, 82:704.

Cohen IR, Wise PM. (1988). Effects of estradiol on the diurnal rhythm of serotonin activity in microdissected brain areas of ovariectomized rats. *Endocrinology*, 122:2619–2625.

Cohen LS, Sichel DA, Robertson LM, Heckscher E, Rosenbaum JF. (1995). Postpartum prophylaxis for women with bipolar disorder. *Am J Psychiatry*, 152:1641–1645.

Cohen P, Cohen J, Kasen S, Velez CN, Hartmark C, Johnson J, et al. (1993). An epidemiological study of disorders in late childhood and adolescence—I. Age- and gender-specific prevalence. *J Child Psychol Psychiatry*, 34:851–867.

Cooper PJ, Murray L. (1995). Course and recurrence of postnatal depression. Evidence for the specificity of the diagnostic concept. *Br J Psychiatry*, 166:191–195.

Costa MM, Reus VI, Wolkowitz OM, Manfredi F, Lieberman M. (1999). Estrogen replacement therapy and cognitive decline in memory-impaired postmenopausal women. *Biol Psychiatry*, 46: 182–188.

Cox JL, Murray D, Chapman G. (1993). A controlled study of the onset, duration and prevalence of postnatal depression. *Br J Psychiatry*, 163:27–31.

Culig Z, Hobisch A, Cronauer MV, Hittmair A, Radmayr C, Bartsch G, Klocker H. (1995). Activation of the androgen receptor by polypeptide growth factors and cellular regulators. *World J Urol*, 13:285–289.

Dean BB, Borenstein JE. (2004). A prospective assessment investigating the relationship between work productivity and impairment with premenstrual syndrome. *J Occup Environ Med*, 46:649–656.

Debus N, Breen KM, Barrell GK, Billings HJ, Brown M, Young EA, Karsch FJ. (2002). Does cortisol mediate endotoxin-induced inhibition of pulsatile LH and GnRH secretion? *Endocrinology*, 143:3748–3758.

Delmas PD, Bjarnason NH, Mitlak BH, Ravoux AC, Shah AS, Huster WJ, et al. (1997). Effects of raloxifene on bone mineral density, serum cholesterol concentrations, and uterine endometrium in postmenopausal women. *N Engl J Med*, 337:1641–1647.

Derman O, Kanbur NO, Tokur TE, Kutluk T. (2004). Premenstrual syndrome and associated symptoms in adolescent girls. *Eur J Obstet Gynecol Reprod Biol*, 116:201–206.

Ditkoff EC, Crary WG, Cristo M, Lobo RA. (1991). Estrogen improves psychological function in asymptomatic postmenopausal women. *Obstet Gynecol*, 78:991–995.

Dorn LD, Chrousos GP. (1997). The neurobiology of stress: understanding regulation of affect during female biological transitions. *Semin Reprod Endocrinol*, 15:19–35.

Dougherty DM, Bjork JM, Moeller FG, Swann AC. (1997). The influence of menstrual-cycle phase on the relationship between testosterone and aggression. *Physiol Behav*, 62:431–435.

Drevets WC, Ongur D, Price JL. (1998). Reduced glucose metabolism in the subgenual prefrontal cortex in unipolar depression. *Mol Psychiatry*, 3:190–191.

Dunn EJ, Steiner M, (2000). The functional neurochemistry of mood disorders in women. In Steiner M, Yonkers KA, Eriksson E. (Eds.), *Mood disorders in women* (pp. 71–82), London, UK:Martin Dunitz Ltd.

Ehlers CL, Frank E, Kupfer DJ. (1988). Social zeitgebers and biological rhythms. A unified approach to understanding the etiology of depression. *Arch Gen Psychiatry*, 45:948–952.

Eley TC, Sugden K, Corsico A, Gregory AM, Sham P, McGuffin P, et al. (2004). Gene-environment interaction analysis of serotonin system markers with adolescent depression. *Mol Psychiatry*, 9:908–915.

Eriksson E, Humble M. (1990). Serotonin psychiatric pathophysiology, a review of data from experimental and clinical research. In Pohl R, Gehrson S. (Eds.), *The Biological basis of psychiatric treatment* (pp. 66–119), Switzerland: Karger, Basel.

Eriksson E, Sundblad C, Landen M, Steiner M. (2000). Behavioral effects of androgens in women. In Steiner M, Yonkers KA, Eriksson E. (Eds.), *Mood disorders in women* (pp. 233–246) London, UK: Martin Dunitz Ltd.

Eriksson E, Sundblad C, Lisjo P, Modigh K, Andersch B. (1992). Serum levels of androgens are higher in women with premenstrual irritability and dysphoria than in controls. *Psychoneuroendocrinology*, 17:195–204.

Fink G, Sumner BE, Rosie R, Grace O,Quinn JP. (1996). Estrogen control of central neurotransmission: effect on mood, mental state, and memory. *Cell Mol Neurobiol*, 16:325–344.

Fink G, Sumner B, Rosie R, Wilson H, McQueen J. (1999). Androgen actions on central serotonin neurotransmission: relevance for mood, mental state and memory. *Behav Brain Res*, 105:53–68.

FitzGerald M, Malone KM, Li S, Harrison WM, McBride PA, Endicott J, et al. (1997). Blunted serotonin response to fenfluramine challenge in premenstrual dysphoric disorder. *Am J Psychiatry*, 154:556–558.

Fleming AS, Corter C. (1988). Factors influencing maternal responsiveness in humans: usefulness of an animal model. *Psychoneuroendocrinology*, 13:189–212.

Fleming AS, Corter C, Steiner M. (1995). Sensory and hormonal control of maternal behavior in rat and human mothers. In Pryce CR, Martin RD, Skuse D. (Eds.), *Motherhood in human and non-human primates*, (pp.106–114) Basel: Karger, Basel.

Fleming AS, Steiner M, Anderson V. (1987). Hormonal and attitudinal correlates of maternal behavior during the early postpartum period in first-time mothers. *J Reprod Infant Psychol*, 5:193–205.

Freedman RR. (2000). Hot flashes revisited. *Menopause*, 7, 3–4.

Freeman EW, Rickels K, Sondheimer SJ. (1993). Premenstrual symptoms and dysmenorrhea in relation to emotional distress factors in adolescents. *J Psychosom Obstet Gynaecol*, 14:41–50.

Freeman EW, Sondheimer S, Weinbaum PJ, Rickels K. (1985). Evaluating premenstrual symptoms in medical practice. *Obstet Gynecol*, 65:500–505.

Freeman EW, Sammel MD, Liu L, Gracia CR, Nelson DB, Hollander L. (2004). Hormones and menopausal status as predictors of depression in women in transition to menopause. *Arch Gen Psychiatry*, 61:62–70.

Garcia-Segura LM, Azcoitia I, DonCarlos LL. (2001). Neuroprotection by estradiol. *Prog Neurobiol*, 63:29–60.

Ge X, Conger RD, Elder GH Jr. (2001). Pubertal transition, stressful life events, and the emergence of gender differences in adolescent depressive symptoms. *Dev Psychol*, 37:404–417.

Glaser J, Russel VA, de Villiers AS, Searson JA, Taljaard JJ. (1990). Rat brain monoamine and serotonin S2 receptor changes during pregnancy. *Neurochem Res*, 15:949–956.

Golub S, Harrington DM. (1981). Premenstrual and menstrual mood changes in adolescent women. *J Pers Soc Psychol*, 41:961–965.

Goodman SH, Gotlib IH. (1999). Risk for psychopathology in the children of depressed mothers: a developmental model for understanding mechanisms of transmission. *Psychol Rev*, 106(3):458–490.

Goodyer IM, Herbert J, Tamplin A, Altham PM. (2000). First-episode major depression in adolescents: affective, cognitive and endocrine characteristics of risk status and predictors of onset. *Br J Psychiatry*, 176:142–149.

Grabe HJ, Lange M, Wolff B, Volzke H, Lucht M, Freyberger HJ, John U, Cascorbi I. (2005). Mental and physical distress is modulated by a polymorphism in the 5-HT transporter gene interacting with social stressors and chronic disease burden. *Mol Psychiatry*, 10:220–224.

Grambsch P, Young EA, Meller WH. (2004). Pulsatile luteinizing hormone disruption in depression. *Psychoneuroendocrinology*, 29:825–829.

Gregoire AJ, Kumar R, Everitt B, Henderson AF, Studd JW. (1996). Transdermal oestrogen for treatment of severe postnatal depression. *Lancet*, 347:930–933.

Guthrie JR, Dennerstein L, Hopper JL, Burger HG. (1996). Hot flushes, menstrual status, and hormone levels in a population-based sample of midlife women. *Obstet Gynecol*, 88:437–442.

Halbreich U, Asnis GM, Schindledecker R, Zurnoff B, Nathan RS. (1985) Cortisol secretion in endogenous depression I. Basal plasma levels. *Arch Gen Psychiatry*, 42:904–908.

Halbreich U, Rojansky N, Palter S, Tworek H, Hissen P, Wang K. (1995). Estrogen augments serotonergic activity in postmenopausal women. *Biol Psychiatry*, 37:434–441.

Hammarback S, Bäckström T, Holst J, von Schoultz B, Lyrenas S. (1985). Cyclical mood changes as in the premenstrual tension syndrome during sequential estrogen-progestagen postmenopausal replacement therapy. *Acta Obstet Gynecol Scand*, 64:393–397.

Hankin BL, Abramson LY, Moffitt TE, Silva PA, McGee R, Angell KE. (1998). Development of depression from preadolescence to young adulthood: emerging gender differences in a 10-year longitudinal study. *J Abnorm Psychol*, 107:128–140.

Hankin BL, Abramson LY, Miller N, Haeffel GJ. (2004). Cognitive vulnerability-stress theories of depression: examining affective specificity in the prediction of depression versus anxiety in three prospective studies. *Cogn Ther Res*, 28:309–345.

Hannah P, Adams D, Glover V, Sandler M. (1992). Abnormal platelet 5-hydroxytryptamine uptake and imipramine binding in postnatal dysphoria. *J Psychiatr Res*, 26:69–75.

Harlow BL, Wise LA, Otto MW, Soares CN, Cohen LS. (2003) Depression and its influence on reproductive endocrine and menstrual cycle markers associated with perimenopause: the Harvard Study of Moods and Cycles. *Arch Gen Psychiatry*, 60: 29–36.

Harris B, Lovett L, Newcombe RG, Read GF, Walker R, Riad-Fahmy D. (1994). Maternity blues and major endocrine changes: Cardiff puerperal mood and hormone study II. *BMJ*, 308:949–953.

Harris B, Othman S, Davies JA, Weppner GJ, Richards CJ, Newcombe RG, et al. (1992). Association between postpartum thyroid dysfunction and thyroid antibodies and depression. *BMJ*, 305:152–156.

Hart S, Field T, del Valle C, Pelaez-Nogueras M. (1998). Depressed mothers' interactions with their one-year-old infants. *Infant Behav Dev*, 21:519–525.

Hay AG, Bancroft J, Johnstone EC. (1994). Affective symptoms in women attending a menopause clinic. *Br J Psychiatry*, 164:513–516.

Hay DF, Pawlby S, Angold A, Harold GT, Sharp D. (2003). Pathways to violence in the children of mothers who were depressed postpartum. *Dev Psychol*, 39:1083–1094.

Heidrich A, Schleyer M, Spingler H, Albert P, Knoche M, Fritze J, Lanczik M. (1994). Postpartum blues: relationship between not-protein bound steroid hormones in plasma and postpartum mood changes. *J Affect Disord*, 30:93–98.

Henderson AF, Gregoire AJ, Kumar RD, Studd JW. (1991). Treatment of severe postnatal depression with estradiol skin patches. *Lancet*, 338:816–817.

Herbison AE, Horvath TL, Naftolin F, Leranth C. (1995). Distribution of estrogen receptor-immunoreactive cells in monkey hypothalamus: relationship to neurones containing luteinizing hormone-releasing hormone and tyrosine hydroxylase. *Neuroendocrinology*, 61:1–10.

Ho H P, Olsson M, Westberg L, Melke J, Eriksson E. (2001). The serotonin reuptake inhibitor fluoxetine reduces sex steroid-related aggression in female rats: an animal model of premenstrual irritability? *Neuropsychopharmacology*, 24:502–510.

Hughes CW, Petty F, Sheikha S, Kramer GL. (1996). Whole-blood serotonin in children and adolescents with mood and behavior disorders. *Psychiatry Res*, 65:79–95.

Hirayasu Y, Shenton ME, Salisbury DF, Kwon JS, Wible CG, Fischer IA, et al. (1999). Subgenual cingulate cortex volume in first-episode psychosis. *Am J Psychiatry*, 156:1091–1093.

Johnson SR. (1987). The epidemiology and social impact of premenstrual symptoms. *Clin Obstet Gynecol*, 30:367–376.

Johnson SR, McChesney C, Bean JA. (1988). Epidemiology of premenstrual symptoms in a nonclinical sample. I. Prevalence, natural history and help-seeking behavior. *J Reprod Med*, 33:340–346.

Josefsson A, Berg G, Nordin C, Sydsjo G. (2001). Prevalence of depressive symptoms in late pregnancy and postpartum. *Acta Obstet Gynecol Scand*, 80:251–255.

Katona CL, Theodorou AE, Missouris CG, Bourke MP, Horton RW, Moncrieff D, et al. (1985). Platelet ^{3}H-imipramine binding in pregnancy and the puerperium. *Psychiatry Res*, 14:33–37.

Kauffman J, Yang BZ, Douglas-Palumberi H, Houshyar S, Lipschitz D, Krystal JH, et al. (2004). Social supports and serotonin transporter gene moderate depression in maltreated children. *Proc Natl Acad Sci USA*, 101:17316–17321.

Kawas C, Resnick S, Morrison A, Brookmeyer R, Corrada M, Zonderman A, et al. (1997). A prospective study of estrogen replacement therapy and the risk of developing Alzheimer's disease: the Baltimore Longitudinal Study of Aging. *Neurology*, 48:1517–1521.

Kendell RE, Chalmers JC, Platz C. (1987). Epidemiology of puerperal psychoses. *Br J Psychiatry*, 150: 662–673.

Kendler KS, Karkowski LM, Corey LA, Neale MC. (1998). Longitudinal population-based twin study of retrospectively reported premenstrual symptoms and lifetime major depression. *Am J Psychiatry*, 155: 1234–1240.

Kendler KS, Kuhn JW, Vittum J Prescott CA, Riley B. (2005). The interaction of stressful life events and a serotonin transporter polymorphism in the prediction of episodes of major depression: a replication. *Arch Gen Psychiatry*, 62:529–535.

Kessler RC, McGonagle KA, Swartz M, Blazer DG, Nelson CB. (1993). Sex and depression in the national comorbidity survey I: lifetime prevalence, chronicity and recurrence. *J Affect Disord*, 29:85–96.

Kessler RC, Walters EE. (1998). Epidemiology of DSM-III-R major depression and minor depression among adolescents and young adults in the National Comorbidity Survey. *Depress Anxiety*, 7:3–14.

Kessler RC, Berglund P, Demler O, Jin R, Koretz D, Merikangas KR, et al. (2003). The epidemiology of major depressive disorder. *JAMA*, 289:3095–3105.

Keverne EB, Kendrick KM. (1994). Maternal behavior in sheep and its neuroendocrine regulation. *Acta Paediatr*, Suppl. 397:47–56.

Kilpatrick LA, Zald DH, Pardo JV, Cahill LF. (2006). Sex-related differences in amygdala functional connectivity during resting conditions. *Neuroimage*, 30: 452–461.

Kim J, Alexander C, Korst L, Agarwal S. (2000). Effects of breastfeeding on hypoestrogenic symptoms in postpartum women. *Obstet Gynecol*, 95(suppl 4): 65S.

Korzekwa MI, Lamont JA, Steiner M. (1996). Late luteal phase dysphoric disorder and the thyroid axis revisited. *J Clin Endocrinol Metab*, 81:2280–2284.

Ladisich W. (1977). Influence of progesterone on serotonin metabolism: a possible causal factor for mood changes. *Psychoneuroendocrinology*, 2:257–266.

Lauber AH, Whalen RE. (1988). Muscarinic cholinergic modulation of hypothalamic estrogen binding sites. *Brain Res*, 443:21–26.

Lewinsohn PM, Rhode P, Seeley JR. (1998). Major depressive disorder in older adolescents: prevalence, risk factors and clinical implications. *Clin Psychol Rev*, 18:765–794.

Lewinsohn PM, Roberts RE, Seeley JR, Rohde P. (1994). Adolescent psychopathology: II. Psychosocial risk factors for depression. *J Abnorm Psychol*, 37:1134–1141.

Lock M. (1994). Menopause in cultural context. *Exp Gerontol*, 29:307–317.

Luine VN, Khylchevskaya RI, McEwen BS. (1975). Effect of gonadal steroids on activities of monoamine oxidase and choline acetylase in rat brain. *Brain Res*, 86:293–306.

MacLusky NJ, Naftolin F, Leranth C. (1988). Immunocytochemical evidence for direct synaptic connections between corticotrophin-releasing factor (CRF) and gonadotrophin-releasing hormone (GnRH)-containing neurons in the preoptic area of the rat. *Brain Res*, 439:391–395.

Maggi A, Perez J. (1985). Role of female gonadal hormones in the CNS: clinical and experimental aspects. *Life Sci*, 37:893–906.

Magiakou MA, Mastorakos G, Rabin D, Dubbert B, Gold PW, Chrouses GP. (1996). Hypothalamic corticotropin-releasing hormone suppression during the post-partum period: implications for the increase of psychiatric manifestations at this time. *J Clin Endocrinol Metab*, 81:1912–1917.

Mani SK, Blaustein JD, O'Malley BW. (1997). Progesterone receptor function from a behavioral perspective. *Horm Behav*, 31:244–255.

McEwen BS. (1988). Genomic regulation of sexual behavior. *J Steroid Biochem*, 30:179–183.

Meller WH, Grambsch PL, Bingham C, Tagatz GE. (2001). Hypothalamic pituitary gonadal axis dysregulation in depressed women. *Psychoneuroendocrinology*, 26:253–259.

Meller WH, Zander KM, Crosby RD, Tagatz GE. (1997). Luteinizing hormone pulse characteristics in depressed women. *Am J Psychiatry*, 154:1454–1455.

Menkes DB, Coates DC, Fawcett JP. (1994). Acute tryptophan depletion aggravates premenstrual syndrome. *J Affect Disord*, 32:37–44.

Millis JB, Kornblith PR. (1992). Fragile beginnings: identification and treatment of postpartum disorders. *Health Soc Work*, 17:92–199.

Mitchell ES, Woods NF. (1996). Symptom experiences of midlife women: observations from the Seattle Midlife Women's Health Study. *Maturitas*, 25:1–10.

Monteleone P, Luisi S, Tonetti A, Bernardi F, Genazzani AD, Luisi M, et al. (2000). Allopregnanolone concentrations and premenstrual syndrome. *Eur J Endocrinol*, 142:269–273.

Moss RL, Gu Q, Wong M. (1997). Estrogen: nontranscriptional signaling pathway. *Recent Prog Horm Res*, 52:33–69.

Mulnard RA, Cotman CW, Kawas C, van Dyck CH, Sano M, Doody R, et al. (2000). Estrogen replacement therapy for treatment of mild to moderate Alzheimer disease. *JAMA*, 283:1007–1015.

Murray L. (1992). The impact of postnatal depression on infant development. *J Child Psychol Psychiatry*, 33: 543–561.

Murray D, Cox JL, Chapman G, Jones P. (1995). Childbirth: Life event or start of a long-term difficulty? Further data on the Stoke-on-Trent controlled study of postnatal depression. *Br J Psychiatry*, 166:595–600.

Nagata C, Takatsuka N, Inaba S, Kawakami N, Shimizu H. (1998). Association of diet and other lifestyle with onset of menopause in Japanese women. *Maturitas*, 29:105–113.

Nilsen J, Mor G, Naftolin F. (1998). Raloxifene induces neurite outgrowth in estrogen receptor positive PC12 cells. *Menopause*, 5:211–216.

Noble RE. (2005). Depression in women. *Metabolism*, 54(5 suppl 1):49–52.

Nolen-Hoeksema S, Girgus JS. (1994). The emergence of gender differences in depression during adolescence. *Psychol Bull*, 115:424–443.

O'Brien, PMS, Abukhalil IEH, Henshaw C. (1995). Premenstrual syndrome. *Curr Obstet Gynecol*, 5:30–37.

O'Brien PMS, Pitt B. (1994). Hormonal theories and therapy for postnatal depression. In Cox JL, Holden J, (Eds.), *Perinatal psychiatry: use and misuse of the Edinburgh postnatal depression scale*, (pp. 103–11). London, UK: Gaskell.

O'Hara MW, Schlechte JA, Lewis DA, Wright EJ. (1991). Prospective study of postpartum blues: Biologic and psychosocial factors. *Arch Gen Psychiatry*, 48:801–806.

Okano T, Nomura J. (1992). Endocrine study of the maternity blues. *Prog Neuropsychopharmacol Biol Psychiatry*, 16:921–932.

Olster DH, Ferin M. (1987). Corticotropin-releasing hormone inhibits gonadotropin secretion in the ovariectomized rhesus monkey. *J Clin Endocrinol Metab*, 65:262–267.

Paganini-Hill A, Henderson VW. (1994). Estrogen deficiency and risk of Alzheimer's disease in women. *Am J Epidemiol*, 140:256–261.

Palinkas LA, Barrett-Connor E. (1992). Estrogen use and depressive symptoms in postmenopausal women. *Obstet Gynecol*, 80:30–36.

Parlee MB. (1976). Social factors in the psychology of menstruation, birth and menopause. *Prim Care*, 3:477–490.

Paykel ES, Emms EM, Fletcher J, Rassaby ES. (1980). Life events and social support in puerperal depression. *Br J Psychiatry*, 136:339–346.

Pearlstein T. (2002). Selective serotonin reuptake inhibitors for premenstrual dysphoric disorder: the emerging gold standard? *Drugs*, 62:1869–1885.

Pecins-Thompson M, Brown NA, Bethea CL. (1998). Regulation of serotonin reuptake transporter mRNA expression by ovarian steroids in rhesus macaques. *Brain Res Mol Brain Res*, 53:120–129.

Pedersen CA, Stern RA, Evans DL, Pate J, Jamison C, Ozer H. (1993). Natural killer cell activity is lower in postpartum dysphorics. *Biol Psychiatry*, 33:85A.

Pedersen CA. (1999). Postpartum mood and anxiety disorders: a guide for the nonpsychiatric clinician with an aside on thyroid associations with postpartum mood. *Thyroid*, 9:691–697.

Petraglia F, Sutton S, Vale W, Plotsky P. (1987). Corticotropin-releasing factor decreases plasma luteinizing hormone levels in female rats by inhibiting gonadotropin-releasing hormone release into hypophysial-portal circulation. *Endocrinology*, 120: 1083–1088.

Pfohl B, Sherman B, Schlechte J, Stone R. (1985) Pituitary-adrenal axis rhythm disturbances in psychiatric depression. *Arch Gen Psychiatry*, 42:897–903.

Polan HJ, Hofer MA. (1999). Maternally directed orienting behaviors of newborn rats. *Dev Psychobiol*, 34: 269–279.

Pop VJ, Essed GG, de Geus CA, van Son MM, Komproe IH. (1993). Prevalence of post partum depression—or is it post-puerperium depression? *Acta Obstet Gynecol Scand*, 72:354–358.

Prior JC. (1998). Perimenopause: The complex endocrinology of the menopausal transition. *Endocr Rev*, 19:397–428.

Purnine D, Frank E. (1996). Should postpartum mood disorders be given a more prominent or distinctive place in DSM-IV? In Widiger TA, Frances AJ, Pincus HA, Ross R, First MB, Davis WW. (Eds.), *DSM-IV Sourcebook*, Vol 2, (pp. 261–279), Washington DC: American Psychiatric Association.

Radovic S, Wondisford FE, Cutler GB. (1988). Isolation of the human gonadotropin gene: analysis of gene structure in isolated hypogonadotropic hypogonadism. Endocrine Society Annual Meeting Abstract #192.

Raja SN, Feehan M, Stanton WR, McGee R. (1992). Prevalence and correlates of the premenstrual syndrome in adolescence. *J Am Acad Child Adolesc Psychiatry*, 31:783–789.

Ramcharan S, Love EJ, Fick GH, Goldfien A. (1992). The epidemiology of premenstrual symptoms in a population based sample of 2650 urban women: attributable risk and risk factors. *J Clin Epidemiol*, 45:377–392.

Rapkin AJ. (1992). The role of serotonin in premenstrual syndrome. *Clin Obstet Gynecol*, 35:629–636.

Rapkin AJ, Morgan M, Goldman L, Brann DW, Simone D, Mahesh VB. (1997). Progesterone metabolite allopregnanolone in women with premenstrual syndrome. *Obstet Gynecol*, 90:709–714.

Rice F, Harold G, Thapar A. (2002). The genetic aetiology of childhood depression: a review. *J Child Psychol Psychiatry*, 43:65–79.

Rivier C, Rivier J, Vale W. (1986). Stress-induced inhibition of reproductive functions: role of endogenous corticotropin-releasing factor. *Science*, 231:607–609.

Rivier C, Vale W. (1984). Influence of corticotropin-releasing factor on reproductive functions in the rat. *Endocrinology*, 114:914–921.

Roca CA, Schmidt PJ, Bloch M, Rubinow DR. (1996). Implications of endocrine studies of premenstrual syndrome. *Psychiatr Ann*, 26:576–580.

Rosenblatt JS, Mayer AD, Giordano AL. (1988). Hormonal basis during pregnancy for the onset of maternal behavior in the rat. *Psychoneuroendocrinology*, 13: 29–46.

Rowe T, Sasse V. (1986). Androgens and premenstrual symptoms—the response to therapy. In Deneerstein L, Frazer I. (Eds.), *Hormones and behavior*, (pp. 160–165). New York: Elsevier Science Publishers.

Rubin RT, Poland RE, Lesser IM, Winston RA, Blodgett AL. (1987). Neuroendocrine aspects of primary endogenous depression I. Cortisol secretory dynamics in patients and matched controls. *Arch Gen Psychiatry*, 44:328–336.

Ryan ND, Varma D. (1998). Child and adolescent mood disorders—Experience with serotonin-based therapies. *Biol Psychiatry*, 44:336–340.

Sachar EJ, Hellman L, Roffwarg HP, Halpern FS, Fukushima DK, Gallagher TF. (1973). Disrupted 24 hour patterns of cortisol secretion in psychotic depression. *Arch Gen Psychiatry*, 28:19–24.

Sakakura M, Takebe K and Nakagawa S. (1975). Inhibition of leutenizing hormone secretion induced by synthetic LRH by long term treatment with glucocorticoids in human subjects. *J Clin Endocrinol Metab*, 40:774–779.

Schmidt PJ, Purdy RH, Moore PH Jr, Paul SM, Rubinow DR. (1994). Circulating levels of anxiolytic steriods in the luteal phase in women with premenstrual syndrome and in control subjects. *J Clin Endocrinol Metab*, 79:1256–1260.

Schmidt PJ, Grover GN, Roy-Byrne PP, Rubinow DR. (1993). Thyroid function in women with premenstrual syndrome. *J Clin Endocrinol Metab*, 76:671–674.

Schmidt PJ, Nieman LK, Danaceau MA, Adams LF, Rubinow DR. (1998). Differential behavioral effects of gonadal steroids in women with and in those without premenstrual syndrome. *N Engl J Med*, 338:209–216.

Schmidt PJ, Neiman L, Danaceau MA, Tobin MB, Roca CA Murphy JH, Rubinow DR. (2000). Estrogen replacement in perimenopause-related depression: a preliminary report. *Am J Obstet Gynecol*, 183:414–420.

Schmidt PJ, Rubinow DR. (1991). Menopause-related affective disorders: a justification for further study. *Am J Psychiatry*, 148:844–852.

Schmidt PJ, Haq NA, Rubinow DR. (2004). A longitudinal evaluation of the relationship between reproductive status and mood in perimenopausal women. *Am J Psychiatry*, 161:2238–2244.

Schmidt PJ. (2005). Depression, the perimenopause, and estrogen therapy. *Ann NY Acad Sci*, 1052:27–40.

Schneider LS, Small GW, Hamilton SH, Bystritsky A, Nemeroff CB, Meyers BS. (1997). Estrogen replacement and response to fluoxetine in a multicenter geriatric depression trial. *Am J Geriatr Psychiatry*, 5:97–106.

Schweiger U, Deuschle M, Weber B, Korner A, Lammers CH, Schmider J, Gotthardt U, Heuser I. (1999). Testosterone, gonadotropin, and cortisol secretion in male patients with major depression. *Psychosom Med*, 61:292–296.

Sherwin BB. (1988). Affective changes with estrogen and androgen replacement therapy in surgically menopausal women. *J Affect Disord*, 14:177–187.

Sherwin BB. (1999a). Can estrogen keep you smart? Evidence from clinical studies. *J Psychiatry Neurosci*, 24:315–321.

Sherwin BB. (1999b). Progestogens used in menopause. Side effects, mood and quality of life. *J Reprod Med*, 44:227–232.

Sherwin BB, Suranyi-Cadotte BE. (1990). Up-regulatory effect of estrogen on platelet 3H-imipramine binding sites in surgically menopausal women. *Biol Psychiatry*, 28:339–348.

Shively CA, Friedman DP, Gage HD, Bounds MC, Brown-Proctor C, Blair JB, et al. (2006). Behavioral depression and positron emission tomography-determined serotonin 1A receptor binding potential in cynomolgus monkeys. *Arch Gen Psychiatry*, 63:396–403.

Sichel DA, Cohen LS, Robertson LM, Ruttenberg A, Rosenbaum JF. (1995). Prophylactic estrogen in recurrent postpartum affective disorder. *Biol Psychiatry*, 38:814–818.

Smith R, Cubis J, Brinsmead M, Lewin T, Singh B, Owens P, et al. (1990). Mood changes, obstetric experience and alterations in plasma cortisol, beta-endorphin and CRH during pregnancy and the puerperium. *J Psychosom Res*, 34:53–69.

Smith SS, Gong QH, Hsu F-C, Markowitz RS, ffrench-Mullen JM, Li X. (1998). GABA$_A$ receptor α4 subunit suppression prevents withdrawal properties of an endogenous steroid. *Nature*, 392:926–930.

Soares CN, Almeida OP, Joffe H, Cohen LS. (2001). Efficacy of estradiol for the treatment of depressive disorders in perimenopausal women: a double blind, randomized, placebo-controlled trial. *Arch Gen Psychiatry*, 58:529–534.

Sohr-Preston SL, Scaramella LV. (2006). Implications of timing of maternal depressive symptoms for early cognitive and language development. *Clin Child Fam Psychol Rev*, 9:65–83.

Steege JF, Stout AL, Knight DL, Nemeroff CB. (1992). Reduced platelet tritium-labeled imipramine binding sites in women with premenstrual syndrome. *Am J Obstet Gynecol*, 167:168–172.

Stein G, Marsh A, Morton J. (1981). Mental symptoms, weight changes, and electrolyte excretion in the first post partum week. *J Psychosom Res*, 25:395–408.

Steiner M, Pearlstein T, Cohen LS, Endicott J, Kornstein SG, Roberts C, et al. (2006). Expert guidelines for the treatment of severe PMS, PMDD, and comorbidities: the role of SSRI's. *J Womens Health*, 15:57–69.

Steiner M. (1998). Perinatal mood disorders: position paper. *Psychopharmacol Bull*, 34:301–306.

Steiner M, Macdougall M, Brown E. (2003). The premenstrual symptoms screening tool (PSST) for clinicians. *Arch Womens Ment Health*, 6:203–209.

Steiner M, Born L. (2000). Advances in the diagnosis and treatment of premenstrual dysphoria. *CNS Drugs*, 13:287–304.

Steiner M, Born L, Marton P. (2000). Menarche and mood disorders in adolescence. In Steiner M, Yonkers KA, Eriksson E. (Eds.), *Mood disorders in women*, (pp. 247–268). London UK: Martin Dunitz Ltd.

Steiner M, Dunn EJ. (1996). The psychobiology of female-specific mood disorders. *Infertil Reprod Med Clin N Am*, 7:297–313.

Steiner M, Fleming AS, Anderson VN, Monkhouse E, Boulter GE. (1986). A psychoneuroendocrine profile for postpartum blues? In Dennerstein L, Fraser I. (Eds.), *Hormones and behavior*, (pp. 327–335) Amsterdam: Elsevier Science Publishers BV (Biomedical Division).

Steiner M, Lepage P, Dunn E. (1997). Serotonin and gender specific psychiatric disorders. *Int J Psych Clin Pract*, 1:3–13.

Steiner M, Tam WYK. (1999). Postpartum depression in relation to other psychiatric disorders. In Miller LJ

(Ed.), *Postpartum mood disorders* (pp. 47–63). Washington DC: American Psychiatric Press.

Steiner M, Wilkins A. (1996). Diagnosis and assessment of premenstrual dysphoria. *Psychiatr Ann*, 26:571–575.

Steiner M, Yatham LN, Coote M, Wilkins A, Lepage P. (1999). Serotonergic dysfunction in women with pure premenstrual dysphoric disorder: is the fenfluramine challenge test still relevant? *Psychiatry Res*, 87:107–115.

Stewart DE, Klompenhouwer JL, Kendell RE, van Hulst Aм. (1991). Prophylactic lithium in puerperal psychosis. *Br J Psychiatry*, 158:393–397.

Stomati, M., Genazzani, AD, Petraglia F, Genazzani AR. (1998). Contraception as prevention and therapy: sex steroids and the brain. *Eur J Contracept Reprod Health Care*, 3:21–28.

Stowe ZN, Cassarella J, Landry J, Nemeroff CB. (1995). Sertraline in the treatment of women with postpartum major depression. *Depession*, 3:49–55.

Su TP, Schmidt PJ, Danaceau M, Murphy DL, Rubinow DR. (1997). Effect of menstrual cycle phase on neuroendocrine and behavioral responses to the serotonin agonist m-chlorophenylpiperazine in women with premenstrual syndrome and controls. *J Clin Endocrinol, Metab*, 82:1220–1228.

Sullivan PF, Neale MC, Kendler KS. (2000). Genetic epidemiology of major depression: review and meta-analysis. *Am J Psychiatry*, 157:1552–1562.

Susman EJ, Dorn LD, Chrousos GP. (1991). Negative affect and hormone levels in young adolescents: concurrent and predictive perspectives. *J Youth Adolesc*, 20:167–190.

Susman EJ, Schmeelk KH, Ponirakis A, Gariepy JL. (2001). Maternal prenatal, postpartum, and concurrent stressors and temperament in 3-year-olds: A person and variable analysis. *Dev Psychopathol*, 13: 629–652.

Sutter DE, Schwartz NB. (1985). Effect of glucocorticoids on secretion of luteinizing hormone and follicle-stimulating hormone by female rat pituitary cells in vitro. *Endocrinology*, 117:849–854.

Tanner JM. (1962). *Growth at adolesence*, 2nd edition. Oxford:Blackwell Scientific Publications.

Tanner JM. (1968). Earlier maturation in man. *Sci Am*, 218:21–27.

Tuiten A, Van Honk J, Koppeschaar H, Bernaards C, Thijssen J, Verbaten R. (2000). Time course of effects of testosterone administration on sexual arousal in women. *Arch Gen Psychiatry*, 57:149–153.

Twenge JM, Nolen-Hoeksema S. (2002). Age, gender, race, socioeconomic status, and birth cohort differences on the children's depression inventory: A meta-analysis. *J Abnorm Psychol*, 111:578–588.

Unden F, Ljunggren JG, Beck-Friis J, Kjellman BF, Wetterberg L. (1988). Hypothalamic-pituitary-gonadal axis in major depressive disorders. *Acta Psychiatr Scand*, 78:138–146.

Vamvakopoulos NC, Chrousos GP. (1993). Evidence of direct estrogenic regulation of human corticotrophin-releasing hormone gene expression. Potential implications for the sexual dimorphism of the stress response and immune/inflammatory reaction. *J Clin Invest*, 92:1896–1902.

Wang M, Seippel L, Purdy RH, Bäckström T. (1996). Relationship between symptom severity and steroid variation in women with premenstrual syndrome: study on serum pregnenolone, pregnenolone sulfate, 5 α–pregnane-3,20-dione and 3 α–hydroxy-5-alpha-pregnan-20-one. *J Clin Endocrinol Metab*, 81:1076–1082.

Waring SC, Rocca WA, Petersen RC, O'Brien PC, Tangalos EG, Kokmen E. (1999). Postmenopausal estrogen replacement therapy and risk of AD: a population-based study. *Neurology*, 52:965–970.

Warnock JK, Bundren JC, Morris DW. (1998). Sertraline in the treatment of depression associated with gonadotropin-releasing hormone agonist therapy. *Biol Psychiatry*, 43:464–465.

Warren MP, Brooks-Gunn J. (1989). Mood and behavior at adolescence: evidence for hormonal factors. *J Clin Endocrinol Metab*, 69:77–83.

Weissman MM, Olfson M. (1995). Depression in women: implications for health care research. *Science*, 269: 799–801.

Whooley MA, Browner WS. (1998). Association between depressive symptoms and mortality in older women. *Arch Intern Med*, 158:2129–2135.

Wieck A, Kumar R, Hirst AD, Marks MN, Campbell IC, Checkley SA. (1991). Increased sensitivity of dopamine receptors and recurrence of affective psychosis after childbirth. *BMJ*, 303:613–616.

Williams CL, Nishihara M, Thalabard JC, Grosser PM, Hotchkiss J, Knobil E. (1990). Corticotropin-releasing factor and gonadotropin-releasing hormone pulse generator activity in the rhesus monkey. Electrophysiological studies. *Neuroendocrinology*, 52:133–137.

Winokur A, Amsterdam J, Caroff S, Snyder PJ, Brunswick D. (1982). Variability of hormonal responses to a series of neuroendocrine challenges in depressed patients. *Am J Psychiatry*, 139:39–44.

Wittchen HU, Becker E, Lieb R, Krause P. (2002). Prevalence, incidence and stability of premenstrual dysphoric disorder in the community. *Psychol Med*, 32:119–132.

Wong M, Thompson TL, Moss RL. (1996). Nongenomic actions of estrogen in the brain: physiological significance and cellular mechanisms. *Crit Rev Neurobiol*, 10:189–203.

World Health Organization. (1981). Research on the menopause. *WHO Techn Rep Ser*, 670:3–120.

World Health Organization. (1996a). Mental, behavioral and developmental disorders. In *Tenth revision of the international classification of diseases* (ICD-10). Geneva: World Health Organization.

World Health Organization. (1996b). Research on the menopause in the 1990s. *WHO Techn Rep Ser*, 866: 1–107.

Yaffe K, Krueger K, Sarkar S, Grady D, Barrett-Connor E, Cox DA, Nickelsen T. (2001). Cognitve function in postmenospausal women treated with raloxifene. N Engl J Med, 344:1207–1213.

Young EA. (1995). Glucocorticoid cascade hypothesis revisited: role of gonadal steroids. Depression, 3:20–27.

Young EA, Carlson NE and Brown, MB. (2001). Twenty-four-hour ACTH and cortisol pulsatility in depressed women. Neuropsychopharmacology, 25:267–276.

Young EA, Midgley AR, Carlson NE, Brown MB. (2000). Alteration in the hypothalamic-pituitary-ovarian axis in depressed women. Archives of General Psychiatry, 57:1157–1162.

Young EA, Ribeiro SC. (2006). Sex differences in the ACTH response to 24H metyrapone in depression. Brain Research, 1126:148–155.

Zacharias L, Wurtman RJ. (1964). Blindness: its relation to age of menarche. Science, 144, 1154–1155.

Zweifel JE, O'Brien WH. (1997). A meta-analysis of the effect of hormone replacement therapy upon depressed mood. Psychoneuroendocrinology, 22: 189–212.

Chapter 22

Sex Differences in Brain Aging and Alzheimer's Disorders

Susan Resnick and Ira Driscoll

Some aspects of behavior, including cognition, tend to be influenced by sex (Maccoby & Jacklin, 1974). For example, men tend to achieve higher scores on some tests of mathematical reasoning ability (Benbow & Stanley, 2000; Benbow et al., 1995) and on tests of spatial ability, especially the ones involving mentally rotating an object in two or three-dimensional space (Voyer et al., 1995). Conversely, women have higher average scores on some language tests, such as verbal fluency (Maccoby & Jacklin, 1974), verbal articulation (Maccoby & Jacklin, 1974), some aspects of verbal memory (Bleecker et al., 1988; Kramer et al., 2003), and tests which assess attention to detail or perceptual speed and accuracy (Maccoby & Jacklin, 1974, Wilson & Vandenberg, 1978). Such findings have led to the hypothesis that there are underlying sex differences in brain anatomy and physiology that subserve sex-influenced aspects of cognition.

Indeed, sex differences in hemispheric specialization have been reported, with men showing greater asymmetry for both verbal and non-verbal material (Harshman et al., 1983; Kimura & Harshman, 1984; McGlone, 1980). Early studies suggested that sex differences in brain lateralization become markedly apparent in certain neurologic disorders, particularly stroke, with men exhibiting more frequent and severe aphasias following left hemisphere stroke (Landsell, 1962; McGlone, 1980). However, such approaches to examine brain sex differences are rather indirect and do not yield consistent evidence of sex differences in the incidence, severity, or type of language disturbance following stroke (Hier et al., 1994; Kersetz & Benke, 1989; Kimura, 1983). When interpreting these findings, it is important to keep in mind that in general there is a high degree of overlap between male and female distributions. The sex differences exist at the population level, and as such they should not be used for making inferences about a single individual.

An understanding of sex differences in brain structure and function is important in defining brain-behavior associations, the neurobiology of these relationships, and how they may be modified by normal aging or disease processes. In this chapter, we discuss the morphological and physiological sex differences in the human brain. Recent progress in neuroimaging technology holds the promise of elucidating the neuroanatomic and neurophysiologic correlates of sex-influenced behavior by offering a direct approach to study the brain non-invasively. The aim is to provide a foundation for understanding the impact of sex on the human brain in the context of aging, be it normal or pathological.

METHODOLOGICAL CONSIDERATIONS RELEVANT TO SEX AND AGE EFFECTS ON BRAIN STRUCTURE AND FUNCTION: MAGNETIC RESONANCE IMAGING (MRI), POSITRON EMISSION TOMOGRAPHY (PET), AND SINGLE PHOTON EMISSION COMPUTED TOMOGRAPHY (SPECT)

Despite the availability and rapid development of sophisticated neuroimaging tools and methodology, the incorporation of imaging techniques into clinical research and mainstream clinical practice has not been without challenges. These challenges arise from the diversity of neuroimaging tools, rapid technical progress leading to changing and often obsolete methodologies for image acquisition and analysis, the need for more sophisticated and less labor-intensive tools for image quantification, and the need to establish clinical relevance of many of the results of these sensitive measures. In the next section, we describe some of the methodological challenges involved in applying the most widely used neuroimaging tools for investigation of brain structure and function.

Magnetic resonance imaging provides morphological parameters of neuroanatomy as well as measures of brain function. While the impact of the specific images acquired is readily appreciated, effects of the approach to image processing on the detection of sex differences are not as apparent, but are equally important. Early studies of structural and functional differences between the male and female brains focused on more global regions or specific brain structures through manual or semi-automated definition of regions of interest (ROIs). This laborious approach requires trained operators using consistent neuranatomical definitions. Somewhat arbitrary boundaries are often employed to achieve acceptable reliability, with the

risk that these arbitrary boundaries may mask a highly local effect.

More recent image analysis methods use automated analysis, most often at the level of individual voxels. These methods are based typically on the registration or warping of each individual brain to a single atlas or template brain followed by varying degrees of spatial smoothing, and they vary greatly with respect to registration accuracy. Automated techniques allow fast and repeatable processing of a large amount of data, but shortcomings may remain in trying to apply these approaches to analysis of smaller areas, especially in regions of high anatomic variability.

Similar issues are also relevant to functional imaging with MRI, PET, and SPECT. Functional magnetic resonance imaging (fMRI) yields measures of brain activation related to changes in cerebral blood flow (CBF), through measurement of the different imaging properties of deoxygenated versus oxygenated hemoglobin which vary as a function of cerebral demand. Images are acquired during different cognitive and affective tasks, in which the hemodynamic response function is estimated, and task activation patterns are investigated for individual and groups of subjects.

Since the statistical analysis of fMRI is based on image subtraction or another form of direct comparison between activation and control tasks, similar to PET, the demands of the latter are as critical in determining the result as the particular activation task itself. The results of these studies must be interpreted within the context of the specific samples studied (e.g., young vs. older) and the particular task demands of the activation *and* control tasks employed in each paradigm.

PET and SPECT allow in vivo imaging of brain physiology and neurochemistry, with the most common applications including studies of regional cerebral oxygen or glucose metabolism, CBF, neurotransmitter function, and more recently, in vivo imaging of amyloid neuropathology. Cerebral blood flow studies are conducted at rest or during the performance of specific tasks to measure regional networks of brain activation in response to a particular cognitive or affective challenge. PET and SPECT are based on the use of a radioactively labeled tracer, which can be oxygen, water, glucose, or another chemical agent, including pharmaceuticals. Although PET technology has been limited by the need for a nearby cyclotron for production of radiotracers with a short half-life, the growing use of this technique in clinical oncology has led to the emergence of regional commercial suppliers that are capable of producing isotopes for other applications. While PET has lower spatial and temporal resolution in comparison with MRI, it provides greater opportunity for investigation of neurotransmission. The limited spatial resolution of each of these techniques must be considered in attempts to resolve small structures. In addition, partial volume effects due to limited resolution or tissue atrophy in a particular region can affect the interpretation of sex differences, particularly in view of the greater overall body and brain size in men.

ASPECTS OF BRAIN STRUCTURE AND FUNCTION THAT DIFFER BETWEEN MEN AND WOMEN

Given the frequency with which morphologic sex differences are observed in the brains of many species, it is not surprising that morphologic sex differences have also been reported in the human brain. More recently, advances in neuroimaging techniques have allowed the non-invasive study of the human brain in vivo, initially using computed tomography (CT); and later, MRI. Magnetic resonance imaging provides excellent resolution and high contrast among gray matter, white matter, and cerebrospinal fluid, permitting quantification of increasing numbers of brain regions and application to large samples, as both image acquisition and processing techniques advance.

Brain Structure

Early studies of neuroanatomic sex differences in humans were based on postmortem examination of gross anatomic differences. For example, males were reported to have a larger preoptic area of the hypothalamus (Allen et al., 1989; Swaab & Fliers, 1985). Males were also more likely to be missing the *massa intermedia*, a midline structure between the right and left thalamus (Allen et al., 1991).

To date, a number of sex differences in brain structure have been reported through quantification of a limited number of brain areas, although several recent studies have examined differences throughout the brain. In this section, we focus primarily on sex differences in the adult brain (see Durston et al., 2001 for a comprehensive review of sex differences earlier in development).

Global Brain Volume and Other Characteristics

Overall, sex differences in brain volume, adjusting for body size, are apparent for the cerebrum, but seem inconsistent for the cerebellum (Nopoulos et al., 2000; Raz et al., 2001). It is now well-accepted that the cerebrum is larger in men (by about 9%), and it also seems larger in boys, despite the fact that there is a great deal of individual variation in human brain morphometry (Giedd et al., 1996).

In general, men seem to have larger brains than women of comparable ages (Nopoulos et al., 2000; Resnick et al., 2000), even after adjusting for variability in height. Nopoulos and colleagues (2000) reported similar sex differences for frontal, parietal, temporal, and occipital lobes in younger individuals. Although not consistent, there is some evidence that this difference is driven by white as opposed to gray matter (Allen et al., 2003; Luders et al., 2005).

Sex differences in other structural characteristics have also been reported. In one study comparing young women and men using proton density and T_2-weighted images, women had a greater percentage of gray matter compared with white matter (Gur et al., 1999), but higher contrast volumetric images did not support this finding in other samples (Resnick et al., 2000; Nopoulos et al., 2001). Sex differences have also been found in tissue contrast and signal intensities (Kim et al., 2002), suggesting qualitative differences in tissue composition. In two large samples of older adults, women had more extensive evidence of white matter signal abnormalities (Yue et al., 1997), and non-significant trends toward more frequent subcortical and periventricular white matter lesions (de Leeuw et al. 2001).

Specific Regions

One region that has received much attention in investigations of morphologic sex differences in the human brain is the corpus callosum, perhaps due to implications of callosal size for interhemispheric transfer of information and hemispheric specialization.

In 1982, DeLacoste-Utamsing and Holloway (1982) reported that adult women had a more bulbous splenium, i.e., the posterior portion of the corpus callosum, in a study based on postmortem samples of 14 brains. The finding of a larger splenial area in females was replicated (Holloway et al., 1993) and extended to the fetal corpus callosum (DeLacoste et al., 1986) by the same research group, but other investigators have been unable to replicate these results in postmortem investigations of either adults (Witelson, 1985; Demeter et al., 1988) or children (Bell & Variend, 1985).

Although the capacity for detailed in vivo visualization of the corpus callosum has led to many more recent studies of sex differences in size of this structure, findings across studies remain inconsistent (Holloway et al., 1993; Parashos et al., 1995). For example, a larger callosal isthmus in females but no sex difference in splenial area was reported in autopsy (Witelson, 1989) and MRI (Steinmetz et al., 1992) studies. Some have suggested that the varied findings across studies may reflect inconsistencies in the way in which sections of the callosum are divided for measurement (Allen et al., 1991; Constant & Ruther, 1996) and that the sex differences are evident in the shape, but not necessarily the size of the corpus callosum (Allen et al., 1991).

Another issue is that not all studies adjust for brain volume when examining sex differences in callosal regions. As males have larger brains than females, it is important to investigate whether there are sex differences in relative size of callosal subunits after adjusting for variability in total brain or callosal volume. A recent study using 3-dimensional morphometry suggests a smaller ratio of corpus callosum to total cerebral volume in men (Allen et al., 2003), consistent with findings suggesting that increased brain size is related to decreased interhemispheric connections (Ringo et al., 1994). More specifically, smaller callosa are found in larger brains of both human (Jancke et al., 1997) and other species (Rilling & Insel, 1999).

In addition, sex differences in neural asymmetry have also been reported in animals and humans (Hines & Gorski, 1985; Hines & Green, 1991). For example, the planum temporale, a superior temporal brain region involved in language function, is thought to be greater on the left than right side of the human brain in right-handed individuals (Galaburda et al., 1978; Geschwind and Levitsky, 1968), and it is believed that this asymmetry may depend on sex (Shapleske et al., 1999; Wada et al., 1976).

In one MRI study of 24 adults (12 male, 12 female), males typically had greater left than right planum temporale area, whereas females showed a more symmetric and less consistent pattern (Kulynych et al., 1994). This finding was not replicated in a study of 40 postmortem brains (20 male, 20 female), which reported sex differences in the bifurcation patterns of the sylvian fissure (Ide et al., 1996).

The availability of high resolution MRI and new image processing techniques has facilitated in recent years the investigation of larger samples to clarify sex differences in brain asymmetries. One such study confirmed the greater leftward asymmetry of tissue volume in the region of Heschl's gyrus and the planum temporale for men versus women in a large sample of participants using a voxel-based analysis (Good et al., 2001b).

Sex differences have also been reported for other specific regions, although they are perhaps even less consistent. In a large study of 465 normal adults, ranging from 18–79 years of age, Good and colleagues (2001b) used voxel-based morphometry (VBM) to examine sex differences throughout the brain.

Significant asymmetry of cerebral grey and white matter was observed in the occipital, frontal, and temporal lobes (including Heschl's gyrus, planum temporale, and the hippocampus). Men had increased leftward asymmetry within Heschl's gyrus and planum temporale, while females had increased grey matter volume adjacent to the depths of both central sulci and the left superior temporal sulcus, in right Heschl's gyrus and planum temporale, in right inferior frontal and frontomarginal gyri, and in the cingulate gyrus. Females also had a significantly higher grey matter concentration in the cortical mantle, parahippocampal gyri, and in the banks of the cingulate and calcarine sulci, while males had increased grey matter volume bilaterally in the mesial temporal lobes, entorhinal and perirhinal cortex, and in the anterior lobes of the cerebellum, but no regions of increased grey matter concentration. Gray and white matter volume sex differences are depicted in Figures 22.1 and 22.2 respectively (reprinted from Good et al., 2001b).

Gur and colleagues (Gur et al., 2002) found larger volumes of orbital frontal regions, but not the hippocampus, amygdala, or dorsal prefrontal cortex, in young women compared with men. Pujol and colleagues (2002) reported that young men had a larger anterior, but not posterior cingulate cortex on the right. Goldstein and colleagues (2001) reported that sexual dimorphisms of adult brain volumes were overall more evident in the cortex relative to cerebrum

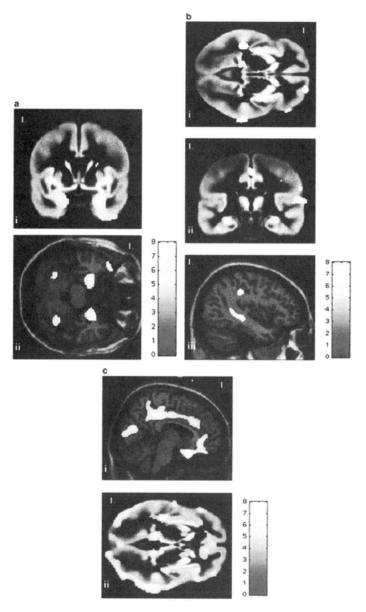

Figure 22.1. (A) Grey matter volume: increases in males vs. females (reprinted from Good et al., 2001b). Significant voxels are seen symmetrically in the mesial temporal lobes, in amygdaloid hippocampal complexes, entorhinal and perirhinal cortex, in the anterior lobes of the cerebellum, and in the left anterior superior temporal gyrus (ii). A few voxels can be seen at the junction of the superior edge of the right putamen and internal capsule (i), which may be misclassified. (B) Grey matter volume: increases in females vs. males. Significant voxels are seen in the right middle temporal gyrus, left parahippocampal gyrus, right lateral orbital, and frontomarginal gyri (i); in the right inferior parietal gyrus, cingulate gyrus and right transverse temporal gyri (Heschl's) gyri/planum temporale (PT) (ii), and within the banks of the left superior temporal and both central sulci (iii). (Significant voxels in the inferior frontal gyri are not shown.) (C) Grey matter concentration: increases in females vs. males. Significant voxels are seen diffusely in the cortical mantle, parahippocampal gyri, and in the banks of the cingulated and calcarine sulci. Significant voxels are also seen around the anterior limbs of the internal capsules, possibly reflecting caudate/lentiform nucleus changes, but probably also misclassification of voxels into grey/white matter.

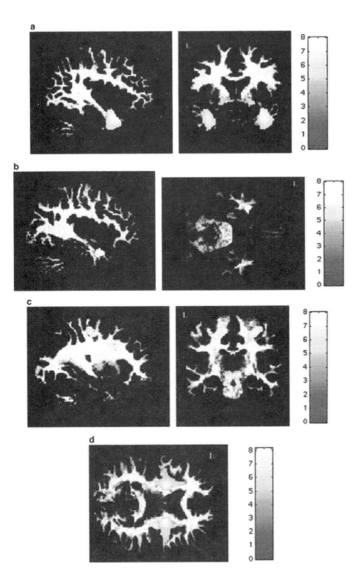

Figure 22.2. (A) White matter volume: increases in males vs. females (reprinted from Good et al., 2001b). Significant voxels are seen in both temporal lobes, extending upwards into the temporal stems and internal capsules. (B) White matter concentration: increases in males vs. females. Significant voxels are seen bilaterally in anterior temporal white matter and adjacent to the central sulcus. (C) White matter volume: increases in females vs. males. Significant voxels are seen bilaterally in posterior frontal white matter, left temporal stem, and optic radiation. (D) White matter concentration: increases in females vs. males. Significant voxels are seen bilaterally in internal and external capsules and optic radiations. A number of voxels are also seen in globus pallidus and putamen on both sides and are probably misclassified voxels owing to poor tissue contrast in these regions. Reprinted with permission from Good CD, et al., (2001). Cerebral asymmetry and the effects of sex and handedness on brain structure: a voxel-based morphometric analysis of 465 normal adult human brains. *Neuroimage*, 14:685–700.

size. Women had larger volumes in frontal and medial paralimbic cortices, while men had larger volumes in frontomedial cortex, the amygdala and hypothalamus.

In addition, there was greater sexual dimorphism among brain areas homologous with those showing greater levels of sex steroid receptors during critical periods of brain development in animals, suggesting mechanisms that relate sex steroid hormones to sexual dimorphisms in humans. Also, there is evidence that the male amygdala undergoes a prolonged growth period in childhood (Merke et al., 2003), is larger in boys (Caviness et al., 1996), and seems to remain

larger in grown men (Goldstein et al., 2001). Sex differences in microarchitecture appear to contribute to these findings, as greater numbers of neurons (Pakkenberg & Gundersen, 1997) and more densely packed neurons (Rabinowicz et al., 2002) have been reported in the cerebral cortex of males in general with some regional differences suggested (Witelson et al., 1995).

Brain Function

A number of physiologic techniques have been employed to assess sex differences in brain function. In this section, we focus on 133-Xenon inhalation and

SPECT measures of regional cerebral blood flow (rCBF), PET measures of regional cerebral glucose metabolism, neuroreceptor distribution, and fMRI to measure task-related brain activation.

Measures of Glucose Metabolism and Blood Flow with PET and SPECT

133-Xenon topographic studies (Gur et al., 1982; Mathew et al., 1988) and SPECT studies of rCBF (DeVoogt & Nottebohm, 1981; Jones et al., 1998) are consistent in reporting higher gray matter CBF in females compared with males. Two studies examining sex differences in regional cerebral glucose metabolism using 18-F-fluorodeoxyglucose (FDG) and PET also suggest increased levels of global brain activity in females (Baxter et al., 1987; Yoshii et al., 1988).

More specifically, women exhibited higher cerebral glucose metabolic rates compared to men in these two studies, although sex differences in brain volume may contribute to sex differences in metabolism (Yoshii et al., 1988). Other investigators have reported no significant sex differences in global cerebral glucose metabolism (Gur et al., 1995; Miura et al., 1990; Murphy et al, 1996) or non-significant trends to higher metabolism in women (Andreason et al., 1994).

Resting Condition Gur and colleagues (1995) reported sex differences in the regional distribution of cerebral metabolic activity during a resting state in a sample of 61 younger individuals (mean ages: 27.3 ± 6.5 and 27.7 ± 7.4 years for 37 males and 24 females, respectively). Relative metabolism (regional radioactivity count rates divided by counts for the whole brain) did not differ between men and women for non-limbic frontal, parietal, and occipital regions. Men, however, had higher relative metabolism in temporal cortex, hippocampus, parahippocampal gyrus, insula, inferior frontal regions, the putamen, and the cerebellum.

Women had higher relative metabolism in the middle and posterior cingulate gyrus. Sex differences in inter-regional correlations of cerebral glucose metabolic rates have also been reported (Azari et al., 1992), suggesting different patterns of neural connectivity during a resting state for men and women.

In addition, recent evidence suggests a sex difference in the patterns of functional connectivity of the amygdala in the resting brain, such that the right amygdala was associated with greater functional connectivity in men while the left amygdala was associated with greater functional connectivity in women. Moreover, the regions that showed stronger functional connectivity with the right amygdala in males (sensorimotor cortex, striatum, pulvinar region) differed from those that had stronger functional connectivity with the left amygdale in females (subgenual cortex, hypothalamus) (Kilpatrick et al., 2006). These finding suggest that sex differences present at rest may not only underlie sex-related differences in the involvement of the amygdala in memory for emotional information, but perhaps more generally in medical and psychiatric disorders.

Activation Studies The examination of sex differences in regional brain activity during the performance of specific cognitive tasks was facilitated by the development of measures to estimate rCBF. In an early study, sex differences in hemispheric activation patterns during the performance of verbal analogies and spatial judgment of line orientation were found with 133-Xenon clearance technique to measure cortical blood flow (Gur et al., 1982).

fMRI

Specific Activation Tasks

A much debated question is whether sex differences exist in the functional organization of the brain for language, and existing evidence suggests that language functions are more likely to be highly lateralized in males while represented in both cerebral hemispheres in females.

Shaywitz and colleagues (1995) used echo-planar fMRI to study 38 right-handed subjects (19 males, 19 females) during orthographic (letter recognition), phonological (rhyme) and semantic (semantic category) tasks. During phonological tasks, brain activation in males was lateralized to the left inferior frontal gyrus regions, while females engaged more diffuse neural systems involving both the left and right inferior frontal gyrus, providing evidence for a sex difference in the functional organization of the brain for language.

The same investigators followed up on the cerebral organization of component processing in reading in the same sample of participants and found significant sex differences in the cerebral organization of reading-related processes as well (Pugh et al., 1996). Similarly, Baxter and colleagues (2003) found, with fMRI, that both males and females displayed activation of left inferior frontal gyrus, left superior temporal gyrus, and cingulate gyrus during a task requiring semantic processing. Females, but not males, showed bilateral inferior frontal and superior temporal gyrus activation, with less diffuse left activation and greater right posterior temporal and insula activation.

Applying an adaptation of the verbal analogies and spatial line orientation tasks for use in an fMRI paradigm, sex differences in hemispheric lateralization were reported in response to the spatial, but not verbal task (Gur et al., 2000). The expected left hemispheric lateralization for the verbal task was found in the inferior parietal and planum temporale regions in both men and women, but only men showed the right lateralized increase in these regions during the spatial task. These findings are somewhat in contrast with the findings of Shaywitz and colleagues (1995) and Baxter and colleagues demonstrating greater bilateral activation during language tasks in young women compared with men. However, the tasks employed across studies have different demands and involve different brain regions.

Other sex differences in aspects of language processing include: more asymmetric activation of the anterior and posterior temporal region (Kansaku et al., 2000; Phillips et al., 2001) in men versus women during passive listening tasks, greater left-lateralized activation in inferior frontal and fusiform gyrus in men, and more symmetric patterns in language-related areas in women during a lexical visual field task (Rossell et al., 2002).

Sex differences have also been reported in the functional organization of the brain for working memory where across a number of tasks women show left lateralization and men show more bilateral or right-sided activation (Speck et al., 2000). During a spatial navigation task, activation is observed in the left hippocampus in men and in right parietal and prefrontal cortex in females (Gron et al., 2000). During odor identification, greater spatial extent of activation of frontal and perisylvian regions is observed in women (Yousem et al., 1999). Sex differences have also been observed in response of primary visual cortex to red and blue light (Cowan et al., 2000).

Differences between men and women have been reported in neural activity during receptive and expressive emotion. Using a mood induction paradigm

and fMRI, Schneider and colleagues (Schneider et al., 2000) found increased right amygdala activity in men but not women during expression of negative affect. Different patterns of brain activation for men and women have also been observed for tasks tapping receptive emotions, with sex differences in activation during the discrimination of happy, sad, and neutral faces (George et al., 1996; Lee et al., 2002), as well as during the retrieval of emotional words (Bremner et al., 2001) and the encoding of emotional pictures (Canli et al., 2002).

In addition to Canli et al. (2002), work by Cahill and colleagues (2001; 2004) provides perhaps some of the most convincing evidence for the existence of a sex-related lateralization of amygdala involvement in emotionally influenced memory processes. For example, Cahill et al. (2004) found that the activity in the left amygdala was associated with encoding of and long-term memory for arousing pictures in women compared to men, while the opposite pattern was seen with the right amygdala whose activity was stronger in men compared to women in relation to encoding and long-term memory for arousing pictures. Hamann and colleagues (2004) found with fMRI that the amygdala and hypothalamus are more strongly activated in men compared to women when viewing the same sexual stimuli regardless of the arousal level, and the sex differences were larger in the left than the right amygdala.

Although sex differences with respect to functional brain imaging can be seen in different regions both during rest and in response to different activation paradigms, the studies are rather few and findings disparate. This is clearly an area where more research is required. At this time caution should be exercised when interpreting, comparing, or generalizing such findings. These studies should be interpreted within the framework of not only the specific sample studied, but perhaps more importantly within the context of methodological and analytical constraints, and the demands of both the control and activation tasks employed by each study.

Neurotransmitter Systems (Young Adults)

There have been few in vivo studies of sex differences of hormone influences on brain neurotransmitter levels and receptor binding distributions. In a preliminary study of dopamine D2 receptors, Wong and colleagues (1988) used 11-C NMSP and PET to show a cyclic variation in D2 receptor binding over the menstrual cycle in a small sample of 6 women, where dopamine receptor binding tended to increase from the follicular to the luteal phase. However, Nordstrom and colleagues (1998) found no differences in raclopride binding to striatal D2-dopamine receptors across the menstrual cycle. Menstrual cycle variation in neurotransmitter receptor binding characteristics is an area which has received little attention, although it has important implications for the efficacy of pharmacotherapies in women.

Sex differences in the dopamine system have been further described in recent years. In a PET study using 18-F Fluorodopa as a radiotracer, women had significantly higher striatal Fluorodopa uptake than men, with the difference more pronounced in the caudate than putamen (Laakso et al., 2002).

Using SPECT and a technetium-99m labeled analog of cocaine (TRODAT-1) to measure availability of the dopamine transporter, women had higher availability than men in the caudate nucleus (Mozley et al., 2001). Moreover, dopamine transporter availability showed associations with executive and motor functioning in women but not men. In another study using a different dopamine transporter radioligand, women had higher uptake than men in the striatum, diencephalon, and brainstem (Staley et al., 2001).

Several more recently developed radiotracers allow visualization of extrastriatal dopamine receptor activity. Using 11-C FLB475, women showed higher D2-like receptor binding potentials than men in the frontal cortex, most pronounced in bilateral anterior cingulate cortex (Kaasinen et al., 2001). Thus, a number of studies support greater dopaminergic activity in both striatal and extrastriatal cortical regions in women, and these sex differences in neurotransmitter activity in healthy individuals may have important implications for the pathophysiology and treatment of neuropsychiatric diseases involving the dopamine system.

Other recent studies indicate that there may also be sex differences in neurotransmitter systems other than dopamine. In a study using PET and 18-F altanserin, greater 5HT2 receptor binding in men than women was found in a number of cortical regions, most pronounced in frontal and cingulate cortex (Biver

et al., 1994). However, using PET and 11-C WAY-100635 to measure serotonin 5-HT$_{1A}$ binding potential, Parsey and colleagues (2002) reported greater binding in women compared with men in the dorsal raphe, amygdala, cingulate gyrus, and prefrontal cortex. Rates of serotonin synthesis, measured with PET and alpha-11-C methyl-trypophan, were higher in men than women (Nishizawa et al., 1997).

Sex differences have also been observed in the regional activation of the mu-opioid system in response to sustained pain (Zubieta et al., 2002). Men had greater activation than women (during follicular phase) in the anterior thalamus, ventral basal ganglia, and amygdala, whereas women showed reduced activation in a basal state during pain in the nucleus accumbens. For comparable levels of pain intensity, men and women differed in the response of the mu-opioid system in specific brain regions. Again, many of the findings on sex differences in neurotransmission are based on single studies. As the implications of these findings for the understanding and treatment of disease are profound, this area clearly merits additional investigation.

SEX DIFFERENCES IN BRAIN AGING: STRUCTURAL AND FUNCTIONAL BRAIN IMAGING

Both postmortem (see Powers, 1994 for a review) and imaging studies (see Coffey, 1994 for a review) provide evidence that aging is associated with decreased brain volume accompanied by increased cerebrospinal fluid volume. In addition to effects of aging, brain size, symmetry, and function seem to be further modified by sex (Gur et al., 1987; Gur & Gur, 1990; Rodriguez et al., 1988; Schlaepfer et al., 1995; Shaw et al., 1984; Witelson, 1992).

It is becoming increasingly important to consider potential sex effects on brain and cognition throughout the lifespan, as different maturational rates for men and women may lead to age-specific findings of sex differences in brain structure and function as well as potentially sex-influenced diagnoses and treatments. To date, relatively few imaging studies have examined the effect of sex on the brain in old age and the results are not easily comparable across different studies due to methodological differences. Although seldom reported, sex-by-age interactions are described

Table 22.1. Sex Differences in Brain Structure and Function: Select Findings in Adult Humans*

Brain Structure:

Cerebrum	- Larger in males
Cerebellum	- Larger in males*
Preoptic area of hypothalamus	- Larger in males
Massa intermedia	- More likely to be missing in males
Corpus Callosum	- Splenium larger in females*
Corpus Callosum	- Isthmus larger in females*
Planum Temporale	- Greater asymmetry in males*
Ventricular Volume	- Relative size larger in men, particularly in elderly*
Sulcal Volume	- Relative size larger in men, particularly in elderly
Atrophy in general	- Greater in elderly men, and may begin earlier than in women
Gray Matter in general	- Greater age-related volume decline in men
Hippocampus	- Greater age-related volume decline in men
Amygdala	- Larger in males#

Brain Function:

PET, SPECT, and 133-Xenon Techniques:

Global cerebral blood flow	- Higher in females
Global cerebral glucose metabolism	- Higher in females*
Regional distribution of glucose metabolism and CBF	- Higher relative activity in males in lateral and ventro-medial temporal lobe, hippocampus, inferior frontal regions, and cerebellum
	- Higher relative activity in females in posterior and middle cingulate and parietal regions
	- Higher absolute glucose metabolic rates in males in hippocampus but lower absolute rates in thalamus#

Functional MRI (most based on single study):

Phonological processing	- Greater left hemisphere lateralization in males and more symmetric activation in females
Passive listening	- Greater asymmetric activation of anterior and posterior temporal regions in men
Lexical visual field task	- Greater left-lateralized activation in inferior frontal and fusiform gyrus in men and more symmetric activation in language areas in women
Working memory	- Women show greater left lateralization and men more bilateral or right-lateralized
Odor identification	- Greater activation of frontal and perisylvian regions in women
Mood induction—negative affect	- Right-lateralized amygdala activation in men but not women

Neurotransmitter systems (most findings based on single study):

Dopamine	- Greater decline of striatal D2 dopamine receptors with age in women
	- Greater striatal uptake of 18-F Fluorodopa in women
	- Greater striatal dopamine transporter availability in women
	- Higher binding potentials for D2-like receptors in the frontal cortex for women
Serotonin	- Greater 5HT2 receptor binding in men than women, most pronounced for frontal and cingulate cortex
	- Greater binding in women for the $5HT_{1A}$ receptor in the dorsal raphe, amygdala, cingulate gyrus and prefrontal cortex
	- Higher rates of serotonin synthesis in men than women
Mu-opioid system	- Men had greater activation in anterior thalamus, ventral striatum, and amygdala in response to sustained pain
	- Women have higher binding in globus pallidus and hypothalamus with aging#

*Findings are often inconsistent but summary statement reflects the direction of effect in studies reporting sex differences
#Results of a single study

when available. Otherwise, we discuss the studies assessing differences in brain structure and function between men and women in samples of older adult participants.

Brain Structure

As seems to be the case with most imaging studies, it is hard to make direct comparisons across studies due to key methodological differences, such as sample size and source of participants, imaging modality, acquisition protocols even when the same imaging modality is employed, and image processing and analysis differences. Most of the studies reporting sex differences in the effects of age on brain structure agree, however, that males show greater age-related structural changes than females (Coffey et al., 1998; Cowell et al., 1994; Gur et al., 1991; Golomb et al., 1993; Kaye et al., 1992; Murphy et al., 1996; Raz et al., 1997).

Global Brain Volume and Measures of Brain Atrophy

The relationship between age and brain volume has been investigated using a variety of methods. Nonetheless, almost all studies converge on the findings that brains become smaller and sulci widen (Raz, 1999). Recent evidence suggests that, although age-related atrophy is clear, it does not occur in a uniform matter. For example, Allen and colleagues (2005) corroborated some earlier findings that gray and white matter do not decline at the same rate with age during adulthood (Bartzokis et al., 2001; Guttman et al., 1998; Jernigan et al., 2001). In this study (Allen et al., 2005), although no sex differences were present for any regions of interest, the gray matter volume decreased linearly with age in adults between the ages of 22 and 88, while white matter volume increased until the mid-50s and then declined at an accelerated rate.

Whether sex differences in brain aging are indeed present remains to be resolved, as the evidence accumulated thus far is equivocal. Many studies have reported sex differences in the patterns of brain aging, for both the whole brain and the specific regions (Coffey et al., 1998; Cowell et al., 1994; Gur et al., 1991; Murphy et al., 1996; Pfefferbaum et al., 2004; Xu et al., 2000), and all such studies with the exception of Murphy and colleagues (1996) show accelerated aging in males compared to females. However, a similar number of studies report the absence of sig-

nificant sex differences (Good et al., 2001a; Jernigan et al., 2001; Raz et al., 2004; Sowell et al., 2003).

Increase in cerebrospinal fluid (CSF) volume is commonly observed with aging and is an indirect measure of tissue loss because intracranial volume remains constant in adulthood (eg. Coffey et al., 1998). Early cross-sectional CT (Barron et al., 1976; Earnest et al., 1979) and MRI (Condon et al., 1988; Grant et al., 1987) studies of adults indicated greater brain atrophy, as indexed by increased cerebrospinal fluid volumes, in older compared with younger individuals and suggested the possibility of greater and earlier increases in atrophy in men compared with women. However, sex differences in age-associated increases in ventricular and/or sulcal volumes were not significant. Although the fact that CSF volume increases with age is undisputed, the data on the effects of sex on CSF change with age remain equivocal. Greater increases in CSF have been reported for older men compared to women (Coffey et al., 1998; Gur et al., 1991).

More recent MRI and CT studies have shown significant sex differences in the effects of age on brain atrophy. Gur and colleagues (1991) reported a significant influence of sex on age differences in MRI-assessed cerebrospinal fluid volumes. Older individuals (aged 55–80 years) had more cerebrospinal fluid than younger individuals (aged 18–54 years), and this difference was greater for men, particularly for sulcal cerebrospinal fluid.

Blatter et al. (1995) also reported higher correlations between age and subarachnoid CSF volume for men, although these correlations were not statistically compared to those found in women. However, there are just as many studies that find no effects of sex on CSF volume (Murphy et al., 1996; Raz et al., 1997; Sullivan et al., 1993). In addition, it is important to consider sex differences in overall brain size and CSF spaces in examining sex as a modifier of age effects, because larger ventricles may appear to change more rapidly. In one study, faster rates of ventricular volume increase in elderly men compared with women were no longer apparent after adjustment for the larger initial size of ventricles in men (Resnick et al., 2003).

In a CT study of ventricular volumes, sex differences in lateral ventricular volume, adjusted for cranial volume, were demonstrated for each decade from the 20s to the 80s (Kaye et al., 1992). MRI-based ratings of ventricular and sulcal atrophy on 3660 community-dwelling individuals aged 65 years and older (Yue et al., 1997) in the Cardiovascular Health

Study are consistent with greater atrophy in older men compared with women.

Kochunov and colleagues (2005) examined the width and depth of 14 prominent sulcal structures per hemisphere with high resolution MRI in 90 individuals age 20–82. In general, sulcal width increased on average 0.7 mm/decade while the depth decreased at a rate of 0.4 mm/decade with age, with sulci located in multimodal cortical areas showing more changes than sulcal structures in unimodal cortical areas. Cortical areas with predominately multimodal function include frontal and parietal lobes, and cingulate gyrus, while occipital and to a lesser degree temporal lobes are considered functionally unimodal. Age-related sulcal changes were highly influenced by sex, where males showed more pronounced age-related changes in the superior temporal, collateral, and cingulate sulci. The decrease in sulcal depth in combination with increasing width observed in this study most likely reflects an opening up of the sulcus with age (Rettmann et al., 2006).

Greater age differences for men compared with women were also reported for quantitative volumes of sulcal and Sylvian fissure CSF in a subgroup of this elderly sample (Coffey et al., 1998). No sex effects on the age-related increase in the volume of lateral or third ventricles were observed (Coffey et al., 1998). These findings are in agreement with many other studies that have examined the lateral ventricles (Coffey et al., 1992; Gur et al., 1991; Kaye et al., 1992; Murphy et al., 1996; Raz et al., 1993; Sullivan et al., 1993; Yoshi et al., 1988; Yue et al., 1997) or the third ventricle (Coffey et al., 1992; Gur et al., 1991; Kaye et al., 1992; Sullivan et al., 1993) volume. Interestingly however, Kaye and colleagues (1991) reported that age-related increase in the volume of the lateral ventricles seems to begin a decade earlier in men compared to women, and Murphy and colleagues (1996) found that women have a greater increase in the ratio of third ventricle volume to intracranial volume compared to men.

In summary, most CT and MRI studies examining cerebrospinal fluid as an index of brain atrophy have found greater age effects on cerebrospinal fluid volumes in men than women. Hence, human brain morphology seems to be sensitive to both the effects of age and sex over a life span. In general, when sex differences in brain changes with age are found, men appear to have greater age-related atrophy. The neurobiological basis for such sex differences remains unknown, although many have suggested varying neuroendocrinological sex differences at different maturational stages as a possible explanation.

Specific Regions

Sex differences in the effects of age on specific brain regions have also been explored and are reported throughout the lifespan. The literature concerning the effects of sex on age-related changes in frontal lobe volumes is conflicting. Although observations of greater volume loss in men for the frontal regions have been reported (Cowell et al., 1994; Murphy et al., 1996; Tisserand et al., 2002). Studies finding no sex effects are ample (Christiansen et al., 1994; Coffey et al., 1992; Cowell et al., 1994; Raz et al., 1993, 1997; Sullivan et al., 1993).

Resnick and colleagues (2000) found that sex differences in older adults were greater for frontal and temporal than parietal and occipital regions. Allen and colleagues (2005) however, investigated gray and white matter aging in the frontal, parietal, temporal, and occipital lobes and in the major sectors of the temporal lobe in 87 adults, ages 22–88. In general, gray matter decreased linearly with age, whereas white matter volume increased until the mid-50s and declined at an accelerated rate thereafter. Overall, frontal gray matter was most strongly associated and occipital gray and white matter were least associated with age. No sex differences in aging were found for any regions of interest.

A recent study by Raz and colleagues (2004) investigated volumes of cerebral hemispheres and 13 regions of interest (ROI) in 200 healthy adults. The pattern of age-related decline resembled those previously reported. There was little evidence for sex-related and hemispheric differences in regional cortical volumes after controlling for body size), except for the increased age-related vulnerability of the lateral prefrontal cortex. However, men had larger volumes in all ROIs except the inferior parietal lobule, and exhibited steeper age-related declines in the volumes of the hippocampus and fusiform gyrus compared to women after controlling for body size.

Similarly, while Coffey and colleagues (1998) found a greater decrease in parieto-occipital regions for men compared to women, other studies did not find the same effect, albeit using slightly different definitions of this brain region (Cowell et al., 1994; Murphy et al., 1996). Raz and colleagues (1993), however, reported that women had a greater volume loss in the visual cortex compared to men. In a large sample of Japanese subjects, men showed greater age-related decreases in tissue volume than women in the posterior right frontal lobe, right temporal lobe, left basal ganglia, and bilaterally in the parietal lobe and the cerebellum (Xu et al., 2000). On the other hand, Lemaitre and colleagues (2005) examined the effects of age and sex on structural brain anatomy of healthy elderly and found that during the seventh and eight decade in life brain atrophy is universal, and does not seem to be modulated by sex.

Consistent with the findings in the Japanese study, there is other evidence that men exhibit greater age-related decrease in the ratio of temporal lobe volume to intracranial volume (Cowell et al., 1994; Murphy et al., 1996) and greater inferior temporal volume loss (Raz et al., 1997) than women. Moreover, age-related hippocampal atrophy seems more pronounced in men than women in some studies (Golomb et al., 1993; Bouix et al., 2005), while another reported the opposite—a greater decrease in hippocampal volume in women with age (Cowell et al., 1994).

It is important to note that the study reporting a greater decrease in hippocampal volume in women (Cowell et al., 1994) also found that the hippocampal volumes were actually greater in younger women than younger men and were not significantly different among older men and women. Overall, there seems to be some evidence to suggest the impact of sex on age-related volume loss in the temporal regions.

Good and colleagues (2001a) reported a linear grey matter volume decrease with age which was more pronounced in males bilaterally in the insula, superior parietal gyri, central sulci, and cingulate sulci. Areas with relative preservation included the amygdala, hippocampus, and entorhinal cortex. Global white matter seemed to remain stable with age, despite the presence of local areas of relative accelerated loss and preservation. There was no interaction of age with sex for regionally specific effects.

Studies of the effects of sex on the association between age and callosal size also yield inconsistent results. In an autopsy sample, Witelson (1991) reported significant negative correlations between age and total callosal area in 23 men age 26–69, but no significant association in 39 women age 35–68. In contrast, other investigators have not found sex differences in the association between age and MRI-assessed callosal size in adults (Johnson et al., 1994; Parashos et al., 1995; Pozilli et al., 1994; Sullivan et al., 2001).

Using MRIs from 8 men and 8 women, age 60–85 years, who are participants in the Baltimore Longitudinal Study of Aging (BLSA), we found significantly larger splenial size in women as well as sex differences in average callosal shape (Davatzikos et al., 1996). This finding was extended and confirmed in a larger sample of 114 right-handed participants in the longitudinal neuroimaging study of the BLSA (Davatzikos & Resnick, 1998).

In the larger sample, we also found significant positive associations between cognitive performance and splenial size in women, but no such associations for men (see Fig. 22.2). Greater interhemispheric connectivity may be more essential to performance in women than men due to their greater reliance on bilateral processing of information. The majority of studies of the influence of sex on brain aging have been cross-sectional, although as noted above, our group at the National Institute on Aging is conducting a longitudinal investigation of brain changes in the BLSA.

It becomes obvious that the findings are largely divergent. The discordance in findings may reflect to some extent methodological differences between the studies. Many of the early studies were based on imaging methodologies with thick slice acquisitions, poor tissue contrast, and image processing strategies limited to large lobar regions of interest. In recent years, there are few new studies and an apparent waning of interest in sex differences. There is a clear need for further delineation of sex differences in age effects on specific regional brain volumes in larger samples with more sophisticated image processing methods that have become available in recent years. It will be critical to characterize any differential effects of age on the male and female brain for diagnosis and treatment of neurodegenerative diseases in the elderly.

Brain Function

Measures of Glucose Metabolism and Blood Flow with PET and SPECT

Murphy and colleagues (1996) found greater hippocampal metabolism in old, but not young men compared with women in a sample of 55 men and 65 women of a broad age range (mean 54 ± 22 years for men and 52 ± 23 years for women), suggesting sex differences in the effect of age on hippocampal glucose metabolism. Using a different approach to image analysis in a study of individuals between the ages of 50 and 92 years, women were found to have higher regional perfusion in the mid-cingulate/corpus callosum, inferior temporal and inferior parietal areas (Pagani et al., 2002). Higher metabolism in women for the cingulate gyrus, but not other regions, is consistent with the findings of Gur et al. (1995) in younger individuals.

Studies using SPECT and ^{99m}Tc-ECD or ^{99m}Tc-HMPAO have demonstrated sex differences in the regional pattern of cerebral perfusion. In a sample of adults ranging in age from 20 to 81 years, voxel-based analysis demonstrated significantly greater perfusion in the right parietal lobe for women and in the anterior temporal, inferior frontal and cerebellar regions for men (Van Laere et al., 2001). To date, there are few studies involving specific activational tasks in the elderly population.

Neurotransmitter Systems
(Elderly Adults)

The majority of in vivo studies of neurotransmission have been performed in younger individuals and do not address sex differences in neurotransmitter systems in older adults or differential aging for men and women. In an early study using PET and 11-C N-methylspiperone (11-C NMSP) as a radiotracer, Wong and colleagues (1984) reported sex differences in the rate of decline with age in D2 dopamine receptor binding. Males had a steeper slope, i.e., decline with age, than females for D2 dopamine receptor binding, but there were no sex differences in associations with age for serotonin binding using this tracer.

One study used [11C] carfentanil PET to establish normative values and assess the effect of age and sex on brain mu-opioid receptor (μ-OR) availability in healthy people, and their implications for neuropsychiatric disease (Ravert et al., 2004). These receptors play a major role in analgesia induced by opioid drugs (Dauge et al., 1987; Fang et al., 1986) and in pain modulation (Martin-Schilds et al., 1999).

Age-related bilateral and symmetrical increase in μ-OR binding were observed in the anterior cingulate, prefrontal, temporal, and parietal cortices. Sex-related differences in μ-OR binding were seen in the hypothalamus and globus pallidus, where females show higher binding than males by about 15% between the 2nd and 8th decade of life. These findings seem consistent with a meta-analysis that concluded that females may be more sensitive to pain, although the effect was relatively small (Riley et al., 1998).

THE RELEVANCE OF SEX DIFFERENCES IN BRAIN STRUCTURE AND FUNCTION TO ALZHEIMER'S DISEASE (AD) AND RELATED DISORDERS

Sex Differences in the Incidence of Alzheimer's Disease

Sex differences in the risk for Alzheimer's disease (AD) have been difficult to establish definitively due to the longer longevity of women compared with men. Although women comprise a large proportion of people with AD, it is not clear whether this is due to higher risk of disease or solely to the larger number of women alive at ages when AD is common. Nevertheless, a number of incidence studies suggest that women are at greater risk for AD especially at the oldest ages. In the EURODEM studies, there was a higher incidence of AD per year for women (2.9%) compared to men (1.6%) at 80–84 years of age (Andersen et al., 1999).

From the Kungsholmen Project (Stockholm), the Swedish study reported slightly higher incidence rates per year for women (2.0) compared to men (1.2) for ages 75–79 while the rate of AD incidence (per 1000 person-years) was much higher for women (8.7%) then men (1.5%) after 90 years of age (Fratiglioni et al., 1997). In the population-based Cache County, Utah study, women had a higher incidence of AD after age 85 (Miech et al., 2002). Data from the Baltimore Longitudinal Study of Aging also were consistent with a trend toward a higher AD incidence per year for women (1.4%) compared to men (1.1%) age 55 and older (Kawas et al., 2000).

However, there are a number of studies that did not find sex differences in the incidence rates for AD in their samples, such as the Cardiovascular Health Cognition Study (Lopez et al., 2003), the Religious Orders Study, a longitudinal, clinical-pathologic study of aging and AD in older Catholic nuns, priests, and brothers in the United States (Barnes et al., 2003), the population-based East Boston, MA study, a site for the Established Populations for Epidemiologic Study of the Elderly (EPESE) Project (Hebert et al., 2001), the long term Framingham Study (Bachman et al.,

1993), and the Canadian Study of Health and Aging which took care to adjust for age and education (Lindsay et al., 2002).

Several meta-analyses indicate that although women are overall not more likely to develop dementia compared to men, they are more likely to develop AD, especially after age 85 (Andersen et al., 1999; Gao et al., 1998; Jorm & Jolley, 1998; Launer et al., 1999). For example, a meta-analysis of the age-specific incidence of all dementias, including AD, found no sex differences in dementia incidence, although women tended to have a higher incidence of AD in very old age, while men tended to have a higher incidence of vascular dementia at younger ages (Jorm & Jolley, 1998). Swedish twin studies investigating sex differences in the incidence of AD as well as in mechanisms underlying dementia and cognitive dysfunction, however, do not find the sex disparity in the risk for developing the disease even though there are hints that different genetic processes may be involved in men and women (Gatz et al., 2003).

There are also several reports on sex differences in the prevalence and risk factors for AD. Meta-analyses suggest that the prevalence of AD is higher for women compared to men (Jorm et al., 1987; Rocca et al., 1991). One should be cautious, however, in interpreting sex differences in prevalence rates, as prevalence rates are confounded by sex differences in longevity, incidence, and post-dementia survival, necessitating adjustment for age of the disease onset among other factors. For example, a direct comparison of AD incidence and prevalence in the Framingham study (Bachman et al., 1992, 1993) indicated that the sex differences in prevalence were not observed when incidence rates were examined. In a mixed community-based study of elderly people, aged 75 years and older and including individuals with and without dementia, a greater risk of death was found for males with AD compared to females (Jagger et al., 1995), which may contribute to the sex differences found in prevalence in the absence of differences in incidence of AD.

Genetic modifiers and how their effects may be influenced by sex have also been evaluated. The presence of the ε4 allele of the apolipoprotein E (APOE) gene constitutes a well established risk factor for AD (Kehoe et al., 1999) and has been associated with increased risk and decreased age of onset for AD (Corder et al., 1993). APOE presents a genetic polymorphism with three common alleles: ε2, ε3, and ε4. People who carry at least one copy of the APOE ε4 allele are at increased risk for both AD and atherosclerosis.

In one study, sex differences in the association of the APOE genotype with risk for AD related β-amyloid plaque accumulation were reported (Johnson et al., 1998). Although the epsilon ε4 allele was associated with earlier deposition of plaques, this association was independent of sex. In contrast, carriers of an epsilon ε2 allele had slower rates of accumulation, with a greater protective effect of the epsilon ε2 allele in men than women. There is evidence that men, but not women, with AD under the age of 80 with higher total cholesterol levels also have the highest ε4 allele frequencies (Jarvik et al., 1995). Thus, the relationship between AD and APOE genotype is complicated not only by age, but additional factors, such as sex and cholesterol levels, may play a role. Moreover, it has been recently suggested that men and women differ in the clinical manifestations of AD pathology, with pathology more likely to be clinically expressed as dementia in women (Barnes et al., 2005).

Furthermore, a study assessing mortality and its predictors in men and women admitted to one of 1500 nursing homes across five states (Kansas, Maine, Mississippi, New York, and South Dakota) found that men with AD seem to have an increased mortality risk compared to women. The best predictors of death in men were those directly related to the disease itself (Lapane et al., 2001), whereas death among women was associated with measures of disability. The impact of other risk factors also appears to be modified by sex. For example, premorbid depressive symptoms are associated with an increased risk for AD in men but not women (Dal Forno et al., 2005). Such findings suggest that the expression of the mechanisms underlying the disease may be somewhat different in men and women and that future study of survival and progression along with new pharmacotherapies of AD should be sufficiently powered for investigations of men and women, separately.

How Sex Differences in Brain Function and Structure May Relate to Sex Differences in Risk for Alzheimer's Disease

Certain aspects of cognition not only decline with normal aging, but are also influenced by sex. For example, spatial ability is a cognitive domain that shows robust sex differences favoring males of both human

(Kimura, 2002) and other mammalian species (Dawson, 1972; Williams et al., 1990; Williams and Meck, 1991). For example, spatial ability declines with age (Driscoll et al., 2003, 2005; Moffat et al., 2001; Moffat and Resnick, 2002), and despite the decline, there is data to suggest that men continue to outperform women throughout adulthood (Driscoll et al., 2003, 2005) on tasks requiring one to navigate in a virtual environment.

To date, there is only limited information on sex differences in various aspects of cognition in people suffering from AD. However, sex differences in cognition have prompted questions regarding biological contributions to sex-influenced behavior. Sex-specific hormonal differences have been proposed as an obvious avenue for exploring the underlying biology of sex-influenced behavior, and as such, may have important implications for understanding Alzheimer's disease.

Given that sex differences have been reported in epidemiological and cognitive studies of aging and AD, it is important to understand whether morphological changes or regional perfusion differ in men and women affected by AD. If AD pathology does not always have the same effect on men and women, it may be important to consider sex differences not only in understanding the disease itself but also when searching for imaging biomarkers. The sex differences may be contributing to the high variability observed in the disease. The fact is that to date there are still relatively few measures that can reliably classify AD patients.

Salat and colleagues (1999) attempted to determine whether AD degeneration of the prefrontal cortex differed between men and women. Using MRI to assess the prefrontal volumes of a group of healthy elderly and AD patients, the expected sex difference in prefrontal volumes, with larger size in men, was observed in healthy elderly but was not sustained in the patients with AD.

Callen and colleagues (2004) used MRI and coregistered SPECT to map the regional volumes and perfusion in the limbic system, which shows substantial pathology in AD (Braak & Braak, 1991, 1998). Many limbic regions were affected in both men and women with AD compared to normal controls. However, men with AD had more atrophy in the orbitofrontal cortex, middle and posterior cingulate cortex, hypothalamus, and mamillary bodies, while women with AD showed exclusive anterior thalamic atrophy.

Men also showed hypoperfusion in the anterior and middle cingulate cortex. No significant sex-differences were observed in limbic volumes or relative perfusion values of the control group, although the control group was relatively small (N = 17). Separating men and women did not significantly improve diagnostic classification in this study. However, the results suggest that AD pathology may be differentially expressed in men and women. The biological mechanisms underlying these differences remain unknown.

Hormones and Risk for AD

Sex differences in cognition have prompted questions regarding the neurobiological differences which may underlie sex-influenced behavior. Sex-specific hormonal differences are an obvious option for exploring the underlying substrates of sex-influenced behavior and related morphology. Both observational (see Maki & Hogervorst, 2003; Maki & Resnick, 2001; Resnick & Maki, 2001; Yaffe et al., 1998) and non-human animal (see Gibbs & Gabor, 2003 for a review) studies suggest that estrogen may protect against age-related memory decline or AD. Such studies have sparked investigations of the effects of estrogen-containing hormone therapy on brain function and anatomy.

The Women's Health Initiative (WHI) clinical trial of hormone supplementation in postmenopausal women, however, was unexpectedly terminated after finding that overall health risks outweighed the benefits (Rossouw et al., 2002). This trial, which evaluated combination hormone therapy in the form of conjugated equine estrogens (CEE) plus medroxyprogesterone acetate in women with a uterus and unopposed CEE in women without a uterus, raised awareness regarding the possible role for hormones in aging and cognition. Recently, the focus has shifted somewhat to the effects of earlier initiation of hormone therapy around the menopausal transition and to the role of testosterone and the andropause in men, as there is an undeniable need for therapies that may improve the quality of life of the aging population.

Understanding neurosteroid action and its role in mediating events during normal brain functioning would yield important information for the development of new therapeutic targets. The specific mechanisms underlying the effects of hormones on cognition remain largely unknown, and research on the effects of steroid manipulation on cognition, although promising, is still in the early stages.

Hormone Therapy and Risk for AD in Elderly Women

Estrogen-containing hormone therapy (HT) is commonly prescribed for treatment of menopausal symptoms and osteoporosis. HT was also widely prescribed for prevention of cardiovascular disease and maintenance of bone density in older postmenopausal women prior to the publication of the reports from the WHI (WHI, 2002; 2004).

Evidence from both randomized clinical trials in younger women following surgical menopause and observational studies of HT in postmenopausal women suggested that estrogen might protect against age-related cognitive decline and Alzheimer's disease (AD; Sherwin, 1997; Henderson, 1997). Such reports of potential protective effects of HT in humans combined with basic science studies showing a similar trend prompted investigations of its role in AD and in brain function in general (LeBlanc et al., 2001; Maki & Hogervorst, 2003; Maki & Resnick, 2001; Yaffe et al.; 1998).

In 2002, the WHI combined CEE plus medoxyprogesterone acetate trial was terminated early due to findings that the overall health risks outweighed the benefits of HT in older women (Rossouw et al., 2002). In addition, CEE with or without progestin appeared to increase the risk for dementia in women initiating HT at age 65 and older in the WHI Memory Study (WHIMS; Shumaker et al., 2002; 2004). Around this time many women either elected or were instructed by their physicians to discontinue hormone therapy. However, the WHIMS study was not designed to address whether earlier initiation of HT around the menopausal transition would be beneficial to cognition, as suggested by some clinical (Carlson et al., 2001; Henderson, 2006; Zandi et al., 2002) and basic science findings (Gibbs & Gabor, 2003). It is clear that the timing, type, and duration of hormone use are important variables that merit additional study.

The importance of these issues has been highlighted by the results of the WHI (Anderson et al., 2004; Stefanick et al., 2006) studies which suggest differences between combination and CEE-alone treatments for some outcomes like cardiovascular health and breast cancer risk, as well as possible effects of timing of exposure with respect to the risk for cardiovascular health. The possibility remains that HT-associated risks are further modulated not only by the type, but also by the dosage, the duration, age and pre-existing pathology of women receiving the treatment; hence, it remains to be determined whether HT may only impose a risk for a subgroup of women.

Furthermore, combination treatment with CEE plus medroxyprogesterone acetate may have different effects on different aspects of cognitive functioning, as suggested by deleterious effects of combination therapy on verbal memory and a trend toward a benefit on figural memory in the WHI Study of Cognitive Aging (WHISCA; Resnick et al., 2006). The large database available through WHIMS (Shumaker et al., 2004) and its ancillary study WHISCA (Resnick et al., 2004) show promise to help in identification of the factors that may predispose some people to ill effects of specific forms of HT on cognitive health.

The fact remains that we still don't have a clear understanding of the mechanisms that mediate the effects of estrogen-containing compounds on brain activity and function. Although estrogen does not prove to be a silver bullet for preventing AD or cognitive decline in older postmenopausal women, its modulatory effects on the brain should not be ignored. It should be recognized that effects of estrogen, including different hormone types and regimens, are more complex than originally anticipated, and efforts should be directed at understanding the mechanisms by which specific types of estrogen treatments exert effects on the brain.

Testosterone and Risk for AD in Elderly Men

Andropause and the role of androgens in cognition and aging are still poorly understood, and the amount of information compared to studies of menopause and modulatory effects of estrogen in women is relatively sparse. Even the healthiest of men experience a decline with age from age 30 on, with 1% decline per year in total testosterone levels (Bardin et al., 1991) and a 2%–3% decline per year in free testosterone (Feldman et al., 2002).

Recent evidence suggests that testosterone loss constitutes a risk for cognitive decline and possibly dementia (Cherrier, 2005; Hogervorst et al., 2005; Janowsky, 2005), and that elderly men might benefit from exogenous supplementation of testosterone (Cherrier, 2005; Tenover, 1994). At the same time, it is possible that low testosterone levels are an outcome of age-related cognitive decline and AD pathology rather than a marker for the disease, although Moffat et al. (2004) found that low free testosterone as long as 10 years prior to diagnosis was associated with increased risk for AD.

It is also unclear whether normal levels of testosterone are required for optimal cognitive performance, and further whether the effects of testosterone on cognition are direct or occur through the conversion to estradiol. One intervention study of elderly men, which included an aromatase inhibitor to block conversion of testosterone to estradiol, indicated that effects on spatial memory were androgen mediated while effects on verbal memory were estrogen mediated (Cherrier, 2005).

Even though a number of studies support the notion that testosterone can enhance cognition in older men, it is imperative to characterize the neural and cognitive effects of testosterone loss, whether these effects are androgen or estrogen mediated, and which specific aspects of cognition may be affected by supplementation. Existing studies indicate that any beneficial effects of testosterone supplementation seem to be selective and present only for certain aspects of cognition.

Results from two large epidemiological studies, although reporting a relationship between testosterone and global measures of cognitive functioning in aging men (Barrett-Connor et al., 1999; Yaffe et al., 2002), also found that higher bioavailable testosterone levels were associated with better long-term verbal memory (Barrett-Connor et al., 1999) and better performance on measures of executive function and attention (Yaffe et al., 2002). Several smaller studies have been less consistent. For example, one study reported a negative relationship between testosterone levels and verbal fluency (Wolf & Kirschbaum, 2002).

Another study found age-related deficits in visual and verbal memory that followed a decrease in bioavailable testosterone with age, but no adjustment was performed to account for the effects of age (Morley et al., 1997). Perhaps the strongest evidence from observational studies supporting a role of testosterone in protecting against age-related cognitive decline and AD comes from the Baltimore Longitudinal Study of Aging (BLSA) (Moffat et al., 2002).

In this study, repeated neuropsychological assessments and morning testosterone levels were obtained from 407 men, 50–91 years of age at baseline, for 10 years on average. The findings suggested that high free (but not total) testosterone at baseline was associated with better visual and verbal memory and visuospatial

functioning, as well as a slower rate of decline in visual memory

It is well known from the non-human animal literature that the effects of testosterone mediated through the androgen receptors are widespread but complex, and as such may have specific effects on certain aspects of cognition. Indeed, studies of exogenous testosterone administration in men have provided mixed results. An early study found that the group receiving testosterone showed an enhancement in spatial cognition, specifically visual perception, and spatial constructional processes as measured by the block design subtest of WAIS-R, but other tested cognitive domains were not affected (Janowsky et al., 1994).

The same group confirmed beneficial effects of testosterone supplementation on spatial cognition and working memory in a subsequent trial (Janowsky et al., 2000). In addition, there are reported improvements in spatial memory (recall of walking routes), spatial ability (block construction), and verbal memory (recall of short story) after treatment compared to both placebo and to baseline performance (Cherrier et al., 2001), in spatial reasoning (Cherrier et al., 2004), and subtle improvements on certain measures of checkerboard test performance (Gray et al., 2005). But not all testosterone intervention studies have produced positive results. For example, two studies reported no beneficial effects of testosterone on aspects of cognition tested in response to an acute testosterone treatment (Sih et al., 1997; Wolf et al., 2000), and another study found no changes in performance on visuospatial test (Haren et al., 2005). A relatively low dose of testosterone compared to non-human animal studies and limited sensitivity of cognitive tests have been suggested as possible contributors to inconsistent findings in human studies of testosterone supplementation.

Despite its widespread use in older men, there are only limited data on the effects of testosterone supplementation on cognitive function and AD. Recently, the effects of testosterone supplementation (hydroalcoholic gel [75 mg] applied daily to the skin) were investigated in 16 male patients with AD and 22 healthy male controls in a 24–week randomized, double-blind, placebo-controlled, parallel-group study (Lu et al., 2006). The findings suggested that although testosterone replacement therapy had minimal effects on cognition, the overall quality of life in patients with AD improved. More specifically, for the testosterone-treated patients with AD the scores on the caregiver version of the quality-of-life significantly improved, and there was a non-significant trend toward greater improvement in self-rated quality of life in the healthy testosterone-treated control group compared with placebo. There were no significant treatment-related group differences in the cognitive scores, although numerically greater improvement or less decline on visuospatial measures was observed with testosterone treatment compared to placebo.

Although there is an undeniable need for therapies that may improve the quality of life of the aging population, and recent findings from observational studies and small-scale testosterone trials in elderly men are promising, additional studies on a much larger scale are required before any conclusions and recommendations for clinical practice can be reached for the use of testosterone in preventing or ameliorating age-related cognitive and neural dysfunction. There are lessons to be learned, not only from the non-human animal studies but also the unexpected results of the WHI studies of hormone therapy with CEE in older women, that caution is warranted without well-designed clinical trials. Furthermore, it will be equally important to consider the safety of any potential treatments.

SUMMARY AND CONCLUSION

We have only recently begun to appreciate the effects of sex, age, and individual differences on brain structure and function. The present overview of sex differences in brain neuroanatomy and neurophysiology and how they impact age-related changes in health and disease highlights findings using neuroimaging tools. In recent years, methods involving image acquisition and processing have advanced tremendously and now allow for a more detailed investigation of morphometric and functional variability in the human brain. The importance of controlling for age and sex in studies of brain morphology is becoming clear. The strength of the imaging approach in investigating the effects of sex differences on brain aging lies in the practicality of the method for testing hypotheses generated from more indirect approaches and from animal models. It is important to realize that each imaging modality comes with its inherent strengths and weaknesses, which must be recognized and considered when interpreting and comparing the results.

As our understanding of sex differences in the human brain across the lifespan advances, the potential contributions of both organizational hormones early in development and activational hormones later in life should be considered. Moreover, it is imperative to emphasize that sex differences in brain and behavior refer to average differences between men and women and that differences between individuals within each sex are much greater than the average differences between sexes.

Cognitive performance of men and women largely overlap; one cannot infer an individual's score for a cognitive test or the volume of a particular brain structure on the basis of sex any more than one can predict someone's blood pressure from group averages. Nonetheless, just as normative values for laboratory tests provide useful clinical guidelines for evaluating patients, sex- and age-specific normative values for brain imaging measures will prove useful. As neurophysiologic techniques assume an increasingly important role in neuroscience and clinical investigations, it is critical to understand the joint effects of sex and age for correct interpretation and application to clinical practice.

Acknowledgments

This research was supported (in part) by the Intramural Research Program of the NIH, National Institute on Aging.

References

Allen JS, Bruss J, Brown CK, Damasio H. (2005). Normal neuroanatomical variation due to age: the major lobes and a parcellation of the temporal region. *Neurobiol Aging*, 26: 1245–1260.

Allen JS, Damasio H, Grabowski TJ, Bruss J, Zhang W. (2003). Sexual dimorphism and asymmetries in the gray-white composition of the human cerebrum. *Neuroimage*, 18:880–894.

Allen LS, Richey MF, Chai YM, Gorski RA. (1991). Sex differences in the corpus callosum of the living human being. *J Neurosci*, 11:933–942.

Allen LS, Hines M, Shryne JE, Gorski RA. (1989). Two sexually dimorphic cell groups in the human brain. *J Neurosci*, 9:497–506.

Andersen K, Launer LJ, Dewey ME, Letenneur L, Ott A, Copeland JR, et al. (1999). Gender differences in the incidence of AD and vascular dementia: The EURODEM Studies. EURODEM Incidence Research Group. *Neurology*, 53:1992–1997.

Anderson GL, Limacher M, Assaf AR, Bassford T, Beresford SA, Black H, et al.(2004). Effects of conjugated equine estrogen in postmenopausal women with hysterectomy: the Women's Health Initiative randomized controlled trial. *JAMA*, 291:1701–1712.

Andreason PJ, Zametkin AJ, Guo AC, Baldwin P, Cohen RM. (1994). Gender-related differences in regional cerebral glucose metabolism in normal volunteers. *Psychiatry Res*, 51:175–183.

Ayoub DM, Greenough WT, Juraska JM. (1983). Sex differences in dendritic structure in the preoptic area of the juvenile macaque monkey brain. *Science*, 219:197–198.

Azari NP, Rapoport SI, Grady CL, DeCarli C, Haxby JV, Schapiro MB, Horwitz B. (1992). Gender differences in correlations of cerebral glucose metabolic rates in young normal adults. *Brain Res*, 574:198–208.

Bachevalier J, Brickson M, Hagger C, Mishkin M. (1990). Age and sex differences in the effects of selective temporal lobe lesion on the formation of visual discrimination habits in rhesus monkeys (Macaca mulatta). *Behav Neurosci*, 104:885–899.

Bachevalier J, Hagger C. (1991). Sex differences in the development of learning abilities in primates. *Psychoneuroendocrinology*, 16:177–188.

Bachman DL, Wolf PA, Linn R, Knoefel JE, Cobb J, Belanger A, et al. (1992). Prevalence of dementia and probable senile dementia of the Alzheimer type in the Framingham Study. *Neurology*, 42:115–119.

Bachman DL, Wolf PA, Linn RT, Knoefel JE, Cobb JL, Belanger AJ, et al. (1993). Incidence of dementia and probable Alzheimer's disease in a general population: the Framingham Study. *Neurology*, 43:515–519.

Bardin CW, Swerdloff RS, Santen RJ. (1991). Androgens: risks and benefits. *J Clin Endocrinol*, 73: 4–7.

Barrett-Connor E, Goodman-Gruen D, Patay B. (1999). Endogenous sex hormones and cognirive function in older men. *J Clin Endocrinol Metab*, 84:3682–3685.

Barron SA, Jacobs L, Kinkel WR. (1976). Changes in size of normal lateral ventricles during aging determined by computerized tomography. *Neurology*, 26:1011–1013.

Barnes LL, Wilson RS, Bienias JL, Schneider JA, Evans DA, Bennett DA. (2005). Sex differences in the clinical manifestations of Alzheimer disease pathology. *Arch Gen Psychiatry*, 62:685–691.

Barnes LL, Wilson RS, Schneider JA, Bienias JL, Evans DA, Bennett DA. (2003). Gender, cognitive decline, and risk of AD in older persons. *Neurology*, 60:1777–1781.

Bartzokis G, Beckson M, Lu PH, Nuechterlein KH, Edwards N, Mintz J. (2001). Age-related changes in frontal and temporal lobe volumes in men: a magnetic resonance imaging study. *Arch Gen Psychiatry*, 58:461–465.

Baxter LR, Mazziotta JC, Phelps ME, Selin CE, Guze BH, Fairbanks L. (1987). Cerebral glucose metabolic rates in normal human females versus normal males. *Psychiatry Res*, 21:237–245.

Baxter LC, Saykin AJ, Flashman LA, Johnson SC, Guerin SJ, Babcock DR, Wishart HA. (2003). Sex differences in semantic language processing: a functional MRI study. *Brain Lang*, 84:264–272.

Bell AD, Variend S. (1985). Failure to demonstrate sexual dimorphism of the corpus callosum in childhood. Journal of Anatomy 143:143–147.

Benbow CP, Stanley JC. (1983). Sex differences in mathematical reasoning ability: more facts. *Science*, 222:1029–1031.

Benbow CP, Lubinski D, Shea DL, Eftekhari-Sanjani H. (2000). Sex differences in mathematical reasoning ability at age 13: their status 20 years later. *Psychol Sci*, 1:474–480.

Biver F, Goldman S, Luxen A, Monclus M, Forestini M, Mendlewicz J, Lotstra F. (1994). Multicompartmental study of fluorine-18 altanserin binding to brain 5HT2 receptors in humans using positron emission tomography. *Eur J Nucl Med*, 21:937–946.

Blatter DD, Bigler ED, Gale SD, Johnson SC, Anderson CV, Burnett BM, et al. (1995). Quantitative volumetric analysis of brain MR: normative database spanning 5 decades of life. *AJNR Am J Neuroradiol*, 16:241–251.

Bouix S, Pruessner JC, Louis Collins D, Siddiqi K. (2005). Hippocampal shape analysis using medial surfaces. *Neuroimage*, 25:1077–1089.

Braak H, Braak E. (1991). Neuropathological staging of Alzheimer-related changes. *Acta Neuropathol*, 82:239–259.

Braak H, Braak E. (1998). Evolution of neuronal changes in the course of Alzheimer's disease. *J Neural Transm Suppl*, 53:127–140.

Breger RK, Yetkin FZ, Fischer ME, Papke RA, Haughton VM, Rimm AA. (1991). T1 and T2 in the cerebrum: correlation with age, gender, and demographic factors. *Radiology*, 181:545–547.

Bremner JD, Soufer R, McCarthy G, Delaney R, Staib LH, Duncan JS, Charney DS (2001). Gender differences in cognitive and neural correlates of remembrance of emotional words. *Psychopharmacol Bull*, 35:55–78.

Cahill L, Haier RJ, White N, Fallon J, Kilpatrick L, Lawrence C, Potkin S, Alkire MT. (2001). Sex-related difference in amygdala activity during emotionally influenced memory storage. *Neurobiol Learn Mem*, 75:1–9.

Cahill L, Uncapher M, Kilpatrick L, ALkire M, Turner J. (2004). Sex-related hemispheric lateralization of amygdala function in emotionally influenced memory: an fMRI investigation. *Learn Mem*, 11:261–266.

Callen DJ, Black SE, Caldwell CB, Grady CL. (2004). The influence of sex on limbic volume and perfusion in AD. *Neurobiol Aging*, 25:761–770.

Canli T, Desmond JE, Zhao Z, Gabrieli JD. (2002). Sex differences in the neural basis of emotional memories. *Proc Natl Acad Sci USA*, 99:10789–10794.

Carlson MC, Zandi PP, Plassman BL, Tschanz JT, Welsh-Bohmer KA, Steffens DC, et al. (2001). Hormone replacement therapy and reduced cognitive decline in older women: the Cache County Study. *Neurology*, 57:2210–2216.

Caviness VS Jr, Kennedy DN, Richelme C, Rademacher J, Filipek PA. (1996). The human brain age 7–11 years: a volumetric analysis based on magnetic resonance images. *Cereb Cortex*, 6:726–736.

Chang L, Ernst T, Poland RE, Jenden DJ. (1996). In vivo proton magnetic resonance spectroscopy of the normal aging human brain. *Life Sci*, 58:2049–2056.

Cherrier MM. (2005). Androgens and cognitive function. *J Endocrinol Invest*, 28:65–75.

Cherrier MM, Asthana S, Plymate S, Baker L, Matsumoto AM, Peskind E, et al. (2001). Testosterone supplementation improves spatial and verbal memory in healthy older men. *Neurology*, 57:80–88.

Cherrier MM, Plymate S, Mohan S, Asthana S, Matsumoto AM, Bremner W, et al. (2004). Relationship between testosterone supplementation and insulin-like growth factor-I levels and cognition in healthy older men. *Psychoneuroendocrinology*, 29:65–82.

Cho S, Jones D, Reddick WE, Ogg RJ, Steen RG. (1997). Establishing norms for age-related changes in proton T1 of human brain tissue in vivo. *Magn Reson Imaging*, 15:1133–1143.

Christiansen P, Larsson HB, Thomsen C, Wieslander SB, Henriksen O. (1994). Age dependent white matter lesions and brain volume changes in healthy volunteers. *Acta Radiol*, 35:117–122.

Clark AS, Goldman-Rakic PS. (1989). Gonadal hormones influence the emergence of cortical function in nonhuman primates. *Behav Neurosci*, 103:1287–1295.

Coffey CE. (1994). Anatomic imaging of the aging human brain: computed tomography and magnetic resonance imaging. In Coffey CE, Cummnings JL (Eds.), *Textbook of geriatric neuropsychiatry* (pp 159–194). Washington, DC: American Psychiatric Press.

Coffey CE, Lucke JF, Saxton JA, Ratcliff G, Unitas LJ, Billig B, Bryan RN. (1998). Sex differences in brain aging: a quantitative magnetic resonance imaging study. *Arch Neurol*, 55:169–179.

Coffey CE, Wilkinson WE, Parashos IA, Soady SA, Sullivan RJ, Patterson LJ, et al. (1992). Quantitative cerebral anatomy of the aging human brain: a cross-sectional study using magnetic resonance imaging. *Neurology*, 42:527–536.

Condon B, Grant R, Hadley D, Lawrence A. (1988). Brain and intracranial cavity volumes: in vivo determination by MRI. *Acta Neurol Scand*, 78:387–393.

Constant D, Ruther H. (1996). Sexual dimorphism in the human corpus callosum? A comparison of methodologies. *Brain Research*, 727:99–106.

Corder EH, Saunders AM, Strittmatter WJ, Schmechel DE, Gaskell PC, Small GW, et al. (1993). Gene dose of apolipoprotein E type 4 allele and the risk of Alzheimer's disease in late onset families. *Science*, 261:921–923.

Cowan RL, Frederick BB, Rainey M, Levin JM, Maas LC, Bang J, et al. (2000). Sex differences in response to red and blue light in human primary visual cortex: a bold fMRI study. *Psychiatry Res*, 100:129–138.

Cowell PE, Turetsky BI, Gur RC, Grossman RI, Shtasel DL, Gur RE. (1994). Sex differences in aging of the human frontal and temporal lobes. *J Neurosci*, 14:4748–4755.

Dal Forno G, Palermo MT, Donohue JE, Karagiozis H, Zonderman AB, Kawas CH. (2005). Depressive symptoms, sex, and risk for Alzheimer's disease. *Ann Neurol*, 57:381–387.

Dauge V, Petit F, Rossignol P, Roques BP. (1987). Use of mu and delta opioid peptides of various selectivity gives further evidence of specific involvement of mu opioid receptors in supraspinal analgesia (tail-flick test). *Eur J Pharmacol*, 141:171–178.

Davatzikos C, Resnick SM. (1998). Sex differences in anatomic measures of interhemispheric connectivity: correlations with cognition in women but not men. *Cereb Cortex*, 8:635–640.

Davatzikos C. (1996). Spatial normalization of 3D brain images using deformable models. *J Comput Assist Tomogr*, 20:656–665.

Davatzikos C, Vaillant M, Resnick SM, Prince JL, Letovsky S, Bryan RN. (1996). A computerized approach for morphological analysis of the corpus callosum. *J Comput Assist Tomogr*, 20:88–97.

Dawson JLM. (1972). Effects of sex hormones on cognitive style in rats and men. *Behav Genet*, 1:21–42.

de Leeuw FE, de Groot JC, Achten E, Oudkerk M, Ramos LM, Heijboer R, et al. (2001). Prevalence of cerebral white matter lesions in elderly people: a population based magnetic resonance imaging study. The Rotterdam Scan Study. *J Neurol Neurosurg Psychiatry*, 70:9–14.

DeLacoste-Utamsing C, Holloway RL. (1982). Sexual dimorphism in the human corpus callosum. *Science*, 216:1431–1432.

DeLacoste MC, Holloway RL, Woodward D. (1986). Sex differences in the fetal corpus callosum. *Human Neurobiology*, 5:93–96.

DeVoogd T, Nottebohm F. (1981). Gonadal hormones induce dendritic growth in the adult avian brain. *Science*, 214:202–204.

Demeter S, Ringo JL, Doty RW. (1988). Morphometric analysis of the human corpus callosum and anterior commissure. *Human Neurobiology*, 6:219–226.

Driscoll I, Hamilton DA, Yeo RA, Brooks WM, Sutherland RJ. (2005). Virtual navigation in humans: the impact of age, sex, and hormones on place learning. *Horm Behav*, 427: 326–335.

Driscoll I, Hamilton DA, Petropoulos H, Yeo RA, Brooks WM, Sutherland RJ. (2003). The aging hippocampus: cognitive, biochemical, and structural findings. *Cereb Cortex*, 13:1344–1351.

Earnest MP, Heaton RK, Wilkinson WE, Manke WF (1979) Cortical atrophy, ventricular enlargement and intellectual impairment in the aged. Neurology 29:1138–1143.

Espeland MA, Rapp SR, Shumaker SA, Brunner R, Manson JE, Sherwin BB, et al. (2004). Conjugated equine estrogens and global cognitive function in postmenopausal women: Women's Health Initiative Memory Study. JAMA, 29:2959–2968.

Fang FG, Fields HL, Lee NM. (1986). Action at the mu receptor is sufficient to explain the supraspinal analgesic effect of opiates. J Pharmacol Exp Ther, 238:1039–1044.

Feldman HA, Longcope C, Derby CA, Johannes CB, Araujo AB, Coviello AD, et al. (2002). Age trends in the level of serum testosterone and other hormones in middle aged men: longitudinal results from the Massachusetts male aging study. J Clin Endocrinol Metab, 87:589–598.

Fratiglioni L, Viitanen M, von Strauss E, Tontodonati V, Herlitz A, Winblad B. (1997). Very old women at highest risk of dementia and Alzheimer's disease: incidence data from the Kungsholmen Project, Stockholm. Neurology, 48:132–138.

Galaburda AM, LeMay M, Kemper TL, Geschwind N. (1978). Right-left asymmetrics in the brain. Science, 199:852–856.

Gao S, Hendrie HC, Hall KS, Hui S. (1998). The relationships between age, sex, and the incidence of dementia and Alzheimer disease: a meta-analysis. Arch Gen Psychiatry, 55:809–815.

Gatz M, Fiske A, Reynolds CA, Wetherell JL, Johansson B, Pedersen NL. (2003). Sex differences in genetic risk for dementia. Behav Genet, 33:95–105.

George MS, Ketter TA, Parekh PI, Herscovitch P, Post RM. (1996). Gender differences in regional cerebral blood flow during transient self-induced sadness or happiness. Biol Psychiatry, 40:859–871.

Geschwind N, Levitsky W. (1968). Human brain: left-right asymmetries in the temporal speech region. Science, 161:186–187.

Gibbs RB, Gabor R. (2003). Estrogen and cognition: applying preclinical findings to clinical perspectives. J Neurosci Res, 74:637–643.

Giedd JN, Snell JW, Lange N, Rajapakse JC, Casey BJ, Kozuch PL, et al. (1996). Quantitative magnetic resonance imaging of human brain development: ages 4–18. Cereb Cortex, 6:551–560.

Giedd JN, Rumsey JM, Castellanos FX, Rajapakse JC, Kaysen D, Vaituzis AC, et al. (1996). A quantitative MRI study of the corpus callosum in children and adolescents. Brain Res Dev Brain Res, 91:274–280.

Giedd JN, Vaituzis AC, Hamburger SD, Lange N, Rajapakse JC, Kaysen D, et al. (1996). Quantitative MRI of the temporal lobe, amygdala, and hippocampus in normal human development: ages 4–18 years. J Comp Neurol, 366:223–230.

Goldman PS. (1975). Age, sex, and experience as related to the neural basis of cognitive development. In

Buchwald NA, Brazier MAB (Eds.), Brain mechanisms in mental retardation (pp 379–392). New York: Academic Press.

Goldman PS, Crawford HT, Stokes LP, Galkin TW, Rosvold HE. (1974). Sex-dependent behavioral effects of cerebral cortical lesions in the developing rhesus monkey. Science, 186:540–542.

Goldstein JM, Seidman LJ, Horton NJ, Makris N, Kenedy DN, Caviness VS Jr, et al. (2001). Normal sexual dimorphism of the adult human brain assessed by in vivo magnetic resonance imaging. Cereb Cortex, 11:490–497.

Golomb J, de Leon MJ, Kluger A, George AE, Tarshish C, Ferris SH. (1993). Hippocampal atrophy in normal aging. An association with recent memory impairment. Arch Neurol, 50:967–973.

Good CD, Johnsrude IS, Ashburner J, Henson RN, Friston KJ, Frackowiak RS. (2001a). A voxel-based morphometric study of ageing in 465 normal adult human brains. Neuroimage, 14:21–36.

Good CD, Johnsrude I, Ashburner J, Henson RN, Friston KJ, Frackowiak RS. (2001b). Cerebral asymmetry and the effects of sex and handedness on brain structure: a voxel-based morphometric analysis of 465 normal adult human brains. Neuroimage, 14:685–700.

Grant R, Condon B, Lawrence A, Hadley DM, Patterson J, Bone I, Teasdale GM. (1987). Human cranial CSF volumes measured by MRI: sex and age influences. Magn Reson Imaging, 5:465–468.

Gray PB, Singh AB, Woodhouse LJ, Storer TW, Casaburi R, Dzekov J, et al. (2005). Dose-dependent effects of testosterone on sexual function, mood, and visuospatial cognition in older men. J Clin Endocrinol Metab, 90:3838–3846.

Gron G, Wunderlich AP, Spitzer M, Tomczak R, Riepe MW. (2000). Brain activation during human navigation: gender-different neural networks as substrate of performance. Nat Neurosci, 3:404–408.

Gur RE, Gur RC. (1990). Gender differences in regional cerebral blood flow. Schizophr Bull, 16:247–254.

Gur RC, Gunning-Dixon FM, Turetsky BI, Bilker WB, Gur RE. (2002). Brain region and sex differences in age association with brain volume: a quantitative MRI study of healthy young adults. Am J Geriatr Psychiatry, 10:72–80.

Gur RC, Alsop D, Glahn D, Petty R, Swanson CL, Maldjian JA, et al. (2000). An fMRI study of sex differences in regional activation to a verbal and a spatial task. Brain Lang, 74:157–170.

Gur RC, Turetsky BI, Matsui M, Yan M, Bilker W, Hughett P, Gur RE. (1999). Sex differences in brain gray and white matter in healthy young adults: correlations with cognitive performance. J Neurosci, 19:4065–72.

Gur RC, Mozley LH, Mozley PD, Resnick SM, Karp JS, Alavi A, et al. (1995). Sex differences in regional cerebral glucose metabolism during a resting state. Science, 267:528–531.

Gur RC, Mozley PD, Resnick SM, Gottlieb GL, Kohn M, Zimmerman R, et al. (1991). Gender differences in age effect on brain atrophy measured by magnetic resonance imaging. *Proc Natl Acad Sci USA*, 88:2845–2849.

Gur RC, Gur RE, Obrist WD, Skolnick BE, Reivich M. (1987). Age and regional cerebral blood flow at rest and during cognitive activity. *Arch Gen Psychiatry*, 44:617–621.

Gur RC, Gur RE, Obrist WD, Hungerbuhler JP, Younkin D, Rosen AD, et al. (1982). Sex and handedness differences in cerebral blood flow during rest and cognitive activity. *Science*, 217:659–661.

Guttmann CR, Jolesz FA, Kikinis R, Killiany RJ, Moss MB, Sandor T, Albert MS. (1998). White matter changes with normal aging. *Neurology*, 50:972–978.

Haacke E. (1999). Magnetic resonance imaging: physical principles and sequence design. New York: John Wiley & Sons.

Hagger C, Bachevalier J. (1991). Visual habit formation in 3-month-old monkeys (*Macaca mulatta*): reversal of sex difference following neonatal manipulations of androgens. *Behav Brain Res*, 45:57–63.

Hamann S, Herman RA, Nolan CL, Wallwn K (2004) Men and women differ in amygdala response to visual sexual stimuli. *Nat Neurosci* 7:411–416.

Haren M, Chapman I, Coates P, Morley J, Wittert G. (2005). Effect of 12 month oral testosterone on testosterone deficiency symptoms in symptomatic elderly males with low-normal gonadal status. *Age Ageing*, 34:125–130.

Harman SM, Metter EJ, Tobin JD, Pearson J, Blackman MR. (2001). Longitudinal effects of aging on serum total and free testosterone levels in healthy men. Baltimore Longitudinal Study of Aging. *J Clin Endocrinol Metab*, 86:724–731.

Harshman RA, Hampson E, Berenbaum SA. (1983). Individual differences in cognitive abilities and brain organization, part I: sex and handedness differences in ability. *Canadian Journal of Psychology*, 37:144–192.

Hebert LE, Scherr PA, McCann JJ, Beckett LA, Evans DA. (2001). Is the risk of developing Alzheimer's disease greater for women than for men? *Am J Epidemiol*, 153:132–136.

Henderson VW. (2006). Estrogen-containing hormone therapy and Alzheimer's disease risk: understanding discrepant inferences from observational and experimental research. *Neuroscience*, 138:1031–1039.

Henderson V. (1997). The epidemiology of estrogen replacement therapy and Alzheimer's disease. *Neurology*, 48:27–35.

Hier DB, Yoon WB, Mohr JP, Price TR. (1994). Gender and aphasia in the Stroke Data Bank. *Brain Lang*, 47:155–167.

Hines M, Gorski RA. (1985). Hormonal influences on the development of neural Asymmetries. In Benson DF, Zaidel E (Eds.), *The dual brain* (pp. 75–96). New York: The Guilford Press.

Hines M, Green R. (1991). Human hormonal and neural correlates of sex-typed behaviors. *Rev Psychiat*, 10:536–555.

Hogervorst E, Bandelow S, Moffat SD. (2005). Increasing testosterone levels and effects on cognitive functions in elderly men and women: a review. *Curr Drug Targets CNS Neurol Disord*, 4:531–540.

Holloway RL, Heilbroner P. (1992). Corpus callosum in sexually dimorphic and nondimorphic primates. *Am J Phys Anthropol*, 87:349–357.

Holloway RL, Anderson PJ, Defendini R, Harper C. (1993). Sexual dimorphism of the human corpus callosum from three independent samples: relative size of the corpus callosum. *Am J Phys Anthropol*, 92:481–498.

Ide A, Rodriguez E, Zaidel E, Aboitiz F. (1996). Bifurcation patterns in the human sylvian fissure: hemispheric and sex differences. *Cereb Cortex*, 6:717–725.

Jagger C, Clarke M, Stone A. (1995). Predictors of survival with Alzheimer's disease: a community-based study. *Psychol Med*, 25:171–177.

Jancke L, Staiger JF, Schlaug G, Huang Y, Steinmetz H. (1997). The relationship between corpus callosum size and forebrain volume. *Cereb Cortex*, 7:48–56.

Janowsky JS. (2006). Thinking with your gonads: testosterone and cognition. *Trends Cogn Sci*, 10:77–82.

Janowsky JS, Chavez B, Orwoll ES. (2000). Sex steroids modify working memory. *J Cog Neurosci*, 12:407–414.

Janowsky JS, Oviatt SK, Orwoll ES. (1994). Testosterone influences spatial cognition in older men. *Behav Neurosci*, 108:325–332.

Jarvik GP, Wijsman EM, Kukull WA, Schellenberg GD, Yu C, Larson EB. (1995). Interactions of apolipoprotein E genotype, total cholesterol level, age, and sex in prediction of Alzheimer's disease: a case-control study. *Neurology*, 45:1092–1096.

Jernigan TL, Archibald SL, Fennema-Notestine C, Gamst AC, Stout JC, Bonner J, Hesselink JR. (2001). Effects of age on tissues and regions of the cerebrum and cerebellum. *Neurobiol Aging*, 22:581–594.

Johnson JK, McCleary R, Oshita MH, Cotman CW. (1998). Initiation and propagation stages of beta-amyloid are associated with distinctive apolipoprotein E, age, and gender profiles. *Brain Res*, 798:18–24.

Jones K, Johnson KA, Becker JA, Spiers PA, Albert MS, Holman BL. (1998). Use of singular value decomposition to characterize age and gender differences in SPECT cerebral perfusion. *J Nucl Med*, 39:965–973.

Johnson SC, Farnworth T, Pinkston JB, Bigler ED, Blatter DD. (1994). Corpus callosum surface area across the human adult life span: effect of age and gender. *Brain Res Bull*, 35: 373–377.

Jorm AF, Korten AE, Henderson AS. (1987). The prevalence of dementia: a quantitative integration of the literature. *Acta Psychiatr Scand*, 76:465–479.

Jorm AF, Jolley D. (1998). The incidence of dementia: a meta-analysis. *Neurology*, 51:728–733.

Kaasinen V, Nagren K, Hietala J, Farde L, Rinne JO. (2001). Sex differences in extrastriatal dopamine d(2)-like receptors in the human brain. *Am J Psychiatry*, 158:308–311.

Kansaku K, Yamaura A, Kitazawa S. (2000). Sex differences in lateralization revealed in the posterior language areas. *Cereb Cortex*, 10:866–872.

Kawas C, Gray S, Brookmeyer R, Fozard J, Zonderman A. (2000). Age-specific incidence rates of Alzheimer's disease: the Baltimore Longitudinal Study of Aging. *Neurology*, 54: 2072–2077.

Kaye JA, DeCarli C, Luxenberg JS, Rapoport SI. (1992). The significance of age-related enlargement of the cerebral ventricles in healthy men and women measured by quantitative computed X-ray tomography. *J Am Geriatr Soc*, 40:225–231.

Kehoe P, Wavrant-DeVrieze F, Crook R, Wu WS, Holmans P, Fenton L, et al. (1999). A full genome scan for late onset Alzheimer's disease. *Hum Mol Gen*, 8:237–245.

Kertesz A, Benke T. (1989). Sex equality in intrahemispheric language organization. *Brain Lang*, 37:401–408.

Kilpatrick LA, Zald DH, Pardo JV, Cahill LF. (2006). Sex-related differences in amygdale functional connectivity during resting conditions. *NeuroImage*, 30:452–461.

Kim DM, Xanthakos SA, Tupler LA, Barboriak DP, Charles HC, MacFall JR, et al. (2002). MR signal intensity of gray matter/white matter contrast and intracranial fat: effects of age and sex. *Psychiatry Res*, 114:149–161.

Kimura D. (2002). Sex hormones influence human cognitive pattern. *Neuro Endocrinol Lett*, 23: 67–77.

Kimura D. (1983). Sex differences in cerebral organization for speech and praxic functions. *Can J Psychol*, 37:19–35.

Kimura D, Harshman RA. (1984). Sex differences in brain organization for verbal and non-verbal functions. In DeVries GJ, et al., (Eds.), *Sex differences in primates* (pp. 423–441). New York:Elsevier.

Kochunov P, Mangin JF, Coyle T, Lancaster J, Thompson P, Riviere D, et al. (2005). Age-related morphology trends of cortical sulci. *Hum Brain Mapp*, 26: 210–220.

Kulynych JJ, Vladar K, Jones DW, Weinberger DR. (1994). Gender differences in the normal lateralization of the supratemporal cortex: MRI surface-rendering morphometry of Heschl's gyrus and the planum temporale. *Cereb Cortex*, 4:107–118.

Laakso A, Vilkman H, Bergman J, Haaparanta M, Solin O, Syvalahti E, et al. (2002). Sex differences in striatal presynaptic dopamine synthesis capacity in healthy subjects. *Biol Psychiatry*, 52:759–763.

Lacreuse A, Diehl MM, Goh MY, Hall MJ, Volk AM, Chhabra RK, Herndon JG. (2005). Sex differences in age-related motor slowing in the rhesus monkey: behavioral and neuroimaging data. *Neurobiol Aging*, 26:543–551.

Lacreuse A, Kim CB, Rosene DL, Killiany RJ, Moss MB, Moore TL, et al. (2005). Sex, age, and training modulate spatial memory in the rhesus monkey (*Macaca mulatta*). *Behav Neurosci*, 119:118–126.

Landsdell H. (1962). Laterality of verbal intelligence in the brain. *Science*, 135:922–923.

Lapane KL, Gambassi G, Landi F, Sgadari A, Mor V, Bernabei R. (2001). Gender differences in predictors of mortality in nursing home residents with AD. *Neurology*, 56:650–654.

Launer LJ, Andersen K, Dewey ME, Letenneur L, Ott A, Amaducci LA, et al. (1999). Rates and risk factors for dementia and Alzheimer's disease: results from EURODEM pooled analyses. EURODEM Incidence Research Group and Work Groups. European Studies of Dementia. *Neurology*, 52: 78–84.

LeBlanc ES, Janowsky J, Chan BK, Nelson HD. (2001). Hormone replacement therapy and cognition: systematic review and meta-analysis. *J Am Med Assoc*, 285:1489–1499.

Lee TM, Liu HL, Hoosain R, Liao WT, Wu CT, Yuen KS, et al. (2002). Gender differences in neural correlates of recognition of happy and sad faces in humans assessed by functional magnetic resonance imaging. *Neurosci Lett*, 333:13–16.

Lemaitre H, Crivello F, Grassiot B, Alperovitch A, Tzourio C, Mazoyer B. (2005). Age- and sex-related effects on the neuroanatomy of healthy elderly. *Neuroimage*, 26:900–911.

Lindsay J, Laurin D, Verreault R, Hebert R, Helliwell B, Hill GB, McDowell I. (2002). Risk factors for Alzheimer's disease: a prospective analysis from the Canadian Study of Health and Aging. *Am J Epidemiol*, 156:445–453.

Lopez OL, Kuller LH, Fitzpatrick A, Ives D, Becker JT, Beauchamp N. (2003). Evaluation of dementia in the cardiovascular health cognition study. *Neuroepidemiology*, 22:1–12.

Lu PH, Masterman DA, Mulnard R, Cotman C, Miller B, Yaffe K, et al. (2006). Effects of testosterone on cognition and mood in male patients with mild Alzheimer disease and healthy elderly men. *Arch Neurol*, 63:177–185.

Luders E, Narr KL, Thompson PM, Woods RP, Rex DE, Jancke L, et al. (2005). Mapping cortical gray matter in the young adult brain: effects of gender. *Neuroimage*, 26:493–501.

Maccoby EE, Jacklin CN. (1974). The psychology of sex differences. Stanford: Stanford University Press.

Maki P, Hogervorst E. (2003). The menopause and HRT. HRT and cognitive decline. *Best Pract Res Clin Endocrinol Metab*, 17:105–122.

Maki PM, Resnick SM. (2001). Effects of estrogen on patterns of brain activity at rest and during cognitive activity: a review of neuroimaging studies. *Neuroimage*, 14:789–801.

Martin-Schild S, Gerall AA, Kastin AJ, Zadina JE. (1999). Differential distribution of endomorphin 1- and endomorphin 2-like immunoreactivities in the CNS of the rodent. *J Comp Neurol*, 405:450–471.

Mathew RJ, Wilson WH, Tant SR, Robinson L, Prakash R. (1988). Abnormal resting regional cerebral blood flow patterns and their correlates in schizophrenia. *Arch Gen Psychiatry*, 45:542–549.

Matthews KA, Shumaker SA, Bowen DJ, Langer RD, Hunt JR, Kaplan RM, et al. (1997). Women's Health Initiative. Why now? What is it? What's new? *American Psychologist*, 52:101–116.

McGlone J. (1980). Sex differences in human brain asymmetry: a critical survey. *Behav Brain Sci*, 3: 215–263.

Merke DP, Fields JD, Keil MF, Vaituzis AC, Chrousos GP, Giedd JN. (2003). Children with classic congenital adrenal hyperplasia have decreased amygdala volume: potential prenatal and postnatal hormonal effects. *J Clin Endocrinol Metab*, 88:1760–1765.

Miura SA, Schapiro MB, Grady CL, Kumar A, Salerno JA, Kozachuk WE, et al. (1990). Effect of gender on glucose utilization rates in healthy humans: a positron emission tomography study. *J Neurosci Res*, 27: 500–504.

Moffat SD, Zonderman AB, Metter EJ, Kawas C, Blackman MR, Harman SM, et al. (2004). Free testosterone and risk for Alzheimer disease in older men. *Neurology*, 62:188–193.

Moffat SD, Zonderman AB, Metter EJ, Blackman MR, Harman SM, Resnick SM. (2002). Longitudinal assessment of serum free testosterone concentration predicts memory performance and cognitive status in elderly men. *J Cin Endocrinol Metab*, 87:5001–5007.

Moffat SD, Resnick SM. (2002). Effects of age on virtual environment place navigation and allocentric cognitive mapping. *Behav Neurosci*, 116:851–859.

Moffat SD, Zonderman AB, Resnick SM. (2001). Age differences in spatial memory in a virtual environment navigation task. *Neurobiol Aging*, 22:787–796.

Morley JE. (2000). Andropause, testosterone therapy, and quality of life in aging men. *Cleve Clin J Med*, 67:880–882.

Morley JE, Kaiser F, Raum WJ, Perry HM 3rd, Flood JF, Jensen J, Silver AJ, Roberts E. (1997). Potentially predictive and manipulable blood serum correlates of aging in the healthy human male: progressive decreases in bioavailable testosterone, dehydroepiandrosterone sulfate, and the ratio of insulin-like growth factor 1 to growth hormone. *Proc Natl Acad Sci USA*, 94:7537–7542.

Mozley LH, Gur RC, Mozley PD, Gur RE. (2001). Striatal dopamine transporters and cognitive functioning in healthy men and women. *Am J Psychiatry*, 158:1492–1499.

Murphy DG, DeCarli C, McIntosh AR, Daly E, Mentis MJ, Pietrini P, et al. (1996). Sex differences in human brain morphometry and metabolism: an in vivo quantitative magnetic resonance imaging and positron emission tomography study on the effect of aging. *Arch Gen Psychiatry*, 53:585–594.

Nishizawa S, Benkelfat C, Young SN, Leyton M, Mzengeza S, de Montigny C, et al. (1997). Differences between males and females in rates of serotonin synthesis in human brain. *Proc Natl Acad Sci USA*, 94:5308–5313.

Nopoulos P, Flaum M, O'Leary D, Andreasen NC. (2000). Sexual dimorphism in the human brain: evaluation of tissue volume, tissue composition and surface anatomy using magnetic resonance imaging. *Psychiatry Res*, 98:1–13.

Nordstrom AL, Olsson H, Halldin C. (1998). A PET study of D2 dopamine receptor density at different phases of the menstrual cycle. *Psychiatry Res*, 83:1–6.

Pagani M, Salmaso D, Jonsson C, Hatherly R, Jacobsson H, Larsson SA, Wagner A. (2002). Regional cerebral blood flow as assessed by principal component analysis and (99m)Tc-HMPAO SPET in healthy subjects at rest: normal distribution and effect of age and gender. *Eur J Nucl Med Mol Imaging*, 29:67–75.

Pakkenberg B, Gundersen HJ. (1997). Neocortical neuron number in humans: effect of sex and age. *J Comp Neurol*, 384:312–320.

Parashos IA, Wilkinson WE, Coffey CE. (1995). Magnetic resonance imaging of the corpus callosum: predictors of size in normal adults. *Journal of Neuropsychiatry*, 7:35–41.

Parsey RV, Oquendo MA, Simpson NR, Ogden RT, Van Heertum R, Arango V, Mann JJ. (2002). Effects of sex, age, and aggressive traits in man on brain serotonin 5-HT1A receptor binding potential measured by PET using [C-11]WAY-100635. *Brain Res*, 54:173–182.

Pfefferbaum A, Sullivan EV, Carmelli D. (2004). Morphological changes in aging brain structures are differentially affected by time-linked environmental influences despite strong genetic stability. *Neurobiol Aging*, 25:175–183.

Phillips MD, Lowe MJ, Lurito JT, Dzemidzic M, Mathews VP. (2001). Temporal lobe activation demonstrates sex-based differences during passive listening. *Radiology*, 220:202–207.

Powers RE. (1994). Neurobiology of aging. In Coffey CE, Cummings JL (Eds.), *Textbook of geriatric neuropsychiatry* (pp. 35–69). Washington, DC: American Psychiatric Press Inc.

Pozzilli C, Bastianello S, Bozzao A, Pierallini A, Giubilei F, Argentino C, Bozzao L. (1994). No differences in corpus callosum size by sex and aging. A quantitative study using magnetic resonance imaging. *J Neuroimaging*, 4:218–221.

Pugh KR, Shaywitz BA, Shaywitz SE, Constable RT, Skudlarski P, Fulbright RK, et al. (1996). Cerebral organization of component processes in reading. *Brain*, 119:1221–1238.

Pujol J, Lopez A, Deus J, Cardoner N, Vallejo J, Capdevila A, Paus T. (2002). Anatomical variability of the anterior cingulate gyrus and basic dimensions of human personality. *Neuroimage*, 15:847–855.

Rabinowicz T, Petetot JM, Gartside PS, Sheyn D, Sheyn T, de CM. (2002). Structure of the cerebral cortex in men and women. *J Neuropathol Exp Neurol*, 61: 46–57.

Ravert HT, Bencherif B, Madar I, Frost JJ. (2004). PET imaging of opioid receptors in pain: progress and new directions. *Curr Pharm Des*, 10:759–768.

Raz N, Gunning-Dixon F, Head D, Rodrigue KM, Williamson A, Acker JD. (2004). Aging, sexual dimorphism, and hemispheric asymmetry of the cerebral cortex: replicability of regional differences in volume. *Neurobiol Aging*, 25:377–396.

Raz N, Gunning-Dixon F, Head D, Williamson A, Acker JD. (2001). Age and sex differences in the cerebellum and the ventral pons: a prospective MR study of healthy adults. *AJNR Am J Neuroradiol*, 22:1161–1167.

Raz N, Gunning FM, Head D, Dupuis JH, McQuain J, Briggs SD, et al. (1997). Selective aging of the human cerebral cortex observed in vivo: differential vulnerability of the prefrontal gray matter. *Cereb Cortex*, 7:268–282.

Raz N, Torres IJ, Spencer WD, Acker JD. (1993). Pathoclisis in aging human cerebral cortex: evidence from in vivo MRI morphometry. *Psychobiology*, 21:151–160.

Resnick SM, Maki PM, Rapp SR, Espeland MA, Brunner R, Coker LH, et al. (2006). Effects of combination estrogen plus progestin hormone treatment on cognition and affect. *J Clin Endocrinol Metab*, 91:1802–1810.

Resnick SM, Coker LH, Maki PM, Rap SR, Espeland MA, Shumaker SA. (2004). The Women's Health Initiative Study of Cognitive Aging (WHISCA): a randomized clinical trial of the effects of hormone therapy on age-associated cognitive decline. *Clin Trials* 1: 440–450.

Resnick SM, Pham DL, Kraut MA, Zonderman AB, Davatzikos C. (2003). Longitudinal magnetic resonance imaging studies of older adults: a shrinking brain. *J Neurosci*, 23:3295–3301.

Resnick SM, Maki PM. (2001). Effects of hormone replacement therapy on cognitive and brain aging. *Ann N Y Acad Sci*, 949:203–214.

Resnick SM, Goldszal AF, Davatzikos C, Golski S, Kraut MA, Metter EJ, et al. (2000). One-year age changes in MRI brain volumes in older adults. *Cereb Cortex*, 10:464–472.

Rettmann ME, Kraut MA, Prince JL, Resnick SM. (2005). Cross-sectional and longitudinal analyses of anatomical sulcal changes associated with aging. *Cereb Cortex*, 2005 Dec 28 [Epub ahead of print].

Riley JL 3rd, Robinson ME, Wise EA, Myers CD, Fillingim RB. (1998). Sex differences in the perception of noxious experimental stimuli: a meta-analysis. *Pain*, 74:181–187.

Rilling JK, Insel TR. (1999). Differential expansion of neural projection systems in primate brain evolution. *Neuroreport*, 10:1453–1459.

Ringo JL, Doty RW, Demeter S, Simard PY. (1994). Time is of the essence: a conjecture that hemispheric specialization arises from interhemispheric conduction delay. *Cereb Cortex*, 4:331–343.

Rocca WA, Hofman A, Brayne C, Breteler MM, Clarke M, Copeland JR, et al. (1991). Frequency and distribution of Alzheimer's disease in Europe: a collaborative study of 1980–1990 prevalence findings. The EURODEM-Prevalence Research Group. *Ann Neurol*, 30:381–390.

Rodriguez G, Warkentin S, Risberg J, Rosadini G. (1988). Sex differences in regional cerebral blood flow. *J Cereb Blood Flow Metab*, 8:783–789.

Rossell SL, Bullmore ET, Williams SC, David AS. (2002). Sex differences in functional brain activation during a lexical visual field task. *Brain Lang*, 80:97–105.

Rossouw JE, Anderson GL, Prentice RL, LaCroix AZ, Kooperberg C, Stefanick ML. (2002). Risks and benefits of estrogen plus progestin in healthy postmenopausal women: principal results from the Women's Health Initiative randomized controlled trial. *J Am Med Assoc*, 288:321–333.

Salat DH, Stangl PA, Kaye JA, Janowsky JS. (1999). Sex differences in prefrontal volume with aging and Alzheimer's disease. *Neurobiol Aging*, 20:591–596.

Schlaepfer TE, Harris GJ, Tien AY, Peng L, Lee S, Pearlson GD. (1995). Structural differences in the cerebral cortex of healthy female and male subjects: a magnetic resonance imaging study. *Psychiatry Res*, 61:129–135.

Schneider F, Habel U, Kessler C, Salloum JB, Posse S. (2000). Gender differences in regional cerebral activity during sadness. *Hum Brain Mapp*, 9:226–238.

Shapleske J, Rossell SL, Woodruff PW, David AS. (1999). The planum temporale: a systematic, quantitative review of its structural, functional and clinical significance. *Brain Res Brain Res Rev*, 29:26–49.

Shaw TG, Mortel KF, Meyer JS, Rogers RL, Hardenberg J, Cutaia MM. (1984). Cerebral blood flow changes in benign aging and cerebrovascular disease. *Neurology*, 34:855–862.

Shaywitz BA, Shaywitz SE, Pugh KR, Constable RT, Skudlarski P, Fulbright RK, et al. (1995). Sex differences in the functional organization of the brain for language. *Nature*, 373:607–609.

Sherwin BB. (1997). Estrogen effects on cognition in menopausal women. *Neurology*, 48:21–26.

Shumaker SA, Legault C, Kuller L, Rapp SR, Thal L, Lane DS, et al. (2004). Conjugated equine estrogens and incidence of probable dementia and mild cognitive impairment in postmenopausal women: Women's Health Initiative Memory Study. *JAMA*, 291:2947–2958.

Shumaker SA, Reboussin BA, Espeland MA, Rapp SR, McBee WL, Dailey M, et al. (1998). The Women's

Health Initiative Memory Study (WHIMS): a trial of the effect of estrogen therapy in preventing and slowing the progression of dementia. *Control Clin Trials*, 19:604–621.

Sih R, Morley JE, Kaiser FE, Perry HM, Patrick P, Ross C. (1997). Testosterone replacement in older hypogonadal men: a 12-month randomized controlled trial. *J Clin Endocrinol Metab*, 82:1661–1667.

Sowell ER, Peterson BS, Thompson PM, Welcome SE, Henkenius AL, Toga AW. (2003). Mapping cortical change across the human life span. *Nat Neurosci*, 6:309–315.

Speck O, Ernst T, Braun J, Koch C, Miller E, Chang L. (2000). Gender differences in the functional organization of the brain for working memory. *Neuroreport*, 11:2581–2585.

Staley JK, Krishnan-Sarin S, Zoghbi S, Tamagnan G, Fujita M, Seibyl JP, et al. (2001). Sex differences in [123I]beta-CIT SPECT measures of dopamine and serotonin transporter availability in healthy smokers and nonsmokers. *Synapse*, 41:275–284.

Steen RG, Gronemeyer SA, Taylor JS. (1995). Age-related changes in proton T1 values of norma human brain. *J Magn Reson Imaging*, 5:43–48.

Stefanick ML, Anderson GL, Margolis KL, Hendrix SL, Rodabough RJ, Paskett ED, et al. (2006). Effects of conjugated equine estrogens on breast cancer and mammography screening in postmenopausal women with hysterectomy. *JAMA*, 295:1647–1657.

Steinmetz H, Jancke L, Kleinschmidt A, Schlaug G, Volkmann J, Huang Y. (1992). Sex but no hand difference in the isthmus of the corpus callosum. *Neurology*, 42:749–752.

Sullivan EV, Rosenbloom MJ, Desmond JE, Pfefferbaum A. (2001). Sex differences in corpus callosum size: relationship to age and intracranial size. *Neurobiol Aging*, 22:603–611.

Sullivan EV, Shear PK, Mathalon DH, Lim KO, Yesavage JA, Tinklenberg JR, Pfefferbaum A. (1993). Greater abnormalities of brain cerebrospinal fluid volumes in younger than in older patients with Alzheimer's disease. *Arch Neurol*, 50:359–373.

Swaab DF, Fliers E. (1985). A sexually dimorphic nucleus in the human brain. *Science*, 228:1112–1115.

Tenover JL. (1994). Androgen administration to aging men. *Clin Androl*, 23:877–892.

The Women's Health Initiative Study Group. (1998). Design of the Women's Health Initiative clinical trial and observational study. *Controlled Clinical Trials*, 19:61–109.

Tisserand DJ, Pruessner JC, Sanz Arigita EJ, van Boxtel MP, Evans AC, Jolles J, Uylings HB. (2002). Regional frontal cortical volumes decrease differentially in aging: an MRI study to compare volumetric approaches and voxel-based morphometry. *Neuroimage*, 17:657–669.

Van Laere K, Versijpt J, Audenaert K, Koole M, Goethals I, Achten E, Dierckx R. (2001). 99mTc-ECD brain perfusion SPET: variability, asymmetry and effects of age and gender in healthy adults. *Eur J Nucl Med*, 28:873–887.

Voyer D, Voyer S, Bryden MP. (1995). Magnitude of sex differences in spatial abilities: a meta-analysis and consideration of critical variables. *Psychological Bulletin*, 117: 250–270.

Wada JA, Clarke R, Hamm A. (1976). Cerebral hemispheric asymmetry in humans. Cortical speech zones in 100 adult and 100 infant brains. *Arch Neurol*, 32:239–246.

Williams CL, Meck WH. (1991). The organizational effects of gonadal steroids on sexually dimorphic spatial ability. *Psychoneuroendocrinology*, 16:155–176.

Williams CL, Barnett AM, Meck WH. (1990). Organizational effects of early gonadal secretions on sexual differentiation in spatial memory. *Behav Neurosci*, 104:84–97.

Wilson JR, Vandenberg SG. (1978). Sex differences in cognition: evidence from the Hawaii Family Study. In McGill TE, Dewsbury DA, Sachs BD (Eds.), *Sex and behavior* (pp. 317–335). New York: Plenum.

Witelson SF, Glezer II, Kigar DL. (1995). Women have greater density of neurons in posterior temporal cortex. *J Neurosci*, 15:3418–3428.

Witelson SF. (1992). Cognitive neuroanatomy: a new era. *Neurology*, 42:709–713.

Witelson SF. (1991). Sex differences in neuroanatomical changes with aging. *N Engl J Med*, 325:211–212.

Witelson SF. (1989). Hand and sex differences in the isthmus and genu of the human corpus callosum: a postmortem morphological study. *Brain*, 112:799–835.

Witelson SF. (1985). The brain connection: the corpus callosum is larger in left-handers. *Science*, 229:665–668.

Wolf OT, Kirschbaum C. (2002). Endogenous estradiol and testosterone levels are associated with cognitive performance in older women and men. *Horm Behav*, 41:259–266.

Wolf OT, Preut R, Hellhammer DH, Kudielka BM, Schurmeyer TH, Kirschbaum C. (2000). Testosterone and cognition in elderly men: a single testosterone injection blocks the practice effect in verbal fluency, but has no effect on spatial or verbal memory. *Biol Psychiatry*, 47:650–654.

Wong DF, Wagner HN Jr, Dannals RF, Links JM, Frost JJ, Ravert HT, et al. (1984). Effects of age on dopamine and serotonin receptors measured by positron tomography in the living human brain. *Science*, 226:1393–1396.

Wong DF, Broussolle EP, Wand G, Villemagne V, Dannals RF, Links JM, et al. (1988). In vivo measurement of dopamine receptors in human brain by positron emission tomography. Age and sex differences. *Ann N Y Acad Sci*, 515:203–214.

Xu J, Kobayashi S, Yamaguchi S, Iijima K, Okada K, Yamashita K. (2000). Gender effects on age-related changes in brain structure. *AJNR Am J Neuroradiol*, 21:112–118.

Yaffe K, Sawaya G, Lieberburg I, Grady D. (1998). Estrogen therapy in postmenopausal women: effects on cognitive function and dementia. *JAMA*, 279: 688–695.

Yaffe K, Lui LY, Zmuda J, Cauley J. (2002). Sex hormones and cognitive function in older men. *J Am Geriatr Soc*, 50:707–712.

Yoshii F, Barker WW, Chang JY, Loewenstein D, Apicella A, Smith D, et al. (1988). Sensitivity of cerebral glucose metabolism to age, gender, brain volume, brain atrophy, and cerebrovascular risk factors. *J Cereb Blood Flow Metab*, 8:654–661.

Yousem DM, Maldjian JA, Siddiqi F, Hummel T, Alsop DC, Geckle RJ, et al. (1999). Gender effects on odor-stimulated functional magnetic resonance imaging. *Brain Res*, 818:480–487.

Yue NC, Arnold AM, Longstreth WT Jr, Elster AD, Jungreis CA, O'Leary DH, et al. (1997). Sulcal, ventricular, and white matter changes at MR imaging in the aging brain: data from the cardiovascular health study. *Radiology*, 202:33–39.

Zandi PP, Carlson MC, Plassman BL, Welsh-Bohmer KA, Mayer LS, Steffens DC, Breitner JC; Cache County Memory Study Investigators. (2002). Hormone replacement therapy and incidence of Alzheimer disease in older women: the Cache County Study. *JAMA*, 288:2123–2129.

Zubieta JK, Smith YR, Bueller JA, Xu Y, Kilbourn MR, Jewett DM, et al. (2002). Mu-opioid receptor-mediated antinociceptive responses differ in men and women. *J Neurosci*, 22(12):5100–5107.

Chapter 23

Sex Differences in Parkinson's Disease

David G. Standaert and Ippolita Cantuti-Castelvetri

Parkinson's disease (PD) is a slow progressing neuro-degenerative disease affecting up to 3% of the population over the age of 65 years, amounting to more than 500,000 individuals in the United States. Clinically it is characterized by rigidity, postural instability, bradykinesia, and resting tremor (Standaert & Young, 2005). The core pathological feature of the disorder is loss of dopaminergic neurons from the substantia nigra pars compacta (SNpc), which innervate the caudate and putamen. Pathological inclusions, known as Lewy bodies, are found within some of the remaining dopaminergic neurons (Forno, 1996).

The destruction of the dopaminergic neurons is very extensive. At the first onset of symptoms of the disease, there is at least 70% depletion of dopaminergic input to the caudate and putamen, and at the end stage of the disease the loss of dopamine neurons can exceed 95% (Forno, 1996). The loss of dopamine is directly related to the characteristic motor features of the disease, including the tremor, bradykinesia, and rigidity.

Therapy for the symptoms of PD is based primarily on replacement or augmentation of dopaminergic function, and can be remarkably effective in alleviating motor symptoms for a number of years (Cantuti-Castelvetri & Standaert, 2004; Standaert & Young, 2005). It is increasingly recognized, however, that as the disease progresses additional, non-motor symptoms develop. These can include sleep and autonomic disorders, impaired postural balance, and dementia. These likely arise from involvement of brain areas outside the SNpc, and in general the dopamine replacement strategies are not helpful in the treatment of the non-motor aspects of the disease (Standaert & Young, 2005).

The etiology of PD is still elusive (Greenamyre & Hastings, 2004), but a long-standing hypothesis is that the disease arises as a result of an inherent or acquired defect in cellular energy metabolism. Central to this idea is the observation that dopamine neurons seem uniquely vulnerable to impairments of energy metabolism, perhaps as a result of the oxidative chemistry which accompanies the catabolism of dopamine and other monoamines (Hastings et al., 1996; Jenner and Olanow, 1996).

Evidence for the contribution of underlying defect in energy metabolism includes the observation that patients with PD have defects in mitochondrial complex I in both brain and circulating platelets (Serra et al., 2001; Swerdlow et al., 2001). In addition, inhibitors of Complex I, such as the toxin MPTP (responsible for the chemically-induced form of PD observed in the "frozen addicts") (Langston, 1996) and the pesticide rotenone (Betarbet et al., 2000) can induce selective destruction of dopaminergic neurons. These observations have led to interest in the possibility that PD may be triggered by an environmental toxin.

Recently, a variety of genetic factors have also been linked to the etiology of PD (Gwinn-Hardy, 2002). The first was the protein alpha-synuclein, an abundant brain protein that appears to be involved in vesicle trafficking and participates in the regulation of dopamine release (Clayton & George, 1998). The first reports to implicate alpha-synuclein to PD described mutations in the protein which cause autosomal dominant forms of the disease (Polymeropoulos et al., 1997; Polymeropoulos, 1998). Subsequent studies revealed that such mutations were exceedingly rare, but also that aggregates of synuclein could be found in all cases of PD (Braak et al., 2003). Even more intriguing was the finding that gene duplication or triplication of alpha-synuclein also causes PD, demonstrating that simple overexpression of the normal protein is sufficient to cause disease (Bradbury, 2003; Singleton et al., 2003; Chartier-Harlin et al., 2004; Farrer et al., 2004; Ibanez et al., 2004; Singleton & Gwinn-Hardy, 2004; Singleton et al., 2004).

Mutations in a number of additional genes have since been identified as causative in PD. Autosomal dominant forms of PD are associated with mutations in LRRK2 (a protein kinase) (Zimprich et al., 2004; Di Fonzo et al., 2005; Gilks et al., 2005; Kachergus et al., 2005; Nichols et al., 2005; Paisan-Ruiz et al., 2005; Skipper et al., 2005), while recessive forms are associated with mutations in parkin (E3 ligase) (Lucking et al., 2000; Hedrich et al., 2001; Hedrich et al., 2002; Kann et al., 2002; Nichols et al., 2002; West et al., 2002; Oliveira et al., 2003a; Oliveira et al., 2003b), PINK1 (a mitochondrial protein kinase) (Valente et al., 2004; Bonifati et al., 2005), and DJ-1 (a protein with antioxidant properties) (Abou-Sleiman

et al., 2003; Eerola et al., 2003; Hague et al., 2003; Macedo et al., 2003; Miller et al., 2003).

The diversity of these different genetic mechanisms, as well as the variable clinical presentation of PD, has led some to question whether in fact it is reasonable to think of PD as a single disease, or whether it is better to view it as a "Parkinson Syndrome," encompassing a spectrum of etiologies and manifestations (Langston, 2006). In any case, it is important to recognize that the genetic mechanisms identified to date are individually rare, and collectively represent only a small fraction of the cases of PD observed by practitioners, probably less than 5% of the total in most clinical settings. This leaves 95% of PD unexplained at present. Until we can account for the mechanism of disease in this broad group, it will be difficult to settle the issue of whether it is best to view PD as a single disease, or a spectrum of disorders.

CLINICAL CHARACTERISTICS OF PD AFFECTED BY GENDER

Gender-specific Incidence and Prevalence

The most clear-cut effect of gender on PD is the marked over-representation of the disease in males. PD is more prevalent in males in nearly every series reported, but such prevalence data must be interpreted cautiously because they may be influenced by a variety of factors including ascertainment bias, the effect of comorbid illnesses, and differing survival among men and women.

There have been several efforts to establish the effect of gender on incidence of PD. The most comprehensive is the study by Van Den Eeden et al., (2003), that used data from the Kaiser Permanente health care system. Investigators found a strong effect of gender on the incidence of PD, with an overall rate for men (19.0 per 100,000 per year) that was 91% higher than that for women (9.9 per 100,000). The incidence of PD increased markedly with age, yet the nearly two-fold increased risk in males was maintained, and at advanced age became even more prominent.

Similar gender differences were observed in surveys of Olmstead County, Minn. (Bower et al., 1999), Italy (Baldereschi et al., 2000), the Netherlands (de Lau et al., 2004) and in a meta-analysis of other studies (Wooten et al., 2004). Interestingly, the elevated prevalence in men is also observed in a cohort of patients with familial forms of PD, suggesting that gender influences the development of PD even when there is also a strong underlying genetic component (Baba et al., 2006).

Age of Onset and Survival

Despite the marked differences in the incidence of PD among men and women, the effect of gender on progression and mortality are less apparent. In several large clinic-based cohorts, both the age of onset and the duration of the disease have been found to be similar in men and women (Diamond et al., 1990; Baba et al., 2005). In a longitudinal study of patients diagnosed at onset (the DATATOP cohort), there was no gender-based difference in survival (Marras et al., 2005). A study of incident cases in Olmsted County, Minnesota found a median survival after disease onset of 10.1 years for men, and 10.3 years for women (Elbaz et al., 2003). Interestingly, the effect of PD on survival seems to override the greater life expectancy of healthy women, leading to higher age-adjusted mortality in women with PD (Diamond et al., 1990; Elbaz et al., 2003). These observations together with the differing incidence of PD suggest that gender has a crucial role in the factors that trigger the development of PD, but that once the disease is established the role of gender is less significant.

Gender Differences in Parkinsonian and Comorbid features

Despite the lack of an effect of gender on the overall rate of progression of PD, the phenotypic features may differ among men and women. The data on these differences are incomplete, because they require longitudinal study and are based for the most part on clinic samples rather than large prospectively studied populations.

Women appear to have more impairment of postural stability and depression appears to be more common in women with PD than men (Fernandez et al., 2000; Rojo et al., 2003; Baba et al., 2005) which may contribute to the lower values on quality of life scales reported in women in some series (Behari et al., 2005). Women have also been reported to have a higher rate of levodopa-related dyskinesia (Lyons et al., 1998) and dystonia (Jankovic & Tintner, 2001).

In contrast, men are more likely to exhibit REM behavior disorders and other sleep disturbances (Scaglione et al., 2005). Women have been reported to have better outcomes after neurosurgical intervention with deep brain stimulation (Hariz et al., 2003), but this may reflect patient selection more than the underlying nature of the disease.

GENDER AND RISK FOR PD

The observation that male gender is among the strongest known risk factors for the occurrence of PD has fueled a search for the underlying mechanisms. It should be noted at the outset that the investigations of this area so far have not revealed a clear-cut answer to the question of why male gender increases risk. It is clear, however, that gender and risk for PD interact on several levels, including genetic, hormonal, and environmental factors.

Interaction of Gender with Genetic Factors

The most direct interaction of gender with genetic factors are the data indicating the presence of genes linked to the occurrence of PD on the X chromosome. A genome-wide linkage study in 362 families revealed evidence for linkage to the X chromosome with a LOD score greater than 3 (Pankratz et al., 2003). Similar results were obtained in a recent genome-wide single nucleotide polymorphism screen in 443 discordant sibling pairs, with linkage to a SNP at Xq28 (Maraganore et al., 2005). At present, the genes responsible for these linkages remain unknown, but polymorphisms in genes present on the X chromosome might provide a direct explanation for some of the gender-related risk of PD.

Gender has also been shown to interact with the risk conferred by several other polymorphisms. An allele of BDNF which is correlated with motor planning ability in PD (presumably a measure of dopaminergic dysfunction), has a greater effect on performance in women than in men (Foltynie et al., 2005). Alleles of monoamine oxidase (MAO) modify the effect that smoking has on PD risk in men, but not in women (Kelada et al., 2002), and gender also influences the risk conferred by alleles of CYP2D6 (Gerard et al., 2002).

Gender may also influence the heritability of PD. In a clinic-based study, 13% of 600 patients with PD had a parent also affected with PD. There was a marked over-representation of maternal, rather than paternal inheritance. This result has been interpreted as evidence for a mitochondrial basis for PD, although it is possible it is due to other gender-specific influences on heritability (Swerdlow et al., 2001).

Role of Estrogen

Estrogen and other gonadal steroid hormones are obvious candidates for modifiers of the risk of PD, and a number of studies have sought a connection between estrogen and injury to dopaminergic systems. Determining the relationship of estrogen to PD is complicated by the long pre-clinical phase of the disease. Most women develop PD after menopause, but it is thought that the degeneration of dopamine neurons begins a decade or more before the symptoms of the disorder appear. Thus the initiation of the degenerative process may well begin during the reproductive years, and yet the presence of the disease only becomes apparent much latter.

The available data on estrogen and human PD suggests that the timing and duration of estrogen depletion and replacement may indeed alter the risk for PD. The largest studies of the effects of estrogen on PD in human populations are analysis of prospective cohorts in which most women experienced late life menopause. In an analysis of the incidence of PD in the Nurses Health Study, a cohort of 77,713 women, Ascherio et al. found that overall that late life post-menopausal estrogen replacement did not alter the risk of PD (Ascherio et al., 2003).

A different result was obtained in studies that focused on women with loss of estrogen earlier in life. In this selected group, increased risk of PD was associated with a fertile life length shorter than 36 years and a cumulative length of pregnancies longer than 30 months (Benedetti et al., 2001; Martignoni et al., 2002; Ragonese et al., 2004). Interestingly, estrogen replacement therapy in women with hysterectomy and/or oophorectomy may increase the risk of PD further, a paradoxical result which has been attributed to the effects of unopposed estrogen treatment without progesterones (Popat et al., 2005). Larger studies will be required to clarify the effects of hormonal status on the biology of PD, which is clearly complex. Nevertheless, the available data do seem to support the view that early life hormonal effects may be more important than late life exposure in influencing the incidence of PD.

Gender and Environmental Factors

The analysis of the role of estrogens in PD is complicated by evidence suggesting an interaction of gender and estrogens with other environmental risk factors. The best studied example is the apparent interaction of estrogen with caffeine.

In men, moderate caffeine consumption (2–4 cups per day) seems to reduce the risk of developing PD. However, in women caffeine is only protective in women who do not use estrogen replacement therapy (Ascherio et al., 2003). This surprising result has been replicated in a second, large prospective population, the Cancer Prevention Study II (Ascherio et al., 2004). Studies in neurotoxin-based animal models of PD also support the view that the presence of estrogen can occlude the neuroprotective effect of caffeine (Xu et al., 2006). Interestingly, caffeine and estrogen are metabolized by the same cytochrome p450 isozyme (CYP1A2) (Abernethy & Todd, 1985; Pollock et al., 1999; Forsyth et al., 2000).

Interaction of gender and environment has also been observed in the effects of non-steroidal anti-inflammatory agents (NSAIDS) in PD. In a large British database, use of NSAIDS other than aspirin was found to be associated with a 20% increase in the risk of PD in women, and a 20% reduction in risk in men (Hernan et al., 2001). These observations point to the importance of considering the role of gender when designing trials of novel protective therapies for PD.

GENDER EFFECTS ON THE BIOLOGY OF CENTRAL DOPAMINERGIC SYSTEMS

Studies of the anatomy and structure of central dopaminergic systems suggest that the effects of gender are pervasive. There are substantial differences in the dopaminergic systems of men and women early in life, and in healthy older adults. Thus, viewing gender solely as a modifier of the disease process responsible for PD is not sufficient; the male and female dopaminergic systems are intrinsically different before the disease develops, and this undoubtedly has an important effect on the outcome.

Morphology and Morphometry of the Substantia Nigra

Most studies of the development of dopaminergic neurons in the substantial nigra have focused on animal models. There is a consistent effect of gender in many species with higher numbers of dopaminergic cells in female than males in African green monkeys (Leranth et al., 2000) and rats (Beyer et al., 1991), although apparently not in mice (Lieb et al., 1996). In rats the higher density in females seems to be determined by factors other than gonadal hormones as it is established before the beginning of the critical period of sexual differentiation (Beyer et al., 1991). In non-human primates, estrogen does seem to have a strong role in maintaining the number of tyrosine hydroxylase (TH) expressing neurons in the SN. In female African Green monkeys, which normally have larger numbers of TH-positive neurons in the SN, ovarectomy reduced the numbers of TH-positive cells to a level comparable to males. Administration of estrogens shortly after the ovarectomy can restore the numbers of TH neurons, but prolonged estrogen deprivation seems to produce irreversible loss of TH neurons (Leranth et al., 2000). This study points to a central role for estrogens in nigral dopaminergic function, but a limitation of the approach is that it cannot distinguish between loss of the TH phenotype and actual cell death related to estrogen depletion.

In vitro systems

Gender-based developmental differences in SN dopaminergic neurons can also be observed using in vitro approaches. Dopaminergic neurons cultured from male and female rat embryos raised in identical hormonal environments show gender-related dimorphism (Reisert & Pilgrim, 1991; Raab, 1995 #491).

Dopaminergic neurons from males and females exhibit differences in dendritic branching and response to exogenous sex steroids (Kuppers et al., 1991; Raab et al., 1995) although these differences may vary with the genetic background of the animals (Sibug et al., 1996). There are also biochemical dimorphisms in animals with differences in dopamine metabolism (Vaccari & Biassoni, 1982b, 1982a). These appear in the rat in the perinatal period between E18 and the end of the first postnatal week, after the morphological differences have been established. These differences in dopamine metabolism can be observed in adult animals using fast cyclic voltammetry, which reveals much greater dopamine release in the striatum of female animals than in males (Walker et al., 2000).

Neurotoxin Models of PD

The basis for the differences observed in the incidence of PD in men and women have been explored in a number of animal and cellular model systems. Both sex-steroid dependent and steroid-independent effects have been observed. A commonly used model of PD is treatment of mice with the neurotoxin MPTP. In most studies, female mice have been reported to be more resistant to the dopamine-depleting effects of the toxin (Dluzen, 1996; Dluzen et al., 1996a; Freyaldenhoven et al., 1996; Miller et al., 1998; Nishino et al., 1998; Disshon & Dluzen, 2000; Dluzen et al., 2003; Tamas et al., 2005). These differences may, however, vary with the strain of mouse and with the MPTP treatment protocol (Hamre et al., 1999). Several studies have documented a protective effect of treatment with estrogens in this system (Dluzen, 1996; Dluzen et al., 1996a, 1996b; Callier et al., 2001; Ramirez et al., 2003; Xu et al., 2006), while testosterones seem to be ineffective (Dluzen, 1996).

An alternative model is the use of the neurotoxic 6-OHDA in rats. In this system, there is also greater susceptibility to toxicity observed in males when measured either by depletion of dopaminergic neurons or by behavioral recovery (Datla et al., 2003; Murray et al., 2003; Gillies et al., 2004; Cass et al., 2005; Tamas et al., 2005). Physiological levels of estrogens appear to be protective in this system as well, at least in female animals (Murray et al., 2003). The effects of estrogens in males is less clear, with some reports suggesting that males may have enhanced, rather than reduced toxicity of 6-OHDA after treatment with estrogens (Gillies et al., 2004). It is also possible to demonstrate more complex interactions between environmental factors, gender, and dopaminergic toxins in animals. For example, prenatal exposure to pesticides enhances the vulnerability of males but not females to dopaminergic neurotoxicants later in life (Barlow et al., 2004).

Gender-based differences in susceptibility to dopaminergic neurotoxins can also be demonstrated using in vitro systems. Neurons from female rodents are more sensitive to the toxic effects of dopamine in culture, and exhibit neuroprotection with NMDA receptor blockade while neurons from male animals do not (Lieb et al., 1995). As in whole animal models, estrogens are neuroprotective in culture systems (Nakamizo et al., 2000; Sawada et al., 2002).

Human Studies: Neuroimaging

Gender-based differences in dopaminergic function can be demonstrated in normal humans by neuroimaging approaches. Using the dopamine transporter PET ligand [123I]FP-CIT, the density of dopamine uptake sites in the caudate and putamen of women is greater than that of men, although both genders show age-related decline (Lavalaye et al., 2000; Staley et al., 2001). Similar results were obtained in a study using the cocaine analog TRODAT-1 (Mozley et al., 2001) and using the dopamine precursor [18F]fluorodopa (Laakso et al., 2002).

Genomics: Effects of Gender on Patterns of Gene Expression

Recent studies of gene expression in SN dopaminergic neurons have revealed additional evidence for fundamental differences in the biology of male and female dopaminergic systems. Using laser capture microdissection and RNA microarray profiling, large-scale differences in the patterns of gene expression in human dopamine neurons can be observed. Functional analysis suggests important gender effects on genes related to oxidative metabolism, vesicle transport, and protein chaperones (Cantuti-Castelvetri et al., 2007). Interestingly, similar differences in gene expression can be observed in male and female C57BL/6J mice (Grammatopoulos et al., 2005).

SUMMARY

Gender has a pervasive effect on the function of the human nigrostriatal dopaminergic system, and its response to disease. Considerable evidence from both animal as well as human studies suggest that the dopaminergic system of healthy males and females are different, both in the anatomical structure of the system as well as in release of dopamine into the striatum. Men clearly have a higher incidence of PD, although once the disease is established the rate of progression and survival are similar in men and women. This points to a crucial role of gender in the factors which are responsible for the initiation of the disease, but only a limited effect on the factors which drive progression once the disease is established. The role of estrogens is complex; in model systems they may be protective, but in humans the data are less clear, perhaps because it is early-life exposure which is most crucial. Identification of the factors which protect women against the occurrence of PD may lead to therapies which are useful in both men and women.

References

Abernethy DR, Todd EL. (1985). Impairment of caffeine clearance by chronic use of low-dose oestrogen-containing oral contraceptives. *Eur J Clin Pharmacol*, 28:425–428.

Abou-Sleiman PM, Healy DG, Quinn N, Lees AJ, Wood NW. (2003). The role of pathogenic DJ-1 mutations in Parkinson's disease. *Ann Neurol*, 54:283–286.

Ascherio A, Chen H, Schwarzschild MA, Zhang SM, Colditz GA, Speizer FE. (2003). Caffeine, postmenopausal estrogen, and risk of Parkinson's disease. *Neurology*, 60:790–795.

Ascherio A, Weisskopf MG, O'Reilly EJ, McCullough ML, Calle EE, Rodriguez C, Thun MJ. (2004). Coffee consumption, gender, and Parkinson's disease mortality in the cancer prevention study II cohort: the modifying effects of estrogen. *Am J Epidemiol*, 160:977–984.

Baba Y, Putzke JD, Whaley NR, Wszolek ZK, Uitti RJ. (2005). Gender and the Parkinson's disease phenotype. *J Neurol*, 252:1201–1205.

Baba Y, Markopoulou K, Putzke JD, Whaley NR, Farrer MJ, Wszolek ZK, Uitti RJ. (2006). Phenotypic commonalities in familial and sporadic Parkinson disease. *Arch Neurol*, 63:579–583.

Baldereschi M, Di Carlo A, Rocca WA, Vanni P, Maggi S, Perissinotto E, et al. (2000). Parkinson's disease and parkinsonism in a longitudinal study: two-fold higher incidence in men. ILSA Working Group. Italian Longitudinal Study on Aging. *Neurology*, 55:1358–1363.

Barlow BK, Richfield EK, Cory-Slechta DA, Thiruchelvam M. (2004). A fetal risk factor for Parkinson's disease. *Dev Neurosci*, 26:11–23.

Behari M, Srivastava AK, Pandey RM. (2005). Quality of life in patients with Parkinson's disease. *Parkinsonism Relat Disord*, 11:221–226.

Benedetti MD, Maraganore DM, Bower JH, McDonnell SK, Peterson BJ, Ahlskog JE, et al. (2001). Hysterectomy, menopause, and estrogen use preceding Parkinson's disease: an exploratory case-control study. *Mov Disord*, 16:830–837.

Betarbet R, Sherer TB, MacKenzie G, Garcia-Osuna M, Panov AV, Greenamyre JT. (2000). Chronic systemic pesticide exposure reproduces features of Parkinson's disease. *Nat Neurosci*, 3:1301–1306.

Beyer C, Pilgrim C, Reisert I. (1991). Dopamine content and metabolism in mesencephalic and diencephalic cell cultures: sex differences and effects of sex steroids. *J Neurosci*, 11:1325–1333.

Bonifati V, Rohe CF, Breedveld GJ, Fabrizio E, De Mari M, Tassorelli C, et al. (2005). Early-onset parkinsonism associated with PINK1 mutations: frequency, genotypes, and phenotypes. *Neurology*, 65:87–95.

Bower JH, Maraganore DM, McDonnell SK, Rocca WA. (1999). Incidence and distribution of parkinsonism in Olmsted County, Minnesota, 1976–1990. *Neurology*, 52:1214–1220.

Braak H, Del Tredici K, Rub U, de Vos RA, Jansen Steur EN, Braak E. (2003). Staging of brain pathology related to sporadic Parkinson's disease. *Neurobiol Aging*, 24:197–211.

Bradbury J. (2003). Alpha-synuclein gene triplication discovered in Parkinson's disease. *Lancet Neurol*, 2:715.

Callier S, Morissette M, Grandbois M, Pelaprat D, Di Paolo T. (2001). Neuroprotective properties of 17beta-estradiol, progesterone, and raloxifene in MPTP C57Bl/6 mice. *Synapse*, 41:131–138.

Cantuti-Castelvetri I, Standaert DG. (2004). *Neuroprotective strategies for Parkinson's disease, Cur Neuropharmacol*, Bentham Science Publishers Ltd., 2: 153–168.

Cantuti-Castelvetri I, Keller-McGandy CE, Bouzou B, Asteris G, Clark TW, Frosch MP, Standaert DG. (2007). Effects of gender on nigral gene expression and parkinson disease. *Neurobiol Dis*, 26:606–614.

Cass WA, Peters LE, Smith MP. (2005). Reductions in spontaneous locomotor activity in aged male, but not female, rats in a model of early Parkinson's disease. *Brain Res*, 1034:153–161.

Chartier-Harlin MC, Kachergus J, Roumier C, Mouroux V, Douay X, Lincoln S, et al. (2004). Alpha-synuclein locus duplication as a cause of familial Parkinson's disease. *Lancet*, 364:1167–1169.

Clayton DF, George JM. (1998). The synucleins: a family of proteins involved in synaptic function, plasticity, neurodegeneration and disease. *Trends Neurosci*, 21:249–254.

Datla KP, Murray HE, Pillai AV, Gillies GE, Dexter DT. (2003). Differences in dopaminergic neuroprotective effects of estrogen during estrous cycle. *Neuroreport*, 14:47–50.

de Lau LM, Giesbergen PC, de Rijk MC, Hofman A, Koudstaal PJ, Breteler MM. (2004). Incidence of parkinsonism and Parkinson disease in a general population: the Rotterdam Study. *Neurology*, 63: 1240–1244.

Di Fonzo A, Rohe CF, Ferreira J, Chien HF, Vacca L, Stocchi F, et al. (2005). A frequent LRRK2 gene mutation associated with autosomal dominant Parkinson's disease. *Lancet*, 365:412–415.

Diamond SG, Markham CH, Hoehn MM, McDowell FH, Muenter MD. (1990). An examination of male-female differences in progression and mortality of Parkinson's disease. *Neurology*, 40:763–766.

Disshon KA, Dluzen DE. (2000). Estrogen reduces acute striatal dopamine responses in vivo to the neurotoxin MPP+ in female, but not male rats. *Brain Res*, 868:95–104.

Dluzen DE. (1996). Effects of testosterone upon MPTP-induced neurotoxicity of the nigrostriatal dopaminergic system of C57/Bl mice. *Brain Res*, 715:113–118.

Dluzen DE, McDermott JL, Liu B. (1996a). Estrogen as a neuroprotectant against MPTP-induced neurotoxicity in C57/Bl mice. *Neurotoxicol Teratol*, 18:603–606.

Dluzen DE, McDermott JL, Liu B. (1996b). Estrogen alters MPTP-induced neurotoxicity in female mice: effects on striatal dopamine concentrations and release. *J Neurochem*, 66:658–666.

Dluzen DE, Tweed C, Anderson LI, Laping NJ. (2003). Gender differences in methamphetamine-induced mRNA associated with neurodegeneration in the mouse nigrostriatal dopaminergic system. *Neuroendocrinology*, 77:232–238.

Eerola J, Hernandez D, Launes J, Hellstrom O, Hague S, Gulick C, et al. (2003). Assessment of a DJ-1 (PARK7) polymorphism in Finnish PD. *Neurology*, 61:1000–1002.

Elbaz A, Bower JH, Peterson BJ, Maraganore DM, McDonnell SK, Ahlskog JE, et al. (2003). Survival study of Parkinson disease in Olmsted County, Minnesota. *Arch Neurol*, 60:91–96.

Farrer M, Kachergus J, Forno L, Lincoln S, Wang DS, Hulihan M, et al. (2004). Comparison of kindreds with parkinsonism and alpha-synuclein genomic multiplications. *Ann Neurol*, 55:174–179.

Fernandez HH, Lapane KL, Ott BR, Friedman JH. (2000). Gender differences in the frequency and treatment of behavior problems in Parkinson's disease. SAGE Study Group. Systematic assessment and geriatric drug use via epidemiology. *Mov Disord*, 15:490–496.

Foltynie T, Lewis SG, Goldberg TE, Blackwell AD, Kolachana BS, Weinberger DR, et al. (2005). The BDNF Va166Met polymorphism has a gender specific influence on planning ability in Parkinson's disease. *J Neurol*, 252:833–838.

Forno LS. (1996). Neuropathology of Parkinson's disease. *J Neuropathol Exp Neurol*, 55:259–272.

Forsyth JT, Grunewald RA, Rostami-Hodjegan A, Lennard MS, Sagar HJ, Tucker GT. (2000). Parkinson's disease and CYP1A2 activity. *Br J Clin Pharmacol*, 50:303–309.

Freyaldenhoven TE, Cadet JL, Ali SF. (1996). The dopamine-depleting effects of 1-methyl-4-phenyl-1,2,3,6-tetrahydropyridine in CD-1 mice are gender-dependent. *Brain Res*, 735:232–238.

Gerard N, Panserat S, Lucotte G. (2002). Roles of gender, age at onset and environmental risk in the frequency of CYP2D6-deficient alleles in patients with Parkinson's disease. *Eur Neurol*, 48:114–115.

Gilks WP, Abou-Sleiman PM, Gandhi S, Jain S, Singleton A, Lees AJ, et al. (2005). A common

LRRK2 mutation in idiopathic Parkinson's disease. *Lancet*, 365:415–416.

Gillies GE, Murray HE, Dexter D, McArthur S. (2004). Sex dimorphisms in the neuroprotective effects of estrogen in an animal model of Parkinson's disease. *Pharmacol Biochem Behav*, 78:513–522.

Grammatopoulos TN, Bouzou B, St. Martin J, Standaert DG. (2005). Microarray analysis of gender-specific gene expression in the substantia nigra of c57bl/6 mice. In: Society for Neuroscience, 35th Annual Meeting, p Program No. 781.711. Washington, D.C.

Greenamyre JT, Hastings TG. (2004). Biomedicine. Parkinson's—divergent causes, convergent mechanisms. *Science*, 304:1120–1122.

Gwinn-Hardy K. (2002). Genetics of parkinsonism. *Mov Disord*, 17:645–656.

Hague S, Rogaeva E, Hernandez D, Gulick C, Singleton A, Hanson M, et al. (2003). Early-onset Parkinson's disease caused by a compound heterozygous DJ-1 mutation. *Ann Neurol*, 54:271–274.

Hamre K, Tharp R, Poon K, Xiong X, Smeyne RJ. (1999). Differential strain susceptibility following 1-methyl-4-phenyl-1,2,3,6-tetrahydropyridine (MPTP) administration acts in an autosomal dominant fashion: quantitative analysis in seven strains of Mus musculus. *Brain Res*, 828:91–103.

Hariz GM, Lindberg M, Hariz MI, Bergenheim AT. (2003). Gender differences in disability and health-related quality of life in patients with Parkinson's disease treated with stereotactic surgery. *Acta Neurol Scand*, 108:28–37.

Hastings TG, Lewis DA, Zigmond MJ. (1996). Reactive dopamine metabolites and neurotoxicity: implications for Parkinson's disease. *Adv Exp Med Biol*, 387:97–106.

Hedrich K, Marder K, Harris J, Kann M, Lynch T, Meija-Santana H, et al. (2002). Evaluation of 50 probands with early-onset Parkinson's disease for Parkin mutations. *Neurology*, 58:1239–1246.

Hedrich K, Kann M, Lanthaler AJ, Dalski A, Eskelson C, Landt O, et al. (2001). The importance of gene dosage studies: mutational analysis of the parkin gene in early-onset parkinsonism. *Hum Mol Genet*, 10:1649–1656.

Hernan MA, Logroscino G, Garcia Rodriguez LA. (2006). Nonsteroidal anti-inflammatory drugs and the incidence of Parkinson disease. *Neurology* 11;66(7):1097–1099.

Ibanez P, Bonnet AM, Debarges B, Lohmann E, Tison F, Pollak P, et al. (2004). Causal relation between alpha-synuclein gene duplication and familial Parkinson's disease. *Lancet*, 364:1169–1171.

Jankovic J, Tintner R. (2001). Dystonia and parkinsonism. *Parkinsonism Relat Disord*, 8:109–121.

Jenner P, Olanow CW. (1996). Oxidative stress and the pathogenesis of Parkinson's disease. *Neurology*, 47:S161-S170.

Kachergus J, Mata IF, Hulihan M, Taylor JP, Lincoln S, Aasly J, et al. (2005). Identification of a novel LRRK2 mutation linked to autosomal dominant parkinsonism: evidence of a common founder across European populations. *Am J Hum Genet*, 76:672–680.

Kann M, Jacobs H, Mohrmann K, Schumacher K, Hedrich K, Garrels J, et al. (2002). Role of parkin mutations in 111 community-based patients with early-onset parkinsonism. *Ann Neurol*, 51:621–625.

Kelada SN, Costa-Mallen P, Costa LG, Smith-Weller T, Franklin GM, Swanson PD, et al. (2002). Gender difference in the interaction of smoking and monoamine oxidase B intron 13 genotype in Parkinson's disease. *Neurotoxicology*, 23:515–519.

Kuppers E, Pilgrim C, Reisert I. (1991). Sex-specific schedule in steroid response of rhombencephalic catecholaminergic neurons in vitro. *Int J Dev Neurosci*, 9:537–544.

Laakso A, Vilkman H, Bergman J, Haaparanta M, Solin O, Syvalahti E, et al. (2002). Sex differences in striatal presynaptic dopamine synthesis capacity in healthy subjects. *Biol Psychiatry*, 52:759–763.

Langston JW. (1996). The etiology of Parkinson's disease with emphasis on the MPTP story. *Neurology*, 47:S153-S160.

Langston JW. (2006). The Parkinson's complex: parkinsonism is just the tip of the iceberg. *Ann Neurol*, 59:591–596.

Lavalaye J, Booij J, Reneman L, Habraken JB, van Royen EA. (2000). Effect of age and gender on dopamine transporter imaging with [123I]FP-CIT SPET in healthy volunteers. *Eur J Nucl Med*, 27:867–869.

Leranth C, Roth RH, Elsworth JD, Naftolin F, Horvath TL, Redmond DE, Jr. (2000). Estrogen is essential for maintaining nigrostriatal dopamine neurons in primates: implications for Parkinson's disease and memory. *J Neurosci*, 20:8604–8609.

Lieb K, Andrae J, Reisert I, Pilgrim C. (1995). Neurotoxicity of dopamine and protective effects of the NMDA receptor antagonist AP-5 differ between male and female dopaminergic neurons. *Exp Neurol*, 134:222–229.

Lieb K, Andersen C, Lazarov N, Zienecker R, Urban I, Reisert I, Pilgrim C. (1996). Pre- and postnatal development of dopaminergic neuron numbers in the male and female mouse midbrain. *Brain Res Dev Brain Res*, 94:37–43.

Lucking CB, Durr A, Bonifati V, Vaughan J, De Michele G, Gasser T, et al. (2000). Association between early-onset Parkinson's disease and mutations in the parkin gene. *N Engl J Med*, 342:1560–1567.

Lyons KE, Hubble JP, Troster AI, Pahwa R, Koller WC. (1998). Gender differences in Parkinson's disease. *Clin Neuropharmacol*, 21:118–121.

Macedo MG, Anar B, Bronner IF, Cannella M, Squitieri F, Bonifati V, et al. (2003). The DJ-1L166P mutant protein associated with early onset Parkinson's disease is unstable and forms higher-order protein complexes. *Hum Mol Genet*, 12:2807–2816.

Maraganore DM, de Andrade M, Lesnick TG, Strain KJ, Farrer MJ, Rocca WA, et al. (2005). High-resolution whole-genome association study of Parkinson disease. *Am J Hum Genet*, 77:685–693.

Marras C, McDermott MP, Rochon PA, Tanner CM, Naglie G, Rudolph A, Lang AE. (2005). Survival in Parkinson disease: thirteen-year follow-up of the DATATOP cohort. *Neurology*, 64:87–93.

Martignoni E, Nappi RE, Citterio A, Calandrella D, Corengia E, Fignon A, et al. (2002). Parkinson's disease and reproductive life events. *Neurol Sci*, 23(Suppl 2):S85-S86.

Miller DB, Ali SF, O'Callaghan JP, Laws SC. (1998). The impact of gender and estrogen on striatal dopaminergic neurotoxicity. *Ann N Y Acad Sci*, 844:153–165.

Miller DW, Ahmad R, Hague S, Baptista MJ, Canet-Aviles R, McLendon C, et al. (2003). L166P mutant DJ-1, causative for recessive Parkinson's disease, is degraded through the ubiquitin-proteasome system. *J Biol Chem*, 278:36588–36595.

Mozley LH, Gur RC, Mozley PD, Gur RE. (2001). Striatal dopamine transporters and cognitive functioning in healthy men and women. *Am J Psychiatry*, 158:1492–1499.

Murray HE, Pillai AV, McArthur SR, Razvi N, Datla KP, Dexter DT, Gillies GE. (2003). Dose- and sex-dependent effects of the neurotoxin 6-hydroxydopamine on the nigrostriatal dopaminergic pathway of adult rats: differential actions of estrogen in males and females. *Neuroscience*, 116: 213–222.

Nakamizo T, Urushitani M, Inoue R, Shinohara A, Sawada H, Honda K, et al. (2000). Protection of cultured spinal motor neurons by estradiol. *Neuroreport*, 11:3493–3497.

Nichols WC, Pankratz N, Uniacke SK, Pauciulo MW, Halter C, Rudolph A, et al. (2002). Linkage stratification and mutation analysis at the Parkin locus identifies mutation positive Parkinson's disease families. *J Med Genet*, 39:489–492.

Nichols WC, Pankratz N, Hernandez D, Paisan-Ruiz C, Jain S, Halter CA, et al. (2005). Genetic screening for a single common LRRK2 mutation in familial Parkinson's disease. *Lancet*, 365:410–412.

Nishino H, Nakajima K, Kumazaki M, Fukuda A, Muramatsu K, Deshpande SB, et al. (1998). Estrogen protects against while testosterone exacerbates vulnerability of the lateral striatal artery to chemical hypoxia by 3-nitropropionic acid. *Neurosci Res*, 30: 303–312.

Oliveira SA, Scott WK, Martin ER, Nance MA, Watts RL, Hubble JP, et al. (2003a). Parkin mutations and susceptibility alleles in late-onset Parkinson's disease. *Ann Neurol*, 53:624–629.

Oliveira SA, Scott WK, Nance MA, Watts RL, Hubble JP, Koller WC, et al. (2003b). Association study of Parkin gene polymorphisms with idiopathic Parkinson disease. *Arch Neurol*, 60:975–980.

Paisan-Ruiz C, Lang AE, Kawarai T, Sato C, Salehi-Rad S, Fisman GK, et al. (2005). LRRK2 gene in Parkinson disease: mutation analysis and case control association study. *Neurology*, 65:696–700.

Pankratz N, Nichols WC, Uniacke SK, Halter C, Murrell J, Rudolph A, et al. (2003). Genome-wide linkage analysis and evidence of gene-by-gene interactions in a sample of 362 multiplex Parkinson disease families. *Hum Mol Genet*, 12:2599–2608.

Pollock BG, Wylie M, Stack JA, Sorisio DA, Thompson DS, Kirshner MA, et al. (1999). Inhibition of caffeine metabolism by estrogen replacement therapy in postmenopausal women. *J Clin Pharmacol*, 39: 936–940.

Polymeropoulos MH. (1998). Autosomal dominant Parkinson's disease and alpha-synuclein. *Ann Neurol*, 44:S63–64.

Polymeropoulos MH, Lavedan C, Leroy E, Ide SE, Dehejia A, Dutra A, et al. (1997). Mutation in the alpha-synuclein gene identified in families with Parkinson's disease. *Science*, 276:2045–2047.

Popat RA, Van Den Eeden SK, Tanner CM, McGuire V, Bernstein AL, Bloch DA, et al. (2005). Effect of reproductive factors and postmenopausal hormone use on the risk of Parkinson disease. *Neurology*, 65:383–390.

Raab H, Pilgrim C, Reisert I. (1995). Effects of sex and estrogen on tyrosine hydroxylase mRNA in cultured embryonic rat mesencephalon. *Brain Res Mol Brain Res*, 33:157–164.

Ragonese P, D'Amelio M, Salemi G, Aridon P, Gammino M, Epifanio A, et al. (2004). Risk of Parkinson disease in women: effect of reproductive characteristics. *Neurology*, 62:2010–2014.

Ramirez AD, Liu X, Menniti FS. (2003). Repeated estradiol treatment prevents MPTP-induced dopamine depletion in male mice. *Neuroendocrinology*, 77:223–231.

Reisert I, Pilgrim C. (1991). Sexual differentiation of monoaminergic neurons—genetic or epigenetic? *Trends Neurosci*, 14:468–473.

Rojo A, Aguilar M, Garolera MT, Cubo E, Navas I, Quintana S. (2003). Depression in Parkinson's disease: clinical correlates and outcome. *Parkinsonism Relat Disord*, 10:23–28.

Sawada H, Ibi M, Kihara T, Honda K, Nakamizo T, Kanki R, et al. (2002). Estradiol protects dopaminergic neurons in a MPP+Parkinson's disease model. *Neuropharmacology*, 42:1056–1064.

Scaglione C, Vignatelli L, Plazzi G, Marchese R, Negrotti A, Rizzo G, et al. (2005). REM sleep behaviour disorder in Parkinson's disease: a questionnaire-based study. *Neurol Sci*, 25:316–321.

Serra JA, Dominguez RO, de Lustig ES, Guareschi EM, Famulari AL, Bartolome EL, et al. (2001). Parkinson's disease is associated with oxidative stress: comparison of peripheral antioxidant profiles in living Parkinson's, Alzheimer's and vascular dementia patients. *J Neural Transm*, 108:1135–1148.

Sibug R, Kuppers E, Beyer C, Maxson SC, Pilgrim C, Reisert I. (1996). Genotype-dependent sex differentiation of dopaminergic neurons in primary cultures of embryonic mouse brain. *Brain Res Dev Brain Res,* 93:136–142.

Singleton A, Gwinn-Hardy K. (2004). Parkinson's disease and dementia with Lewy bodies: a difference in dose? *Lancet,* 364:1105–1107.

Singleton A, Gwinn-Hardy K, Sharabi Y, Li ST, Holmes C, Dendi R, et al. (2004). Association between cardiac denervation and parkinsonism caused by alpha-synuclein gene triplication. *Brain,* 127:768–772.

Singleton AB, Farrer M, Johnson J, Singleton A, Hague S, Kachergus J, et al. (2003). alpha-Synuclein locus triplication causes Parkinson's disease. *Science,* 302:841.

Skipper L, Shen H, Chua E, Bonnard C, Kolatkar P, Tan LC, et al. (2005). Analysis of LRRK2 functional domains in nondominant Parkinson disease. *Neurology,* 65:1319–1321.

Staley JK, Krishnan-Sarin S, Zoghbi S, Tamagnan G, Fujita M, Seibyl JP, et al. (2001). Sex differences in [123I]beta-CIT SPECT measures of dopamine and serotonin transporter availability in healthy smokers and nonsmokers. *Synapse,* 41:275–284.

Standaert GS, Young AB. (2005). Treatment of the central nervous system degenerative disorders. In Brunton LL (Ed.), *Goodman & Gilaman's the pharmacological basis of therapeutics,* 11th Edition (pp 527–545). New York, NY: McGraw-Hill.

Swerdlow RH, Parks JK, Cassarino DS, Binder DR, Bennett JP, Jr., Di Iorio G, et al. (2001). Biochemical analysis of cybrids expressing mitochondrial DNA from Contursi kindred Parkinson's subjects. *Exp Neurol,* 169:479–485.

Tamas A, Lubics A, Szalontay L, Lengvari I, Reglodi D. (2005). Age and gender differences in behavioral and morphological outcome after 6-hydroxydopamine-induced lesion of the substantia nigra in rats. *Behav Brain Res,* 158:221–229.

Vaccari A, Biassoni R. (1982a). Constancy of adult hypothalamic tyrosine hydroxylase after gonadal steroid treatment during development. *J Neurosci Res,* 8:21–25.

Vaccari A, Biassoni R. (1982b). Gonadal influences on the inhibition of monoamine oxidase type B activity. *J Neurosci Res,* 8:13–19.

Valente EM, Abou-Sleiman PM, Caputo V, Muqit MM, Harvey K, Gispert S, et al. (2004) Hereditary early-onset Parkinson's disease caused by mutations in PINK1. *Science,* 304:1158–1160.

Van Den Eeden SK, Tanner CM, Bernstein AL, Fross RD, Leimpeter A, Bloch DA, Nelson LM. (2003). Incidence of Parkinson's disease: variation by age, gender, and race/ethnicity. *Am J Epidemiol,* 157:1015–1022.

Walker QD, Rooney MB, Wightman RM, Kuhn CM. (2000). Dopamine release and uptake are greater in female than male rat striatum as measured by fast cyclic voltammetry. *Neuroscience,* 95:1061–1070.

West A, Periquet M, Lincoln S, Lucking CB, Nicholl D, Bonifati V, et al. (2002). Complex relationship between Parkin mutations and Parkinson disease. *Am J Med Genet,* 114:584–591.

Wooten GF, Currie LJ, Bovbjerg VE, Lee JK, Patrie J. (2004). Are men at greater risk for Parkinson's disease than women? *J Neurol Neurosurg Psychiatry,* 75:637–639.

Xu K, Xu Y, Brown-Jermyn D, Chen JF, Ascherio A, Dluzen DE, Schwarzschild MA. (2006). Estrogen prevents neuroprotection by caffeine in the mouse 1-methyl-4-phenyl-1,2,3,6-tetrahydropyridine model of Parkinson's disease. *J Neurosci,* 26:535–541.

Zimprich A, Biskup S, Leitner P, Lichtner P, Farrer M, Lincoln S, et al. (2004). Mutations in LRRK2 cause autosomal-dominant parkinsonism with pleomorphic pathology. *Neuron,* 44:601–607.

Index